The Health of
Sexual Minorities

Edited by
Ilan H. Meyer, PhD,
and
Mary E. Northridge, PhD, MPH
Mailman School of Public Health, Columbia University
New York, New York, USA

The Health of Sexual Minorities

Public Health Perspectives on
Lesbian, Gay, Bisexual
and Transgender Populations

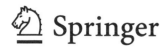

Ilan H. Meyer, PhD
Mary E. Northridge, PhD, MPH
Department of Sociomedical Sciences
Mailman School of Public Health
Columbia University
New York, NY 10032
USA

Library of Congress Control Number: 2005939066

ISBN-10: 0-387-28871-6   e-ISBN-10: 0-387-31334-6
ISBN-13: 978-0-387-28871-0   e-ISBN-13: 978-0-387-31334-4

Printed on acid-free paper.

Portions of Chapter 10 are adapted from Meyer I.H. Prejudice, social stress, and mental health in lesbian, gay, and bisexual populations: conceptual issues and research evidence. *Psychol. Bull.* 2003;129:674–697. Copyright © 2003 by the American Psychological Association. Adapted with permission.

Chapter 14 is adapted from Sell, R.L. Defining and measuring sexual orientation: a review. *Archives of Sexual Behavior* 1997;26:643–658.

9 8 7 6 5 4 3 2 1

springer.com

Preface

Our collaboration on the editing of this book revives an earlier joint effort. In June 2001, we teamed up on the first issue of the *American Journal of Public Health*, devoted to lesbian, gay, bisexual, and transgender (LGBT) health (Northridge, 2001). Five years later, we reunited to conceptualize, coordinate, and oversee the compilation of this volume on the health of sexual minorities. In both the special issues and this volume, we sought a public health perspective that was broad enough to encompass the diverse populations and communities that comprise LGBT people, yet recognized the similarities in the experiences they share across cultures and locales—often related to stigma, discrimination, rejection, and violence but also resilience and resistance (Meyer, 2001). An overarching goal for this book is that careful treatment afforded to issues such as the impact of prejudice on the health of LGBT people may thoughtfully inform research and practice on other stigmatized groups and thereby help advance civil society.

The Institute of Medicine (1988) defined the mission of public health as fulfilling society's interest in ensuring conditions in which people can be healthy. When conceptualizing this book, we invoked this broad definition of public health to mean, quite literally, the health of the public. How are we to advance conditions in which LGBT people can be healthy? To seek answers, we called on leading researchers who are conducting formative and applied research on LGBT health for their contributions derived from empirical studies and critical analysis in the form of peer-reviewed chapters. The result is this comprehensive and rigorous text.

Conceptual Approach to Editing This Volume

Our aim from the outset when commissioning chapters was to be inclusive but not exhaustive. That is, we did not aim for an encyclopedic book that covers all the areas of interest to LGBT populations. Rather, we aimed for a book that would rely on the best available thought on issues of concern to LGBT health. We sought a cross-disciplinary approach. Anthropology, biology, law, medicine, psychology, and sociology are among the disciplines represented in this volume in addition to public health. They are interwoven in interdisciplinary and intersectional works that are at the forefront of formative and applied LGBT public health research today. In addition, we invoked an ecological, multilevel approach by ensuring that structural determinants of LGBT health as well as individual-level specific health concerns of sexual minorities were covered.

When choosing chapter contributors and editing the chapters, we did not impose an editorial ideology other than what is described above and implied in the organization of this book. That is, we did not seek uniformity among authors in definitions of the populations of interest, the approaches they have taken to investigate these populations, or the types of solutions sought. Rather, we allowed—indeed aimed for—the book to reflect current ideologic and conceptual controversies and debates at the cost of introducing incongruities among chapters. Thus, a reading of different chapters may give a better appreciation of the current state of LGBT public health research than would any single chapter.

We also sought to represent the concerns of various groups among LGBT populations—but not by paying lip service to representation at the expense of significant content. Rather, we sought areas of strong research in various specific populations (e.g., American Indians, Latinos, women, transgender individuals) with the expectation that conceptual work and certain findings from such works would be transferable across populations. Finally, although this text is based in the United States, we provoked inquiry into global health issues because they provide an important perspective on LGBT health relevant both to U.S. and global populations.

Tour of the Book

Some chapters of this book are largely theoretical, others synthesize empirical research, and still others are especially hands-on. Each chapter in this volume may be read independently and understood without reference to the rest of the book. A real advantage of this text, however, is the interchange among chapters. We deliberately included different perspectives on the core topics presented. Together, their purpose is to inform readers committed to understanding and addressing social disparities in health for LGBT populations.

Careful readers will discern that, despite broad areas of agreement, contributors differ with regard to the definition of populations of interest, research methodologies employed, and health concerns targeted. Rather than censor points of view, we championed a more provocative, comprehensive, and in-depth understanding of the central themes deliberated within the text toward evolving the field of LGBT health. We urge the reader to expand her/his scope when searching for insights in this book by exploring chapters even if their relevance to a specific population or a narrow public health question of interest is not superficially apparent. To gain the most from this volume, we believe it is advantageous to compare and contrast chapters within and across sections.

Although this volume was not intended to be read in order from cover to cover, the sequence and organization of its parts were purposeful, moving from overarching issues including conceptual and definitional frameworks; legal, social, and cultural perspectives and methodologic approaches; through specific health issues among LGBT populations; and concluding with an examination of health systems and institutions through which LGBT health is (or is not) addressed.

First, "Who Are LGBT Individuals?" By examining populations of interest, the chapters included in this part wrestle with topics such as definitions of identity; intersections across sexual, race/ethnicity, and gender identities; sexual development across the life course; and social and biologic constructs of sexuality. The following part, "LGBT Health and the State," takes on legal, ethical, and political dilemmas as well as opportunities for policy, research, and advocacy on sexual minorities. Next, the part entitled "Prejudice and Pride in Health" investigates the relations between societal structures and individual health, including the impact of structural violence, stigma, prejudice, and discrimination on the health of LGBT people.

Part IV, "Research Methodologies," sets about honing the processes and means for understanding and addressing disparities in LGBT health. It is incumbent on researchers to ensure that methodologic refinements and exquisite sensitivity are employed when bringing LGBT issues into public health focus. The chapters in this part cover a variety of methodologic issues that require special attention in studies of LGBT populations, including definitions, measurement, and sampling as well as quantitative, qualitative, and community-based participatory research approaches.

Rather than try to cover the entire spectrum of health needs, we elected to include a diversity of health issues, with particular attention to areas that have not received much attention in books and compilations to date. In the part entitled "Health Concerns," we included the following three categories of LGBT issues: (1) areas in which LGBT people are at increased risk for disease because of unique exposures (e.g., use of hormones by trans-people undergoing sex change procedures); (2) areas in which LGBT people have a high prevalence of exposure and/or disease that are not caused by unique exposures (e.g., methamphetamine use and risk of HIV infection among gay men); and (3) areas in which LGBT people are not at increased risk for disease but that nevertheless require specialized, culturally appropriate approaches (e.g., general health concerns of lesbian and bisexual women, including cancer prevention and treatment).

Finally, no public health text would be complete absent a look at "Healthcare Systems and Services." The final part of this book accordingly covers the issues of accessing and ensuring respectful health care for LGBT groups that have traditionally experienced the greatest barriers in U.S. systems: racial/ethnic minorities, transgender people, and youths. We end with an inspiring chapter on Fenway Community Health, a model of integrated community-based LGBT care, education, and research that serves as a beacon for other locales, both within the United States and abroad.

Areas and Topics Not Included in This Book

Despite the breadth of this book, there are many areas that it does not cover. These areas can be divided into two general types: The first includes work we omitted because there are many other resources to which the reader can turn. In this, we include HIV/AIDS and psychological/mental health issues. HIV/AIDS has been a major, and predominant, area of investigation in gay men's health research. Many books have been published to provide the reader good reviews of various areas of research within public health work on HIV/AIDS. These resources include books that provide comprehensive coverage of HIV/AIDS and sexually transmitted diseases (STDs) (e.g., Holmes, 1999; Emini, 2002) as well as books that address specific aspects of public health, such as HIV prevention (Peterson & DiClemente, 2000) and specific issues affecting HIV-positive and HIV-negative gay and bisexual men (Halkitis et al., 2005; Kalichman, 2005). Similarly, the area of mental health has been the topic of many books that provide an excellent discussion of psychological development across the life-span and mental health problems related to LGB populations (D'Augelli & Patterson, 1996, 2001; Garnets & Kimmel, 2002; Omoto & Kurtzman, 2006).

The second area of interest excluded from this volume includes many emerging areas. We omitted them because we assessed that based on the existing research we could not commission reviews that were sufficiently comprehensive. To pursue such areas, the reader would be better served by searching scientific journals that can provide more timely coverage of emerging research areas. Such areas include topics that have not been fully developed in public health work to date. For example, the discussion of family levels of influence within the conceptual model that guided the organization of this book. Many important issues face LGBT individuals as they form families. Such a chapter might have covered issues related to conception, adoption, child rearing, cohabitation, and marriage among others. Notwithstanding notable works describing anthropologic and psychological perspectives on LGB families (Weston, 1991; Patterson & D'Augelli, 1998), public health research in this area is still forming, and links to health issues have not yet been carefully explicated, evaluated, and published in the peer-reviewed literature. The need for such work is particularly heightened as debate is growing on access for LGBT individuals to civil marriage and its public health implications (Herdt & Kertzner, 2006). There are also specific health concerns that have not received sufficient research attention (Dean et al., 2000)—for example, gay men may be at risk for anal cancer unrelated to HIV/AIDS—but the lack of research on such topics make them unsuitable for coverage in a book chapter.

References

D'Augelli, A.R., and Patterson, C.J. (1996) *Lesbian, gay, and bisexual identities over the lifespan: psychological perspectives.* Oxford University Press, New York.

D'Augelli, A.R., and Patterson, C.J. (2001) *Lesbian, gay, and bisexual identities and youth: psychological perspectives.* Oxford University Press, New York.

Dean, L., Meyer, I.H., Robinson, K., Sell, R.L., Sember, R., Silenzio, V.M.B., Bowen, D.J., Bradford, J., Rothblum, E., Scout, White, J., Dunn, P., Lawrence, A., Wolfe, D., and Xavier, J. (2000) Lesbian, gay, bisexual, and transgender health: findings and concerns. *Journal of the Gay and Lesbian Medical Association* 4: 102–151.

Emini, E. (2002) *The human immunodeficiency virus: biology, immunology, and therapy.* Princeton University Press, Princeton, NJ.

Garnets, L., and Kimmel, D. (2002) *Psychological perspectives on lesbian, gay, and bisexual experiences.* Columbia University Press, New York.

Halkitis, P.N., Gomez, C.A., and Wolitski, R.J. (2005) *HIV + sex: the psychosocial and interpersonal dynamics of HIV-seropositive gay and bisexual men's relationships.* American Psychological Association, Washington, DC.

Herdt, G., and Kertzner, R. (2006) I do, but I can't: the impact of marriage denial on the mental health and sexual citizenship of lesbians and gay men in the United States. *Sexuality Research & Social Policy* 3: 33–49.

Holmes, K. (1999) *Sexually transmitted diseases,* 3rd ed. McGraw-Hill, New York.

Institute of Medicine. (1988) *The future of public health.* National Academy Press, Washington, DC.

Kalichman, S.C. (2005) *Positive prevention: reducing HIV transmission among people living with HIV/AIDS.* Springer, New York.

Meyer, I.H. (2001) Why lesbian, gay, bisexual, and transgender public health? *American Journal of Public Health* 91: 856–859.

Northridge, M.E. (2001) Editor's note: advancing lesbian, gay, bisexual, and transgender health. *American Journal of Public Health* 91: 855–856.

Omoto, A.M., and Kurtzman, H.S. (2006) *Sexual orientation and mental health: examining identity and development in lesbian, gay, and bisexual people.* American Psychological Association, Washington, DC.

Patterson, C.J., and D'Augelli, A.R. (1998) *Lesbian, gay, and bisexual identities in families: psychological perspectives.* Oxford University Press, New York.

Peterson, J.L., and DiClemente, R.J. (2000) *Handbook of HIV prevention.* Springer, New York.

Weston, K. (1991) *Families we choose.* Columbia University Press, New York.

New York, New York, USA
Ilan H. Meyer
Mary E. Northridge

Acknowledgments

As we embarked on this project, we relied on established, busy researchers and public health professionals who have dedicated their work to LGBT health issues. The unanimous endorsement of this undertaking among the many researchers we approached is a remarkable testament to the devotion of contemporary public health scientists and scholars to LGBT health, to one another, and to collaborative undertakings. We thank the authors of the chapters for their dedication and trust. We also thank the following individuals for providing invaluable advice at various stages and various aspects of the book: Gabriel Galindo, Michael Gross, Dawn Harbatkin, Linwood Lewis, John Peterson, Lauren Porsch, Randall Sell, and Donna Shelley. Finally, we thank Bill Tucker, our editor at Springer, for believing in this project and for his continued support and help in seeing this project to fruition.

We hope that this book helps encourage researchers and public health professionals to direct their attention to LGBT health. Despite the formidable challenges ahead, the future looks bright for LGBT public health. We have come too far to turn back, and we will not. The lives and welfare of too many of us hang in the balance.

New York, New York, USA

Ilan H. Meyer
Mary E. Northridge

Contents

Contributors

Jan Baer, Research Foundation for Mental Hygiene, New York State Psychiatric Institute, New York, New York, USA

Juan Battle, Department of Sociology, The Graduate Center, City University of New York; and Hunter College, New York, New York, USA

Diane Binson, Center for AIDS Prevention Studies, University of California–San Francisco, San Francisco, California, USA

Johnny Blair, Abt Associates, Inc., Bethesda, Maryland, USA

Ulrike Boehmer, School of Public Health, Boston University, Boston, Massachusetts, USA

Deborah J. Bowen, School of Public Health and Community Medicine, University of Washington, Seattle, Washington, USA

Judith B. Bradford, School of Medicine and L. Douglas Wilder School of Government and Public Affairs, Virginia Commonwealth University, Richmond, Virginia; and The Fenway Institute, Fenway Community Health, Boston, Massachusetts, USA

William Byne, Mount Sinai School of Medicine, New York; and Bronx Veterans Affairs Medical Center, Bronx, New York, USA

Regina Chopp, Department of Psychology, University of California–Davis, Davis, California, USA

Kenneth M. Cohen, Gannett Health Center, Cornell University, Ithaca, New York, USA

Martha Crum, Department of Sociology, The Graduate Center, City University of New York, New York, New York, USA

Rafael M. Diaz, César E. Chávez Institute, San Francisco State University, San Francisco, California, USA

Gary W. Dowsett, Australian Research Centre in Sex, Health and Society, La Trobe University, Melbourne, Australia

Michele J. Eliason, Institute for Health and Aging, University of California–San Francisco, San Francisco, California, USA

Steven Epstein, Department of Sociology, University of California–San Diego, La Jolla, California, USA

Stefano Fabeni, School of Law, Columbia University, New York, New York, USA

Karen C. Fieland, School of Social Work, University of Washington, Seattle, Washington, USA

Hilary Goldhammer, The Fenway Institute, Fenway Community Health, Boston, Massachusetts, USA

Gregory L. Greenwood, Behavioral Health Sciences, United Behavioral Health, San Francisco, California, USA

Elisabeth P. Gruskin, Kaiser Permanente, Oakland, California, USA

Gregory M. Herek, Department of Psychology, University of California–Davis, Davis, California, USA

David M. Huebner, Center for AIDS Prevention Studies, University of California–San Francisco, San Francisco, California, USA

Joyce Hunter, HIV Center for Clinical and Behavioral Studies, New York State Psychiatric Institute and Department of Psychiatry; and Department of Psychiatry, Columbia University, New York, New York, USA

Christy M. Isler, Brody School of Medicine, East Carolina University, Greenville, North Carolina, USA

Robert M. Kertzner, Department of Psychiatry, Columbia University, New York, New York, USA

Sam Quan Krueger, United Way of New York, New York, New York, USA

Anne A. Lawrence, Seattle, Washington, USA

Emilia Lombardi, Graduate School of Public Health, University of Pittsburgh, Pittsburgh, Pennsylvania, USA

David Malebranche, School of Medicine, Emory University, Atlanta, Georgia, USA

Kenneth H. Mayer, Medicine and Community Health, Brown University, Providence, Rhode Island; and The Fenway Institute, Fenway Community Health, Boston, Massachusetts, USA

Brian P. McGrath, Graduate School of Architecture, Planning and Preservation, Columbia University, New York, New York, USA

Ilan H. Meyer, Mailman School of Public Health, Columbia University, New York, New York, USA

Alice M. Miller, Mailman School of Public Health, Columbia University, New York, New York, USA

Gregorio A. Millett, Centers for Disease Control and Prevention, Atlanta, Georgia, USA

Matthew J. Mimiaga, The Fenway Institute, Fenway Community Health, Boston, Massachusetts, USA

Mary E. Northridge, Mailman School of Public Health, Columbia University, New York, New York, USA

Katherine A. O'Hanlan, Gynecologic Oncology Associates, Portola Valley, California, USA

Mark B. Padilla, Mailman School of Public Health, Columbia University, New York, New York, USA

Richard G. Parker, Mailman School of Public Health, Columbia University, New York, New York, USA

John L. Peterson, Department of Psychology, Georgia State University, Atlanta, Georgia, USA

Jesus Ramirez-Valles, School of Public Health, University of Illinois–Chicago, Chicago, Illinois, USA

Esther D. Rothblum, Women's Studies Department, San Diego State University, San Diego, California, USA

Marla Russo, School of Public Health and Community Medicine, University of Washington, Seattle, Washington, USA

Ritch C. Savin-Williams, Department of Human Development, Cornell University, Ithaca, New York, USA

Robert Schope, Department of Social Work, The University of Wisconsin Oshkosh, Oshkosh, Wisconsin, USA

Randall L. Sell, School of Public Health, Drexel University, Philadelphia, Pennsylvania, USA

Jane M. Simoni, Department of Psychology, University of Washington, Seattle, Washington, USA

Edward Stein, Benjamin N. Cardozo School of Law, New York, New York, USA

Darryl Strohl, Department of Psychology, University of California–Davis, Davis, California, USA

Rodney VanDerwarker, The Fenway Institute, Fenway Community Health, Boston, Massachusetts, USA

Ernesto Váquez del Aguila, Mailman School of Public Health, Columbia University, New York, New York, USA

Karina L. Walters, School of Social Work, University of Washington, Seattle, Washington, USA

Patrick A. Wilson, Yale University School of Medicine, New Haven, Connecticut, USA

William J. Woods, Center for AIDS Prevention Studies, University of California–San Francisco, San Francisco, California, USA

Hirokazu Yoshikawa, Harvard Graduate School of Education, Cambridge, Massachusetts, USA

Part I

Who Are LGBT Individuals?

Shifting Sands or Solid Foundation? Lesbian, Gay, Bisexual, and Transgender Identity Formation

Michele J. Eliason and Robert Schope

1 Introduction

How do some individuals come to identify as lesbian, gay, bisexual, and/or transgender? Is there a static, universal process of identity formation that crosses all lines of individual difference, such as sexual identities, sex/gender, class, race/ethnicity, and age? If so, can we describe that process in a series of linear stages or steps? Is identity based on a rock-solid foundation, stable and consistent over time? Or are there many identity formation processes that are specific to social and historical factors and/or individual differences, an ever-shifting landscape like a sand dune? The field of lesbian/gay/bisexual/transgender (LGBT) studies is characterized by competing paradigms expressed in various ways: nature versus nurture, biology versus environment, and essentialism versus social constructionism (Eliason, 1996b). Although subtly different, all three debates share common features. Nature, biology, and essentialistic paradigms propose that sexual and gender identities are "real," based in biology or very early life experiences and fixed and stable throughout the life span. These paradigms allow for the development of linear stages of development, or "coming out," models. On the other hand, nurture, environment, and social constructionist paradigms point to sexual and gender identities as contingent on time and place, social circumstances, and historical period, thus suggesting that identities are flexible, variable, and mutable. "Queer theory" conceptualizations of gender and sexuality as fluid, "performative," and based on social-historical contexts do not allow for neat and tidy stage theories of identity development. Most of the linear stage models today are based on the assumption of an essential sexual orientation, but moving through the stages is predicated on responses from the social and cultural environment.

This chapter critically reviews research and theory on LGBT identity development, considering the positive aspects of both social construction and essentialist paradigms. We propose that the field needs theories that are broad, inclusive, and interactionist, taking into account potential biologic, psychological, historical, and sociocultural factors. We briefly review early research/theory on sexual identity formation, and the plethora of stage theories that appeared during the 1980s and 1990s, choosing a few of these models to describe in more detail to highlight the key features or themes of stage models. Other models are presented in a table for the reader's convenience. These models generally focused on gay and lesbian identity. There has been much less work on bisexual and transgender identities, but the little theory available often provides a challenge to gay and lesbian identity models. We also summarize some of the major challenges to linear stage models, propose a compromise model, and suggest some future directions for theory and research.

Before proceeding, it is important to address changes in language: In the years since identity models began to appear, there have been staggering changes in Western society. Those changes include the language we use to describe gender and sexuality. Early theories describe "homosexual" identity formation and are often focused on the (white) gay male experience. Later theories are somewhat more inclusive and describe "gay and lesbian" identities, or even lesbian, gay, and bisexual identities (theories have not advanced to include transgender identities as of yet). Most of the theories are derived from a Eurocentric, Western science perspective and thus are not inclusive of all the people who develop minority sexual and gender identities. We use the terms "sexual identities" or "sexualities" in the place of "homosexuality" here unless quoting from one of the earlier works. Early theories also used language that seems dated or even offensive today, such as "gay life-styles." We try to avoid this language but recognize that any attempts to find inclusive language are bound to fail in these ever-changing times. There is no consensus about the best terms to describe gender or sexual identities. Ringo (2002) found that 19 female-to-male trans-men used 33 combinations of labels to describe themselves. The terms gay, lesbian, and bisexual are equally contested terms.

2 Identity Development Models

2.1 In the Beginning

One of the most important early works dealing with minority self-identity is Erving Goffman's (1963) *Stigma: Notes on the Management of Spoiled Identity*. Social stigma, which is learned and internalized through childhood socialization, shapes the minority individual's identity. Because of this internalization, Goffman proposed that minority individuals share the majority's belief that they are a failure and abnormal. This knowledge leads to self-hate and self-derogation. Because they are stigmatized persons, minority individuals are uncomfortable during interactions with the majority and often try to limit such contacts. The formation of the minority sexual identity involves dealing with social expectations of what is normal.

Dennis Altman and Ken Plummer were among the first to offer explanations for the development of a stable "homosexual" identity. Altman (1971) discussed the potential costs and benefits of disclosing one's homosexuality in a hostile environment. Although perhaps giving too much emphasis to the role of sexual encounters, he was one of the first to describe coming out as a long process where one has to weigh satisfying emotional and physical needs with the resulting stigmatization. Altman suggested that coming out involved dealing with the socially learned "internalization of oppression." Society might for some time remain hostile to homosexuality and homosexuals, but the author believed that individuals could and should seek "liberation" from their own internalized oppression.

Plummer (1975) went further, using symbolic interactionism as his theoretical basis for examining homosexuality (at least in men). Unfortunately, much of his work remains rigidly mired in the sociology of deviance of his time. Thus he talks of individuals adopting a "homosexual way of life" or a "career type" of sexuality. Plummer did recognize, however, that homosexuality was a social construct developed by the majority to restrict and pathologize a sexual minority. He argued that all forms of deviancy need to be viewed within a historical and cultural context. Moreover, he stated that current social hostility to homosexuality (homophobia) was responsible for many of what he labeled "pathologies," such as promiscuity and exaggerated effeminacy.

Plummer's advice for "sexual deviants" was that they should find acceptance and support from others within the "gayworld." The author was one of the first to present a process of identifiable stages. In his first two stages, the homosexual individual moves from pondering sexual identity (sensitization) to accepting the deviant label with all the potential social consequences (significance and disorientation). Plummer argued that social oppression creates disequilibrium where the homosexual becomes stalled (perhaps for the rest of his life) in this second stage. In Plummer's third stage (coming out), the homosexual individual "goes public" with his rebuilt sexual identity. Disclosure, however, was specifically linked by the author to the person's willingness and ability to join the homosexual community. When the homosexual person no longer even questions his homosexual identity, he has reached Plummer's last stage (stabilization). Plummer stressed that the individual is now trapped in this deviant sexual identity by his own continued desire for sexual pleasure and by pressure from the homosexual community itself. Like all groups, the gayworld protects its boundaries by trying to prevent any attempt by members to "retrace their steps" back to heterosexuality or even bisexuality. Thus the author concluded that the homosexual individual who makes it to the last stage finds himself imprisoned by his deviancy and suffering a new form of oppression by his own sexual subgroup.

2.2 Plethora of Stage Models

Building on Plummer and others, the 1980s saw the creation of a variety of models of sexual identity based on the individual's progression through specific stages. Fortunately, most of these theories moved away from the deviance model of Plummer and focused on the healthy consequences of accepting one's sexuality. Most stage model authors assumed that one is or is not gay or lesbian; thus they embrace the argument through an Essentialist lens. The question for them is the individual's recognition of one's own sexuality and the building of a stable sexual identity based on one's innate physical or emotional attractions. Most of the stage models incorporate both the individual's psychological development and real or expected societal reactions to the individual's sexuality. Stage model authors explored the variety of social factors affecting the individual and the enormous choices the individual could make based on those factors. Table 1 summarizes some of the stage models that have appeared in the literature. Most of the models are based on a review of the literature, but they are not empirically tested or are based on only a single, small sample of participants. Stage theories are clearly still at a formative stage and much work needs to be done to validate the processes that lead toward adoption of a gender or sexual identity. The models in Table 1 describe anywhere from three to fourteen stages, phases, or cycles of identity formation and have a great deal of overlap. A few of these theories are described in more detail in the sections that follow.

2.2.1 Eli Coleman

Coleman (1982) presented a five-stage model but rejected the idea that gay individuals all move predictably through the process stage by stage. Rather, the author contended that each person works on the tasks that seem most pressing, which could include working on tasks from two or three stages at the same time. Although Coleman adhered to some linearity (his stages are clearly presented as movement toward a psychologically healthy self-identity), he proposed that individuals in the final stage may still be working on tasks from earlier stages.

In Coleman's model, individuals move through stages driven by an ever clearer awareness of their same-sex feelings. His first stage (before coming out) is characterized by the individual's sense of being different and that others sense this differentness. Unsure what this difference is, the individual often develops low self-esteem and behaviorally acts out trying to avoid dealing with the real cause of the difference. Failure to resolve this growing crisis could result in mental illness or suicide, whereas resolution of the conflict leads the person into Coleman's second stage (coming out).

Coming out to self is clearly the most important task of the second stage. Disclosure to others is also a task of this stage, but to Coleman coming out does not necessarily lead to adopting an openly gay life. Many authors have been critical of stage models that include the necessity of disclosure to others, but Coleman countered that an individual needs the acceptance of others to build self worth and self acceptance. A positive reaction to disclosure provides support against the unending assault by a homophobic society. Coleman suggested that acceptance by heterosexual friends may be more valuable in the struggle to reverse negative self images than acceptance from sexual minorities.

Table 1. Summary of Stage Theories

Study	Basis of stages	Stages or phases of identity formation
Plummer (1975)	Theory about gay men	Sensitization Significance Coming out Stabilization
Ponse (1978)	Interviews with 75 lesbians	*"Gay trajectory"* Subjective feeling of difference from sexual/emotional desire for women Understanding feelings as "lesbian" Assuming a lesbian identity Seeking the company of lesbians Engaging in lesbian relationship (sexual and/or emotional)
Cass (1979, 1996)	Gay and lesbian development; some empirical validation (Cass, 1984)	Confusion Comparison Tolerance Acceptance Pride Integration
Coleman (1982)	No empirical validation	Pre-coming out Coming out Exploration First relationship Integration
Minton & McDonald (1984)	From ego development theory; surveys of 199 gay men	Egocentric Sociocentric Universalistic
Faderman (1984)	Lesbian feminist identity; no empirical validation	Critical evaluation of societal norms and acceptance of lesbian identity Encounters with stigma Lesbian sexual experience (optional)
Sophie (1985/1986)	Lesbian identity; interviews with 14 women	First awareness Testing/exploration Acceptance Integration
Chapman & Brannock (1987)	Lesbian identity; surveys of 197 lesbians	Same-sex orientation Incongruence Self-questioning Identification Choice of life-style
Troiden (1989)	Gay and lesbian development: interviews with 150 men (Troiden, 1979)	*Spirals rather than linear* Sensitization Confusion Assumption Commitment
Morales (1989)	Racial/ethnic minority LGB; no empirical validation	Denial of conflicts Bisexual vs. gay/lesbian identity Conflicts in allegiances Establish priorities in allegiances Integrate various communities
Reynolds & Pope (1991)	Multiple identity formation; no empirical validation	Passive acceptance of society's expectations for one aspect of self Conscious identification with one aspect of self

Table 1. *Continued*

Study	Basis of stages	Stages or phases of identity formation
		Segmented identification with multiple aspects of self
		Intersection identities with multiple aspects of self
Isaacs & McKendrick (1992)	Gay male identity; no empirical validation	Identity diffusion Identity challenge Identity exploration Identity achievement Identity commitment Identity consolidation
Siegel & Lowe (1994)	Gay male identity; no empirical validation	Turning point 　Aware of difference 　Identify source of difference Coming out 　Assumption 　Acceptance 　Celebration Maturing phase 　Reevaluation 　Renewal 　Mentoring
Fox (1995)	Bisexual identity formation; no empirical validation	First opposite sex attractions, behaviors, relationships First same-sex attractions, behaviors, relationships First self-identification as bisexual Self-disclosure as bisexual
McCarn & Fassinger (1996); Fassinger & Miller (1996)	Lesbian and gay identity; study of 34 gay men and 38 lesbians	Awareness Exploration Deepening/commitment Internalization/synthesis
Eliason (1996a)	Lesbian identity; no empirical validation	*Cycles/not linear* 　Preidentity 　Emerging identity 　Recognition/experiences with oppression 　Reevaluation/evolution of identities
Nuttbrock et al. (2002)	Transgender identity; no empirical validation	Awareness Performance Congruence Support
Devor (2004)	Transgender identity; no empirical validation	Abiding anxiety Confusion Comparison (birth sex/gender) Discover trans identity Confusion (trans) Comparison (trans) Tolerance (trans) Delay before acceptance Acceptance Delay before transition Transition Acceptance of posttransition gender/sex Integration Pride

Forming positive self concepts is needed (or is highly desirable) as one moves into and through the third stage (exploration).

Having accepted the label "homosexual," the person in this stage sets out to discover what it means. Often for gay men, it means having sexual contact with many partners. Coleman, however, does not present this stage as simply one of fun and sexual adventure. Frequently individuals during this period may turn to drug use to cope with the stress. Although many of the person's behaviors in this stage may be judged as age-inappropriate, Coleman argued that they are working through issues that most heterosexuals addressed as adolescents. At some point, the individual starts to contemplate the possibility of more serious connections and relationships with others. Coleman's fourth stage (first relationships) is relatively unique among stage models and answers the call that identity development should focus more on relationship development (e.g., DeCecco & Shively, 1984). Coleman emphasized that many early relationships flounder because the individual is controlled by internalized homophobia. The lack of a stable self identity may mean the individual has yet to develop empathy and social skills. Moreover, being in a relationship may "out" the person before he or she is prepared to deal with the consequences. Pressures resulting from these early relationships may make the adventures of sexual experimenting sound enticing, and there may be movement back into the previous stage.

In Coleman's last stage (integration), the individual consolidates private self with public self. This task is highly stressful, and many do not succeed. Unlike many stage theorists, Coleman does not believe that reaching this stage means all the tasks of the previous stages have been resolved. However, he states that it is unlikely that one could achieve identity integration with the early crises still in conflict. Reaching the integration stage opens up the possibility of more successful relationships and the exploration of new and potentially more satisfying social networks.

2.2.2 Richard Troiden

Troiden (1988, 1989) firmly stated that sexual identities are socially learned, although he did not completely dismiss biology. His emphasis was on how social scripts of gender role behavior affect adoption of a sexual identity. Troiden stressed that individuals are not fixed into neat categories of "homosexual" or "heterosexual" but develop sexual identities along any point on Kinsey's scale; thus theoretically this theory can accommodate bisexual identities. Sexual identities form as individuals learn to interpret what their sexual feelings mean to themselves and to society as a whole. Troiden emphasized that no one fits perfectly into any one stage, that his stages are only clusters of characteristics; he rejected linear stage models, stressing that the process is more like a "horizontal spiral" where individuals move in all sorts of directions. Troiden's first stage (sensitization) refers to feelings of being different during puberty, focusing on gender difference, such as not fitting into typical boy and girl behaviors or interests. These feelings of being different are not understood by the child as implying a sexual differentness. When the feelings do start signifying the sexual aspect, one has entered Troiden's second stage (identity confusion). Troiden emphasized that as gender roles become more rigid during adolescence the teen, overwhelmed by guilt, usually desperately tries to hide his or her feelings. Like Plummer and Coleman, Troiden used "coming out" as a stage (his third) but not necessarily in the same way. In Troiden's coming out stage, individuals accept their self identity and presented identity as being the same. This acceptance often results in a new sense of belonging to a group, with possible anger against those in the heterosexual group. Troiden also included sexual experimentation (for gay men) and emotionally charged relationships (for lesbians) in this stage. He argued that these different gender behaviors come out of one's socialization of males as seekers of quick gratification and females as seekers of emotional security. When the individual firmly adopts this new identity and is willing to disclose this identity to others, he or she enters Troiden's last stage (commitment). Although the author contended that persons in this stage most likely disclose to a large number of people in their environment, he also discussed strategies used to evade detection by others. Troiden proposed that even individuals who have stable sexual identities may have to remain hidden because their particular social environment is especially homophobic. Moreover, the formation of a sexual identity is never fully complete as new challenges may strengthen or weaken the individual's commitment to the sexual identification.

2.2.3 *Vivienne Cass*

Vivienne Cass (1979, 1990, 1996) has become one of the most often cited stage model theorists. The author repeatedly emphasizes the importance of the interaction between the individual and the environment. Her six stages have become more and more elaborate as she seeks to demonstrate the impact of family, friends, and other social players on the individual's movement through the stages. In response to the multitude of studies and critiques since her 1979 model was unveiled, Cass clearly has recognized that what is regarded as a gay, lesbian, or bisexual identity is rooted in the culture and history of Western society.

The six stages developed by Cass are levels through which the individual moves, driven by incongruence between self-perception, sexual behaviors, and the perception of how others would view the person if they knew of those behaviors. Each stage is characterized by a struggle to find an acceptable balance but does not necessarily lead to further growth and the next stage. Identity foreclosure is a possibility in every stage as the individual evaluates the costs of continuing the process. According to Western psychologies, the healthiest response at each stage is to meet the challenges involved and evolve into a stable, openly gay individual who is at peace with self and society. Cass's own testing has only partially validated the six stages (Cass, 1984). Still, even those stages with less empirical support, especially her pride stage, make sense as they often are included in other minority identity models (e.g., Cross, 1991).

The individual remains to a large extent in the closet through the first four of Cass's stages. In the first stage (identity confusion), the individual has become aware that he or she has thoughts or has acted in ways that may be identified as "homosexual." This prompts the person to recognize a need to redefine either one's identity or behavior. The reaction to this incongruence leads either to identity foreclosure or movement into the second stage (identity comparison), where the individual accepts that his or her behavior is indeed homosexual in nature. Redefining the behavior is no longer a viable option. Most important, the person is aware of the gap between identity as seen by oneself and identity as presented to others. In stage three (identity tolerance), the individual grudgingly adopts a gay, lesbian, or bisexual self-concept but remains resistant to this identity because of the internalized stigma and fear of negative reactions from others. The individual's options include identity foreclosure, living a life of self-hatred, or movement into the fourth stage (identity acceptance). During this last closeted stage, the individual learns to accept the sexual identity as positive but is still well aware of the social stigmatization. Passing often becomes a more conscious act to avoid the social costs of disclosure. Membership in gay organizations and frequenting of gay bars is now more acceptable as one builds a "second" life rather than the secret life of previous stages.

Incongruence in identity acceptance may lead to Cass's first "open" stage (identity pride). In this stage, the individual determines to reconcile identity as seen by self with identity presented to others through extensive self-disclosure. Cass stresses that this stage may include a rejection of heterosexual society, a reflection of one's anger toward having to bear the burden of the stigma for years. Individuals in this stage also tend to make their sexuality the center of their lives, making it (to use Goffman's words) as obtrusive as possible. Identity foreclosure may leave the individual continually struggling against society. Movement into the sixth stage (identity synthesis) brings balance and peace as the individual becomes more accepting of others and of self, and one's sexuality is no longer the central focus of life. Because the anger over the social stigma is no longer overwhelming, one is equally comfortable around heterosexual and sexual minority individuals.

2.2.4 A Few Other Theories
South African authors Isaacs and McKendrick (1992) presented a different twist on gay male identity formation by emphasizing sexual behaviors and feelings. They based their stages of identity growth on ego development in response to the presence of male and female sexual images. They provided prospective ages for each of their six stages. The first two stages, identity diffusion (age 0 to 9) and identity challenge (age 10 to 15), are characterized by primitive, unclear sexual fantasies, resulting in confused self-esteem. Stage three, identity exploration (age 16 to 19) is a testing phase with confusion over which sexual fantasies to use for masturbation. Beginning identity achievement (age 19 to 65)

finds the individual fixating on same-sex fantasies, resulting in a "coming out crisis." Self-acceptance develops during the identity commitment stage (age 19 to 65), which also includes new and open participation in the "homosexual" subculture. Isaacs and McKendrick emphasized the critical role of this subculture and its power over its members. In the last stage, identity consolidation (age 19 to 65), there is full ownership of one's sexual fantasies. Moreover, the subculture becomes even more important, demanding behavioral changes in accordance with shifting norms. In some ways, the authors see the individual as being victimized by the need to adapt oneself continually to subcultural roles and values, reminiscent of Plummer's model.

In stark contrast to Isaac and McKendrick, Lillian Faderman (1984) discussed the lesbian feminist identity, whereby women can come to identify as lesbians through politics, rather than any innate feelings, drives, or sexual experiences. Indeed, the lesbian feminist may never have a sexual experience with another woman at all. Faderman described three stages that are the reverse of Minton and McDonald's (1984) stages, beginning with a commitment to a lesbian identity and progressing to possibly having a sexual relationship with a woman (although it is not required for a lesbian feminist identity).

Fassinger and Miller (1996) and McCarn and Fassinger (1996) presented a stage model with familiar stages: awareness, exploration, deepening/commitment, and internalization/synthesis. What makes their theory different is that they hypothesize two "branches" to the model. The stages can describe a person's individual process of grappling with internal feelings, behaviors, and attractions; and/or it can describe a process of adopting a group membership, stages toward defining oneself as a member of an oppressed minority group.

Devor (2002) proposed one of the few theories to explore transgender identity formation, basing the stages on Cass's model. Devor's sociological work has focused primarily on female-to-male transsexuals (Devor, 1997). With 14 stages, the theory explores identity comparisons with one's birth sex followed by identity comparisons with a transgender notion; it identifies certain stalled or arrested developmental stages as "delay" stages. Although the stages themselves may or may not be inclusive of lesbian, gay, and bisexual individuals, Devor notes two concepts that underlie all identity formation: witnessing and mirroring. Witnessing refers to the longing we all have to be witnessed by others for who we believe ourselves to be. Witnesses are objective, external validation of the self. Mirroring involves seeing oneself in the eyes of someone who is similar, a person with an insider perspective on the group with which we identity. Identity formation hinges on these two social processes. For transgender or transsexual to be social categories at all, societal assumptions must hold that there are two clearly distinct categories called male and female. The transgender individual must traverse two of society's deeply entrenched belief systems: that men and women are distinct and mutually exclusive categories, and that sex/gender determines sexuality. Coleman et al. (1993) also studied a small group of female-to-male transsexuals who identified as gay men after transition. These authors suggested that transgender individuals go through two developmental stage processes: first for gender identity and then for sexual identity.

2.3 Common Themes of Stage Models

It is clear that linear stage models have a number of similarities and differ primarily in the subtle details. Some of the common themes are described below.

2.3.1 Identity Development Begins with a Feeling of Differentness

The differentness varies somewhat from one theory to another, ranging from gender role deviations (Troiden; Devor) to same-sex attractions (Cass; Chapman & Brannock) to gender of sexual fantasy objects (Isaacs & McKendrick). For all theorists, the difference is motivated by comparison to others or social norms. At first, there is no language for the difference. Rarely do the stage theorists speculate as to the origins of this difference, whether it is innate, generated from early life experiences, the result of name-calling on the playground, or other beginnings.

2.3.2 Identity Formation Is Developmental

The stages are a journey from lack of identity (with poor psychological adjustment) to solid identity and acceptance of one's identity (with good psychological adjustment). That is, later stages are healthier or more advanced than earlier stages. Many theorists refer to the coming out process, whenever it occurs, as similar to adolescence in that the individual must learn dating norms and explore their sexuality and/or gender. In general, the stage models describe a sequence from immaturity and unhealthy adjustment to maturity and good health.

2.3.3 People Need to Disclose

A common belief among many of the stage theorists is that the closeted individual is less healthy than the open individual, who has successfully achieved the ability to live openly and comfortably with his or her sexuality. In Cass's last closeted stage (identity acceptance), the fear of exposure remains for many the focus of their lives, and the person often is dominated by self-hatred. Wells and Kline (1987), like many stage theorists, argued that disclosure to others is an essential part of the coming out process because "each time homosexuals deny their sexual orientation, they hurt themselves slightly, which has a cumulative effect" (p. 192).

2.3.4 The Need for a Stage of Pride/Cultural Immersion

Cass's identity pride stage is perhaps her most controversial because it focuses on the initial anger felt by many LGB individuals against heterosexual society (see also Plummer and Troiden). Before coming out, much time and energy has been lost grappling with society's prejudice. Long forced to pretend to be someone they were not, LGB individuals often respond with rejection of heterosexual society and even most heterosexual persons. For many, coming out feels like the world has become open to them. According to Cass, though, it may at the same time shrink because the initial phase of coming out most often involves a submersion in gay society. Heterosexual friends are often abandoned as untrustworthy; and, ironically, as it has since early childhood, the individual's sexuality or gender continues to dominate his or her life. Now, however, the driving force is to affirm one's identity rather than to desperately hide it.

According to many stage theorists, the pride stage often involves behaviors that would have been considered quite outrageous and unthinkable before coming out. Sexual promiscuity may become a way of constantly reaffirming one's sexuality, especially for men. It also confirms that one no longer accepts society's right to set the rules of behavior. This may be when one is more likely to become involved in political organizations that directly challenge or even threaten the dominant system. Most authors believe that these later stages of coming out force the discomfort in social situations and the psychological work of adjustment from the gay person to the heterosexual person (Brooks, 1981). Certainly, gay individuals in the pride stage are determined to force heterosexuals to feel the discomfort that had long been oppressing the gay person. Goffman (1963) stressed that coming out is a movement from being "discreditable" to "discredited" (openly stigmatized). Yet, although the pride stage is where the person has become discredited in the eyes of society, it is also when the individual is unwilling to accept the stigma as his or her problem. Without confronting the pain of stigma, homophobia will continue to damage society as a whole (Blumenfeld, 1992). Not surprisingly, individuals in the pride stage are most criticized not only by heterosexual persons but also many LGBT individuals, who are uncomfortable forcing the majority to share the discomfort. Heterosexual individuals may express bewilderment at the term "gay pride," arguing that they do not talk about "straight pride," whereas some LGBT people urge their more visible counterparts to try to blend in and "act normal."

2.3.5 Need for Identity Integration/Synthesis

The final or highest stage of most models requires that gender and sexual identities become integrated into the whole personality, so they are no more and no less important than any other aspect of identity. Integration means lessening of the anger against societal norms and a greater emotional balance. According to McCarn and Fassinger (1996), achieved lesbian development means that, "she will have traversed the path from rage, anxiety, insecurity, and rhetoric to directed anger, dedication, and self-love as a lesbian woman" (p. 525). Loiacano (1989) also stressed the need to integrate identities in African American gays and lesbians, citing the struggle for validation of both stigmatized identities as a "challenge to sanity" (p. 23).

3 Challenges to Linear-Stage Models of Identity

Throughout the 1980s to the present, there have been challenges to stage model theories of sexual or gender identity formation. The critics noted that sexual identities are cultural constructs of fairly recent origin and are not universal. There are a wide variety of cultural views of gender and sexuality that differ from our Western notions. Even in Western societies such as the United States, there are subcultural differences based on race/ethnicity, religion, or even age that demonstrate the shaky ground of social identities. For example, many middle-aged and older lesbians have difficulty understanding why many young women are hesitant to call themselves lesbians, preferring instead to call themselves "fluid" or defy categories. As another example, the concept of two-spirit in Native American communities is not synonymous with gay, lesbian, bisexual, or transgender concepts in Western society. Many subcultural groups continue to define sexual identity by active/passive terms rather than gender of partner—that is, the passive or receptive partner is "gay" but not the active or dominant partner. Most of the stage theories do not account for bisexual identity formation, as they are based on the assumption of same-sex desires in opposition to other-sex desires (an exception is Fox, 1995, who provided a stage model of bisexual identity). Finally, few theories have attempted to include transgender identity or theorize the role of gender in identity processes in a more sophisticated manner (Devor, 1993). This section describes some of the major categories of challenges to linear stage models.

3.1 Changes in Social Context

There have been enormous changes in pop culture and media images of gender and sexuality during the past three decades, with an explosion of images and information about alternative gender and sexual roles that the early stage theorists scarcely could have imagined. The youth's of today have access to unlimited information on the Internet and are exposed to a plethora of sexual styles and behaviors. These changes are bound to affect identity formation models in a variety of ways, from earlier age of labeling one's difference to the wider variety of ways gender and sexuality can be expressed. These changes are evident when 7-year-olds "come out" as transgendered on Oprah, junior high kids identify as "genderqueer," straight men allow themselves to be "made over" by a team of gay men, and books proclaim, *The End of Gay* (Archer, 2002). Theoretical models of sex and gender need to accommodate these changes in the culture.

Furthermore, one has to consider the influence of research on the biological underpinnings of gender and sexuality. How is the debate about biology related to cultural notions of sexual and gender identity and to societal attitudes? The question of whether one is born with a sexual orientation or acquires it later needs to figure into discussions of identity formation. Whisman (1996) found that lesbian and bisexual women were more likely to think their sexuality was a choice than men. Many identity models presuppose an innate sexual orientation and have little room for choice, except whether to express sexuality.

3.2 Changing Notions of Sex/Gender

Some stage theorists spend considerable time discussing gender-atypical behavior or feelings during childhood (most notably, Troiden), which leaves out LGBT people who had gender-conforming childhoods, and dismisses the possibility of transgender identity in some individuals who do have gender-atypical childhoods. The role of sex/gender has been debated. It is widely recognized that women and men are socialized differently in most cultures and that gender has different meanings in different cultural groups. Even within LGBT communities, gender has quite varied meanings. Consider a femme lesbian, a transgender woman, a drag queen, and a butch lesbian. Are these all separate identities or variations on the theme of "woman?" Do butch lesbians have the same identity formation processes as femme lesbians (e.g., Levitt, 2003)?

Bisexual identities challenge the foundation of gay and lesbian identities on the sex/gender of the sexual partner, creating anxieties in lesbian and gay communities. How does bisexuality, having a physical attraction to, or choosing sexual or romantic partners on the basis of some characteristic other than their sex/gender, disrupt monosexual identities that are firmly defined by the sex/gender of partners? Most linear stage theories are unable to accommodate the flexibility of a bisexual identity (Horowitz & Newcomb, 2001).

Transgender identities challenge the stability of biologic categories such as sex, which underlie gay and lesbian identity. Kate Bornstein astutely pointed out: "What makes a man—testosterone? What makes a woman—estrogen? If so, you could buy your gender over the counter at any pharmacy" (Bornstein, 1994, p. 56). Other "biologic" markers of sex, such as chromosomes, genitals, and reproductive capabilities, are similarly ambiguous. Again, transgender identities challenge the viability of an identity based on the sex/gender of partners.

Finally, male and female socialization about sex/gender and sexuality in most cultures is quite different and challenges the idea of whether one could ever develop a model of sexual identity formation that captures the experiences of women and men (or even more difficult, people who never felt comfortable in the roles assigned to women and men). In a culture that devalues women and femininity, prejudice against "effeminacy" in men exists in both the dominant culture and in LGBT subcultures (Taywaditep, 2001); and it must play a role in individual development of men. The very different ways that men and women in Western society are socialized about sex and love may affect the trajectories their sexual identity formation may take. Men may be more likely to experiment sexually and define themselves in terms of their sexual behavior, whereas women may define themselves in terms of love relationships, regardless of whether they are sexual. Much of the criticism of linear stages theories has come from women, and there is growing evidence that men experience their sexuality as more linear and less fluid than do women.

3.3 Challenges to the Stability of Identity

Queer theory, an increasingly influential theoretical framework in the humanities, has begun to filter more into the social sciences (it has had a minority voice there all along—see Mary McIntosh, 1968, and various sociologists through the years). These frameworks view social identities of all kinds as contingent on time, place, and circumstances. According to queer theory, identities are always tentative, fragmented, and essentially figments of our imagination attempting to create some order out of the chaos of our lives (Fuss, 1991).

Identities can create problems for individuals when the categories, labels, or stages they choose are too confining and rigid to contain their individual differences. LGBT communities are often shocked when one of their members "leaves the fold." Identity change is threatening to the whole community as it challenges the stability of gender and sexuality (Rust, 1993). The literature is full of stories of rejection when lesbians have relationships with men, when gay men transition to women, when butch lesbians identify as trans-men, and so on. These events are only unsettling if we make the assumption that gender and sexual identities are fixed and stable.

3.4 Challenges to the Developmental Sequence of Stage Theories

Do people have to pass through a series of stages, or can they experience only one stage? Can they go through stages in different orders? Skip stages? Regress? Joan Sophie (1985/1986) reported that women who were questioning their sexual identities often did not fit into stage theories—they skipped stages or went through stages in different orders. Because many of the theories parallel developmental theories of child and adolescent development, they may not be as applicable to adults who adopt a different gender or sexual identity when they are older. The focus on childhood and adolescent experiences leaves out those who form an LGBT identity later in life, who may have never struggled with identity issues during adolescence or young adulthood.

Cox and Gallois (1996) noted that the highest or final stage of many linear stage theories is integration, consolidation, or synthesis of sexuality with other identities, such as gender, race, and age. This privileging of integration as the ultimate state "suggests the existence of a best identity, specifically, an identity that supports the dominant heterosexual hegemony, or at least, is not antagonist to it" (p. 9). Other commentators (Celia Kitzinger, 1987, in particular) have pointed out the apolitical nature of sexual identity stage models in that they focus on individual adjustment so the person can ultimately "fit in" society rather than alter it.

McCarn and Fassinger (1996) noted that most identity models focus on the individual's internal developmental processes; but if sexual identity is socially constructed in response to societal oppression and stigma, it can also be a political identity. Theories that focus on the personal tend to emphasize erotic desires and intimacy needs, where disclosure may be less important. If the theory focuses on social group membership, identity disclosure is a key element. This schism in the definition of identity can also be seen in individuals. In one study, lesbians were asked to define what it meant to be a lesbian. Thirty-five percent gave a nonpolitical, personal definition, such as to love or have sex with women or sexuality is a part of core personality, whereas 65%

gave a political definition, such as to be a lesbian is to have a world-view associated with feminism or civil rights issues (Eliason & Morgan, 1998). Stage theorists often equate sexual identity formation with other developmental processes in humans, such as cognitive and affective development. Some internal processes, such as motor development, perception, sensation, and cognition, are more biologically hard-wired and may unfold in predictable patterns. However, social identities are much more context-bound and may not follow any "rules" of development.

Another issue has to do with the retrospective nature of most research—asking people with variant sexual or gender identities to recall their childhood, adolescence, or feelings/attitudes that occurred in the past. As humans, we tend to reconstruct our past to make sense of our current situations, and so we may impose an order on our lives that is not actually present. This makes it difficult to understand what the early phases/stages of the process might have been like, as most research has focused on people who have already accepted a sexual or gender identity. Swann and Anastas (2003) tried to capture data from young women who were earlier in the developmental process, and they identified three dimensions of lesbian identity. The early phase seemed to be associated with consideration of new identity possibilities, and the later phases were associated with identity consolidation and stigma management.

3.5 Need to Disclose

Goffman (1963) noted that "because of the great rewards in being considered normal, almost all persons who are in a position to pass will do so on some occasion by intent" (p. 74). The individual sees how society treats those who are discredited, such as racial minorities, and may choose not to expose oneself to such pain. Disclosure is not a simple matter of being in or out of the closet. LGBT people are out to some but not to others; out in some situations but not in others (Eliason & Schope, 2001; Schope, 2002). Disclosure is a complicated phenomenon. Schope (2004) reported that some gay men who were closeted did report experiencing less discrimination—realistically, withholding disclosure can be safer. As Fassinger and Miller (1996) suggested, "disclosure is so profoundly influenced by contextual oppression that to use it as an index of identity development directly forces the victim to take responsibility for his or her own victimization" (p. 56). Examples of groups or individuals who may have same-sex relationships or different gender identities and not publicly disclose them may include older individuals who were socialized to consider "passing" as a sign of identity competence (Grossman, 1997; Rosenfeld, 1999); members of racial/ethnic groups who need the support of their families and communities to sustain them in a racist world (Loiacano, 1989; Conerly, 1996; Rosario et al., 2004); and deeply religious individuals whose churches would reject them if they disclosed or whose religious value systems cannot incorporate an LGBT identity (Yarhouse, 2001).

3.6 Rigidity of Labels

Kristin Esterberg (1997) noted, "identities are coercive; they pin people down in both intended and unintended ways . . . identities are accompanied by a freight of social baggage, some of which—perhaps for some women, much of which—may be undesired" (p. 170). She pointed out that identities provide an anchor for some women, a stability and a social validation they need. Identities are particularly useful for political organizing. A main challenge to postmodern theory has been its lack of any solid foundation for political organizing around gender and sexuality (Beemyn & Eliason, 1996). However, for the individual, identities can be restrictive. Paula Rust (1993, 1996b) pointed out the fluidity of sexual identification, particularly in women, as they move between lesbian and bisexual identities. She argued, contrary to stage model theorists, that identity flexibility is more psychologically healthy than identity stability. Rigid identification does not allow adaptations to changes in one's "sexual landscape."

3.7 Role of Other Cultural Identities

Many individuals have dual or multiple social identities that intersect in diverse ways. Those other social identities may involve belief systems that view gender and sexuality differently than Eurocentric Western world views. For example, the term "two-spirit," adopted at a conference in 1990 as a "pan-Indian" term that encompasses both contemporary forms of gender and sexualities in Native American people and traditions of multiple gender and sexuality categories. The term privileges the spiritual aspect of life over the sexual (Jacobs et al., 1997). The term was deliberately selected to distance from non-Native American LGBT individuals who view gender and sexuality differently, although the term does not have universal acceptance.

Other writers have discussed various cultural differences in LGBT identities, such as how butch/femme identities are expressed in Asian American women (Lee, 1996), and how African Americans answer the question, "Are you black first or gay?" (Conerly, 1996). Conerly noted that "there are a multiplicity of potentially valuable black lesbigay identities, rather than just one 'right' one" (p. 141). These, and other authors, discuss the impact of race, class, gender, (dis)ability, and other factors on the development of sexual identities, noting that a model that describes only sexual identity formation in isolation of these other cultural identities is bound to be limiting (Chan, 1989; Espin, 1987; Alonso & Koreck, 1993; Eliason, 1996a; Rosario et al., 2004; Dube & Savin-Williams, 1999). Some cultural values that may affect how an individual defines or expresses his or her gender and/or sexuality may include whether the culture focuses on the individual or the group (family or larger group); how acceptable it is to talk openly about sexuality; the degree of separation of public and private realms; the social organization and definitions of gender; the role of religion within their own culture; and the degree of assimilation into the dominant society (Rust, 1996a).

4 Conclusions and Future Directions

Stage theories have been very popular among human service professionals, such as teachers, social workers, and psychologists who work with LGBT individuals because they provide guidelines for what interventions the individual in therapy may need. They are simplifications of complex developmental processes. However, rigid linear stage models are unlikely to apply to all or even most LGBT people. What are the potential effects on clients in emotional distress who learn that they did not even "come out" right according to the therapist's favorite stage model? How can the challenges to linear stage models be addressed in ways that are still helpful to treatment providers who must deal with real-world concerns of people who choose to use the labels of lesbian, gay, bisexual, or transgender or some variation of these terms? Instead of using linear stage theories, the best parts of these stage models could be combined to produce a series of processes or common themes that individuals may or may not experience at some point in their identity evolution. Identity formation is a lifelong process, rather than some discrete event with a clear beginning, middle, and endpoint. Some potential themes of identity evolution are presented below as a starting point for developing a more flexible and inclusive, nonlinear model of sexual and gender identity formation.

Differences: Many LGBT people report feeling "different" as children or adolescents. However, the difference can take many forms such as gender atypical interests, not feeling like they fit into any peer group, or not meeting parents' or society's expectations. A common experience is a lack of language to describe the difference. Feeling different often results in alienation and isolation.

Confusion: Many LGBT people report feeling confused at some point. The confusion can be because of incongruence between internal feelings and how one is perceived by others, and/or it can be related to gender-role behaviors, physical appearance, sexual or emotional attractions, mannerisms (such as the way one moves one's hands). Confusion can be an unsettling emotional state.

Exploration: Individuals use many methods of identity comparison to others in the mainstream or to those with sexual/gender minority identities, including reading, surfing the Internet, using chat rooms, cruising for sex, joining a social support group or political organization, watching pornography, trying out new hair styles, experimenting with clothing choices, hanging out in gay neighborhoods or bars, learning to ride a motorcycle, or practicing walking in high heels. There are no right or wrong ways to explore, but some forms of exploration carry greater risks than others, for example unsafe sexual practices and making one's difference more obvious to others, which increases risk for violence.

Disclosure: All LGBT people must make some conscious decisions about whether to disclose information about their gender or sexuality to others, and they must consciously weigh the risks and benefits of disclosure in each new situation. The costs of disclosure may be too great. For example, some racial/ethnic minority LGBT people need the support of their families and/or racial/ethnic communities to survive and do not risk disclosure of sexual/gender identities. The adolescent who still depends on family emotional and financial support may not be able to risk rejection. These decisions must be respected. Disclosure decisions can be separate from internal identity processes.

Labeling: Some individuals ultimately decide on an identity label such as lesbian, gay, bisexual, or transgender, whereas others choose queer, genderqueer, fluid, kinky, two-spirit, or other designation; or they refuse to engage in labeling at all. There is no empirical evidence that adopting a label for one's gender or sexuality is more psychologically healthy than not adopting a label. Labels are culture-bound concepts. Whereas white mainstream individuals may use, and find comfort in, labels such as gay and lesbian, others may not relate to these terms at all.

Cultural Immersion: Some individuals who live in sufficiently large cities may immerse themselves in LGBT communities. Although commonly reported in identity models, this option is not available to most LGBT people, who must live in many worlds and communities. Rather than cultural immersion, some individuals may experience cognitive and emotional immersion in their identities that manifests as a preoccupation with identity issues. James Marcia (1987), describing adolescent identity, suggested that people often enter an intense period of thinking about identity options (moratorium) before adopting an identity. One problem that can arise is when the psychological establishment mislabels this immersion as "egocentric," "narcissistic personality disorder," or some other pathologic condition without examining the context in which the preoccupation occurs.

Distrust of the Oppressor: Part of developing a political awareness of sexual and gender identities involves recognizing the role of oppression on the group and the individual. Many individuals react with anger, distrust, disappointment, or rejection of groups that have acted in a discriminatory way toward them. LGB people in general may distrust heterosexuals; transgender and bisexual individuals may distrust gays and lesbians; LGBT people of color may distrust white LGBT individuals; lesbians may distrust gay men; and so on. The oppressor and the oppressed are changing social phenomenon, dependent on context. Of course, it is possible to develop a personal sexual or gender identity without a group membership or political identity at all and not recognize the impact of societal oppression.

Degree of Integration: Although most identity models end with integration of sexual identity into the personality as a seamless whole, the reality is that our social circumstances change constantly; and experiences of oppression, discrimination, and violence may trigger the privileging of certain identities at certain times. To be acutely aware of one's sexual identity when a string of murders of LGBT people has occurred is normal. For LGBT people of color, racism may be a much stronger force in their lives, leading to a privileging of racial identity. For some women, sexism is the salient factor. All people have multiple intersecting identities, and full integration all the time is unrealistic. Most people, however, seek validation of all parts of their identity and do not want to be seen as only one facet of who they are.

Internalized Oppression: All members of stigmatized groups are exposed to negative stereotypes and internalize them to some degree. Overcoming the effects of racism, sexism, homophobia, biphobia, transphobia, ableism, classism, and so on, are lifelong processes in many people's lives. Assisting clients to recognize that some of their problems are due to systemic oppression (developing a political consciousness) often helps to relieve the guilt, shame, anxiety, and fear about personal responsibility for victimization. The political awareness is empowering.

Managing Stigma: LGBT people must learn to negotiate their social contexts. Attitudes about LGBT people are influenced by many types and degrees of stigma, which may vary considerably in an individual's life or over time. For example, attitudes in the general public are influenced by beliefs about whether sexuality is chosen. Public opinion polls show a positive correlation between the belief that sexuality is chosen and homophobic attitudes. Other public discourses that shape attitudes are notions of sick/healthy, unnatural/natural, abnormal/normal, and secrecy/openness. A given individual may experience more of one type of attitude in the family, another in the military, and yet another in the streets outside the gay bar. In addition, the individual's personal beliefs about the causation of gender or sexuality may influence their own identity processes. Those who believe they were "born this way" seem to offer more coherent, continuous stories of having always been LGBT and learning to come to grips with it. Those who believe they chose their gender or sexuality may offer more discontinuous narratives, with more heterosexual and gender-conforming behavior in their younger days.

Identity Transformation: Change is difficult for individuals and their social networks no matter the direction of the change, whether from heterosexual to gay, from lesbian to bisexual, from bisexual to transgender, or more controversially from gay to heterosexual. Although there is no evidence that reparative therapies are effective in changing one from gay to straight, there are individuals who do perceive that their sexuality changed. As Paula Rust (1996b) noted, changes in our sexual landscapes do occur; and to be psychologically healthy we must learn to adapt to these changes.

Authenticity: For many individuals, the identity formation process means moving from a position of hiding, secrecy, and denying to being able to fully accept and express oneself. That expression of authenticity may involve the choice of sexual and/or life partners, dressing or appearing the way one feels inside, or choosing hobbies, jobs, and interests according to one's likes and dislikes rather than the expectations of family or society. Living in an authentic manner does not necessarily require labeling oneself in any particular way but follows the philosophy "to thine own self be true."

We have provided a critique of linear stage models that have appeared in the social science literature since the mid-1970s and explored the challenges to these theories. Stage models have been enormously valuable during the early years of LGBT studies by beginning to explore how sexual and gender identities may form. These linear stage models are less useful, however, as the field evolves. We have presented an approach that blends the best of the stage model theories with the critiques they have engendered, proposing that sexual and gender identity formation is a highly individual process with many components. Recognition of these diverse components allows a more flexible identity model that can adapt to the changing times. Research using these themes could explore how often they present overall or in specific subsets of the LGBT population. Perhaps some themes are more often found in biologic women's identity development and others cluster together for male-to-female transgenders. Maybe some aspects of the themes are developmental and/or linear in nature, whereas others are tied to specific life circumstances that can occur at any point.

In conclusion, the impetus toward linear stage models of sexual and gender identities have stimulated interesting and challenging questions about the nature of identities and have been extremely useful to clinicians who work with LGBT clients. We have proposed a way of retaining the best elements of stage models while at the same time addressing some of the more serious challenges to them.

References

Alonso, A.M., and Koreck, M.T. (1993) Silences: "Hispanics," AIDS, and sexual practices. In: Abelove, H., Barale, M., and Halperin, D.M. (eds) *The lesbian and gay studies reader*. Routledge, New York, pp. 110–126.

Altman, D. (1971) *Homosexual: oppression and liberation*. E.P. Dutton, New York.

Archer, B. (2002) *The end of gay and the death of heterosexuality*. Fusion Press, London.

Beemyn, B., and Eliason, M. (1996) *Queer studies: a lesbian, gay, bisexual, and transgender anthology*. New York University Press, New York.

Blumenfeld, W. (1992) Squeezed into gender envelopes. In: Blumenfeld, W. (ed) *Homophobia: how we all pay the price*. Beacon Press, Boston, pp. 23–38.

Bornstein, K. (1994) *Gender outlaw: on men, women, and the rest of us*. Routledge, New York.

Brooks, V. (1981) *Minority stress and lesbian women*. Lexington Books, Lexington, MA.

Cass, V. (1979) Homosexual identity formation: a theoretical model. *Journal of Homosexuality* 4:219–235.

Cass, V. (1984) Homosexual identity formation: testing a theoretical model. *Journal of Sex Research* 20(2):143–167.

Cass, V. (1990) The implications of homosexual identity formation for the Kinsey model and scale of sexual preference. In: Saunders, S., and Reinisch, J. (eds) *Homosexuality/heterosexuality: concepts of sexual orientation*. Oxford University Press, New York, pp. 239–266.

Cass, V. (1996) Sexual orientation identity formation: a Western phenomenon. *Journal of Homosexuality* 9(2/3):227–251.

Chan, C.S. (1989) Issues of identity development among Asian-American lesbians and gay men. *Journal of Counseling and Development* 68:16–20.

Chapman, B., and Brannock, J. (1987) Proposed model of lesbian identity development: an empirical examination. *Journal of Homosexuality* 14(3/4):69–80.

Coleman, E. (1982) Developmental stages of the coming-out process. In: Paul, W., Weinrich, J.D., Gonsiorek, J.C., and Hotvedt, M.E. (eds) *Homosexuality: social, psychological and biological issues*. Sage Publications, Beverly Hills, CA, pp. 149–158.

Coleman, E., Bockting, W., and Gooren, L. (1993) Homosexual and bisexual identity in sex-reassigned female to male transsexuals. *Archives of Sexual Behavior* 22(1):37–50.

Conerly, G. (1996) The politics of black lesbian, gay, and bisexual identity. In: Beemyn, B., and Eliason, M. (eds) *Queer studies: a lesbian, gay, bisexual, and transgender anthology*. NYU Press, New York, pp. 133–145.

Cox, S., and Gallois, C. (1996) Gay and lesbian identity development: a social identity perspective. *Journal of Homosexuality* 30(4):1–30.

Cross, W. (1991) *Shades of black: diversity of African-American identity*. Temple University Press, Philadelphia.

DeCecco, J.P., and Shively, M.G. (1984) From sexual identity to sexual relationships: A contextual shift. *Journal of Homosexuality* 9(2/3):1–26.

Devor, H. (1997) *FTM: female-to-male transsexuals in society*. Indiana University Press, Bloomington, IN.

Devor, A.H. (2002) Who are "We?" Where sexual orientation meets gender identity. *Journal of Gay and Lesbian Psychotherapy* 6(2):5–21.

Devor, A.H. (2004) Witnessing and mirroring: a fourteen stage model of transsexual identity formation. *Journal of Gay and Lesbian Psychiatry* 8(1/2):41–67.

Devor, H. (1993) Toward a taxonomy of gendered sexuality. *Journal of Psychology and Human Sexuality* 6(1):23–55.

Dube, E.M., and Savin-Williams, R. (1999) Sexual identity development among ethnic sexual-minority male youth. *Developmental Psychology* 35(6):1389–1398.

Eliason, M.J. (1996a) An inclusive model of lesbian identity. *Journal of Gay Lesbian and Bisexual Identity* 1(1):3–19.

Eliason, M.J. (1996b) Identity formation for lesbian, bisexual, and gay persons: beyond a minoritizing view. *Journal of Homosexuality* 30(3):35–62.

Eliason, M.J., and Morgan, K. (1998) Lesbians define themselves: diversity in lesbian identification. *Journal of Gay Lesbian and Bisexual Identities* 3(1):47–63.

Eliason, M.J., and Schope, R. (2001) Does "don't ask, don't tell" apply to health care? Lesbian, gay, and bisexual people's disclosure to health care providers. *Journal of the Gay and Lesbian Medical Association* 5(4):125–134.

Espin, O. (1987) Issues of identity in the psychology of Latina lesbians: explorations and challenges. In: Boston Lesbian Psychology Collective (eds) *Lesbian psychologies*. University of Illinois Press, Urbana, pp. 35–51.

Esterberg, K.G. (1997) *Lesbian and bisexual identities: constructing communities, constructing selves*. Temple University Press, Philadelphia.

Faderman, L. (1984) The "new gay" lesbians. *Journal of Homosexuality* 10(3/4):65–75.

Fassinger, R.E., and Miller, B.A. (1996) Validation of an inclusive model of sexual minority formation on a sample of gay men. *Journal of Homosexuality* 32(2):53–78.

Fox, R.C. (1995) Bisexual identities. In: D'Augelli, A.R., and Patterson, C.J. (eds) *Lesbian, gay, and bisexual identities over the lifespan: psychological perspectives*. Oxford University Press, New York, pp. 48–86.

Fuss, D. (1991) *Inside/out: lesbian theories, gay theories*. Routledge, New York.

Goffman, E. (1963) *Stigma: notes on the management of spoiled identity*. Simon & Schuster, New York.

Grossman, A.H. (1997) The virtual and actual identities of older lesbians and gay men. In: Duberman, M. (ed) *A queer world: the Center for Lesbian and Gay Studies reader*. NYU Press, New York, pp. 615–626.

Horowitz, J.L., and Newcomb, M.D. (2001) A multidimensional approach to homosexual identity. *Journal of Homosexuality* 42(2):1–19.

Isaacs, G., and McKendrick, B. (1992) *Male homosexuality in South Africa: identity formation, culture, and crisis*. Oxford University Press, Capetown.

Jacobs, S.E., Thomas, W., and Lang, S. (1997) *Two-spirit people: Native American gender identity, sexuality, and spirituality*. University of Illinois Press, Urbana.

Kitzinger, C. (1987) *The social construction of lesbianism*. Sage, London.

Lee, J.Y. (1996) Why Suzie Wong is not a lesbian: Asian and Asian American lesbian and bisexual women and femme/butch gender identities. In: Beemyn, B., and Eliason, M. (eds) *Queer studies: a lesbian, gay, bisexual, and transgender anthology*. NYU Press, New York, pp. 115–132.

Levitt, H. (2003) The misunderstood gender: A model of modern femme identity. *Sex Roles* 48(3/4):99–113.

Loiacano, D.K. (1989) Gay identity issues among black Americans: racism, homophobia, and the need for validation. *Journal of Counseling and Development* 68:21–25.

Marcia, J. (1987) Identity in adolescence. In: Adelson, J. (ed) *Handbook of adolescent psychology*. Wiley, New York.

McCarn, S.R., and Fassinger, R.E. (1996) Re-visioning sexual minority identity formation: a new model of lesbian identity and its implications for counseling and research. *The Counseling Psychologist* 24(3):508–534.

McIntosh, M. (1968) The homosexual role. *Social Problems* 16:182–193.

Minton, H.L., and McDonald, G.J. (1984) Homosexual identity formation as a developmental process. *Journal of Homosexuality* 8(1):47–60.

Morales, E.S. (1989) Ethnic minority families and minority gays and lesbians. *Journal of Homosexuality* 17:217–239.

Nuttbrock, L., Rosenblum, A., and Blumenstein, R. (2002) Transgender identity affirmation and mental health. *International Journal of Transgenderism* 6(4).

Plummer, K. (1975) *Sexual stigma: an interactionist account*. Routledge & Kegan Paul, Boston.

Ponse, B. (1978) *Identities in the lesbian world: the social construction of self*. Greenwood Press, London.

Reynolds, A.I., and Pope, R.L. (1991) The complexities of diversity: exploring multiple oppressions. *Journal of Counseling and Development* 70:174–180.

Ringo, P. (2002) Media roles in female-to-male transsexual and transgender identities. *International Journal of Transgenderism* 6(3).

Rosario, M., Schrimshaw, E.W., and Hunter, J. (2004) Ethnic/racial differences in the coming-out process of lesbian, gay, and bisexual youths: a comparison of sexual identity development over time. *Cultural Diversity and Ethnic Minority Psychology* 10(3):215–228.

Rosenfeld, D. (1999) Identity work among lesbian and gay elderly. *Journal of Aging Studies* 13(2):121–144.

Rust, P. (1993) Coming out in the age of social constructionism: sexual identity formation among lesbian and bisexual women. *Gender and Society* 7:50–77.

Rust, P. (1996a) Managing multiple identities: diversity among bisexual women and men. In: Firestein, B. (ed) *Bisexuality: the psychology and politics of an invisible minority*. Sage, Thousand Oaks, CA, pp. 53–83.

Rust, P. (1996b) Sexual identity and bisexual identities: the struggles for self-description in a changing landscape. In: Beemyn, B., and Eliason, M. (eds)

Queer studies: a lesbian, gay, bisexual, and transgender anthology. NYU Press, New York, pp. 64–86.

Schope, R.D. (2002) The decision to tell: factors influencing the disclosure of sexual orientation by gay men. *Journal of Gay and Lesbian Social Services* 14(1):1–22.

Schope, R.D. (2004) Practitioners need to ask: culturally competent practice requires knowing where the gay male client is in the coming out process. *Smith College Studies in Social Work* 74(2):257–270.

Siegel, S., and Lowe, R., Jr. (1994) *Uncharted lives: understanding the life passages of gay men.* Dutton, New York.

Sophie, J. (1985/1986) A critical examination of stage theories of lesbian identity development. *Journal of Homosexuality* 12:39–51.

Swann, S.D., and Anastas, J.W. (2003) Dimensions of lesbian identity during adolescence and young adulthood. *Journal of Gay and Lesbian Social Services* 15(1/2):109–125.

Taywaditep, K.J. (2001) Marginalization among the marginalized: gay men's anti-effeminacy attitudes. *Journal of Homosexuality* 42(1):1–28.

Troiden, R. (1988) *Gay and lesbian identity: a sociological analysis.* General Hall, Dix Hills, NY.

Troiden, R. (1989) The formation of homosexual identities. *Journal of Homosexuality* 17:43–73.

Wells, J., and Kline, W. (1987) Self-disclosure of homosexual orientation. *Journal of Social Psychology* 127(2):191–197.

Whisman, V. (1996) *Queer by choice: lesbians, gay men, and the politics of identity.* Routledge, New York.

Yarhouse, M.A. (2001) Sexual identity development: the influence of valuative frameworks on identity synthesis. *Psychotherapy* 38(3):331–341.

2

Development of Same-Sex Attracted Youth

Ritch C. Savin-Williams and Kenneth M. Cohen

1 Construction of "Gay Youth"

1.1 The Beginnings

Although youthful homoeroticism has been documented by artisans, poets, and historians for thousands of years, it was not until the early 1970s that American scientists—primarily medical researchers and mental health professionals—began systematically studying a newly recognized clinical group they classified as "gay youth." Casting doubt on earlier interpretations that adolescent same-sex encounters were experimental events that were temporary derailments from inevitable heterosexuality, they acknowledged that these youth comprised a unique grouping with their own exceptional experiences, needs, and risks. Not surprisingly, early sources of information about gay youth were comprised mostly of the adolescents who investigators could unquestionably identify and entice to participate in gay research: male prostitutes, runaways, and delinquents. Their early findings consequently highlighted the lives of specific adolescents who were, by definition, in physical, psychological, and social peril.

As information accumulated from studies drawn from similar populations, the accepted portrait of gay youth narrowed to a simplistic, monolithic life representation. These depictions warned that adolescents necessarily suffered miserable, rejected, and risk-filled existences. Dissemination of this "truth" through mental health alerts, advocacy tracts, and policy proposals achieved an intended outcome—eliciting the aid of social service and educational agencies, which created support groups and mental health guidelines (Jones, 1978; Tartagni, 1978; Coleman, 1981/1982; Malyon, 1981; Martin, 1982; Remafedi, 1985). One such agency, the Institute for the Protection of Lesbian and Gay Youth (IPLGY), was established in New York City in 1979 (Martin and Hetrick, 1988). Renamed for its founders, the Hetrick-Martin

Manuscript based in part on Savin-Williams and Cohen (2004), Cohen and Savin-Williams (2004), and Savin-Williams (2005).

Institute and its affiliated Harvey Milk School committed themselves to addressing the heretofore ignored physical, social, educational, and therapeutic needs of gay youth. Social services and community support groups in other large urban centers (e.g., Horizons in Chicago) opened shortly thereafter. Comprising an easily identifiable population of homoerotic youth, the attendees were repeatedly tapped by investigators as a primary pool of research subjects. Drawing conclusions from a sample that was composed, by definition, of troubled and help-seeking individuals, researchers perhaps unwittingly further perpetuated a particular negative characterization of gay youth.

Few researchers at the time questioned whether these youth group members were representative or even characteristic of other youth with same-sex attractions and behavior. The mere fact that any gay teenagers were located was itself cause for celebration and publication. For example, the first empirical study included 60 young men, many of whom were Seattle hustlers (Roesler and Deisher, 1972). Predictably, many recounted high numbers of sexual encounters, with one young man logging 3000+ partners. Furthermore, many participants had visited a gay bar, and nearly half had sought mental health counseling. These boys perceived homosexuals as inherently distraught, desperate misfits *because* of their homosexuality and the stereotyped life script they were destined to follow. Many were suicidal, lived on the fringes of society, and felt rejected and disdained. These youth needed rescuing, and researchers advocated for them with data highlighting societal contributions to their destitute lives.

Subsequent research explored the social stressors that placed gay (male) youth at high risk for physical and psychological problems (Remafedi, 1987a,b). Indeed, most participants reported emotional difficulties, poor grades, school truancy, and substance abuse. Many had consulted a psychiatrist or psychologist. Almost one in two had contracted a sexually transmitted infection, had committed a crime, or had run away from home; and nearly one in three had attempted suicide and had been hospitalized for psychological difficulties. Most of the other youth reported that they would likely attempt suicide in the future. Despite this morbid profile, Remafedi concluded that it was "unlikely" that his adolescent sample was biased because "the very experience of acquiring a homosexual or bisexual identity at an early age [adolescence] places the individual at risk for dysfunction" (Remafedi, 1987a, p. 336). Similarly, after identifying numerous mental health problems (e.g., suicidality) and a history of running away, unsafe sexual behaviors, and drug use among IPLGY clientele, another research team concluded that there was "no evidence that the agency attracts primarily troubled youth" (Rotheram-Borus et al., 1995, p. 77).

The legacy of these research efforts left an indelible impression on health care providers, educators, parents, and youth: Being young, gay, and *troubled* were intrinsically linked. One positive outcome was that as mental health professionals became increasingly sensitized to the needs of these disenfranchised teenagers who often led challenging lives, vital attention and support were provided. Research data were embraced to buttress arguments for the inclusion of gay youth in services provided by physicians, therapists, and educators. One clinician implored mental health professionals to help gay youth to transcend their "impoverished socialization" so they can adjust "to a stigmatized identity [that] is inherently problematic" (Malyon, 1981, p. 321). Similarly, an early sexologist argued that therapists should "assist homosexual individuals to recognize and accept their sexual identity, improve interpersonal and social functioning, and value and integrate this identity while living in a predominantly heterosexual society" (Coleman, 1981/1982, p. 42).

1.2 Methodologic Problems

There were other ways in which gay youth were marginalized and thus removed from mainstream developmental considerations. Even as journal articles about gay youth substantially increased from several during the 1970s to almost 40 during the 1980s to more than 120 during the 1990s (Ryan, 2000), few of the early empirical investigations were published in prestigious, peer-reviewed social science journals or cited in adolescent textbooks. Reasons for this exclusion from adolescent behavioral scholarship were likely the following:

1. Early studies failed to meet the stringent methodologic requirements of scholarly research; were based on flawed research designs; and sampled small, usually biased, populations of help-seeking youth.
2. Manuscripts were likely to be rejected by journal reviewers and editors, who believed that preadult homoeroticism did not exist or was a transient, experimental phase.
3. Researchers did not submit manuscripts to top-tier journals because they feared that their scholarship would not be respected or judged with dispassion.
4. Most of the researchers were physicians and clinicians who submitted their work to specialty journals beyond the usual purview of mainstream social and behavioral scientists.
5. Some of the most innovative research was produced by graduate students who shunned publishing their findings because they feared being labeled a "gay researcher" or because they pursued nonacademic, often clinical vocations.

In defense of the early heroic research efforts, access to gay youth was severely limited to a fraction (the homeless, hustlers, "sissy boys") of this largely invisible population. Investigators and clinicians who recognized these methodologic limitations justifiably reasoned that to present *any* information on gay youth was a worthy achievement. Indeed, research-generated guidelines for health care practitioners and policy-oriented recommendations regarding the treatment of gay youth proved invaluable in elevating public and professional awareness of these young people. However, the generalizability of the research findings and clinical insights to the much larger population of nongay-identified, invisible youth with same-sex attractions who did not volunteer for these early studies was rarely considered inappropriate.

Although later investigators claimed to reduce sample bias drastically by soliciting school-based populations across numerous states (DuRant et al., 1998; Faulkner and Cranston, 1998; Garofalo et al., 1998, 1999; Remafedi et al., 1998), it is almost certain that most same-sex attracted youth remained unwilling to endorse the socially stigmatized identity label "gay," even on anonymous questionnaires. As a result, even though these studies corrected some of the methodologic problems of earlier research, they too failed to elicit a representative or even diverse sample of adolescents with same-sex attractions. The 1% to 2% of the total adolescent population who reported being gay in these studies is not likely to be orthogonal from the earlier 1980s youth participants: the "out," visible, early identifying, help-seeking teens. This nonrepresentative 1% to 2% is substantially below population estimates (10% to 20%) of young adults who have some degree of same-sex attractions (Savin-Williams, 2005).

Investigators were, however, beginning to sample from broader venues and were thus recruiting ethnically diverse teenagers, young women, bisexuals, and international gays (e.g., Australia, Brazil, England, France, Mexico, Sweden). Youth populations were solicited from a range of public settings, including gay community picnics, collegiate meetings, friendship networks, and activist conferences. Research efforts were also being directed less to psychosocial stressors and psychopathology and more to normative developmental milestones. Similar to heterosexual youth, it was shown that gay youth experienced sexual attractions and behaviors starting at an early age, talked to friends and parents about their sexuality, and established committed romantic relationships (Herdt, 1989; Savin-Williams, 1990; D'Augelli, 1991; Herdt and Boxer, 1993).

Because most studies, including these later investigations, included only youth who freely volunteered for *gay-specific* research, little is known about teenagers who have same-sex attractions but who, for unknown reasons, do not willingly participate. In addition, population-based (e.g., school) investigations that sample youth of all sexual orientations provide limited information because they fail to elicit gay identity labels from many homoerotic youth. Both gay-specific and population-based investigations do not adequately sample the full range of same-sex attracted youth. The reasons are overlapping. Particularly in the former studies, *nonparticipating* youth may be unaware or uncertain of their sexuality, perhaps because they have not yet had a sexual experience (the proof). Also, they may not volunteer for the same reasons others do not participate in scientific sexuality studies: They have little sexual experience, hold traditional sexual attitudes and beliefs, have low levels of sexual sensation-seeking (low sexual libido), and excessively self-monitor their expressive (e.g., sexual) behavior (Wiederman, 1999). Among the latter population-based studies, participating but *nondisclosing* homoerotic youth may be reluctant or unwilling to assume a socially stigmatized identity label during adolescence. Nondisclosure may also reflect personal or political resistance to being categorized or defined by their sexuality (Savin-Williams, 2005). The consequence of these limitations is that little is known about homoerotic persons "who are *not* linked, either superficially or strongly, to the gay world" (Sandfort, 1997, p. 265, emphasis added). Accordingly, caution is advised when appraising the scientific merit of research on gay youth (Boxer and Cohler, 1989; Savin-Williams, 1990).

Despite this limited research foundation, general consensus exists regarding the lives of same-sex attracted youth. This information is ordered here according to the average age of acquired developmental milestones. After addressing the elusive issue of estimating the prevalence of youth with same-sex attractions, we review that which is known about early feelings of differentness, the onset of same-sex attractions, initial indications one might not be heterosexual, first sexual experiences, the recognition (self-label) of homosexuality, and the disclosure of this information to others.

2 Prevalence of Gay Youth

The number of youth with same-sex attractions far exceeds those who engage in same-sex behavior or who identify as gay. This fact is consistent with the findings of a national study of adults in which the proportion of individuals with same-sex attractions (8%) was far greater than the fraction who identified as gay, lesbian, or bisexual (2%) and was slightly higher than those who engaged in same-sex behavior (7%) (Laumann et al., 1994); these findings are congruent with data from other countries (Sell et al., 1995). In early investigations of youth, discrepancies among these domains of same-sex sexuality (attractions, identity, behavior) were also evident. For example, whereas nearly 5% of youth in a school-based study reported same-sex fantasies or had predominant same-sex attractions, slightly more than 1% had same-sex behavior or a sexual identification (Remafedi et al., 1992). Indeed, most anonymous surveys of representative samples of U.S. adolescents reveal that fewer than 2% *identify* as gay/bisexual (Garofalo et al., 1999). The propensity toward greater same-sex attractions than sexual identification has also been observed in other countries (van Griensven et al., 2004).

Recent surveys of adolescents and young adults document significantly higher prevalence rates for same-sex attractions, behavior, and identity, although the discrepancies among them remain. Eleven percent of students at one high school self-ascribed one or more attributes of a same-sex sexuality, whereas fewer than 3% identified as gay (Orenstein, 2001). In another high school sample, 6% acknowledged that they "know that I am homosexual or bisexual" and an additional 13% "frequently or sometimes wonder" if they are homosexual (Lock and Steiner, 1999). Among college students, 10% of males and 12% of females reported "neutral" to "strong" attractions to members of the same sex, two to four times as many as those who identified as gay/bisexual (Lippa, 2000).

Self-identified gay youth could conceivably represent as little as 10% of all youth who have same-sex attractions or who engage in same-sex behavior. Whether these adolescents differ from nongay-identified homoerotic youth in important ways remains unknown. So long as research participation necessitates identifying oneself as gay, investigators will overlook many youth who ultimately identify as gay after adolescence and nearly all who will never identify as gay but who nonetheless have a homoerotic orientation.

Before proceeding to a discussion of typical developmental milestones among same-sex attracted youth, several cautionary notes must be advanced. First, despite the seemingly continuous progression of developmental milestones that are based on the average age for reaching particular events, *same-sex development does not proceed in an orderly, invariant, or universal manner or occur within a set, or even typical, time frame* (Savin-Williams, 2005). For example, although most adolescents self-identify as gay or bisexual prior to disclosing this information to others or dating a same-sex partner, some youth enter a committed romantic relationship before self-labeling. Unlike previous cohorts of gay men, an equal proportion of contemporary young men recognize that they are gay *before* engaging in homoerotic sex as *after* (Dubé, 2000). Whereas it is typical to recollect initial same-sex attractions prior to pubertal onset, it is not uncommon for attractions to first surface in high school. Indeed, the variability among developmental milestones is so large that in one study the age range among all 10 identified milestones overlapped (Floyd and Stein, 2002). Thus, sweeping assumptions about "normal" or "typical" developmental trajectories should be rejected.

Second, the unfolding of homoerotic development has been deeply influenced by the sexual revolution that has both normalized and destigmatized same-sex sexuality, particularly among youth. One consequence has been an accelerated evolution in which developmental cohorts, or generations, transform every 5 years and contain greater intragroup variability than during any preceding era (Savin-Williams, 2005). The increasing acceptance of sexual diversity and mainstreaming, rather than ghettoizing, homoeroticism have allowed contemporary cohorts of same-sex attracted youth to incorporate and express life-styles, perspectives, and languages that are similar to those embraced by heterosexual youth. Stereotypes have dwindled as gay youth increasingly reveal that they vary among themselves in much the same way as heterosexual youth vary—shaped more by their gender, ethnicity, physical attributes, personality, and economic class than by their sexuality. Thus, it is essential to acknowledge that past research on gay youth development has limited generalizability to today's same-sex attracted teens. The findings recounted below may better serve as guideposts than definitive maps.

3 Feeling Different

Research frequently documents that gay adults recall growing up feeling different from same-sex peers. However, many nongay children also feel estranged, and many children who eventually identify as gay do not feel different. Furthermore, children of all sexual orientations may feel different because of their physical appearance, race/ethnicity, religious affiliation, personality characteristics, or sex-atypical motor behavior rather than because of their sexuality. One investigation found that regardless of sexual orientation, only a small number of adults, about one in five, recalled feeling "not at all" different from childhood peers (Bell et al., 1981). Among the remaining participants, gays were three times more likely than heterosexuals to feel "very much" different as children, and they more often felt dissimilar primarily because of their sex-atypical behavior and interests. However, nearly one-fourth of heterosexual men also felt different due to their low interest in masculine sports. A second major reason for feeling different, reported by one in five lesbians and gays but only 1 in 50 heterosexuals, was undeniable homoerotic interest and heteroerotic indifference.

Additional research confirmed that gay adult recollections of marginalization were predominantly related to personality variables and behavioral sex atypicality rather than libidinal desires per se (Troiden, 1979). Almost half of the adult gay men attributed their initial feelings of differentness to gender inadequacies, effeminacy, and lack of masculine interests. Other reasons included general alienation and experiences of warmth and excitement in the company of males. Most asserted that their "inappropriate" sexual longings were less influential than the shame associated with gender ineptitude. Children seemingly develop awareness of the ways in which members of their sex are supposed to act at an earlier age than they come to understand what it means to be gay or straight. By their teenage years, however, 99% of the homoerotic men reported that they had come to feel *sexually* different because of erotic interest in boys, diminishing or absent sexual longings for girls, and same-sex sexual activities with peers. Adult lesbians share similar developmental memories. Whereas 75% felt different, only half attributed this distinction to their sexuality (Schneider, 2001).

In a youth-based study, the mean age of first feeling different among gay youth was 8 years (D'Augelli and Grossman, 2001). Half of all boys and two-thirds of all girls remembered being called sissy or tomboy, respectively. Just over half reported that they had been directly told by others that they *were* different, and about one-third recalled that at around age 10 or 11 their parents had attempted to prevent them from behaving like a sissy or tomboy. Thus, although many homoerotic youth feel at odds with peers for reasons common to other adolescents (e.g., appearance, abilities), they are more likely to identify sex-atypical behavior and interests, including same-sex attractions, as a basis for their feelings of estrangement.

4 Same-Sex Attractions

Investigators frequently propose that the manifestation of same-sex attractions is the earliest and most reliable predictor of adult homosexuality. Across studies there is considerable diversity in the age of reported first same-sex attractions, from the very first memories onward. Furthermore, averages have been steadily declining over the last four decades, especially among girls, closing the gap between the sexes. This ongoing diminution among successive cohorts in recognition of homoeroticism cannot be attributed to an earlier pubertal onset but to cultural shifts in awareness of same-sex attractions. Labels and meanings have been given to previously unspecified and seemingly inconsequential desires (Knoth et al., 1988; Rosario et al., 1996; Savin-Williams and Diamond, 2000, 2004; Baumeister et al., 2001).

Regardless of these cohort changes, boys usually report becoming cognizant of their same-sex erotic interests and impulses at an earlier age than do girls. This is not because boys are sexual and girls are not but because the eroticism girls recall is usually thought to be romantic rather than physical. Girls' greater attention to romanticism is related to the greater extent to which they are erotically aroused by psychological rather than physical stimulation (Kinsey et al., 1948, 1953), a trend no doubt reinforced by cultural values. Girls do, however, engage in sexual behavior such as petting and masturbation, but these activities are only minor manifestations of their first erotic arousal. Later research confirmed this sex difference: Girls are more likely to recall their first same-sex attraction as an emotional attachment or crush, whereas boys recall a sexual thought, arousal, or behavior (Herdt and Boxer, 1993).

These sex differences support the hypotheses that female sexual attractions are more contextual than male attractions and more dependent on interpersonal relationships. Central for young women is the desire to form pair bonds, for romantic intimacy, and for emotional responsiveness (Weinberg et al., 1994; Golden, 1996; Peplau et al., 1999). The origin of these sex differences remains uncertain and raises fundamental questions about the relative roles of biology and environment. One uncontested fact is that, relative to male sexuality, female sexuality is considerably more responsive to cultural and social factors, more subject to change in response to external circumstances, and more variable within a particular life course (Baumeister, 2000; Diamond, 2003b).

Several research findings raise questions about portraying the onset of same-sex attractions as necessarily the earliest or best developmental indicator of gayness. First, quite often same-sex attractions do not proceed but are contemporaneous with other developmental milestones, such as feeling different, first sex, or first romance. Second, some heterosexuals, especially females, experience same-sex attractions. Across cultures, girls are less likely than boys to have exclusive heterosexual attractions (Storms, 1981; Rosario et al., 1996; Hillier et al., 1998). Third, most gay youth experience opposite-sex attractions, sometimes prior to same-sex attractions. In several studies, more than 80% of same-sex attracted girls and 60% of the boys acknowledged opposite-sex attractions, fantasies, and/or arousals; in addition, boys reported the onset of heterosexual attractions at the same age, on average, as same-sex attractions—a year or two earlier than girls (Rosario et al., 1996; Savin-Williams, 1998; D'Augelli and Grossman,

2001). Two thirds of adult heterosexual females and nearly half of adult lesbians in another study reported romantic/sexual attractions counter to their sexual orientation—at 18 years for heterosexual females but at 13 years for lesbians (Pattatucci and Hamer, 1995). That lesbians report attractions counter to their sexual orientation at an earlier age could represent cultural pressure to conform to social expectations, leading some girls to recognize or perhaps misinterpret heteronormative feelings. Alternatively, it may represent authentic attractions to both females and males. For both sexes, sexual/romantic attractions consistent with one's sexual orientation appear to emerge first, prior to or during early pubertal development, whereas attractions that are inconsistent surface later, following pubertal onset.

Early sexual attractions are relatively unrelated, however, to the timing at which same-sex attracted young adults eventually self-label, disclose to others, enter a romantic relationship, or experience a positive or negative same-sex identity. Whether the attractions are general or specific, emotional or sexual, they are similarly unrelated. They appear to stand alone; they are highly personally significant but not necessarily connected to subsequent aspects of a youth's sexuality. It remains empirically unknown why some youth with same-sex attractions do not identify as lesbian or gay, although it is conceivable that those who do identify may experience same-sex attractions with greater frequency or intensity (Savin-Williams, 2005).

Regardless of the specific memory of same-sex attractions or its timing, most youth recount that they were not troubled by their early homoeroticism because it felt natural, pleasurable, and mysterious (Savin-Williams, 2005). Eventually, however, a significant number of youth question the meaning of their homoeroticism.

5 Doubting One's Heterosexuality

Simultaneously or years after the onset of same-sex attractions, some youth begin to entertain the notion that they are not heterosexual. They question the implications of their homoerotic attractions or behavior for their adult sexual status. Most homoerotic youth recall same-sex attractions, fantasies, and arousal several years prior to examining the meaning of these feelings. Challenging one's assumed heterosexuality rarely occurs among preteenagers but is more often a milestone achieved during adolescence proper (Rosario et al., 1996; Frankel, 2003). The process can lead to rejection or acceptance of a sexual-minority identity label.

Some youth report they never had such a phase because they immediately understood the meaning of their homoeroticism. The most common precursors to questioning among females in several studies were awareness of same-sex attractions, encounters with a facilitating environment (e.g., peer conversations, university courses, movies), or an exceedingly intimate, emotional same-sex bond (Savin-Williams and Diamond, 2000; Diamond, 2003a,b; Savin-Williams, 2005). Males usually first doubted their heterosexuality subsequent to homoerotic arousal or same-sex sexual experiences, unusually low heterosexual libido, or same-sex romantic crushes (Troiden, 1979; Hillier et al., 1998; Savin-Williams, 1998).

The fact that some youth interpret their homoerotic experiences as a phase or normal experimentation may prevent them from immediately progressing from sexual questioning to gay identification. Others may need further evidence before self-defining because they have not yet had gay sex or they believe that they do not act "stereotypically gay." However, sex as a testing ground for a gay identity is increasingly becoming a relic of previous generations (Dubé, 2000).

6 Same-Sex Behavior

A same-sex encounter can be the earliest, intermediate, or final milestone. Indeed, among contemporary cohorts of same-sex attracted youth, approximately 5% to 10% of boys and 20% of girls identify as gay without having had gay sex. By contrast, most of the youth who engage in gay sex do not identify as gay; some do not even acknowledge their same-sex attractions (Savin-Williams, 1998, 2005). A recent review of the empirical literature concluded that some homoerotic youth are not sexually active (heterosexually and homosexually virgins), that some homoerotic youth are same-sex virgins but heterosexually experienced, that some heteroerotic youth have gay sex, that most homoerotic and an unknown number of heteroerotic youth have both homosexual and heterosexual sex, and that some youth only have sexual encounters consistent with their sexual orientation (Savin-Williams, 2005).

Challenging popular beliefs in childhood sexual latency, Kinsey and colleagues (1948, 1953) demonstrated that humans are naturally sexual throughout childhood. Sex play was a source of erotic arousal for both sexes, consisting of genitalia exhibition, examination, and mutual manipulation among peers. Accessibility to same-sex peers facilitated widespread homosexual encounters, which declined dramatically with age due to repressive socialization that caused heterosexually conditioned adolescents to renounce same-sex behavior. By age 20 years, 17% of women and 37% of men had had at least one homosexual experience to the point of orgasm. Altogether, 10% of boys and 2% of girls were judged almost entirely or exclusively homosexual in overt sexual activities by age 15. Recent research documents a lower percentage of the population engages in same-sex behavior: Approximately 3% of British, Greek, and U.S. adult and adolescent populations had a history of same-sex activities (Garofalo et al., 1999; Papadopoulos et al., 2000; Copas et al., 2002). Diamond's (1993) cross-cultural review concluded that 2% to 3% of females and 5% to 6% of males had engaged in homoerotic behavior since the onset of adolescence.

Nonetheless, most of the adolescents and young adults with same-sex behavior *identify* as heterosexual and most of the gay/bisexual males (averaging 60%) and lesbian/bisexual females (averaging 80%) are heterosexually experienced (Remafedi et al., 1992; Garofalo et al.,

1999; Savin-Williams, 2005). Thus, only a small proportion of gay-identified youth engages *solely* in homoerotic behavior and some homoerotic youth (especially females) have significantly more opposite-sex than same-sex encounters (D'Augelli, 1991; D'Augelli and Hershberger, 1993; Hillier et al., 1998). These data imply that neither preadult opposite-sex nor same-sex behavior necessarily predicts heterosexual or homosexual identification. These "aberrations" are most likely to occur under the pretense of adolescent or young adult "experimentation" when same-sex encounters "mean" the least (Diamond, 1993).

Although adolescents of all sexual orientations seemingly share same-sex experiences, there are notable differences in the extent to which particular youth consistently and fervently pursue homoerotic encounters, the significance they ascribe to same-sex and opposite-sex behavior, and the emotional and physical satisfaction derived from these interactions. For example, in contrast to heterosexual or bisexual youth, opposite-sex activities may be mandatory and yet relatively unappealing to gay youth. A comparative investigation of young women's sexual experiences found that the degree, proportion, and level of sexual arousal and behavior most differentiated homoerotic from heteroerotic women. The former had sex with men, but they had it less often, had it later, and enjoyed it less than did the heteroerotic women (Goode and Haber, 1977). Similarly, compared to heterosexual youth, gay-identified and bisexual-identified male youth reported far more homoerotic contact, by ratios of nearly 40:1 and 20:1, respectively, as well as fewer opposite-sex experiences (Remafedi et al., 1992; DuRant et al., 1998; Garofalo et al., 1999). Whereas having many same-sex partners best predicted homoerotic orientation among males, the only significant predictor of future identity among females was initial greater relative proportions of same-sex to opposite-sex *attractions* (Diamond, 2000, 2003a,b).

The source of greatest intrapopulation variation among many studies is the subject's biologic sex. There are sex differences in the number and sequence of same-sex and opposite-sex encounters, mean age of initial sexual encounters, and context for sexual behavior (Remafedi et al., 1992; D'Augelli and Hershberger, 1993; Rosario et al., 1996; Kryzan, 1997; DuRant et al., 1998; Saewyc et al., 1998; Garofalo et al., 1999; Savin-Williams, 2005). Compared to females, homoerotic males were more likely to participate in homosexual activity and to report more same-sex partners; homoerotic females were more likely to engage in heterosexual behavior. In one study, young women had more total same-sex encounters even though they had fewer sex partners, suggesting that they may forgo casual sex in favor of frequent sexual contact with a single partner (Rosario et al., 1996).

The mean age of first sexual experience was reported in these studies to be later (adolescence proper) for females than males, resulting in fewer early sexual contacts. Males were more likely to experience a same-sex before an opposite-sex encounter, whereas females reported the reverse pattern. This likely reflects the greater incidence of girls as "invitee" rather than "inviter" in heterosexual dating/sex and the greater likelihood that females are genuinely attracted to both sexes. The initial opposite-sex experiences for both sexes usually occurred in the context of a dating relationship (Weinberg et al., 1994; Baumeister, 2000; Diamond, 2003b).

Contexts for first same-sex sexual behavior also reveal sex differences. Most young women (two thirds in one study) had their initial same-sex contact within a friendship or dating relationship (Herdt and Boxer, 1993). Whereas one-third of males also preferred "relationship sex," their most common first context was a purely sexual encounter. Overall, females are more likely than males to attach emotional and romantic meaning to their same-sex relationship prior to engaging in sexual behavior. These sex differences, however, are a matter of degree, not of kind (Savin-Williams and Diamond, 2004).

7 Self-Identification

"Coming out to self," or self-labeling, is perhaps the most personally significant developmental milestone. A historically recent construction (Foucault, 1978), prior to the twentieth century people seldom thought of their sexuality as a basis for their personal identity. Other historic developments are the escalating prevalence of individuals who identify as a sexual minority, the decreasing age at which this occurs, and the social visibility afforded to those who self-label. Nonetheless, despite ever-increasing numbers of self-identified gays, lesbians, and bisexuals, most of the same-sex attracted individuals have not, and likely will never, identify as gay. This issue and the increasing cultural visibility of sexual minorities are addressed elsewhere (Savin-Williams, 2005).

In the past, identification as a sexual minority occurred following adolescence, often well into young adulthood (mid-twenties). In sharp contrast, increasingly contemporary youth are self-labeling while still in high school, often by age 15 (Savin-Williams, 2005). Furthermore, fewer females than males ever label their feelings but not themselves as gay; they more often transition immediately from labeling attractions to labeling self. The developmental lag from first same-sex attractions, behaviors, and questioning to identification might span months, years, or decades and is briefer among females than males (Sears, 1991; D'Augelli and Hershberger, 1993; D'Augelli and Grossman, 2001). One study reported that the average girl required a little more than 3 years to progress from first same-sex attractions to self-labeling compared to 5 years for the average boy (Savin-Williams, 2005). Additionally, the factors that inspire adolescents to embrace a socially stigmatized label remain mostly unexamined. In one study girls credited a fascination with other girls, a same-sex romantic involvement, or a facilitative event (book, academic course, movie); boys attributed sexual thoughts, arousals, and sexual experiences (Savin-Williams and Diamond, 2000). These factors mirror those reviewed above that lead to questioning one's assumed heterosexuality.

Although considerable research documents diversity between the sexes, few empirical investigations address variations among ethnic/racial groups in identity formation (Ryan, 2002). Contingent on their degree of enculturation into mainstream society and their corresponding identification and immersion into their own ethnic culture, young Latinos, Asians, and African Americans face "social suicide" if they adopt an identity closely associated with White decadence—homosexuality (Manalansan, 1996; Savin-Williams, 1996). Because homosexuality is characterized by some ethnic groups as a White disease, identifying as homosexual is interpreted as a rejection of one's ethnic community. Thus, compared to Whites, it would be expected that these youth would identify at later ages. However, the limited empirical evidence does not support this conclusion. Among college men, Latinos were aware of their same-sex attractions at an early age and Asian Americans engaged in sex at a late age. Yet, compared to the total sample, both groups self-labeled as gay/bisexual at about the same age, 15 to 16 years (Dubé and Savin-Williams, 1999). African American young men were less likely than White men to label their same-sex feelings and behavior as gay, but those who did self-labeled at the same age as Whites (Edwards, 1996; Dubé and Savin-Williams, 1999). Reluctance to self-identify is particularly prevalent among African American men who are on the "down low," highly masculine, secretive, gay identity-rejecting individuals who engage in overt heterosexual and covert homosexual behavior within a context of a heterosexual identity (Denizet-Lewis, 2003). Native American Indian youth were less likely than Whites to identify as exclusively heterosexual and more likely to label themselves as bisexual or homosexual, consistent with cultural norms regarding the fluidity or flexibility of gender and sexuality (Saewyc et al., 1998).

Bisexuals, especially females, comprise a sizable portion of most studies and generate further intrapopulation variability. In extensive reviews of the empirical literature, Rodríguez Rust (2000, 2002) found that, in contrast to gays, bisexuals tend to recall heteroerotic before homoerotic attractions, perhaps reflecting memory bias for socially sanctioned sexuality. They are less likely than gays to maintain a consistent sexual identity and thus tend to reach developmental milestones at later ages. Over time, bisexuals often gravitate toward involvement with one sex only and to have fewer same-sex partners than gays but not necessarily fewer other-sex partners than heterosexuals.

Although the empirical data are scant, contemporary youth appear to be more fully embracing bisexuality and other nontraditional expressions of sexuality, including sexual fluidity, gender-based sexual categories, and identity refusal. The only prospective study of sexual fluidity among same-sex attracted young women found frequent changes in identity over 8 years (Diamond, 1998, 2000, 2003a). Most (63%) women transitioned among several identities from childhood through young adulthood, with many considering their sexuality fluid (e.g., love depends on the person and not gender, labels are limiting).

Some reclaimed a heterosexual label, whereas others dispensed with labels altogether. Notably, they were relinquishing their sexual identification, not their sexual orientation (attractions to women).

One implication of these findings is that because sexual identities are socially constructed and personally chosen, they might not reflect underlying biologic or psychogenic sexual orientation or match previous and ongoing sexual contact. Thus, research designs that operationalize sexual identity in a unidimensional, fixed, limited, forced-choice manner omit most of the homoerotic youth who assume unspecified sexual identities (e.g., two-spirit, boydyke, omnisexual, trans-boi), bridge multiple identities (e.g., bi-lesbian, half-dyke), claim no sexual label (e.g., unlabeled, "I love Jen"), and remain fluid in their sexuality. These individuals remain undetectable to investigators who depend on self-identifying populations.

Researchers, however, do not yet understand the reasons some youth acknowledge their same-sex attractions yet fail to self-ascribe a sexual identity label or whether this incongruence reflects sexual developmental delay or rejection of sexual classification schemes. Savin-Williams (2005) postulated several practical, philosophical, and sexual explanations for this inconsistency. For some individuals, sexual attractions and desires may be especially broad and thus transcendent of any single sexual identity category. Others forgo sexual-minority self-labeling for cultural reasons, such as unwillingness to risk or invite rejection by religious institutions or conservative ethnic or cultural affiliations. Still others eschew identification because they repudiate social or political definitions of what it means to be gay or believe prevailing sexual labels are excessively simplistic or reductionistic to represent the magnitude of their sexuality. Sexual categories unnecessarily condense a complex aspect of the self, which some youth believe is less relevant than other facets of their identity (e.g., ethnicity, career, religion). Thus, youth may conclude that they have same-sex attractions and behavior but that they are not "gay."

8 Disclosure

The disclosure of one's homoeroticism is often an arduous and protracted process. The endpoint of complete revelation may never be reached as new individuals who are naive about a youth's same-sex sexuality continually enter a youth's life. The process of "coming out" to others is thus seldom a single event but requires vigilance and persistence; individuals must constantly negotiate their ambivalence about the extent to which they want others to know about their sexuality. Whereas coming out can generate ridicule that imperils a youth's physical and psychological safety, it can also enhance personal integrity, identity synthesis, and psychological health—although the latter is of some dispute (Cohen and Savin-Williams, 1996). Few researchers have explored other essentials of this milestone, including disclosure outcomes and the people to whom it is most important and most difficult to disclose.

Disclosure to others can immediately follow self-disclosure, or it may be deferred for years or decades, though the average interval between the two milestones is 1 to 2 years for boys and somewhat less for girls. It is especially noteworthy that many contemporary adolescents disclose while living at home. The first person told is usually a best friend, often a female, and increasingly, as more gay youth are visible, another same-sex attracted peer. Rarely told first are parents, extended family members, and health care or pastoral care professionals. Despite stereotypes, the reaction received from the first disclosure to a friend or sibling is usually positive, and to parents, more accepting than rejecting (Savin-Williams, 1990, 1998, 2001a).

Incentives and deterrents for coming out to others are inadequately understood. Motivations for *not disclosing* include fear of negative reprisals, fear of the unknown, desire not to hurt or disappoint others, and wish for privacy (Savin-Williams, 1998). Impetus *for disclosing* can be fueled by a desire to preserve or intensify a friendship—either by augmenting communication and trust or by attenuating miscommunication, especially if the potential recipient of the disclosure is an opposite-sex peer thought to have romantic or sexual interest in the youth. Other reasons for coming out are to elicit sympathy and acceptance, to determine whether the recipient of the news is similarly homoerotic and/or interested in a sexual or romantic relationship, to compel oneself to be more sexually honest, to relieve the stress of maintaining a shameful and potentially dangerous secret, and to make a political statement.

It is particularly noteworthy that many youth postpone coming out to parents, the likely consequence of its developmental importance (signifying a commitment to homoerotic sexuality) or dreaded outcomes (fearing rejection and homelessness) (Savin-Williams, 2001a). However, adolescents are increasingly coming out to a parent (usually the mother) while living at home and only infrequently receive a severely negative response. Reasons to disclose to parents are mostly unknown but include internal factors (e.g., mounting comfort with one's sexuality) and external factors (e.g., escalating desire for a homoerotic romantic relationship). In one study, most youth disclosed to parents because they longed to share this aspect of themselves or because a parent, unable to ignore the many subtle and blatant gestures by the child, directly inquired (Savin-Williams, 2001a). Parents responded with a range of reactions, from celebration to rejection, but most eventually accepted what many had suspected for years.

9 Acceptance

Developmental pathways from first feeling different or recognizing same-sex attractions to eventually accepting a same-sex sexuality are seldom linear or universal. Neither is it necessarily the case that milestones, such as coming out to self and others and feeling positive about one's identity, are inevitably linked. For example, one qualitative study found that many adolescents felt positive about their sexuality *the same year* they identified as homosexual, some felt good *before* they identified, and some felt fine but *never* identified (Sears, 1991).

Most investigations report that participants recount feeling good about their sexuality and their identity, although this may be the consequence of biased research samples in which only happy youth volunteer or report a homoerotic identity. In several studies, 75% of adolescents reported feeling very good, good, or okay/indifferent about being gay; fewer than 10% wished they were not gay (Kryzan, 1997, 2000; Hillier et al., 1998; D'Augelli and Grossman, 2001). These data contradict research documenting the supposed ubiquity of suicidality among gay youth (reviewed in Savin-Williams, 1994, 2001b; Savin-Williams and Ream, 2003). Young women are usually more positive than young men about their sexuality and develop this attitude at a younger age, perhaps because they experience less sexual orientation victimization, including verbal harassment, physical abuse, and sexual abuse (D'Augelli and Grossman, 2001; Savin-Williams, 2001b).

10 Conclusions

Since the "construction" of the gay youth during the 1970s, considerable research has focused on their mental health status and, to a lesser extent, their developmental trajectories. The accumulated findings present two significant limitations. First, the issues addressed have been restricted to "negative" life scripts. Indeed, according to one recent review, topics most frequently published have been related to gay youth's poor physical and sexual health, counseling and mental health, risky behaviors, (poor) school performance, and (no) family support (Ryan, 2000). This focus on pathology has tainted the perception of same-sex attracted youth, characterizing them as necessarily troubled individuals destined to lead sad, risky lives.

A second constraint on our knowledge has resulted from reducing youth samples to a narrow band of individuals: those who volunteer for gay research or who identify as gay in sexual research. This subset of homoerotic individuals certainly deserves attention, as many undergo unique experiences that place their health in jeopardy. However, they should not be recognized as "typical" lest they eclipse the needs and challenges of the broader community of same-sex attracted youth who are strong and resilient. The challenge of future research is identifying and sampling this larger population from which more representative conclusions can be drawn. Until such time, research on "gay youth" must be interpreted with caution.

The start of the twenty-first century has seen prolific increases in gay youth research and exposure. The media is increasingly celebrating their culture and characterizing them as any youth (i.e., the girl/boy next door). Charting their development by identifying and describing milestones is one way in which their presence is validated and normalized. It escorts them into the realm of "human development" rather than child development gone awry.

References

Baumeister, R.F. (2000) Gender differences in erotic plasticity: the female sex drive as socially flexible and responsive. *Psychological Bulletin* 126:247–374.

Baumeister, R.F., Catanese, K.R., and Vohs, K.D. (2001) Is there a gender difference in strength of sex drive? Theoretical views, conceptual distinctions, and a review of relevant evidence. *Personality and Social Psychology Review* 5:242–273.

Bell, A.P., Weinberg, M.S., and Hammersmith, S.K. (1981) *Sexual preference: its development in men and women.* Indiana University Press, Bloomington.

Boxer, A.M., and Cohler, B.J. (1989) The life course of gay and lesbian youth: an immodest proposal for the study of lives. *Journal of Homosexuality* 17:315–355.

Cohen, K.M., and Savin-Williams, R.C. (1996) Developmental perspectives on coming out to self and others. In: Savin-Williams, R.C., and Cohen, K.M. (eds) *The lives of lesbians, gays, and bisexuals: children to adults.* Harcourt Brace College Publishing, Forth Worth, TX, pp. 113–151.

Cohen, K.M., and Savin-Williams, R.C. (2004) Growing up with same-sex attractions. *Current Problems in Pediatric and Adolescent Health Care* 34(10): 361–369.

Coleman, E. (1981/1982) Developmental stages of the coming out process. *Journal of Homosexuality* 7:31–43.

Copas, A.J., Wellings, K., Erens, B., Mercer, C.H., McManus, S., Fenton, K.A., Korovessis, C., Macdowall, W., Nanchahal, K., and Johnson, A.M. (2002) The accuracy of reported sensitive sexual behaviour in Britain: exploring the extent of change 1990–2000. *Sexually Transmitted Infections* 78:26–30.

D'Augelli, A.R. (1991) Gay men in college: identity processes and adaptations. *Journal of College Students Development* 32:140–146.

D'Augelli, A.R., and Grossman, A.H. (2001, August) Sexual orientation victimization of lesbian, gay, and bisexual youths. Paper presented at the American Psychological Association, San Francisco.

D'Augelli, A.R., and Hershberger, S.L. (1993) Lesbian, gay, and bisexual youth in community settings: personal challenges and mental health problems. *American Journal of Community Psychology* 21:421–448.

Denizet-Lewis, B. (2003, August 3) Double lives on the down low. *New York Times Magazine,* pp. 28–33, 48, 52–53.

Diamond, L.M. (1998) The development of sexual orientation among adolescent and young adult women. *Development Psychology* 34:1085–1095.

Diamond, L.M. (2000) Sexual identity, attractions, and behavior among young sexual-minority women over a two-year period. *Development Psychology* 36:241–250.

Diamond, L.M. (2003a) Was it a phase? Young women's relinquishment of lesbian/bisexual identities over a 5-year period. *Journal of Personality and Social Psychology* 84:352–364.

Diamond, L.M. (2003b) What does sexual orientation orient? A biobehavioral model distinguishing romantic love and sexual desire. *Psychological Review* 110:173–192.

Diamond, M. (1993) Homosexuality and bisexuality in different populations. *Archives of Sexual Behavior* 22:291–310.

Dubé, E.M. (2000) The role of sexual behavior in the identification process of gay and bisexual males. *Journal of Sex Research* 37:123–132.

Dubé, E.M., and Savin-Williams, R.C. (1999) Sexual identity development among ethnic sexual-minority male youths. *Development Psychology* 35:1389–1399.

DuRant, R.H., Krowchuk, D.P., and Sinal, S.H. (1998) Victimization, use of violence, and drug use at school among male adolescents who engage in same-sex sexual behavior. *Journal of Pediatrics* 132:113–118.

Edwards, W.J. (1996) Operating within the mainstream: coping and adjustment among a sample of homosexual youths. *Deviant Behavior Interdisciplinary Journal* 17:229–251.

Faulkner, A.H., and Cranston, K. (1998) Correlates of same-sex sexual behavior in a random sample of Massachusetts high school students. *American Journal of Public Health* 88:262–266.

Floyd, F.J., and Stein, T.S. (2002) Sexual orientation identity formation among gay, lesbian, and bisexual youths: multiple patterns of milestone experiences. *Journal of Research on Adolescence* 12:167–191.

Foucault, M. (1978) *The history of sexuality*. Pantheon, New York.

Frankel, L.B. (2003) Do heterosexual men have a sexual identity? An exploratory study. Doctoral dissertation, Cornell University, Ithaca, NY.

Garofalo, R., Wolf, R.C., Kessel, S., Palfrey, J., and DuRant, R.H. (1998) The association between health risk behaviors and sexual orientation among a school-based sample of adolescents. *Pediatrics* 101:895–902.

Garofalo, R., Wolf, R.C., Wissow, L.S., Woods, E.R., and Goodman, E. (1999) Sexual orientation and risk of suicide attempts among a representative sample of youth. *Archives of Pediatric and Adolescent Medicine* 153:487–493.

Golden, C. (1996) What's in a name? Sexual self-identification among women. In: Savin-Williams, R.C., and Cohen, K.M. (eds) *The lives of lesbians, gays, and bisexuals: children to adults*. Harcourt Brace College Publishing, Fort Worth, TX, pp. 229–249.

Goode, E., and Haber, L. (1977) Sexual correlates of homosexual experience: an exploratory study of college women. *Journal of Sex Research* 13:12–21.

Herdt, G. (ed) (1989) *Gay and lesbian youth*. Harrington Park Press, New York.

Herdt, G., and Boxer, A.M. (1993) *Children of horizons: how gay and lesbian teens are leading a new way out of the closet*. Beacon Press, Boston.

Hillier, L., Dempsey, D., Harrison, L., Beale, L., Matthews, L., and Rosenthal, D. (1998) *Writing themselves in: a national report on the sexuality, health and well-being of same-sex attracted young people*. Monograph series 7. Australian Research Centre in Sex, Health and Society, National Centre in HIV Social Research, La Trobe University, Carlton, Australia.

Jones, G.P. (1978) Counseling gay adolescents. *Counselor Education and Supervision* 18:149–152.

Kinsey, A.C., Pomeroy, W.B., and Martin, C.E. (1948) *Sexual behavior in the human male*. W.B. Saunders, Philadelphia.

Kinsey, A.C., Pomeroy, W.B., Martin, C.E., and Gebhard, P.H. (1953) *Sexual behavior in the human female*. W.B. Saunders, Philadelphia.

Knoth, R., Boyd, K., and Singer, B. (1988) Empirical tests of sexual selection theory: predictions of sex differences in onset, intensity, and time course of sexual arousal. *Journal of Sex Research* 24:73–89.

Kryzan C. (1997) OutProud/Oasis Internet survey of queer and questioning youth. Sponsored by OutProud, The National Coalition for Gay, Lesbian, Bisexual and Transgender Youth and *Oasis Magazine*. Contact: survey@outproud.org.

Kryzan, C. (2000) OutProud/Oasis Internet survey of queer and questioning youth. Sponsored by OutProud, The National Coalition for Gay, Lesbian, Bisexual and Transgender Youth and *Oasis Magazine*. Contact: survey@outproud.org.

Laumann, E.O., Gagnon, J., Michael, R.T., and Michaels, S. (1994) *The social organization of sexuality: sexual practices in the United States*. University of Chicago Press, Chicago.

Lippa, R.A. (2000) Gender-related traits in gay men, lesbian women, and heterosexual men and women: the virtual identity of homosexual-heterosexual diagnosticity and gender diagnosticity. *Journal of Personality* 68:899–926.

Lock, J., and Steiner, H. (1999) Gay, lesbian, and bisexual youth risks for emotional, physical, and social problems: results from a community-based survey. *Journal of the American Academy of Child Adolescent Psychiatry* 38:297–304.

Malyon, A.K. (1981) The homosexual adolescent: developmental issues and social bias. *Child Welfare* 60:321–330.

Manalansan, M.F. (1996) Double minorities: latino, Black, and Asian men who have sex with men. In: Savin-Williams, R.C., and Cohen, K.M. (eds) *The lives of lesbians, gays, and bisexuals: children to adults*. Harcourt Brace College Publishing, Forth Worth, TX, pp. 393–415.

Martin, A.D. (1982) Learning to hide: the socialization of the gay adolescent. *Adolescent Psychiatry* 10:52–65.

Martin, A.D., and Hetrick, E.S. (1988) The stigmatization of the gay and lesbian adolescent. *Journal of Homosexuality* 15:163–183.

Orenstein, A. (2001) Substance use among gay and lesbian adolescents. *Journal of Homosexuality* 41:1–15.

Papadopoulos, N.G., Stamboulides, P., and Triantafillou, T. (2000) The psychosexual development and behavior of university students: a nationwide survey in Greece. *Journal of the Psychology of Human Sexuality* 11:93–110.

Pattatucci, A.M.L., and Hamer, D.H. (1995) Development and familiality of sexual orientation in females. *Behavior Genetics* 25:407–420.

Peplau, L.A., Spalding, L.R., Conley, T.D., and Veniegas, R.C. (1999) The development of sexual orientation in women. *Annual Review of Sex Research* 10:70–99.

Remafedi, G. (1985) Adolescent homosexuality: issues for pediatricians. *Clinical Pediatrics* 24:481–485.

Remafedi, G. (1987a) Adolescent homosexuality: psychosocial and medical implications. *Pediatrics* 79:331–337.

Remafedi, G. (1987b) Male homosexuality: the adolescent's perspective. *Pediatrics* 79:326–330.

Remafedi, G., Resnick, M., Blum, R., and Harris, L. (1992) Demography of sexual orientation in adolescents. *Pediatrics* 89:714–721.

Remafedi, G., French, S., Story, M., Resnick, M.D., and Blum, R. (1998) The relationship between suicide risk and sexual orientation: results of a population-based study. *American Journal of Public Health* 88:57–60.

Rodríguez Rust, P.C.R. (2000) *Bisexuality in the United States: a social science reader*. Columbia University Press, New York.

Rodríguez Rust, P.C.R. (2002) Bisexuality: the state of the union. *Annual Review of Sex Research* 13:180–240.

Roesler, T., and Deisher, R.W. (1972) Youthful male homosexuality: homosexual experience and the process of developing homosexual identity in males aged 16 to 22 years. *Journal of the American Medical Association* 219(8):1018–1023.

Rosario, M., Meyer-Bahlburg, H.F.L., Hunter, J., Exner, T.M., Gwadz, M., and Keller, A.M. (1996) The psychosexual development of urban lesbian, gay, and bisexual youths. *Journal of Sex Research* 33:113–126.

Rotheram-Borus, M.J., Rosario, M., Van Rossem, R., Reid, H., and Gillis, J.R. (1995) Prevalence, course, and predictors of multiple problem behaviors among gay and bisexual male adolescents. *Developmental Psychology* 31:75–85.

Ryan, C. (2000, March 15) An analysis of the content and gaps in the scientific and professional literature on the health and mental concerns of lesbian, gay and bisexual youth. Paper prepared for the American Psychological Association Healthy LGB Students Project.

Ryan, C. (2002) *A review of the professional literature and research needs for LGBT youth of color*. National Youth Advocacy Coalition, Washington, DC.

Saewyc, E.M., Skay, C.L., Bearinger, L.H., Blum, R.W., and Resnick, M.D. (1998) Demographics of sexual orientation among American Indian adolescents. *American Orthopsychiatric Association* 68:590–600.

Sandfort, T.G.M. (1997) Sampling male homosexuality. In: Bancroft, J. (ed) *Researching sexual behavior: methodological issues*. Indiana University Press, Bloomington, pp. 261–275.

Savin-Williams, R.C. (1990) *Gay and lesbian youth: expressions of identity*. Hemisphere, Washington, DC.

Savin-Williams, R.C. (1994) Verbal and physical abuse as stressors in the lives of sexual minority youth: associations with school problems, running away, substance abuse, prostitution, and suicide. *Journal of Consulting and Clinical Psychology* 62:261–269.

Savin-Williams, R.C. (1996) Ethnic- and sexual-minority youth. In: Savin-Williams, R.C., and Cohen, K.M. (eds) *The lives of lesbians, gays, and bisexuals: children to adults*. Harcourt Brace College Publishing, Fort Worth, TX, pp. 152–165.

Savin-Williams, R.C. (1998) *"... And then I became gay": young men's stories*. Routledge, New York.

Savin-Williams, R.C. (2001a) *"Mom, Dad. I'm gay: how families negotiate coming out*. American Psychological Association, Washington, DC.

Savin-Williams, R.C. (2001b) Suicide attempts among sexual-minority youth: population and measurement issues. *Journal of Consulting and Clinical Psychology* 69:983–991.

Savin-Williams, R.C. (2005) *The new gay teenager*. Harvard University Press, Cambridge, MA.

Savin-Williams, R.C., and Cohen, K.M. (2004) Homoerotic development during childhood and adolescence. *Child and Adolescent Psychiatric Clinics of North American* 13:529–549.

Savin-Williams, R.C., and Diamond, L.M. (2000) Sexual identity trajectories among sexual-minority youth: gender comparisons. *Archives of Sexual Behavior* 29:419–440.

Savin-Williams, R.C., and Diamond, L.M. (2004) Sex. In: Lerner, R.M., and Steinberg, L. (eds) *Handbook of adolescent psychology*, 2nd ed. John Wiley, New York, pp. 189–231.

Savin-Williams, R.C., and Ream, G.L. (2003) Suicide attempts among sexual-minority male youth. *Journal of Clinical Child Adolescent Psychology* 32:509–522.

Schneider, M.S. (2001) Toward a reconceptualization of the coming-out process for adolescent females. In: D'Augelli, A.R., and Patterson, C.J. (eds) *Lesbian, gay, and bisexual identities and youth: psychological perspectives*. Oxford University Press, New York, pp. 71–96.

Sears, J.T. (1991) *Growing up gay in the South: race, gender, and journeys of the spirit*. Harrington Park Press, New York.

Sell, R.L., Wells, J.A., and Wypij, D. (1995) The prevalence of homosexual behavior and attraction in the United States, the United Kingdom and France: results of national population-based samples. *Archives of Sexual Behavior* 24:235–248.

Storms, M.D. (1981) A theory of erotic orientation development. *Psychological Review* 88:340–353.

Tartagni, D. (1978) Counseling gays in a school setting. *School Counselor* 26:26–32.

Troiden, R.R. (1979) Becoming homosexual: a model of gay identity acquisition. *Psychiatry* 42:362–373.

Van Griensven, F., Kilmarx, P.H., Jeeyapant, S., Manopaiboon, C., Korattana, S., Jenkins, R.A., Uthaivoravit, W., Limpakarnjanarat, K., and Mastro, T.D. (2004) The prevalence of bisexual and homosexual orientation and related health risks among adolescents in northern Thailand. *Archives of Sexual Behavior* 33:137–147.

Wiederman, M.W. (1999) Volunteer bias in sexuality research using college student participants. *Journal of Sex Research* 36:59–66.

Weinberg, M.S., Williams, C.J., and Pryor, D.W. (1994) *Dual attraction: understanding bisexuality*. Oxford University Press, New York.

3

Developmental Issues in Lesbian and Gay Adulthood

Robert M. Kertzner

1 Introduction

The developmental issues of adulthood for lesbians and gay men are poorly characterized compared with descriptions of adolescent development in sexual minority persons, on the one hand, and adult development in the U.S. general population, on the other hand. As Harry (1993) noted, "Coming out has little to say to adults and life seems to end at about age twenty-five with the rest of the life span left unanalyzed and unexplained" (p. 38). Yet examining the rest of the life span is likely to yield important information about how sexual minority status shapes adult experience and the ongoing revision of personal identity in the context of cumulative life history, an increasing awareness of less time remaining in life, and social and cultural norms that define what it means to be an adult (Erikson, 1959; Neugarten, 1968; Levinson, 1980; Colarusso and Nemiroff, 1981).

This chapter, accordingly, explores lesbian and gay development as revealed through revisions in personal identity and life narrative throughout the years of adulthood. The adult modification of identity and narrative is a central concern of life span psychology with interesting but relatively unexplored implications for sexual minority persons (Cornett and Hudson, 1987). There are several reasons for the relatively limited though increasing literature on adult development in lesbian and gay lives. Perhaps most importantly, examining how sexual minority status informs the subjective appraisal of life experience requires consideration of a great diversity of factors such as gender and gender role attributes, race and ethnicity, class, historical age cohort effects, the experience of and response to stigmatization of homosexuality, and variability in the meaning and expression of nonconventional sexualities (Herdt et al., 1997). Consequently, most reports on sexual minority adulthood focus on specific topics in specific populations, for instance, concerns about aging in gay men (Mennigerode, 1976; Berger, 1982), relationships among midlife lesbians (Adelman, 2000), or social support in the lives of older lesbians and gay men (Grossman et al.,

2000). This selectivity of focus also reflects the paucity of theoretical work integrating theories of homosexual identity maintenance with theories describing the psychological and socialization processes of aging (Kimmel, 2004), methodologic problems when conducting systematic research on lesbian and gay populations (see Section IV), and difficulties inherent in the multidisciplinary study of adulthood where social, cultural, historical, and psychological perspectives all contribute to a greater understanding of lesbian and gay lives.

In focusing on revisions of personal identity and life narrative, this chapter emphasizes a psychological approach and an individual level of analysis, mindful that individual experience cannot be divorced from the sociocultural context. Within the psychological domain, I focus on identity and narrative because of two compelling sets of stories that, despite their overlap, are usually told separately: stories about being lesbian or gay and stories about becoming older. This chapter considers the potential heuristic and clinical significance of an adult developmental approach that attempts to integrates both sets of stories.

2 Developmental Versus Life Course Models

At the outset, it is important to acknowledge that the frame of adult development is one of several approaches to understanding subjective experience during adulthood, each of which is associated with advantages and limitations. Developmental approaches emphasize intrinsic and idiosyncratic factors associated with the evolution of individual capacity to understand and be engaged in the world. Thus, the continuing maturation of the brain into the fifth decade of life (Bartzokis et al., 2001), the ability to utilize higher level coping mechanisms and engage in more complex patterns of thought characteristic of adults (Stevens-Long, 1990; Vaillant, 1993), and the increasing tendency during adulthood to interpret present experience through the lens of what has been learned in the past (Neugarten, 1968) influence how identity and life narrative are fashioned and refashioned. In addition, developmental models posit that adult experience is strongly shaped by innate and early life factors (i.e., the interaction of heritable traits, childhood environment, and idiosyncratic life events) that create a psychological template upon which adult identity and narrative are constructed.

In contrast, other approaches to understanding adult subjective experience place equal or greater emphasis on social, cultural, and historical forces (Neugarten, 1970; Cohler and Galatzer-Levy, 2000). Life course perspectives on adulthood, for instance, highlight socially defined age norms and a social schedule of expectable life transitions as major determinants of the subjective experience of adulthood and aging (Neugarten, 1970). Whether one feels old, from this perspective, is determined more by social convention than by any intrinsic sense of aging. A life course approach also suggests that identity and personal narratives are best understood as constructions of meaning shaped by culture in a specific historical context (Herdt, 1997). As seen from this approach, the seemingly linear order of adult development is better understood as an artifact of individual efforts to impose a sense of narrative coherence on a series of random and disruptive events that occur throughout any individual life course (Cohler and Galatzer-Levy, 1990). These perspectives have implications for how lesbian and gay adulthood is understood and described. Psychologically based models of development do not fully consider sociocultural and historical influences, including those that define what is valued and devalued during adulthood. Such models also overlook the intersectionality of multiple identities and the pluralism of meanings inherent in subjective representations of self (Simon, 1996). These models, moreover, are greatly influenced by dominant cultural values in the West of personal autonomy and self-sufficiency and, in earlier conceptualizations, by an overrepresentation of relatively affluent, White male respondents in study samples (Kimmel, 1978; Gilligan, 1982; Kimmel and Sang, 1995; Cass, 1996).

Life course models based on social determinism, on the other hand, overlook the influence of developmental change that seems at least partially rooted in changing physical and psychological capacities of individuals. Nor do they speak to the idiosyncrasies of individual lives that influence how social and cultural cues are incorporated into personal identity and narrative. As already suggested, these idiosyncrasies include individual factors such as temperament and disposition, the microenvironment of early family life, psychiatric vulnerability, and specific life events that shape personal biography.

A more specific dualism of psychological and social perspectives central to this chapter is how lesbian and gay identity is defined and shaped during adulthood. The chapter emphasizes meaning-making by individuals with a focus on what lesbian and gay identity signifies for a key task of adulthood: revising representations of the self and reshaping life narrative as informed by a changing sense of time left remaining in life, on the one hand, and an accumulating dossier of life experience on the other. I am interested in personal identity as a psychological construct, recognizing that individuals borrow heavily from shared social and cultural vocabularies of meaning. Herdt (1997), for example, believes that the concept of lesbian and gay identity erroneously emphasizes conscious choice rather than identification with culturally defined sexual lifeways. Furthermore, Herdt and Boxer (1992) argue that age in lesbian and gay lives is best understood on two levels: (1) within the social experience of individuals and (2) the implicit cultural practices of institutions and organizations in sexual minority cultural communities. In keeping with my comments on the idiosyncrasies of meaning-making, however, this chapter retains a focus on how men and women selectively incorporate social meanings of a minority sexual identity in their personal reckoning with time, age, and the specific lives they have lived.

Bisexuality as realized and expressed during adulthood introduces additional complexity to the discussion of adult development in sexual minority lives; bisexual identity can represent, for example, transitional, historical, sequential, or concurrent identities (Fox, 1996), all of which suggest different developmental trajectories of life experience. Despite this heterogeneity of experience, research on adult development, aging, and mental health in older sexual minority persons aggregates bisexuals and homosexuals together and therefore does not address the question of how bisexuals differ from homosexuals in revision of personal identity and life narrative. Nonetheless, recent studies suggest that bisexuals may be at greater risk for adverse life events and psychological distress (Jorm et al., 2002), perhaps because of social isolation and additional stigma bisexual men and women experience as adults who self-identify as neither heterosexual nor homosexual (for a review of mental health research on bisexual individuals, see Dodge and Sandfort, 2006). Yet, although adult development has not yet been systematically studied in bisexuals per se, it seems likely that stigmatization of same-sex desire and nonconventional lifeways would impart important similarities to the adult development of homosexual and bisexual persons.

Knowledge of adult development in sexual minority persons is also limited by the underrepresentation of ethnic minority adults in related research. Little is known about the reciprocal influences on self-representation of aging and ethnic minority identity. Is the importance of family ties and minority community identity as identified by Greene (1990), for example, modified for African American, Latino, and Asian American lesbians and gay men during the second half of life? If so, in what ways? How do persons with multiple minority identities take on another stigmatized identity (i.e., that of being old) in terms of identity management and mental health? These questions reflect a broader need to understand better how multiple minority identities intersect to shape self-representation, response to stigmatization, and mental health (Stewart and McDermott, 2004).

With these caveats in mind, I focus my comments on the large population of adults self-identified as lesbian or gay since adolescence or early adulthood to gauge the impact of a sustained sexual minority identity on the developmental issues of adulthood. Adults who develop or enact a lesbian or identity for the first time in midlife are characterized by different life trajectories that often include prior heterosexual marriage and parenthood, belated entry into gay social worlds, and specific challenges to integrate a new or a more public sexual minority identity with established family or community identities (Galatzer-Levy and Cohler, 2002).

3 Themes of Adult Development

To consider possible differences in adult development by sexual orientation, I first highlight several themes of the adult development literature pertinent to the constructs of identity and narrative. This literature encompasses a multitude of theoretical models and a wide range of interests including subjective and objective well-being (Ryff, 1989), intrapsychic change (Colarusso and Nemiroff, 1981), psychosocial identity (Erikson, 1959), the maintenance of meaning and morale (Cohler and Galatzer-Levy, 1990), processes of emotional regulation (Carstensen et al., 2000), and structural properties of thought (Neugarten, 1968).

A brief synthesis of this literature suggests that adulthood, particularly midlife, is a time of greater introspection, "interiority," and reappraisal of what is possible and desirable in life given the greater salience of personal mortality (Neugarten, 1968; Chiraboga, 1981). This reappraisal is, in turn, linked to a reprioritization of commitments and interests and, on a more abstract level, a rethinking of one's place in the world and a more nuanced understanding of how individuals are shaped by the worlds in which they live (Levinson, 1980; Vaillant, 1993). Middle-aged adults, for example, reshape identity and personal narratives to incorporate a greater awareness of ambiguity, complexity, and uncertainty about their lives (McAdams, 1993; Stevens-Long, 1990; Helson, 1997). They develop a deeper empathy for and identification with other persons previously regarded as too different to permit these considerations (Levinson, 1978). In addition, they are increasingly likely to universalize certain aspects of the life experience and believe that their existence transcends the particulars of individual biography (Erikson, 1959).

By middle age, adults begin to lessen their psychological identification with the world of the young while maintaining an active portfolio of social roles that involve interactions with the young as exemplified by parenting, coaching, mentoring, or leadership responsibilities at work (Neugarten, 1968). Despite their numerous social and public roles, midlife adults become more inclined to resist conventional social norms to create more authentic, personally meaningfully lives (Kernberg, 1989). In the conduct of sexual lives, there may be an especially pronounced disjunction between social mores and private conduct. As adults age, for instance, they contend with social norms that stigmatize sexuality in older persons and devalue their desirability (Schiavi, 1999). Older adults also cultivate alternate expressions of sexual intimacy. Many psychologically based discussions of older adults' sexuality stress the importance of ongoing intimacy as it shifts away from genitally based sex toward greater flexibility in gender roles as they are expressed in intimate relationships and the vital importance of maintaining attachments despite loss and disappointment in self and in others (Colarusso and Nimeroff, 1981; Schiavi, 1999).

4 Circumstances of Gay and Lesbian Lives

When applying the above descriptions of adult development to lesbians and gay men, three factors require consideration. First, many children and adolescents who go on to develop homosexual identities contend with stigmatization of atypical gender role attributes and same-gender romantic and sexual longings; this stigmatization has implications for early psychosocial development and for later psychological health and life narrative. Second, lesbians and gay men create nonconventional family structures and adult lifeways that receive little social, legal, or cultural recognition. Social institutions and cultural rites lend psychosocial support to adults undergoing life transitions, serve as reference points for the revision of identity throughout adulthood, define age norms, and enhance a sense of meaning in life. Third, the human immunodeficiency virus (HIV) epidemic shattered expectations of a normal life span for several generations of gay men and, for much of the past 25 years, obscured the possibility that adult development might extend into later decades of life. These three factors are here explored in greater depth.

4.1 Stigmatization

Stigmatization and discrimination related to sexual orientation remain salient forces in the lives of many lesbian and gay adults and affect expectations of what is desirable and possible to achieve. For instance, legally and socially defined structures such as civil marriage or second-parent adoption enhance, or when denied undermine, an assumption of adult roles and responsibilities and their psychological dividend: discovering new capacities within oneself, experiencing new sources of meaning in life, and being regarded as a full person (Meyer, 1995). Furthermore, the harmful effects of sexual orientation discrimination on self-esteem and health behaviors cast long shadows on adult trajectories of psychological and social well-being. Drescher (1998), for instance, describes the lifelong hazards of psychological dissociation when sexual identity is repressed and individuals are burdened with feelings of shame, secrecy, and inauthenticity.

Overt discrimination and stigmatization of homosexuality may be waning in certain quarters of the United States, but the lack of social recognition of life experience continues to affect the adult development of many lesbian and gay persons. Writing from the perspectives of self psychology and social theory, Cohler and Galatzer-Levy (1990) argue that adults need psychological valuation of life experience by others to maintain a sense of meaning and morale throughout adulthood. Many of the fundamental expressions of lesbian and gay lives evident over the life span, such as long-term partnerships, families composed of nonbiologic kin, and nontraditional configurations of sexual and emotional intimacy, receive little if any social valuation and are unsupported by law or public policy, cultural rites marking life transitions, or social roles that allow individuals to integrate their homosexuality with identities based in community or civic life.

The stigmatization of homosexuality also creates an altered timing of life transitions for lesbians and gay men. Limited opportunities for dating and role playing during adolescence, little if any access to positive lesbian and gay adult role models, and delays in consolidation of sexual identity because of time needed to overcome stigma and find appropriate partners result in later ages at which lesbians and gay men initiate relationships or undertake parenthood compared with heterosexual peers (Maylon, 1982; Coleman, 1985). Consequently, lesbians and gay men may begin to feel "off schedule" in their twenties or thirties as they make social comparisons to heterosexual peers who have married, started traditional families, or established community identities (Cohler and Galatzer-Levy, 2000). This nontraditional schedule has implications for how some lesbians and gay men experience a sense of aging.

4.2 The Structure of Lesbian and Gay Adult Lives

Lesbian and gay adulthood is characterized by greater proportions of single and childless adults, different configurations of family life, and different relationship dynamics compared to heterosexual couples (Blumstein and Schwartz, 1983; Weston, 1993). Until the recent legalization of marriage in Massachusetts, same-sex couple co-parenting always occurred outside the institution of marriage in the United States. Excluding parenting that arose in earlier heterosexual marriages, most lesbian and gay parenting is achieved through means of adoption, foster parenting, surrogacy, assisted reproduction, or co-parenting agreements between men and women who may be heterosexual or homosexual. Many of these arrangements are socially unheralded and unprotected by law and public policy.

The coupling of two same-gender persons creates unique dynamics and narratives compared with heterosexual relationships; for instance, the convergence of gender roles described in long-term heterosexual marriages is not found in homosexual relationships (Chiraboga, 1981). Compared with heterosexual couples, lesbian and gay male couples are more likely to include ex-lovers as friends or family members and place a greater premium on an equitable division of responsibilities throughout the course of relationships (Blumstein and Schwartz, 1983). Lesbians and gay male couples are also more likely than heterosexual couples to change concordantly in their expectations of how much time partners should spend with each other as they grow old together (Blumstein and Schwartz, 1983).

Hostetler and Cohler (1997) have called for greater study of single lesbian and gay lives across adulthood, citing the lack of research that describes ways in which relational status influences lived experience, identity, and development. Single status in homosexual lives is likely to have different meanings and mental health significance than that observed in single heterosexual lives, reflecting different norms about being partnered, opportunities for friendship and sexual intimacy that are structured differently in gay social worlds, and the historical absence of legal recognition of same-sex unions (Blumstein and Schwartz, 1983; Fowlkes, 1994).

4.3 HIV

As a final consideration of life circumstances that shape identity and narrative in sexual minority adults, the experience of multiple acquired immunodeficiency syndrome (AIDS) bereavements, occurrence of new infections among gay men, and improved but not insignificant course of HIV infection have all contributed to a personalization of mortality that occurs at earlier ages for some lesbians and gay men than for their heterosexual peers (Hopcke, 1992; Cohler and Galatzer-Levy, 2000). Cumulative mortality from AIDS has resulted in an inestimable loss of past, present, and future partners, friends, co-parents, protégés, and mentors. Opportunities for maintaining long-term friendships, sustaining intergenerational ties, and creating new families have been lost. Although the galvanizing effects of HIV on many gay men's lives may be receding, it is important to remember the critical impact of AIDS on the adult development of currently middle-aged and old gay men (Kertzner, 1997). In particular, the voices of a significant number of men who would have otherwise contributed to the anthology of growing older as openly gay adults have been silenced by AIDS.

5 Developmental Themes of Lesbian and Gay Adulthood

Beyond issues of stigma, family life, and HIV, lesbians and gay men face more universal issues related to the meaning of becoming older. These issues include the recontexualization of sexual identity in the larger frame of cumulative biography; the reassessment of social, community, and intergenerational identity; and change in relationships with families of origin. In this section, I highlight several prominent themes of adult development that, although not limited to lesbians and gay men, assume nuances that reflect differences in the social configuration and regard of sexual minority lives.

5.1 Age and Aging

Although earlier studies based on convenience samples describe a premature sense of aging among gay men (Mennigerode, 1976) and more negative attitudes toward aging among older gay men compared to older lesbians (Herdt et al., 1997), there is no evidence from systematic study to suggest that lesbian and gay persons are more likely than heterosexuals to endorse a sense of accelerating aging or experience a crisis of aging. Lesbians and gay men, for instance, do not differ from heterosexuals in their perception of chronological age at which midlife begins and ends (Kertzner, 2001). As is true of adults in general, disruptive life transitions are more likely to occur during the early decades of life. In heterosexual lives, young adulthood is associated with a peak incidence of emotionally difficult life transitions (Wethington et al., 2004); three-fourths of lifetime psychiatric disorders in the United States have their onset by age 24 (Kessler et al., 2005). In lesbian and gay lives, the process of coming out during adolescence or young adulthood is associated with more than psychological difficulty than adjustments later in life (Kimmel, 1978; Weinberg and Williams, 1974). This observation is supported by recent data suggesting that older gay men have fewer depressive symptoms than younger gay men (Mills et al., 2004).

Although aging per se does not appear to be associated with increased psychological distress, lesbians and gay men may experience a sense of "agelessness" reflecting the diminished applicability of conventional age markers, such as entry into marriage or becoming a parent (Kertzner, 1999). Coupled with late starts in consolidating sexual identity, exploring sexuality, or initiating partnerships, while sometimes living with illness or caring for those who with illnesses such as AIDS, lesbians and gay men may experience a disjunction in their chronological, sexual, social, and existential sense of how old they are (Kooden & Flowers, 2000). Moreover, heteronormative culture confers full adult status to men and women only when they marry and become parents (Herdt, 1997). Correspondingly, the nonrecognition of lesbian and gay unions, family structures, and friendship networks contributes to a sense of developmental limbo or incomplete adulthood that may be experienced by sexual minority persons.

5.2 Salience of Homosexual Identity in Life Narratives

Change in the centrality, salience, and regard of homosexual identity by lesbians and gay men throughout adulthood is highly variable reflecting different life circumstances, context, and concurrent identities. Reflecting this complexity and related methodological issues, there are few extant data describing change in the signification of homosexual identity across adulthood (Troiden, 1984; Adelman, 1991). Cohler and Galatzer-Levy (2000) speculated that with increasing age, lesbians and gay men may be less concerned with the opinions of others, including conventional attitudes about homosexuality. In a small qualitative study of midlife gay men, Kertzner (1999) found that most respondents regarded their homosexual identity as becoming less central to their sense of self as they became older; it was still regarded as essential but no longer as central. These observations, of course, could reflect idiosyncratic elements of individual experience, psychological change characteristic of midlife such as an increased sense of personal autonomy and environmental mastery (Ryff, 1989), change intrinsic to the process of homosexual identity formation that culminates in greater integration of lesbian and gay identity with other aspects of the self (Cass, 1996), historical change in the social tolerance of homosexuality, or some combination of all these elements. It seems likely, however, that the meaning and significance of homosexual identity is dynamic across individual lives and inseparable from other elements of individual biography.

As described above, adults continually reshape individual biography reflecting cumulative life experience, changing psychological attributes associated with aging, and change in social and historical context, although this process has been less studied in lesbians and gay men. McAdams (1993) notes that the ongoing revision of personal narrative is a key developmental task of adulthood as individuals seek to integrate self-representations that have become increasingly diverse, elaborate, and contradictory with age. For lesbians and gay men, life narratives can illuminate the extent to which themes of homosexual minority identity are interwoven with other strands of biography and the dynamic process whereby this occurs.

Several studies of lesbian and gay adult adjustment, for instance, emphasize a lifelong task of overcoming stigmatization of homosexuality and other social prejudices. In work that examined adult narratives of gay identity, Berger (1982) described the emblematic story of midlife and older gay men who took a "long and tortuous road" toward self-acceptance. In a study of lesbians 55 years of age and older, Jones and Nystrom (2002) noted themes of personal and professional success despite numerous obstacles, including discrimination based on gender, sexual orientation, and age. Many respondents in this study conveyed their belief that these hardships and adversity made them stronger. Galatzer-Levy and Cohler (2002) summarized other studies of life narrative including descriptions of contemporary young lesbian and gay adults who were more likely than preceding generations to accept contradiction and inconsistencies in their story of unfolding sexual identity.

Two recent studies of narratives examined attitudes toward sexual minority identity, future orientation, and psychological well-being. King and Smith (2004) found that acceptance of one's gay or lesbian identity and pursuit of goals centered in this identity were associated with subjective well-being, but that the capacity to elaborate a possible but unrealized heterosexual life was associated with personality development over time as defined by Loevinger's measure of ego development (Loevinger & Wessler, 1970). They concluded that there is value in being able to acknowledge what is regrettable in life without being consumed by regret and to be able to see the multitude of best possible lives that may be sources of fulfillment. Although this study included young as well as older adults, it suggests that the complex cognitive appraisal of identity that is a hallmark of adult maturity is important to the ongoing psychological growth of lesbians and gay men beyond that which is provided by coming out and self-acceptance of homosexual identity.

In a second study of identity and life story, Kertzner (2001) described several themes among midlife gay men that expressed varying interpretations of sexual minority identity in personal narrative. These themes were recovery from stigmatization of same sex desire, pride in identity consolidation, a sense that being different was an inextricable and valued source of opportunity in life, an accommodation of homosexuality as something neither desired nor rejected, and a problematic view of lesbian and gay identity as an encumbrance causing a series of hardships in life history. None of these themes was uniquely associated with psychological well-being, except the theme of encumbrance that was associated with depression and substance use.

Though potentially rich in implications, this line of research is subject to cohort bias in terms of respondents most inclined and able to tell life stories; life history study, for instance, is time-consuming and dependent on participants' abilities to articulate their experiences (Ryff, 1984). In addition, historical age cohort effects render narratives generation-specific and favor certain "stories" about the process and meaning of becoming gay (Plummer, 1995), which in turn influence the content of individual narratives.

5.3 Commitments and Community

Several reports describe change in orientation toward work, friendship, and relationships as lesbians and gay men enter middle age. Many lesbians and gay men value vocational identity as a means of ensuring self-sufficiency and enhancing self-esteem in a variably tolerant world; by midlife, this prioritization may begin to shift as other needs ascend in importance. Sang (1991), for instance, found that middle-aged lesbians sought to strike a new balance between work and family life with friends and partners. Weinstock (2000) reported that the search for a long-term partner and plans for parenting become more important for midlife lesbians.

Clinical and research reports describe a reexamination of sexuality and sexual culture by gay men as they approach midlife. Isensee (1999) describes the changing meaning of sex for many gay men as they age: Whereas earlier in life, sexuality consolidates personal identity and defines social identity, these functions become less relevant in middle age. Gagnon and Simon (1973) and Weinberg and Williams (1974) found that men nearing their forties began to withdraw from gay social worlds that emphasize youthful desirability in sex partners and shun older men. Although lesbians are also influenced by prevailing cultural values that emphasize the desirability of youthfulness in partners and exalt an idealized body, lesbians may perceive themselves as less influenced by these norms (Barker, 2004). Lesbians may be more likely to maintain intergenerational ties throughout the life span and partake of long-standing traditions within the lesbian culture of political advocacy, community, and friendship that are less generationally bound (Weinstock, 2000). It is important to note, however, that new institutions in sexual minority communities and a greater acceptance of openly gay and lesbian adults in certain spheres of public life have increased opportunities for intergenerational involvement (Boxer, 1997).

5.4 Family Relations and Social Support

Many traditional models of adult development suggest that adults widen their radius of social concern and commitment to include members of younger generations as expressed in such activities as parenting, teaching, mentoring, and advocacy (McAdams et al., 1998). Although systematic data describing the prevalence of these commitments in sexual minority populations is lacking, many lesbians and gay men undertake these roles (Cohler et al., 1998). Lesbian and gay parenting, for instance, has increased over recent years with an estimated 34% and 22% of female and male same-sex-coupled households, respectively, raising children under the age of 18 (U.S. Census Bureau, 2000). The boom in parenting has two important implications for purposes of the present discussion. First, parenting is likely to shape the psychological and social experience of adulthood, as has been well described in heterosexual populations (Marks et al., 2004). As parenting becomes a more common experience and one that is undertaken at earlier ages, it may decrease the sense among lesbian and gay men of being "off schedule," as described earlier. Second, the possibility of parenting influences the life expectations of younger lesbians and gay men. Contemporary generations of gay adolescents and young adults, for instance, may be increasingly apt to envision their adulthood as parents or grandparents and to imagine a greater blending of families of origin with families of choice (Boxer, 1997).

In perspective, however, it seems likely that many lesbians and gay men will continue to traverse midlife and old age without children and feel, as they grow older, increasingly free of conventional expectations of parenting (Weinstock, 2000). The extent to which norms favoring parenthood will become established in gay and lesbian social worlds remains to be seen.

Little is known about lesbians' and gay men's changing identity as adult children of aging parents or as adult siblings. Greater social tolerance of homosexuality and a greater sense of personal independence may permit disclosure of sexual identity to parents that was previously unthinkable; conversely, some lesbians and gay men find that their parents' increasing infirmity or inflexibility precludes this disclosure. The death of parents, particularly in the lives of childless adults, may be a milestone in one's own sense of aging and increase a sense of intergenerational and family isolation. Of note, Adelman et al. (2006) reported that only 15% of gay men and 2% of lesbians over 65 years of age recruited in a community survey said that they would turn to siblings during a time of crisis; this could reflect the absence, death, or unavailability of siblings or a greater inclination to turn to friends and partners for help.

Maintaining social support is a vital task for lesbians and gay men throughout adulthood, given the greater likelihood during middle age and late life they will be unpartnered and without children to provide care compared to heterosexual peers (Adelman et al., 2006). In a landmark study of lesbians and gay men 60 years of age and older, Grossman et al. (2000) found that the size of support networks was associated with satisfaction with social support, and that this satisfaction was associated with less loneliness and more positive appraisals of mental health. Those living with partners were less lonely and reported being in better physical and mental health.

6 Discussion

This chapter explores how sexual minority identity shapes and is shaped by the developmental tasks of revising personal identity and narrative throughout the adult years. This exploration does not yield easy answers given the great heterogeneity of sexual minority lives, the multiplicity of identities that characterize any individual, and the dynamic interaction of historical change, social context, and idiosyncrasies of personal history and psychology that shape life stories. For these reasons, life course approaches that emphasize social, cultural, and historical vectors may seem more appealing in the study of homosexual adulthood, a phenomenon that is in large part socially constructed.

A focus on idiosyncratic meaning-making over the course of life trajectories, however, has much to yield. By studying lives over time, we can understand the significance of lesbian and gay identity for the task of creating a sense of coherence, reconciliation, and transcendence in life review. For instance, is the increasing tendency of adults to view the world with a sense of paradox and complexity particularly relevant to sexual minority men and women as they consider and reconsider the meaning of being homosexual in the larger context of life experience? This is suggested by King and Smith's (2004) observation that some aspects of a lesbian or gay man's journey toward maturity may entail the sacrifice of wholly positive feelings and the ability to accommodate a measure of regret.

A perspective that considers the modifying effect of adulthood on lesbian and gay experience also addresses a shortcoming of the clinical literature on sexual minority mental health. Although making vital contributions to an understanding of how stigma shapes mental health (Cohen and Stein, 1986; Isay, 1989; Drescher, 1998), this literature is less explicitly concerned with how psychological and social processes associated with adult development modify issues arising from childhood, adolescence, or early adulthood. Given reports of increased risks of depression and anxiety disorders in sexual minority populations and the effects of minority stress on these disorders (Mays and Cochran, 2001; Sandfort et al., 2001; Meyer, 2003), it would be helpful to know how lesbians and gay men apply cumulative life experience and the resources of adulthood to decrease distress and maximize psychological well-being. An adult developmental perspective illuminates pathways of such resilience.

7 Conclusions

This chapter focuses on revisions in personal identity and life narrative, two key tasks of adult development that have relatively unexplored salience in sexual minority lives. Whereas there are other aspects of adult development and models of life course change that can be considered, a psychological inquiry into the stories of lesbians and gay men as they are modified across the life span is compelling. The longitudinal perspective of adult development has heuristic value for an understanding of how homosexual identity is maintained and modified during adulthood. Moreover, this perspective helps clarify the extent to which sexual minority lives are characterized by unique values and norms regarding sexuality, intimacy, and, more generally, human existence and purpose as revealed over the individual life span (Meyer, 1995). Just as importantly, understanding the trajectories of lesbian and gay lives broadens and enriches an understanding of how adults come to terms with the human predicament of living full and meaningful lives while incorporating the idiosyncracies of identity and history that shape any individual life.

References

Adelman, M. (1991) Stigma, gay lifestyles, and adjustments to aging: a study of later-life gay men and lesbians. In: Lee, J.A. (ed) *Gay midlife and maturity.* Harrington Park Press, New York, pp. 7–32.

Adelman, M. (2000) *Midlife lesbian relationships: friends, lovers, children, and parents.* Harrington Park Press, New York.

Adelman, M., Gurevitch, J., de Vries, B., and Blando, J. (2006) Openhouse: community building and research in the LGBT aging population. In: Kimmel, D., Rose, T., and David, S. (eds) *Lesbian, gay, bisexual, and transgender aging: research and clinical perspectives.* Columbia University Press, New York, pp. 247–264.

Barker, J.C. (2004) Lesbian aging: an agenda for social research. In: Herdt, G., and de Vries, B. (eds) *Gay and lesbian aging: research and future directions.* Springer Publishing Company, New York, pp. 29–72.

Bartzokis, G., Beckson, M., Lu, P.H., Nuechterlein, K.H., Edwards, N., and Mintz, J. (2001) Age-related changes in frontal and temporal lobe volumes in men: a magnetic resonance imaging study. *Archives of General Psychiatry* 58:461–465.

Berger, R.M. (1982) *Gay and gray: the older homosexual man.* Alyson Publications, Boston.

Blumstein, P., and Schwartz, P. (1983) *The American couple.* Simon & Schuster, New York.

Boxer, A.M. (1997) Gay, lesbian, and bisexual aging into the twenty-first century: an overview and introduction. *Journal of Gay Lesbian and Bisexual Identity* 2(4):187–197.

Carstensen, L.L., Mayr, U., Pasupathi, M., and Nesselroade, J.R. (2000) Emotional experience in everyday life across the life span. *Journal of Personality and Social Psychology* 79(4):644–655.

Cass, V. (1996) Sexual orientation identity formation. In: Cabaj, R.P., and Stein, T.S. (eds) *Textbook of homosexuality and mental health.* American Psychiatric Press, Washington, DC, pp. 227–251.

Chiraboga, D.A. (1981) The developmental psychology of middle age. In: Howells, J.G. (ed) *Modern perspectives in the psychiatry of middle age.* Brunner/Mazel, New York, pp. 3–25.

Cohen, C.J., and Stein, T.S. (1986) Reconceptualizing individual psychotherapy with gay men and lesbians, In: Stein, T.S., and Cohen, C.J. (eds) *Contemporary perspectives on psychotherapy with gay men and lesbians.* Plenum Medical, New York, pp. 27–53.

Cohler, B., and Galatzer-Levy, R. (1990) Self, meaning, and morale across the second half of life. In: Nemiroff, R.A., and Colarusso, C.A. (eds) *New dimensions in adult development.* Basic Books, New York, pp. 214–220.

Cohler, B.J., and Galatzer-Levy, R.M. (2000) *The course of gay and lesbian lives: social and psychoanalytic perspectives.* University of Chicago Press, Chicago.

Cohler, B.J., Hostetler, A.J., and Boxer, A.M. (1998) Generativity, social context, and lived experience: narratives of gay men in middle adulthood. In: McAdams, D.P., and de St. Aubin, E. (eds) *Generativity and adult development.* American Psychological Association, Washington, DC, pp. 265–310.

Colarusso, C.A., and Nemiroff, R.A. (1981) *Adult development: a new dimension in psychoanalytic theory and practice.* Plenum Press, New York.

Coleman, E. (1985) Developmental stages the coming out process. In: Gonsiorek, J.C. (ed) *Homosexuality and psychotherapy: a practitioner's handbook of affirmative models.* Haworth Press, New York, pp. 31–44.

Cornett, C.W., and Hudson, R.A. (1987) Middle adulthood and the theories of Erikson, Gould, and Valliant: where does the gay man fit in? *Journal of Gerontological Social Work* 10(3/4):61–73.

Dodge, B., and Sandfort, T.G.M. (2006) Mental health among bisexual individuals when compared to homosexual and heterosexual individuals. In: Firestein, B.A. (ed) *Becoming visible: counseling bisexuals across the lifespan.* Columbia University Press, New York, pp. 16–32.

Drescher, J. (1998) *Psychoanalytic therapy and the gay man.* Analytic Press, Hillsdale, NJ.

Erikson, E.H. (1959) Identity and the life cycle. *Psychological Issues* 1(1):50–100.

Fowlkes, M. (1994) Single worlds and homosexual lifestyles: patterns of sexuality and intimacy. In: Rossi, A.S. (ed) *Sexuality across the life course.* University of Chicago Press, Chicago, pp. 151–186.

Fox, R. (1996) Bisexuality: an examination of theory and practice. In: Cabaj, R.P., and Stein, T.S. (eds) *Textbook of homosexuality and mental health.* American Psychiatric Press, Washington, DC, pp. 147–172.

Gagnon, J.H., and Simon, W. (1973) *Sexual conduct: the social sources of human sexuality.* Aldine Publishing, Chicago.

Galatzer-Levy, R., and Cohler, B. (2002) Making a gay identity: coming out, social context, and psychoanalysis. In: Winer, J.A., and Anderson, J.W. (eds) *Rethinking psychoanalysis and the homosexualities.* Analytic Press, Hillsdale, NJ, pp. 255–286.

Gilligan, C. (1982) *In a different voice: psychological theory and women's development.* Harvard University Press, Cambridge, MA.

Greene, B. (1990) Ethnic-minority lesbians and gay men: mental health and treatment issues. *Journal of Consulting and Community Psychology* 62:243–251.

Grossman, A.H., D'Augelli, A.R., and Hershberger, S.L. (2000) Social support networks of lesbian, gay, and bisexual adults 60 years of age and older. *Journal of Gerontology Series B Psychological Sciences and Social Sciences* 55B(3):171–179.

Harry, J. (1993) Being out: a general model. *Journal of Homosexuality* 26(1):25–40.

Helson, R. (1997) The self in middle age. In: Lachman, M.E., and James, J.B. (eds) *Multiple paths of midlife development.* Chicago University Press, Chicago, pp. 21–44.

Herdt, G. (1997) *Same sex different cultures: exploring gay and lesbian lives.* Westview Press, Boulder, CO.

Herdt, G., and Boxer, A. (1992) Introduction: culture, history, and life course of gay men. In: Herdt, G. (ed) *Gay culture in America: essays from the field.* Beacon Press, Boston, pp. 1–28.

Herdt, G., Beeler, J., and Rawls, T.W. (1997) Life course diversity among older lesbians and gay men: a study in Chicago. *Journal of Gay Lesbian and Bisexual Identity* 2(3/4):231–246.

Hopcke, R.H. (1992) Midlife, gay men, and the AIDS epidemic. *Quadrant* 35(1):101–109.

Hostetler, A.J., and Cohler, B.J. (1997) Partnership, singlehood, and the lesbian and gay life course: a research agenda. *Journal of Gay Lesbian and Bisexual Identity* 2(3/4):199–219.

Isay, R.A. (1989) *Being homosexual: gay men and their development.* Farrar, Straus, & Giroux, New York.

Isensee, R. (1999) *Are you ready? The gay man's guide to thriving at midlife.* Alyson Books, Los Angeles.

Jones, T.C., and Nystrom, N.M. (2002) Looking back . . . looking forward: addressing the lives of lesbians 55 and older. *Journal of Women and Aging* 14(3–4):59–76.

Jorm, A.F., Korten, A.E., Rodgers, B., Jacomb, P.A., and Christensen, H. (2002) Sexual orientation and mental health: results from a community survey of young and middle-aged adults. *British Journal of Psychiatry* 188:423–427.

Kernberg, O.F. (1989) The interactions of middle age and character pathology: treatment implications. In: Oldham, J.M., and Liebert, R.S. (eds) *The Middle Years.* Yale University Press, New Haven, pp. 209–223.

Kertzner, R.M. (1997) Entering midlife: gay men, HIV and the future. *Journal of the Gay and Lesbian Medical Association* 1:87–95.

Kertzner, R.M. (1999) Self-appraisal of life experience and psychological adjustment in midlife gay men. *Journal of Psychology and Human Sexuality* 11:43–64.

Kertzner, R.M. (2001) The adult life course and homosexual identity in midlife gay men. *Annual Review of Sex Research* 12:75–92.

Kessler, R.C., Berglund, P., Demler, O., Jin, R., and Walters, E.E. (2005) Life prevalence and age-of-onset distributions of DSM-IV Disorders in the National Comorbidity Survey Replication. *Archives of General Psychiatry* 62:593–602.

Kimmel, D.C. (1978) Adult development and aging: a gay perspective. *Journal of Social Issues* 34(3):113–130.

Kimmel, D.C. (2004) Issues to consider in studies of midlife and older sexual minorities. In: Herdt, G., and de Vries, B. (eds) *Gay and lesbian aging: research and future direction.* Springer, New York, pp. 265–283.

Kimmel, D.C., and Sang, B.E. (1995) Lesbians and gay men in midlife. In: D'Augelli, D., and Patterson, C.J. (eds) *Lesbian, gay, and bisexual identities over the lifespan: psychological perspectives.* Oxford University Press, New York, pp. 190–214.

King, L.A., and Smith, N.G. (2004) Gay and straight possible selves: goals, identity, subjective well-being, and personality development. *Journal of Personality* 72(5):967–994.

Kooden, H., and Flowers, C. (2000) *Golden men: the power of midlife.* Avon Books, New York.

Levinson, D.J. (1978) *The seasons of a man's life.* Alfred Knopf, New York.

Levinson, D.J. (1980) Conception of the adult life course. In: Smelser, N.J., and Erikson, E.H. (eds) *Themes of work and love in adulthood.* Harvard University Press, Cambridge, pp. 265–283.

Loevinger, J., and Wessler, R. (1970) *Measuring ego development. Vol. 1. Construction and use of a sentence completion test.* Jossey-Boss, San Francisco.

Marks, N.F., Bumpass, L.L., and Heyjung, J. (2004) Family roles and well-being during the middle life course. In: Brim, O.G., Ryff, C.D., and Kessler, R.C. (eds) *How healthy are we? A national study of well-being at midlife.* University of Chicago Press, Chicago, pp. 514–549.

Maylon, A. (1982) Biphasic aspects of homosexual identity formation. *Psychotherapy Theory Research and Practice* 19(3):355–240.

Mays, V.M., and Cochran, S.D. (2001) Mental health correlates of perceived discrimination among lesbian, gay, and bisexual adults in the United States. *American Journal of Public Health* 91:1869–1876.

McAdams, D.P. (1993) *The stories we live by: personal myths and the making of the self.* Guilford Press, New York.

McAdams, D.P., Hart, H.M., and Maruna, S. (1998) The anatomy of generativity. In: McAdams, D.P., and de St. Aubin, E. (eds) *Generativity and adult development.* American Psychological Press, Washington, DC, pp. 7–44.

Mennigerode, F.A. (1976) Age-status labeling in homosexual men. *Journal of Homosexuality* 1(3):273–276.

Meyer, I.H. (1995) Minority stress and mental health in gay men. *Journal of Health and Social Behavior* 36:339–367.

Meyer, I.H. (2003) Prejudice, social stress, and mental health in lesbian, gay, and bisexual populations: conceptual issues and research evidence. *Psychological Bulletin* 129:674–697.

Mills, T.C., Paul, J., Stall, R., Pollack, J., Canchola, J., Chang, Y.J., Moskowitz, J.T., and Catania, J.C. (2004) Distress and depression in men who have sex with men: the Urban Men's Health Study. *American Journal of Psychiatry* 161:278–285.

Neugarten, B. (1970) Adaptation and the life cycle. *Journal of Geriatric Psychiatry* 4:71–87.

Neugarten, B.L. (1968) The awareness of middle age. In: Neugarten, B. (ed) *Middle age and aging*, University of Chicago Press, Chicago, pp. 93–98.

Plummer, K. (1995) *Telling sexual stories*. Routledge, London.

Ryff, C.D. (1984) Personality development from the inside: the subjective experience of change in adulthood and aging. *Lifespan Development and Behavior* 6:243–279.

Ryff, C.D. (1989) Happiness is everything, or is it? Explorations on the meaning of psychological well-being. *Journal of Personality and Social Psychology* 57(6):1069–1081.

Sandfort, T.M., de Graaf, R., Bijl, R.V., and Schnabel, P. (2001) Same-sex behavior and psychiatric disorders. *Archives of General Psychiatry* 58:85–91.

Sang, B. (1991) Moving toward balance and integration. In: Sang, B., Warshow, J., and Smith, A.J. (eds) *Lesbians at mid-life: the creative transition*. Spinster Books, San Francisco, pp. 206–214.

Schiavi, R.C. (1999) *Aging and male sexuality*. Cambridge University Press, Cambridge, UK.

Simon, W. (1996) *Postmodern sexualities*. Routledge, New York.

Stevens-Long, J. (1990) Adult development: theories past and present. In: Nemiroff, R.A., and Colarusso, C.A. (eds) *New dimensions in adult development*. Basic Books, New York, pp. 125–164.

Stewart, A.J., and McDermott, C. (2004) Gender in psychology. *Annual Review of Psychology* 55:519–544.

Troiden, R.R. (1984) Self, self-concept, identity, and homosexual identity: constructs in need of definition and differentiation. *J Homosexuality* 10(3/4): 97–109.

U.S. Census Bureau National Population Estimates (2000) www.census.gov/population/estimates/nation/intfile2-1.txt.

Vaillant, G.E. (1993) *The wisdom of the ego*. Harvard University Press, Cambridge, MA.

Weinberg, M.S., and Williams, C.J. (1974) *Male homosexuals: their problems and adaptations*. Penguin, New York.

Weinstock, J.S. (2000) Lesbian friendships at midlife: patterns and possibilities for the 21st century. In: Adelman, M. (ed) *Midlife lesbian relationships: friends, lovers, children, and parents*. Harrington Park Press, New York, pp. 1–32.

Weston, K. (1993) *Families we choose*. Columbia University Press, New York.

Wethington, E., Kessler, R.C., and Pixley, J.E. (2004) Turning points in adulthood. In: Brim, O.G., Ryff, C.D., and Kessler, R.C. (eds) *How healthy are we? A national study of well-being at midlife*. University of Chicago Press, Chicago, pp. 586–614.

Biology and Sexual Minority Status

William Byne

1 Introduction

The purpose of this chapter is to provide clinicians with an overview of current knowledge pertaining to the biology of sexual minority status. Under the umbrella of sexual minority are included homosexuals, bisexuals, transgenders and intersexes. The most developed biologic theory pertaining to sexual minority status is the *prenatal hormonal hypothesis*. According to this hypothesis, prenatal hormones act (primarily during embryonic and fetal development) to mediate the sexual differentiation not only of the internal and external genitalia but also of the brain. The sexually differentiated state of the brain then influences the subsequent expression of gender identity and sexual orientation. Intersexuality results from variation in the normative course of somatic sexual differentiation, and homosexuality and bisexuality have been proposed to reflect variant sexual differentiation of hypothetical neural substrates that mediate sexual orientation. Similarly, transgenderism has been conjectured to reflect variant differentiation of hypothetical neural substrates that mediate gender identity. Some of the same hormones and hormonal receptors mediate the sexual differentiation of both the brain and the genitalia. Thus, the brains, as well as the genitalia, of intersexes may exhibit sexual differentiation that is intermediate between that of normatively developed males and females.

The chapter begins with clarification of terminology and then an overview of the genetics and neuroendocrinology of sexual differentiation. The prenatal hormonal hypothesis is then elaborated and evaluated in light of current evidence. Genetic and other salient biologic evidence is then summarized. Models are examined for considering how biologic factors, in concert with experiential factors, might influence sexual minority status.

2 Terminology

In this chapter, *sex* refers to the status of biologic variables that can be described as either male-typical or female-typical in normatively developed individuals (e.g., genes, chromosomes, gonads, internal and external genital structures, hormonal profiles). Particular features of the human brain also appear to be sexually dimorphic, at least in a statistical sense, and should perhaps also be considered among the variables of sex (Collaer et al., 2003). *Gender* refers to social categories (e.g., man or woman, boy or girl) or to factors related to living in the social role of a man or a woman. *Gender identity* refers to one's sense of belonging to the male or female gender category, whereas *gender role* refers to behaviors (e.g., mannerisms, style of dress, activities) that convey to others one's membership in one of those categories (Money & Ehrhardt, 1972). *Sexual orientation* refers to one's pattern of erotic responsiveness and is described here as *androphylic* (attracted to men), *gynephilic* (attracted to women), or *bisexual* (attracted to both).

The course of normative development culminates in full concordance among all of the biologic variables of sex (i.e., either all male or all female). In intersexed individuals, however, one or more of those variables is discordant with the others, or its differentiation is intermediate between male and female norms. The fact that gender identity and role may be discordant with one or more of the biologic variables of sex underscores the social basis of gender categories.

Intersex has become the preferred term to encompass a variety of syndromes previously classified on the basis of gonadal histology as *true hermaphroditism*, in which both testicular and ovarian tissue are present in a single individual, and *pseudohermaphroditism*, in which only one type of gonadal tissue is present. In that system of taxonomy, precedence was given to gonadal histology as the arbiter of "true sex" upon which gender assignment should be based. With the advent of karyotype analysis, chromosomal sex became viewed as the arbiter of "true sex" (Zucker, 1999). When the sexual variables are not fully concordant in a given individual, there is no reason to insist that one variable should hold precedence over the others. Instead, the status of each variable must be stated to describe accurately the sex of the individual. In the *Diagnostic and Statistical Manual of Mental Disorders* (4th edition), the presence of an intersex disorder excludes the diagnosis of a gender identity disorder (American Psychiatric Association, 1994).

3 Overview of Sexual Differentiation

The mammalian embryo is initially sexually bipotential (Collaer et al., 2003; Arnold et al., 2004). During the usual course of male differentiation a testis determining gene, *SRY*, which is normally on the Y chromosome, directs the development of testes from the fetal gonadal precursor. Subsequently, testicular secretions orchestrate differentiation of the male genitalia and brain. Initially, both male and female embryos possess two sets of primordial internal genital duct systems: one (the müllerian, or paramesonephric, duct system) is capable of developing into female internal genital structures and another (the woffian, or mesonephric, duct system) is capable of developing into the male internal genitalia. A secretion from the testis, müllerian inhibitory substance, induces regression of the müllerian (i.e., female) duct system, and the 5α-reduced derivative of testosterone, 5α-dihydrotestosterone (DHT), stimulates the development of male internal genital structures. DHT also stimulates both the growth and differentiation of the embryonic phallus into a penis and fusion of the labioscrotal folds to form the scrotum into which the testes later descend. In the absence of testes or müllerian inhibitory factor, the internal female genital system fails to regress. In the complete absence of testosterone, the 5α-reductase enzyme that converts it to DHT, or functional androgen receptors, the male internal genital structures fail to develop, the phallic rudiment develops into a clitoris rather than a penis, and the labioscrotal folds develop into labia instead of a scrotum. Intermediate levels of androgenic exposure result in intermediate development of internal male genital structures and differentiation of the external genital structures that are intermediate between those of normatively developed males and females.

Work in laboratory animals suggests that sexual differentiation of the brain is analogous to sexual differentiation of the internal genitalia, where separate male and female primordia are involved, and thus fully developed male and female structures can theoretically exist in the same individual. Extending this analogy, sexual differentiation can be conceptualized as involving processes of defeminization (i.e., suppression of female characteristics—analogous to regression of the müllerian ducts) and masculinization (i.e. the development of male characteristics—analogous to development of the male internal genitalia). In rats, the most studied aspects of brain defeminization include suppression of the brain's potential to mediate a stereotypically female mating posture called lordosis, and its ability to orchestrate the neuroendocrine response necessary for normal ovarian function. Both defeminization and masculinization of the rodent brain are brought about by testosterone and its derivatives. Testosterone acts on the brain by two primary pathways: (1) an androgen pathway in which either testosterone or DHT interacts with androgen receptors on target cells and (2) an estrogen pathway in which testosterone is converted to estrogen by aromatase enzymes in the brain. In the latter pathway the brain-derived estrogen interacts with estrogen receptors. In laboratory rodents, the androgen pathway contributes to masculinization of the brain, and the estrogen pathway contributes to both defeminization and masculinization (Goy & McEwen, 1980; Olsen, 1983). In addition to having different hormonal requirements, animal work suggests that the various aspects of somatic and brain sexual differentiation occur during different periods of development in a sequence of temporally overlapping steps (Goy & McEwen, 1980; Byne & Kemether, 2000). In the absence of the cascade set in motion by the testis-determining gene, female development ensues, at least to a first approximation.

3.1 Timing of Sexual Differentiation in the Human

Human testes begin to secrete androgens by the seventh or eighth week of gestation (Siiteri & Wilson, 1974), a process initially regulated by human chorionic gonadotropin secreted by the placenta (Moore, 1982).

By the 15th week of gestation the regulation of androgen secretion is taken over by gonadotropin from the fetal pituitary, which is regulated by the fetal hypothalamus. Genital differentiation occurs largely during the period when androgen secretion is regulated by the placenta rather than by the fetal pituitary. Gonadotropin secretion decreases toward the end of gestation presumably due to the development of inhibitory inputs to the hypothalamus in addition to the onset of negative feed-back of androgen on gonadotropin release. Thus, fetal androgen in males is elevated between weeks 8 to 24 of gestation, with peak levels occurring between weeks 14 and 16 (Smail et al., 1981). In males, the level of testosterone increases from birth to a peak at 1 to 3 months and then decreases to prepubertal levels by ages 4 to 6 months (Hrabovsky & Hutson, 2002). The ovary is believed to be relatively quiescent pre-natally but secretes substantial levels of estradiol during the first 6 to 12 months after birth. A sharp reduction of gonadal activity then occurs in both sexes until 10 to 12 years of age when sex-characteristic adult hormonal profiles emerge and trigger the development of secondary sexual characteristics. Thus, hormonal influences could conceivably influence psychosexual differentiation prenatally (8 to 24 weeks of gestation), during the first 6 to 12 months postnatally, and again at puberty.

4 Prenatal Hormonal Hypothesis

4.1 Sexual Orientation

From the turn of the century into the 1970s, a popular hypothesis held that the amount of androgens or estrogens in the bloodstream of adult men and women might influence or determine their sexual orientation. That hypothesis is no longer viewed favorably because most studies failed to demonstrate a correlation between sexual orientation and adult hormone levels (Meyer-Bahlburg, 1977, 1984). In fact, androgens have been found to increase libido in adults of both sexes but not to alter sexual orientation (Glass & Johnson, 1944; Sherwin, 1991). Simi-larly, alterations in adult hormone levels resulting from gonadal malig-nancies, trauma, or surgical removal do not alter sexual orientation (Gooren, 1990).

Research currently focuses on the potential role of prenatal hormonal influences on the brain. The prenatal hormonal hypothesis posits that: (1) the brains of heterosexual men and women differ from each other both structurally and functionally; (2) those differences result from early hormonal influences on the developing fetus; and (3) sexual ori-entation is derivative of a hormonally mediated developmental process leading to sexual differentiation of the brain. Consequently, the brains of homosexual individuals are expected to exhibit characteristics that would be considered more typical of the other sex or intermediate between male and female norms (Byne & Parsons, 1993). The expecta-tion that sexual minorities should have brains that are in some ways intermediate between those of normatively developed heterosexual men and women may be referred to as the "intersex hypothesis of homosexuality, bisexuality, and transgenderism."

The "prenatal hormonal hypothesis" draws upon observations of rodents in which the balance between male and female patterns of mating behaviors is strongly influenced by the amount and timing of early androgen exposure (Meyer-Bahlburg, 1984; Gooren, 1990; Byne & Parsons, 1993). The period of maximal sensitivity to these organizing effects of androgen varies from one species to the next (Goy & McEwen, 1980). The rat has been employed extensively in such research because the period of brain sexual differentiation extends into the early postnatal period (which corresponds to the midtrimester of human gestation). Thus, the hormonal exposure of the rat's brain can be experimentally manipulated by perinatal gonadectomy and injection of various hormones.

It is problematic to make assumptions about human sexual psychology based on extrapolations from rodent behaviors caused by experimental endocrine manipulations. For example, a neonatally castrated male rat that shows lordosis—a receptive posture to permit mounting—when mounted by another male is sometimes considered homosexual, as is the perinatally androgenized female rat that mounts others. The male that mounts another male is sometimes considered heterosexual, as is the female that displays lordosis when mounted by another female. Thus, in this particular laboratory paradigm, sexual orientation is defined in terms of specific behaviors and postures. In contrast, human sexual orientation is defined not by the motor patterns of copulation but by one's pattern of erotic responsiveness and the gender of one's preferred sex partner.

Because of the problems when equating rodent mating behavior with human sexual orientation, researchers have begun to employ a variety of strategies to assess partner preference in animals. This is sometimes done by seeing whether a test animal chooses to approach a male or a female stimulus animal placed in opposite arms of a T-maze (Paredes & Baum, 1995). Although some unaltered laboratory animals spontaneously direct most of their sexual behaviors toward their own sex (Bagemihl, 1999), animal studies of sexual orientation are usually carried out on animals that have been experimentally manipulated (Hennessey et al., 1986; Paredes and Baum, 1995). For example, a genetically male rodent may either be castrated as a neonate, depriving his developing brain of androgens, or particular androgen-responsive regions of his brain may be destroyed. To activate the display of female-typical behaviors and preferences in such male animals, estrogen injections are also required during adulthood. Because adult homosexual men and women have hormonal profiles that are indistinguishable from those of their heterosexual counterparts, it remains unclear how findings based on such hormonally abnormal animals pertain to human sexual orientation.

4.2 Gender Identity

Early hormonal exposure is widely believed to influence subsequent gender identity (Zhou et al., 1995). This possibility is potentially relevant not only to the etiology of transgenderism but also to early gender assignment in intersexes. Among male-to-female transgenders who elect sex-change surgery, most are sexually attracted primarily to men; but a substantial minority (perhaps 40%) are attracted either exclusively to women or to both women and men. Similarly, most but not all female-to-male transgenders are sexually attracted to women (Zucker, 1995). Because sexual orientation and gender identity can vary independently of one another, in keeping with the prenatal hormonal hypothesis one must propose either that gender identity and sexual orientation would be sensitive to the organizing effects of androgens during different periods of development or that they would be influenced by different androgens or their metabolites. Similarly, because testosterone and its metabolites are responsible for masculinization of the external genitalia, the absence of genital anomalies in most homosexuals and transgenders suggests that genital differentiation occurs during a different developmental period or is sensitive to different metabolites compared to the neural substrates that mediate sexual orientation and gender identity.

5 Testing the Prenatal Hormonal Hypothesis

Tests of the prenatal hormonal hypothesis have been reviewed extensively elsewhere with respect to both sexual orientation (Byne & Parsons, 1993) and gender identity (Gooren, 1986a,b, 1990). Here we review the search for correlates of sexual orientation and gender identity and then focus on outcome studies of individuals with known endocrine anomalies and/or gender reassignment during childhood.

5.1 Neuroendocrinologic Studies

One of the most-studied sex differences in the rat brain pertains to its role in regulating the secretion of luteinizing hormone (LH) from the pituitary gland. In brief, the brain of a normal female rat responds to an injection of a large amount of estrogen by signaling the pituitary gland to secrete large amounts of LH, a phenomenon referred to as the positive feedback effect of estrogen on LH release. This positive feedback effect is a measure of the brain's ability to support normal cyclic ovarian function in females. In contrast, the male brain, in response to the same injection that produced positive feedback in the female, signals the pituitary gland to decrease its secretion of LH. This is because in the course of normative male development testosterone defeminizes the feedback mechanism.

Many textbooks and popular accounts suggest that defeminization of the positive feedback mechanism also occurs during human male development; however, several lines of evidence suggest that it does not. In fact, laboratory work carried out on nonhuman primates suggests that defeminization of the positive feedback mechanism may not occur in any primate. Prolonged developmental exposure to testosterone does not defeminize the feedback mechanism in genetic female monkeys (Resko & Phoenix, 1972) or in human females with congenital virilizing adrenal hyperplasia (Wilkins, 1952). Moreover, ovarian tissue continues its cyclic pattern of hormonal secretion when transplanted into male monkeys that were castrated as adults (Norman & Spies, 1986). Developmental studies suggest that the positive feedback system matures during puberty in boys as well as in girls (Kulin & Reiter, 1976).

Despite the lack of evidence for sexual differentiation of the feedback mechanism in humans, there has been considerable speculation that male homosexuals should exhibit feminized feedback responses to estrogen. As a direct test of that hypothesis, Gooren and collaborators (Gooren, 1986a, 1986b) examined the positive feedback response in normal men and women and in transgendered individuals (homosexual and heterosexual) both before and after surgical and hormonal reassignment. Those studies suggested that in humans, in contrast to laboratory rats, the neuroendocrine response in question depends on the hormonal status of the individual at the time of the estrogen challenge and that it is independent of sex, gender identity, or sexual orientation.

5.2 Neuroanatomic Studies

Over the past two decades, sex differences have been confirmed by the size of several brain structures in a variety of laboratory animals. These findings have generated speculation concerning the existence of parallel differences in the human brain associated not only with sex but also with gender identity and sexual orientation (Swaab & Fliers, 1985; Allen et al., 1989; Levay, 1991; Byne et al., 2001). Several of the structural sex differences identified in animals involve specific cell groups in a broad region of the rodent hypothalamus that participates in regulating a variety of functions including sexually dimorphic copulatory behaviors. Several structur sex differences in the rodent brain have been demonstrated to develop in response to sex differences in early androgen exposure (Collaer et al., 2003; Arnold et al., 2004). The best-studied anatomic sex difference in the rodent brain involves a cell group straddling the medial preoptic and anterior regions of the hypothalamus—the sexually dimorphic nucleus of the preoptic area (SDN-POA). In the rat this structure is five to eight times larger in males than in females. Damage to the preoptic region decreases mounting behavior in laboratory animals, whereas electrical stimulation of the region elicits mounting behavior. These observations and the finding that the size of the SDN-POA correlates positively with the frequency of mounting behavior displayed by male rats have established the belief that the SDN-POA participates in regulating male sex behavior. However, electrolytic lesions in the region of the SDN-POA of male rats do not disrupt mounting behavior. Instead, they allow male rats (castrated as adults and therefore having fully defeminized and masculinized brains) to exhibit lordosis if they are given injections of estrogen and progesterone (Hennessey et al., 1986). Thus, rather than regulating male behavior in rats, the SDN-POA may act to inhibit the display of female mating behavior.

The belief that the SDN-POA participates in regulating sex behavior in rats has led to the search for a comparable nucleus in humans. The human third interstitial nucleus of the anterior hypothalamus (INAH3) has been identified as the most promising candidate (Byne et al., 2001). This nucleus is much larger (Allen et al., 1989; Levay, 1991) and contains substantially more neurons in presumed heterosexual men than in women (Byne et al., 2001). By extrapolation from animal work, this human sex difference is widely believed to reflect sex differences in early hormone exposure. The acquired immunodeficiency syndrome (AIDS) epidemic has made it possible to study this nucleus in individuals whose medical records indicated homosexual behavior as the risk factor for contracting AIDS. (Unless someone dies from complications of AIDS there is usually no documentation of sexual orientation in the medical records available for autopsy studies. To date, therefore, postmortem studies on the brains of gay men without AIDS and lesbians have not been possible.) These studies suggest that the volume of INAH3 may be smaller in homosexual men than in heterosexual men but that the number of neurons in the nucleus does not vary with sexual orientation (Levay, 1991; Byne et al., 2001). The suggestion of volume reduction must be viewed skeptically for a variety of technical reasons, including the confounding of sexual orientation and AIDS in the execution of the research (i.e., all of the brains of gay men were from AIDS victims). In addition, tissue shrinks in the process of fixation for histologic analysis. This shrinkage influences measures of size but not measures of cell number. Thus, the finding of equal numbers of neurons in homosexual and heterosexual men may be a more reliable finding than the suggestion of a difference in the volume of the nucleus between the two groups. Alternatively, a difference in the volume of the nucleus between groups could reflect a difference in the volume of neuropil, the brain substance surrounding neuronal cell bodies, which includes neuronal fibers and synapses. A similarly appearing nucleus has been identified in sheep and has been reported to be larger in those male sheep that preferentially mount females than in those that preferentially mount other males (Roselli et al., 2004). Although that study is intriguing, it has yet to be subjected to independent replication attempts.

Another putatively sexually dimorphic hypothalamic nucleus, the central part of the bed nucleus of the stria terminalis (BSTc), has been investigated in a small number of postmortem brains for variation with both gender identity and sexual orientation (Zhou et al., 1995). That study measured the BSTc in postmortem tissue from 6 male-to-female transsssexuals (2 of whom were exclusively androphilic, 3 of whom were gynephilic, and 1 bisexual), 12 presumed heterosexual men, 11 presumed heterosexual women, and 9 homosexual men. The BSTc was found to be statistically significantly larger in both homosexual and heterosexual nontransgendered men than in women; however, among the male-to-female transgenders, the nucleus was the same size as in the heterosexual women. In the transgendered group, the size of the nucleus did not appear to vary with sexual orientation. The suggestion that this nucleus varies with gender identity (but not with sexual orientation) in men must be viewed cautiously given the absence of replication studies and the small sample size. Moreover, five of the six transgenders had been orchiectomized, raising the possibility that the observed difference in this androgen-responsive nucleus reflected hormonal status rather than gender identity.

In addition to the hypothalamus, researchers have sought to identify variation with sex and sexual orientation in the brain commissures, the fiber bundles that connect the left and right hemispheres of the brain (Lasco et al., 2002). These studies have produced conflicting results regarding variation with both sex and sexual orientation. Thus, to date there is no compelling evidence of sexual atypicality in the cerebral commissures of homosexuals. The commissures have not been investigated with regard to gender identity.

5.3 Anthropometric Characteristics

Several anthropometric characteristics have been explored in relation to sexual orientation. Most of these studies have been executed with the expectation that homosexual individuals would exhibit characteristics intermediate between those of heterosexual men and women or more typical of heterosexuals of the other sex. Such measures have included not only height and weight but also the amount and distribution of facial hair, the ratio of shoulder width to hip width, the size of the genitalia, and more recently dermatoglyphic (fingerprint) characteristics, and finger length ratios (ratio of the length of the index finger to that of the ring finger). Most of these studies have been flawed in one or more ways, making their findings difficult to interpret. Some of these flaws include reliance on self-reports of small self-selected samples or on measures obtained by raters who were not blind to the sexual orientation of the subjects. The finger length ratio appears to be a sexually dimorphic phenomenon, but whether it truly varies with sexual orientation remains to be established by further investigation (Williams et al., 2000). It also remains to be demonstrated that the sex difference in the finger length ratio is a function of early androgen exposure. Recent research suggests that cell autonomous mechanisms (e.g., sex differences in gene dosing due to incomplete inactivation of one X chromosome in female cells) contributes more to the establishment of sexual dimorphisms than previously appreciated (Arnold et al., 2004). Finally, one laboratory (Loehlin and McFadden, 2003) has reported that lesbian women exhibit masculinized otoaccoustic emissions (an echo-like waveform emitted by the inner ear response to brief sounds). Replication by independent laboratories is required to substantiate those results.

5.4 Outcome Studies Following Childhood Gender Reassignment

Beginning in the 1950s, John Money and colleagues (Money et al., 1957) observed that because intersexes are neither completely male nor completely female they "are likely to grow up with contradictions existing between the sex of assignment and rearing, on the one hand, and various physical sexual variables, singly or in combination, on the other." They therefore collected data on the psychosexual development of children born with various intersex conditions to determine whether their gender role and identity are more likely to be concordant with the sex of assignment and rearing or with one or another of the physical variables of sex. Of 105 intersexes studied, they reported that only 5 had a gender role or identity that was "ambiguous and deviant from the sex of assignment and rearing." Thus, they concluded, as had Ellis a dozen years previously (Ellis, 1945), that the sex of assignment and rearing is a much better predictor of gender role and identity than the biologic variables of sex. The brain was not counted among those variables.

Evidence for the early malleability of gender identity instigated a shift away from prior attempts to assign gender to intersexes on the basis of their "true sex." Instead, as detailed by Zucker (1999) and Meyer-Bahlburg (1994), an "optimal gender policy for psychosocial and medical management" was developed by Money and his collaborators. This policy aimed to optimize the prognosis with respect to six variables: reproductive potential, sexual function, minimization of medical procedures, gender-appropriate appearance, stable gender identity and psychological well-being. Widespread implementation of this optimal gender policy eventuated in the assignment of most intersexed infants to the female gender because, compared to phalloplasty, vaginoplasty produces superior cosmetic and functional results (Fausto-Sterling, 2000) and because it has been believed that a small or absent penis would be a tremendous psychosocial burden for a boy (Zucker, 1999). The surgical policy was premised on the untested assumption that gender-appropriate genitals are necessary not only to convince the affected child that he/she is truly a member of the assigned gender but also to convince the parents whose job it is to unambiguously rear the child in a manner consistent with that gender assignment (Zucker, 1999). Prompt surgical attention to the genital anomalies of intersexed infants was viewed as necessary to establish the dominance of social influences over biologic predispositions on gender identity. Under the optimal gender policy, many 46XY infants with normally functioning testes but with a stretched phallus length less than 2 cm have been surgically reassigned to the female gender (Zucker, 1999; Fausto-Sterling, 2000), as have some normal male infants who suffered traumatic loss of the penis (Diamond & Sigmundson, 1997; Bradley et al., 1998; Zucker, 1999). The indications for early feminizing genitoplasty have been called into question on a variety of grounds (Schober, 1999), including the possibility that gender identity has been substantially organized by hormonal influences prior to birth (Reiner, 1997).

Various intersex and related syndromes have been reviewed extensively with regard to gender identity and sexual orientation (e.g., Zucker, 1999; Byne & Sekaer, 2004). Below is a selective review of those syndromes most frequently cited with reference to gender minority status.

5.4.1 Ablatio Penis
Zucker (1999) reviewed six cases of normal males who suffered accidental or traumatic loss of the penis during infancy and were

reassigned to the female gender prior to 2 years of age. The brains of such female-assigned individuals would have been exposed to the full complement of defeminizing and masculinizing hormones prenatally. Although they are not intersexes, such cases are informative with respect to the question of gender neutrality at birth. These cases would provide a stringent test of the hypothesis of gender neutrality at birth if the female reassignments had been made at birth. Contrary to popular accounts of some of these cases (e.g., Diamond and Sigmundson, 1997), however, gender reassignment has not been made at birth.

Of the six cases reviewed by Zucker (1999), at least two (orchiectomized at 6 and 21 months, respectively) had switched to a male gender identity by or during puberty, whereas two (orchiectomized at 2 and 6 months, respectively) had retained a female identity at last follow-up (one at age 17 and the other in her mid-twenties); no reliable information was available concerning the gender development of the other two. As described below, detailed information is available for only two cases. Although these two detailed cases differed with respect to ultimate gender identity, both exhibited tomboyism during childhood and described predominant or exclusive gynephilia as adults.

In the first detailed case, Money and Ehrhardt (1972) reported on a case of ablatio penis that continues to receive widespread attention. The case involved a pair of normal monozygotic 46XY twins, one of whom suffered accidental penile ablation at the age of 7 months. After much debate, the decision for gender reassignment was made at 17 months, with orchiectomy and preliminary vaginoplasty occurring at 21 months (Diamond & Sigmundson, 1997; Zucker, 1999). Follow-up when the twins were 7 years old suggested that the patient had accepted the female gender identity and that the twin brother was a normal male (Money & Ehrhardt, 1972). Two years later, the patient was described as having many tomboyish traits but that "Her activity is so normally that of an active little girl. . . ." (Money, 1975). Thus, it was concluded that "gender identity is sufficiently incompletely differentiated at birth as to permit successful assignment of a genetic male as a girl . . . and differentiates in keeping with the experiences of rearing." This case was lost to follow-up for many years, and for approximately two decades that conclusion was cited in innumerable medical review articles and textbooks, forming the crux of theories concerning the malleability of gender and gender reassignment in intersexed individuals (Reiner, 1997). Follow-up when the patient was in his early thirties, however, suggested that he had rejected the female identity, had resisted feminizing estrogen therapy, and had begun to live as a male by the age of 14 (Diamond & Sigmundson, 1997). At the age of 14, he underwent a mastectomy and began testosterone replacement therapy and surgical procedures for phallus reconstruction. At the age of 25, he married a woman and adopted her children. At last follow-up, prior to his suicide in 2004, he reported a history of exclusive gynephilic orientation.

A second detailed case of ablatio penis was reported by Bradley et al. (1998). This normal 46XY patient's penis was destroyed during an electrocautery circumcision at 2 months. At 7 months the patient was admitted to the hospital for orchiectomy and initial feminizing surgery, but the decision for gender reassignment had been made previously. Feminizing hormone therapy was initiated at 11 years. At age 16 she reported being a tomboy but denied uncertainty about her female gender identity. At age 26 she remained confident of her female gender. Although at that time she was sexually active with a man, she reported primarily gynephilic fantasies and described her sexual orientation as bisexual.

5.4.2 Congenital Virilizing Adrenal Hyperplasia

With congenital virilizing adrenal hyperplasia an enzymatic abnormality in cortisol synthesis results in an overproduction of androgens beginning during the fetal period (New and Levine, 1981). In genetic males, no genital abnormality ensues; however, in genetic females varying degrees of external genital masculinization can occur ranging from mild clitoral enlargement to complete fusion of the labioscrotal folds with a phallic urethra. Consequently, there is sometimes uncertainty regarding gender assignment at birth. Cortisol replacement therapy can minimize further virilization after birth and allow normal ovarian function and fertility to emerge with puberty. In one large cohort, 9% of genetic females were assigned and reared as males without reported complications (Mulaikal et al., 1987). It is likely that as early detection and diagnosis improve the proportion assigned male will decrease in keeping with the optimal gender policy that places emphasis on female reproductive potential.

Affected individuals with this condition who were reared as females have been studied extensively with regard to cognitive profiles (Berenbaum, 2001), childhood gender conformity (Reinisch & Sanders, 1984), gender identity (Hines, 1998), and sexual orientation (Money, 2002). Most affected individuals are believed to retain their female gender identity into adulthood although with a statistically increased incidence of gender nonconformity (Reinisch & Sanders, 1984; Hines, 1998), gender dysphoria (Slijper et al., 1998) or ambivalence about gender (Ehrhardt et al., 1968) during childhood and gynephilia during adulthood (Hines, 1998; Money, 2002). The retention of female gender identity appears to be the rule even when treatment is delayed resulting in heavy postnatal virilization and lack of feminine secondary sexual characteristics. Meyer-Bahlburg et al. (1996), however, described four cases in which a male identity emerged gradually between late adolescence and adulthood despite having been assigned female within a few weeks of birth. Gender dysphoric subjects appear to be less willing to participate in follow-up studies than are subjects without gender dysphoria (Zucker, 1999), making the proportion of affected individuals who change from female to male gender identity difficult to know with any degree of certainty. In one study that figure was approximately 1 of 50, statistically significantly higher than the rate (approximately 1 per 34,000) of transgenderism among nonintersex females (Zucker, 1999).

5.4.3 Complete Androgen Insensitivity

With complete androgen insensitivity, 46XY individuals develop normally functioning testis but lack functional androgen receptors. Thus, their tissues are unable to respond to androgens, and they develop normal female external genitalia. Because they are capable of responding to müllerian inhibitory substance, however, internal female genital structures regress. Untreated, they develop breasts and female-typical fat distribution at puberty in response to estrogens derived from testosterone synthesized by their testes. Historically, these individuals were assumed to be normal females at birth and did not come to medical attention until testes descended into the labia, or until they failed to menstruate or conceive children. According to Meyer-Bahlburg (1998), the literature does not contain any reports of affected individuals changing to a male gender identity. Thus, in the absence of functional androgen receptors, female gender identity appears to be the rule in individuals with an XY karyotype and normally functioning testes. Although it has been suggested that in the absence of functioning androgen receptors these individuals would have female-typical brain differentiation (Collaer & Hines, 1995), in laboratory rodents androgens appear to orchestrate differentiation of the male brain primarily by interaction with estrogen receptors after conversion to estrogen by aromatase enzymes in the brain (Goy & McEwen, 1980). For example, mice with complete androgen insensitivity appear to be female physically but exhibit defeminized and masculinized behavior, including mating behavior (Olsen, 1983). It has therefore been suggested that humans, in contrast to rodents, require functional androgen receptors for male brain development (Goy & McEwen, 1980). From a psychosocial standpoint, however, one might suggest that gender outcome in humans with complete androgen insensitivity is due to the fact that they were assigned unequivocally to the female gender at birth and were subjected to the same gender socialization as unaffected girls.

5.4.4 Partial Androgen Insensitivity

Partial androgen insensitivity refers to disorders in which there is only partial resistance to androgens at the cellular or receptor level. The testes are believed to function normally, and there is no deficiency of 5α-reductase enzymes; however, the partial insensitivity to androgens results in external genitalia that are only partially masculinized. The degree of masculinization of the external genitalia varies according to the degree of androgen resistance. Affected individuals have been assigned and reared as males or females depending in part on the degree of external genital virilization. Zucker (1999) reviewed six cases in which individuals with partial androgen insensitivity were reared as girls (although one was initially assigned male until 13 days after birth). Among them, five retained a female gender identity into adulthood (ages 19 to 30 at follow-up), even though one remained gonadally intact into adulthood and experienced marked postnatal virilization. The sixth patient was reassigned female 5 days after birth and was reared as a girl. At age 30 he requested sex reassignment following a long history of masculine gender role interests and gynephilia.

Data are available on an additional 18 subjects from two group studies. The first of these studies involved 10 patients of whom 8 were reared as boys, 1 as a "hermaphroditic girl," and 1 as a girl (Chase,

1998). At follow-up between 13 and 39 years it was concluded that gender identity differentiated in accordance with the gender of rearing. The second study included eight patients, seven of whom were assigned female at birth (Slijper et al., 1998). Details on gender identity were not provided at follow-up (at ages 6 to 23 years); however, the authors concluded that the female assignment had been wrong on the basis of the patients' "boyish behavior. . . . In particular, the wild, rough play . . . [which was] difficult for their parents to regulate."

5.4.5 5α-Reductase Deficiency

Deficiency of the enzyme 5α-reductase affects 46XY individuals. During fetal development the gonads differentiate into normal testes and secrete appropriate amounts of testosterone; however, because of the deficiency of 5α-reductase, affected individuals are unable to convert testosterone to dihydrotestosterone in amounts sufficient for the external genitalia to masculinize normally. Consequently, the newborn may have a phallus that more closely resembles a clitoris than a penis and unfused labioscrotal folds resembling labia majora. In the absence of sophisticated diagnostic testing, affected individuals have often been assumed to be females at birth and have been reared accordingly (Imperato et al., 1974; Imperato-McGinley et al., 1979). At puberty, however, testosterone, not dihydrotestosterone, is the essential androgen for growth of the male external genitalia and the emergence of male secondary sex characteristics (Wilson, 2001). Thus, masculinizing puberty ensues: The phallus markedly enlarges, the testes descend into the bifid labioscrotal folds, the beard grows, the voice deepens, and a masculine habitus develops (Imperato et al., 1974; Imperato-McGinley et al., 1979).

This condition began to receive much attention a quarter of a century ago with a report on a cohort of affected individuals in a region of the Dominican Republic (Imperato et al., 1974; Imperato-McGinley et al., 1979) where the prevalence of the condition is unusually high due to consanguineous marriages. Of 18 individuals who reportedly had been assigned and reared as females from birth, 17 changed to a male gender identity and 16 to a male gender role at puberty. The authors concluded that male gender identity and gynephilia "appear to be testosterone and not dihydrotestosterone related . . . and that sex of rearing as females . . . appears to have a lesser role in the presence of two masculinizing events—testosterone exposure in utero and again at puberty with the development of a male phenotype."

Because the studied individuals came from interrelated families living in the same village, questions were raised about the initial gender assignments as females. Specifically, it was wondered if, despite being declared female and issued a female birth certificate, would parents "rear their child as one of ambiguous sex, not knowing what to expect at puberty" (Money, 1976). Imperato-McGinley et al. (1979) deny that this was the case for their subjects, although they state that now that the villagers are familiar with the condition, they "raise the subjects as boys from birth, rear them as boys as soon as the problem is recognized in childhood or raise them ambiguously as girls."

Similar accounts of gender change from female to male have been made in cohorts from Mexico, Papua New Guinea, and Brazil (Herdt, 1990; Zucker, 1999; Wilson, 2001). Herdt (1990) questioned the lack of ambiguity in the female gender assignments in the New Guinea cohort. Al-Attia (1997) reported on a cohort of six affected Omani Arabs who had been assigned as females at birth, 4 of whom (ages 16 to 28 years) had reached puberty prior to the last assessment. Among them, only one individual (Allen et al., 1989) was unequivocally male in identity and role. One (age 28) was unequivocally female in identity and role. The other two individuals were ambivalent in identity and role: One (age 16) expressed erotic interest in females and requested gender reassignment but refused to declare as a male publicly and "continued the role of a conservative female." The final subject "engaged in sexual activity as a male" but would dress as a male only when away from his home community.

5.4.6 Summary

Review of the clinical data leads to a conclusion similar to that suggested by Money et al. (1957) nearly half a century ago. By and large, individuals with functional androgen receptors and prenatal exposure to elevated levels of androgens appear to have the capacity at birth to develop either a male or a female gender identity in response to gender assignment and rearing. When assigned female, these individuals nevertheless have an increased likelihood of exhibiting masculinized play preferences, gender dysphoria, and gynephilia; and a small number ultimately reject the female identity and role. The proportion that ultimately rejects the female assignment is unknown, as it can occur quite late in life, and relatively few studies have followed and adequately assessed affected individuals during adulthood. The data on individuals with 5α-reductase suggest that the probability of switching to a male gender identity and role after female assignment is increased in androgen-sensitive individuals whose testes are left in place until puberty. The data do not justify the conclusion that prenatal androgen exposure produces a brain that is hardwired for male gender identity at birth. A more conservative interpretation of the data is that prenatal androgens may bias particular behavioral propensities in a manner that facilitates acquisition of a male identity. This effect of prenatal androgens might be reinforced by the elevated androgen secretion that occurs during the neonatal period and again at puberty. At puberty, the psychological impact of somatic virilization in response to elevated androgens must be considered in addition to the possibility of physiologic effects on the brain. The data suggest that among prenatally virilized individuals who were assigned female in infancy the proportion who subsequently exhibit gynephilia is greater than the proportion who reject the female gender assignment. Thus, any effect of prenatal hormones may be greater for sexual orientation than for gender identity.

Data from the studies of intersex disorders also suggest which pathways of androgen action may contribute to psychosexual differentiation of the brain. Although individuals with complete androgen insensitivity have normal testes and all the hormones and metabolic machinery necessary to masculinize the rodent brain (i.e., testosterone, aromatase enzyme, estrogen receptors), all reported cases have been reared unambiguously as females, have retained that identity into adulthood, and are described as having stereotypically feminine interests and behaviors as children (Zucker, 1999). Thus, if prenatal hormones exert an organizing influence on the human brain with respect to gender, masculinization of the brain in this regard must be mediated primarily via androgen receptors. The evolution of masculine behavior and male identity among individuals with 5α-reductase deficiency suggests that those androgen receptors may be activated by testosterone in the absence of 5α-reduction. Moreover, as reviewed by Byne and Sekaer (2004) the gender and sexual orientation outcomes among individuals with very little testosterone production in utero suggest that very little testosterone is required to bias psychosexual development in the male direction. As discussed below, however, the mechanism through which such a bias might be exerted is far from clear. The variability of gender outcomes even among related intersexed individuals known to share identical genetic mutations suggests the importance of psychological, social, and cultural factors as co-mediators of gender development (Wilson, 2001).

6 Genetic Studies

As in neuroendocrinologic research, some genetic studies of sexual orientation have been premised on the intersex hypothesis. To date there have been no such studies of transgenderism perhaps because of its relatively lower prevalence. Genetic studies include (1) attempts to show that homosexuals have opposite-sex chromosomal material in their cells (Money & Ehrhardt, 1972) and (2) studies seeking to link homosexuality with genetically controlled aberrations in the process of sexual differentiation (Macke et al., 1993). None of those studies has met with success. More recent genetic studies (discussed below) are not necessarily based on the intersex assumption and are compatible with a variety of more diverse and complex pathways.

6.1 Heritability Studies

Although studies have suggested that homosexuality runs in families (Pillard & Weinrich, 1986; Bailey & Pillard, 1991), such studies are not helpful for distinguishing between genetic and environmental influences because most related individuals share environmental influences as well as genes. Disentangling genetic and environmental influences often involves comparisons between identical and fraternal twins. The most thorough study of this sort was conducted by Bailey and Pillard (1991). Their study assessed sexual orientation in identical and fraternal twins, nontwin biologic brothers, and unrelated adopted brothers of gay men. The concordance rate for identical twins (52%) in that study was much higher than the rate for the fraternal twins (22%). The higher concordance rate for the identical twins is consistent with a genetic effect because identical twins share all of their genes whereas fraternal twins, on average, share only half of their genes. These studies assume that environmental influences would be the same for all brothers.

It would be a mistake, however, to attribute the increased concordance rate in identical twins to increased gene sharing alone. If there were no environmental effect on sexual orientation, the rate of homosexuality among the adopted brothers should have equaled the rate of homosexuality in the general population. Recent studies place the rate of homosexuality in men between 2% and 5% (Hamer et al., 1993; Bailey et al., 1994). The fact that the concordance rate in adopted brothers was eleven percent (two to five times higher than in the general population) suggests a major environmental contribution. The rate for homosexuality among non twin biologic brothers was only 9%, a figure statistically indistinguishable from the 11% recorded for adopted brothers. If the concordance rate for homosexuality among nontwin brothers is the same regardless of whether the brothers are genetically related, the concordance rate cannot be explained exclusively by genetics.

When considered together, the data from the twins and the adopted brothers suggest that the increased concordance in the identical twins may be due to the combination of both genetic and environmental influences. Perhaps the most interesting finding to emerge from twin studies is that approximately 50% of identical twins are discordant for sexual orientation even when they are reared together. This finding, which has been consistent across studies, underscores just how little we actually know about the origins of sexual orientation.

6.2 Linkage Studies

In 1993 a highly publicized study (Hamer et al., 1993) presented statistical evidence that genes influencing sexual orientation reside on a portion of the X chromosome known as the q28 region. Contrary to some media reports and popular belief, that study did not claim to discover any particular gene or sequence of DNA associated with homosexuality. That is not the aim of linkage studies. The aim of such studies is merely to identify chromosomal regions in which such genes might reside. It is important to understand that the statistical significance of genetic linkage studies depends on assumptions about the rate of homosexuality in the population (Risch et al., 1993). Problems involved in calculating this rate have been reviewed elsewhere (McGuire, 1995). Hamer's conclusions rest on the assumption that the rate of male homosexuality in the population at large is 2%; however, if the base rate is actually 4% or higher, the results that he reported are not statistically significant. One leading geneticist argues that Hamer's own data support a 4% estimate (Risch et al., 1993). A Canadian team has been unable to duplicate the Xq28 finding in men using a comparable experimental design (Rice et al., 1999), and Hamer's team found no evidence that Xq28 is linked to sexual orientation in women (Hu et al., 1995).

6.3 "Gay Genes"

It cannot be overemphasized that "gay genes" are not required for homosexuality to run in families or for researchers to determine that it is "heritable." This is because, to geneticists, heritability has a precise technical meaning. It is defined as the ratio between genotypic variation (genetic variation) and phenotypic variation (observable expressed variation in a trait). Thus, heritability reflects only the degree to which a given trait is associated with genetic factors. It says nothing about the specific genetic factors involved or about the mechanisms through which they exert their influence. Furthermore, heritability gives no information about how a particular trait might change under different environmental conditions. Therefore, as described in the next section, homosexuality could be highly heritable even if genes influenced sexual orientation entirely through indirect pathways.

7 Models for Conceptualizing the Role of Biology

Most efforts to explain the development of gender identity and sexual orientation have focused exclusively on either biologic or psychosocial factors. Three models for integrating biologic and psychosocial contributions are considered here. The first model is the permissive effects model in which biology primarily provides the neural substrate on which gender identity and sexual orientation are inscribed by formative experience (i.e., at birth the brain would be viewed as a blank slate). In this model, genes or other biologic factors could also delimit the period during which the relevant formative experience(s) must occur. By analogy, some song birds can only learn their species' song by hearing it sung during a relatively restricted period of early development. If they hear the song of another species during that time, they may learn it instead (Nottenbohm, 1972). Once a song has been learned, that is the bird's song for life. The bird can neither unlearn that song nor learn another. Whereas the song is clearly acquired through experience, biology determines when during development that experience must occur.

In the second, direct effects, model, biologic factors exert their influence through the organization of hypothetical brain circuits that mediate gender identity and sexual orientation. The fact that sexual orientation and gender identity can vary independently suggests different, though perhaps overlapping, circuits. This model is called "direct" because the arrows of causation point directly from discrete biologic factors such as genes or hormones to gender identity and sexual orientation. This model allows for the possibility that direct biologic effects could be subsequently modified by experience. For example, some have speculated that most women who were exposed as fetuses to masculinizing hormones become heterosexual because "social factors override their biological predisposition toward lesbianism" (Money & Ehrhardt, 1972). Thus, direct model effects could be either determinative or predisposing. They could also be graded in magnitude such that exposure to graded amounts of androgen would produce correspondingly graded degrees of brain masculinization.

In the third, indirect effects, model, the arrow of causation does not lead from biologic factors directly to gender identity or sexual orientation. Instead, biologic factors would directly influence other personality traits or temperamental characteristics that would then influence not only how the environment is experienced internally but how one interacts with and modifies the environment in shaping the relationships and experiences that influence the development of gender identity and sexual orientation. This model is similar to the permissive effects model but goes beyond that model by including the possibility that the relevant formative experiences may themselves be strongly affected by hormonally or genetically influenced personality variables.

7.1 Gender Identity

The direct model with respect to gender identity is best exemplified by the work of Swaab and collaborators who suggested that gender identity is difficult to change because it is fixed in brain structure as a consequence of gender differences in developmental androgen exposure (Zhou et al., 1995). As discussed above, they identified the BSTc as a component of the hypothetical gender identity circuit. Exactly how such a hypothetical brain circuit could act, independent of experience, to cause the child to feel or say "I am a boy" or "I am a girl" is unknown. Moreover, it remains to be explained how such a circuit could be sex-reversed in transsexuals who have no demonstrable genetic or endocrine abnormality.

Irene Fast's (1984) work exemplifies the permissive effects model. She suggests that gender identity in both sexes begins by building self-representations by identification with others. At first these self-representations are over-inclusive such that the toddler is not aware that all sex and gender characteristics are not open to him (e.g., he does not realize that he cannot grow up to be both a mommy and a daddy). Upon recognizing sex differences, the toddler moves from this assumption to a recognition of limits imposed by the reality of his body structure and function. Relinquishing attributes of the over-inclusive self-representation does not involve suppression of biologically based gender constructs, as in the direct model, but the abandonment of self-representations acquired by identification. For example, the child realizes he is a boy and therefore cannot become a mommy. Under normative circumstances the formative experiences that shape gender identification would be consistent with one's gender assignment, which in turn would be in accord with all biologic variables of sex. The psychic pain (narcissistic injury) in response to relinquishing valued but cross-gendered aspects of the over-inclusive self-representation would be mitigated in environments in which the assigned gender is valued.

Conflicts might arise in environments in which the child perceives that the gender to which he has been assigned is not valued as highly as the other or where being one gender is perceived as unsafe. In such environments, the child might cling tenaciously to identification of the over-inclusive gender self-representation that corresponds to the favored gender. During early stages of cognitive development (perhaps up to the age of 4 to 6 years) when the child believes that he could become the other gender merely by dressing or behaving as that gender (for references see Byne and Sekaer, 2004), he might then resolve conflicts in the arena of gender by identifying with the gender contrary to that assigned. It is also easy to imagine how difficulties could occur in the case of intersexes where parents might be ambivalent about the gender assignment and communicate their ambivalence (consciously or unconsciously) to their child. Thus, in the permissive effects model, cognitive limitations interacting with relational and emotional issues (e.g., identification and the shaping influences of parental behavior) could account for the development of normative and variant gender identities without requiring a brain circuit dedicated specifically to gender identity. Moreover, according to Fast's model, one's gender identity consists of those aspects of the over-inclusive gendered self that one retains rather than relinquishes during the course of development. Thus, one would not necessarily develop either an exclusively male or an exclusively female identity but could retain elements of both genders in the self-representation.

In an indirect effects model, the relational issues and identifications that influence gender identity would be biased by inborn behavioral or temperamental traits. The propensity to engage in rough and tumble play is an example of a temperamental variant that may be influenced by early androgen exposure (Goy & McEwen, 1980) and that may act as a mediating factor in the formation of gender identity. For example, children who exhibit gender-atypical levels of rough and tumble play (e.g., the extreme tomboy, the boy who avoids all such activities) might prefer playmates of the other gender with similar activity levels and play interests and identify with them as well as with adults of that gender. The gender-atypical play would elicit reactions from peers and adults that might take the form of teasing, reprimands, or efforts to change the behaviors. Thus, the child's brain-driven propensities would elicit particular responses from his environment that would in turn modify his identifications and self-perceptions.

Attempts by parents or clinicians to modify the gender-inappropriate behaviors might unwittingly reinforce the opposite-gender identification. For example, prior to the mastery of the concepts of gender stability and constancy at 6 to 7 years of age (for references see Byne and Sekaer, 2004), a boy who is repeatedly reprimanded or shamed for acting like a girl might conclude (on some less than fully conscious level) that it would be easier to become a girl than to act like a boy. Or, more simply, he might conclude, "I act like a girl; therefore, I am a girl." Similarly, during the vulnerable period of development, a girl who is told she does not behave like a girl might conclude that she must therefore be a boy. This dynamic could be particularly relevant in the development of gender identity in intersexes if, perhaps owing to sexually intermediate hormonalization of their brains, their behavioral propensities were androgenous. Regardless of which gender they were assigned, such individuals might be perceived as gender-atypical in environments that demand conformity to strict gender role stereotypes.

7.2 Sexual Orientation

Traditional psychoanalytic models exemplify the model of permissive biologic effects. According to the psychoanalytic view, the sexual instinct is biologically based but neutral with respect to sexual orientation. Sexual orientation is determined by whether the child navigates the oedipal conflict by identifying with the father or mother. The psychoanalytic view is compatible with the model of indirect biologic effects if one supposes that inborn temperamental factors influence the dynamics of the oedipal triad.

The existing data relevant to sexual orientation are equally compatible with both the direct and indirect models of biologic influence. The distinction between these models can be appreciated in their differing interpretations of three of the more robust findings in the sexual orientation literature. The first of these findings is that the propensity to engage in rough-and-tumble play appears to be influenced by prenatal exposure to androgens (Goy & McEwen, 1980). Second, compared to heterosexual men, more, but not all, homosexual men recall a childhood aversion to competitive rough-and-tumble play (Bell et al., 1981). Third, compared to heterosexual men, more, but not all, homosexual men recall their fathers as having been distant or rejecting (Bell et al., 1981; Isay, 2004).

In the direct model interpretation, the aversion to rough-and-tumble play represents the childhood expression of a brain that has been prewired for homosexuality. This is the position of Richard Isay (Isay, 2004), a psychoanalyst who suggests that biologic factors wire the brain for sexual orientation and consequently reverse the polarity of the oedipal complex. According to this model, in addition to shunning rough-and-tumble play, prehomosexual boys are erotically interested in their fathers during the oedipal period. Fathers might recoil from their prehomosexual sons' gender nonconformity or sexual inclinations. Even if the father did not recoil, Isay speculates that during adulthood gay men might nevertheless recall their fathers as having been cold or distant to avoid conscious awareness of their earlier sexual attractions to them (Isay, 2004).

According to the indirect model, the biologically influenced aversion to rough and tumble play does not imply prewiring for homosexuality at all. Instead, this aversion would become a potent factor predisposing to homosexual development only in particular environments, perhaps where such an aversion is stigmatized as "sissy" behavior and causes a boy to see himself as being different from his father and male peers. This early sense of difference from other males might contribute to the subsequent consolidation of a homosexual identity (Bem, 1996). A father might withdraw from a son he views as a "sissy" or a disappointment. Thus, the father's withdrawal would contribute to his son's homosexuality rather than result from it. Importantly, this temperamental variant would arguably have different consequences in environments where the boy's aversion to rough and tumble play is socially acceptable, perhaps making no contribution to the development of sexual orientation at all. The above example should not be taken to imply that either an aversion to sports or a rejecting father is a feature of all or even most of the pathways to male homosexuality. Using the indirect model, one could conjecture how any number of temperamental variants might have an impact on the development of sexual orientation (Byne & Parsons, 1993). A given variant might predispose to homosexuality in one environment, to heterosexuality in another, and have no contribution to sexual orientation in others.

References

Al Attia, H.M. (1997) Male pseudohermaphroditism due to 5 alpha-reductase-2 deficiency in an Arab kindred. *Postgraduate Medical Journal* 73:802–807.

Allen, L.S., Hines, M., Shryne, J.E., and Gorski, R.A. (1989) Two sexually dimorphic cell groups in the human brain. *Journal of Neuroscience* 9:497–506.

American Psychiatric Association (1994) *Diagnostic and statistical manual of mental disorders.* APA, Washington, DC.

Arnold, A.P., Agate, R.J., and Carruth, L.L. (2004) Hormonal and cell autonomous mechanisms of sexual differentiation of the brain. In: Legato, M. (ed) *Principles of gender specific medicine.* Elsevier Science, San Diego, pp. 84–96.

Bagemihl, B. (1999) *Biological exuberance: animal homosexuality and natural diversity.* St. Martin's Press, New York.

Bailey, J.M., and Pillard, R.C. (1991) A genetic-study of male sexual orientation. *Archives of General Psychiatry* 48:1089–1096.

Bailey, J.M., Gaulin, S., Agyei, Y., and Gladue, B.A. (1994) Effects of gender and sexual orientation on evolutionarily relevant aspects of human mating psychology. *Journal of Personality and Social Psychology* 66:1081–1093.

Bell, A.P., Weinberg, M.S., and Hammersmith, S.K. (1981) *Sexual preference: its development in men and women.* Indiana University Press, Bloomington.

Bem, D.J. (1996) Exotic becomes erotica developmental model of sexual orientation. *Psychology Review* 103:320–335.

Berenbaum, S.A. (2001) Cognitive function in congenital adrenal hyperplasia. *Endocrinology and Metabolism Clinics of North America* 30:173.

Bradley, S.J., Oliver, G.D., Chernick, A.B., and Zucker, K.J. (1998) Experiment of nurture: ablatio penis at 2 months, sex reassignment at 7 months, and a psychosexual follow-up in young adulthood. *Pediatrics* 102:e9.

Byne, W., and Kemether, E. (2000) The sexual brain. In: Bittar, E., and Bittar, N. (eds) *Biological psychiatry.* JAI Press, Greenwich, CT, pp. 59–86.

Byne, W., and Parsons, B. (1993) Human sexual orientation: the biologic theories reappraised. *Archives of General Psychiatry* 50:228–239.

Byne, W., and Sekaer, C. (2004) The question of psychosexual neutrality at birth. In: Legato, M. (ed) *Principles of gender specific medicine.* Elsevier Science, San Diego, pp. 155–167.

Byne, W., Tobet, S., Mattiace, L.A., Lasco, M.S., Kemether, E., Edgar, M.A., Morgello, S., Buchsbaum, M.S., and Jones, L.B. (2001) The interstitial nuclei of the human anterior hypothalamus: an investigation of variation with sex, sexual orientation, and HIV status. *Hormones and Behavior* 40:86–92.

Chase, C. (1998) Surgical progress is not the answer to intersexuality. *Journal of Clinical Ethics* 9:385–392.

Collaer, M.L., and Hines, M. (1995) Human behavioral sex-differences: a role for gonadal hormones during early development. *Psychological Bulletin* 118:55–107.

Collaer, M.L., Tory, H.O., and Valkenburgh, M.C. (2003) Do steroid hormones contribute to sexual differentiation of the human brain? In: *Principles of gender specific medicine.* Elsevier Science, San Diego, pp. 71–84.

Diamond, M., and Sigmundson, H.K. (1997) Sex reassignment at birth: long-term review and clinical implications. *Archives of Pediatric and Adolescent Medicine* 151(3):298–304.

Ehrhardt, A.A., Evers, K., and Money, J. (1968) Influence of androgen and some aspects of sexually dimorphic behavior in women with late-treated adrenogenital syndrome. *Johns Hopkins Medical Journal* 123:115.

Ellis, A. (1945) The sexual psychology of human hermaphrodites. *Psychosomatic Medicine* 7:108–125.

Fast, I. (1984) *Gender identity: a differentiation model.* Analytic Press, Hillsdale, NY.

Fausto-Sterling, A. (2000) *Sexing the body.* Basics Books, New York.

Glass, S.J., and Johnson, R.W. (1944) Limitations and complications of organotherapy in male homosexuality. *Journal of Clinical Endocrinology and Metabolism* 4:550–554.

Gooren, L. (1986a) The neuroendocrine response of luteinizing hormone to estrogen administration in heterosexual, homosexual, and transsexual subjects. *Journal of Clinical Endocrinology and Metabolism* 63:583–588.

Gooren, L. (1986b) The neuroendocrine response of luteinizing hormone to estrogen administration in the human is not sex specific but dependent on the hormonal environment. *Journal of Clinical Endocrinology and Metabolism* 63:589–593.

Gooren, L. (1990) Biomedical theories of sexual orientation: a critical examination. In: McWhirter, D.P., Sanders, S.A., and Reinisch, J.M. (eds) *Homosexuality/heterosexuality: concepts of sexual orientation.* Oxford University Press, New York, pp. 71–87.

Goy, R.W., and McEwen, B.S. (1980) *Sexual differentiation of the brain.* MIT Press, Cambridge, MA.

Hamer, D.H., Hu, S., Magnuson, V.L., Hu, N., and Pattatucci, A.M.L. (1993) A linkage between DNA markers on the X-chromosome and male sexual orientation. *Science* 261:321–327.

Hennessey, A.C., Wallen, K., and Edwards, D.A. (1986) Preoptic lesions increase the display of lordosis by male rats. *Brain Research* 370:21–28.

Herdt, G. (1990) Mistaken gender: 5-alpha-reductase hermaphroditism and biological reductionism in sexual identity reconsidered. *American Anthropologist* 92:433–446.

Hines, M. (1998) Abnormal sexual development and psychosexual issues. *Baillieres Clinical Endocrinology and Metabolism* 12:173–189.

Hrabovsky, Z., and Hutson, J.M. (2002) Androgen imprinting of the brain in animal models and humans with intersex disorders: review and recommendations. *Journal of Urology* 162:2142–2148.

Hu, S., Pattatucci, A.M.L., Patterson, C., Li, L., Fulker, D.W., Cherny, S.S., Kruglyak, L., and Hamer, D.H. (1995) Linkage between sexual orientation and chromosome Xq28 in males but not in females. *Nature Genetics* 11:248–256.

Imperato, J., Guerrero, L., Gautier, T., and Peterson, R.E. (1974) Steroid 5alpha-reductase deficiency in man: inherited form of male pseudohermaphroditism. *Science* 186:1213–1215.

Imperato-McGinley, J., Peterson, R.E., Teofilo, G., and Sturla, E. (1979) Androgens and the evolution of male-gender identity among pseudohermaphrodites with 5-alpha-reductase deficiency. *New England Journal of Medicine* 300:1233–1237.

Isay, R. (2004) *Being homosexual: gay men and their development.* Avon Press, New York.

Kulin, H.E., and Reiter, E.O. (1976) Gonadotropin and testosterone measurements after estrogen administration to adult men, prepubertal and pubertal boys, and men with hypogonadotropism: evidence for maturation of positive feedback in male. *Pediatric Research* 10:46–51.

Lasco, M.S., Jordan, T.J., Edgar, M.A., Petito, C.K., and Byne, W. (2002) A lack of dimorphism of sex or sexual orientation in the human anterior commissure. *Brain Research* 936:95–98.

Levay, S. (1991) A difference in hypothalamic structure between heterosexual and homosexual men. *Science* 253:1034–1037.

Loehlin, J.C., and McFadden, D. (2003) Otacoustic emissions, auditory evoked potentials, and traits relating sex and sexual orientation. *Archives of Sexual Behavior* 32(2):115–127.

Macke, J.P., Hu, N., Hu, S., Bailey, M., King, V.L., Brown, T., Hamer, D., and Nathans, J. (1993) Sequence variation in the androgen receptor gene is not a common determinant of male sexual orientation. *American Journal of Human Genetics* 53:844–852.

McGuire, T.R. (1995) Is homosexuality genetic? A critical review and some suggestions. *Journal of Homosexuality* 28:115–145.

Meyer-Bahlburg, H.F. (1994) Intersexuality and the diagnosis of gender identity disorder. *Archives of Sexual Behavior* 23:21–40.

Meyer-Bahlburg, H.F. (1998) Gender assignment in intersexuality. *Journal of the Psychology of Human Sexuality* 10:1–21.

Meyer-Bahlburg, H.F., Gruen, R.S., New, M.I., Bell, J.J., Morishima, A., Shimshi, M., Bueno, Y., Vargas, I., and Baker, S.W. (1996) Gender change from female to male in classical congental adrenal hyperplasia. *Hormones and Behavior* 30:19–32.

Meyer-Bahlburg, H.F.L. (1977) Sex hormones and male homosexuality in comparative perspective. *Archives of Sexual Behavior* 6:297–325.

Meyer-Bahlburg, H.F.L. (1984) Psychoendocrine research on sexual orientation: current status and future options. *Progression Brain Research* 71:375–397.

Money, J. (1975) Ablatio penis: normal male infant sex-reassigned as a girl. *Archives of Sexual Behavior* 4:65–71.

Money, J. (1976) Gender identity and hermaphroditism. *Science* 191:872.

Money, J. (2002) Amative orientation: the hormonal hypothesis examined. *Journal of Pediatric Endocrinology and Metabolism* 15:951–957.

Money, J., and Ehrhardt, A.A. (1972) *Man and woman, boy and girl.* John Hopkins University Press, Baltimore.

Money, J., Hampson, J.G., and Hampson, J.L. (1957) Imprinting and the establishment of gender role. *Archives of Neurology and Psychiatry* 77:333–336.

Moore, K.L. (1982) *The developing human.* W.B. Saunders, Philadelphia.

Mulaikal, R.M., Migeon, C.J., and Rock, J.A. (1987) Fertility rates in female patients with congenital adrenal hyperplasia due to 21-hydroxylase deficiency. *New England Journal of Medicine* 316:178–182.

New, M.L., and Levine, L.S. (1981) Adrenal hyperplasia in intersex states. *Pediatric and Adolescent Endocrinology* 8:51–64.

Norman, R.L., and Spies, H.G. (1986) Cyclic ovarian function in a male macaque: additional evidence for a lack of sexual-differentiation in the physiological mechanisms that regulate the cyclic release of gonadotropins in primates. *Endocrinology* 118:2608–2610.

Nottenbohm, F. (1972) The origins of vocal learning. *American Naturalist* 105: 116–140.

Olsen, K.L. (1983) Genetic determinants of sexual differentiation. In: Balthazart, J., Prove, E., and Gilles, R. (eds) *Hormones and behavior in higher vertebrates.* Springer-Verlag, Heidelberg.

Paredes, R.G., and Baum, M.J. (1995) Altered sexual partner preference in male ferrets given excitotoxic lesions of the preoptic area anterior hypothalamus. *Journal of Neuroscience* 15:6619–6630.

Pillard, R.C., and Weinrich, J.D. (1986) Evidence of familial nature of male homosexuality. *Archives of General Psychiatry* 43:808–812.

Reiner, W. (1997) To be male or female—that is the question. *Archives of Pediatrics and Adolescent Medicine* 151:224–225.

Reinisch, J.M., and Sanders, S.A. (1984) Prenatal gonadal steroidal influences on gender-related behavior. *Progress in Brain Research* 61:407–416.

Resko, J.A., and Phoenix, C.H. (1972) Sexual behavior and testosterone concentrations in plasma of rhesus monkey before and after castration. *Endocrinology* 91:499.

Rice, G., Anderson, C., Risch, N., and Ebers, G. (1999) Male homosexuality: absence of linkage to microsatellite markers at Xq28. *Science* 284:665–667.

Risch, N., Squireswheeler, E., and Keats, B.J.B. (1993) Male sexual orientation and genetic evidence. *Science* 262:2063–2065.

Roselli, C.E., Larkin, K., Resko, J.A., Stellflug, J.N., and Stormshak, F. (2004) The volume of a sexually dimorphic nucleus in the ovine medial preoptic area/anterior hypothalamus varies with sexual partner preference. *Endocrinology* 145(2):478–483.

Schober, J.M. (1999) Quality-of-life studies in patients with ambiguous genitalia. *World Journal of Urology* 17:249–252.

Sherwin, B.B. (1991) The psychoendocrinology of aging and female sexuality. *Annual Review of Sexual Research* 2:181–198.

Siiteri, P.K., and Wilson, J.D. (1974) Testosterone formation and metabolism during male sexual differentiation in human embryo. *Journal of Clinical Endocrinology and Metabolism* 38:113–125.

Slijper, F.M.E., Drop, S.L.S., Molenaar, J.C., and Keizer-Schrama, S.M.P.F. (1998) Long-term psychological evaluation of intersex children. *Archives of Sexual Behavior* 27:125–144.

Smail, P.J., Reyes, F.I., Winter, J.S., and Faiman, C. (1981) The fetal hormonal environment and its effect on the morphogenesis of the genital system. In: Kogan, S.J., and Hafez, E.S.E. (eds) *Pediatric anthology.* Martinus Nijhoff, The Hague.

Swaab, D.F., and Fliers, E. (1985) A sexually dimorphic nucleus in the human brain. *Science* 228:1112–1115.

Wilkins, L. (1952) Treatment of congenital adrenal hyperplasia with cortisone. *Pediatrics* 9:338.

Williams, T.J., Pepitone, M.E., Christensen, S.E., Cooke, B.M., Huberman, A.D., Breedlove, N.J., Breedlove, T.J., Jordan, C.L., and Breedlove, S.M. (2000) Finger-length ratios and sexual orientation. *Nature* 404:455–456.

Wilson, J.D. (2001) Androgens, androgen receptors, and male gender role behavior. *Hormones and Behavior* 40:358–366.

Zhou, J.N., Hofman, M.A., Gooren, L.J.G., and Swaab, D.F. (1995) A sex difference in the human brain and its relation to transsexuality. *Nature* 378:68–70.

Zucker, K.J. (1995) *Gender identity disorder.* Gilford Press, New York.

Zucker, K.J. (1999) Intersexuality and gender identity differentiation. *Annual Review of Sex Research* 10:1–69.

Part II

LGBT Health and the State

The Importance of Being Perverse: Troubling Law, Identities, Health and Rights in Search of Global Justice

Stefano Fabeni and Alice M. Miller

1 Why Should Sexual Health Policy Makers and Practitioners Be Concerned with Contemporary Struggles in Human Rights?

The premise of this chapter is that policy makers and practitioners concerned with sexual health or with the health of persons of diverse sexualities can and should be part of a global struggle for justice and rights. At the same time, because rights claims for gay-identified or sexually and gender-nonconforming persons do not automatically encompass broader justice claims in health, we seek to explore the tools and principles in health, rights, law, and sexuality that open or close down a connection to broader justice. We suggest that the process of theorizing and practicing an integrated approach to sexuality—critiquing and linking the worlds of health, law, and human rights—can result in practices and positions that are more than mere sums of our current understanding and thus contribute to politically strategic and self-conscious strategies of coalition with others seeking greater justice in health.

We argue this because of a belief that health and law are in themselves sites of practice and experiences of social justice—or injustice—at local and global levels. Health systems and all the players and forces in them can be analyzed for their impact on human dignity, equality, and freedom as well as for their effectiveness in preventing or treating ill-health or disease. Linking health with human rights has become a key for many variously empowered people demanding change in the structures that provide health services and care globally (Freedman, 1995b; Farmer, 1999; Yamin, 2002). More than that, however, linking health systems with justice claims requires health policy makers to assess the power structures within which they operate and use even as they "do good" by organizing or delivering health care (Mackintosh, 2001; Gilson, 2003).

Law plays a significant role with respect to health as well as to sexuality. The discourse around law, health, and sexuality is not simple, however, as there is rarely a direct relationship among the three, although they intersect in ways that produce multiple meanings. The rights and law discourse, for example, includes the notion of identities, behavior, and expression; individuals and groups; claims of actors and responses of states (and supranational organisms). Law is then functionally linked as a tool for respecting, protecting, and fulfilling rights. As for the field of health, the questions of (human) rights and (social) justice vis-à-vis health requires a discussion of principles, policies, and practices. The emergence of sexual rights as an overarching category of rights claiming—encompassing lesbian/gay/bisexual/transgender (LGBT) claims, sexual and reproductive health, responses to sexual harm and other linked claims—demands similar, careful analysis, especially regarding its connection to law.

Moreover, rights work and law-as-rights practice demand an understanding of how gender, race, and sexual power structures are linked—connections that are revealed in national discourses of anxiety arising in South and North. Sexual rights claims have generated some affirmative responses in international, regional, and national law and standards. However, progress has been uneven and inconsistent, such as between same-sex and different-sex sexual rights, across genders, among ages, and between nations and global regimes. There have been varied deployments of the rights claims based on identity, personhood, equality, privacy, freedom, autonomy, health, and dignity (Fried & Landsberg-Lewis, 2000; Miller, 2000; Katyal, 2004; Saiz, 2004), with limited success vis-à-vis the rights recognition of diversity of gender expression. We argue in this chapter that an aspect of that incoherence in sexual rights—especially its exclusionary tendencies—is linked to the qualities of law as a system of categorization, in this case through binaries and rigid group line drawing.

Thus, for persons interested in how rights-oriented work in health can serve the health, dignity, and respect for sexually diverse persons, understanding the current status and context of sexual rights claiming as well as its inner fault lines and biases, especially as linked to the domains of law and health is critical. Although the conversation about sexuality and rights, health, and law is global, the nature and impact of the specific local/international interaction varies: There is no "global gay" with the power to compel identity formation, but there are hegemonic terms, variable portals of entry, and mechanisms of inclusion and exclusion linked to health and law (media, markets, travel/migration, and advocacy campaigns to name a few) interacting with widely divergent local interests and stratifications across gender, race, class, age, religious, rural/urban, and linguistic exchanges—sets of variables that help determine the shape of claims, practices, and identities.

1.1 Using or Avoiding Convenient and Politically Adept Shorthand for Sexual and Gender Claims?

We sometimes use several less common terms here to speak of the galaxy of *nonnormative sexualities* and *gender roles*, rather than the widely used acronym LGBT or the convenient shorthand "sexual minorities." We are aware our longer phrases may be disorienting, but as the primary thrust of our inquiry challenges the way law, rights, and health have arrived at fixed categories of sexuality, we cannot make use of the very definitions we are problematizing. During various political struggles, locally and globally, the terms have functioned as dual-edged swords, often progressively cutting through thickets of opposition to the rights claims of sexually marginalized persons and at times cutting out others from the benefits of the rights claims (Rubin, 1984).

Thus, we do not use terms such as "sexual minorities," which often appears to be good shorthand, laying claim to an existing, apparently analogous system of antidiscrimination. Yet "sexual minorities" does not delimit a meaningful group—By what set of criteria are members of this minority defined? Is it identity-based or practice based? When do we deem sexual identities sufficiently coherent and practices sufficiently nonmajoritarian? Women who have sex outside marriage are deemed a member of a sexual minority if they are same-sex loving but not a member of a sexual minority if they have sex with men outside marriage, with or without pay, even though globally such women are stigmatized and legally and nonlegally attacked. Is a sexual minority permanent/rigid/embodied? Cultural/temporary/flexible? Life and harm is most often experienced as intersectional; and people (both as individuals and groups) fit many and diverse categories shaped across differently functioning axes of gender, sexuality, race, age, health, and religion. If a sociolegal system does not respond to the barriers and inequalities experienced together (intersectional) or separately, as Crenshaw shows, it perpetuates the mechanisms of subordination instead of producing social justice (Crenshaw, 1991). Thus we are left with ungainly phrases: nonheteronormative sexual behavior; locally self-identified gay and lesbian, among others.

1.2 Why Investigate Health and Sexual Rights So Skeptically?

During the last decade, one of the greatest areas of progress for sexual rights has been in health—the right to health specifically but also in regard to the various health effects of sexual acts: the human immunodeficiency virus/acquired immunodeficiency syndrome (HIV/AIDS) pandemic and responses to sexual violence against women being among the most generative of these conversations (Miller, 2001). The focus on sexual health as a strategy to develop and claim "sexual rights" has been important: nonetheless, although it appears politically tempting to claim more aspects of sexual rights through this approach (as it sidesteps certain condemnations based on religion, culture, or morals), we should be wary of over-medicalizing a constellation of social and biologic processes that encompass domains of imagination, expression, and communication, law, religion, and economics as well as the body (Vance, 1999; Miller, 2000). Health cannot be presumed to be a benign site for sexuality, especially homosexuality. Through knowing the history of medical and psychological interventions that oppress lesbians, gay men, and bisexual persons, including the very naming of "homosexuality" as a disease, and the complicated relation between transsexuality and medical intervention, progressive strategies for better care and services for persons of disparate sexualities face the reality that medicine can also function as a regime of control, alone or in partnership with law including criminal laws and public health legislation (Miller, 2001). This reality links to our interrogation of law and rules. How diverse sexualities face inclusion, regulation, and/or exclusion in health bolsters our concern with health systems as a site of social transformation or continued exclusion and therefore becomes a topic of broader global justice.

Concepts of "sexual health" and "healthy sexuality" have dangerous tendencies to slide from denoting sexual behaviors carried out without coercion, violence, or exposure to disease to connoting "normal, naturalized" sex, creating a hierarchy that excludes diverse—or to some, perverse—sexualities (Miller, 2001; Miller & Vance, 2004). Moreover, this slide alerts us to the many valences of sexual judgment in health, and that talking about sexuality within the context of health should not imply that all of the demands of sexuality are encompassed in the domain of health. Conversely, one's sexuality is not the only aspect of identity or behavior affecting health status; a "sexual health and rights" approach should constantly explore and relink the focus on sexuality and health to the many social determinants (e.g., occupational environment, job and social security, poverty, housing, education) factored across other key variables, such as race and sex, that affect health status. Although access to health care does not equal good health, good health nonetheless requires available, accessible, acceptable, quality health services.

The picture for sexual rights is further complicated by the fact that the sociolegal paradigm of identity should not be tethered only to sexual behavior, however much the health lens tends toward that bias. Other elements play important roles: Expression encompasses political, cultural, or personal expression and physical (nonsexual) expression. Expression is also relational, functioning in regard to seeing and being seen by another in both intimate and social contexts. Expression, behavior, and the social and political linkage of these factors to an identity can generate both solidarity and discriminatory conduct or policies. Under these circumstances and in the context of health, we are always asking, then, for what reason do we want to identify a person: to better protect a category of persons or to understand their probable sexual behaviors? These can be related or noncontiguous concerns. Thus, the law's language needs to be shaped in ways that elucidate rather than obscure the understanding necessary to reach these goals.

1.3 Themes and a Road Map

We thus perversely unsettle language and overly neat claims about health, rights, law, and sexuality as part of a project to use these same concepts to increase both the well-being of specific marginalized persons and overall global well-being and justice. In the sections that follow, we enumerate some of the specific principles that underlie rights claims, map the current status of (predominantly homo) sexual rights claiming and geopolitics, and finally set out the geopolitical context of sexual rights claiming. We pay particular attention to the operation of health systems on the one side and law on the other as we argue for rights-based approaches to sexual and gender diversity in health settings.

At the same time, our concern with the impact of the connected but distinct systems of principles and rules (or rights and regulation) suggests the multiple domains where we must look to view these connections between health, sexuality, and rights. The application of principles in health and rights sometimes produces rules on sexual rights, such as through national or international judicial processes, and can be found in diverse branches of law (e.g., criminal, family, citizenship/immigration, labor/employment); it sometimes produces policies that affect sexual health, which must be sought in health law/administration of public health or the practice of health institutions. The forms and effects of such policies and regulations are multiple and massive: As Meyer (2001) points out, due concern by persons in public health with just LGBT sexuality (leaving aside other forms of marginalized sexual behavior or heteronormative sexuality) encompass attention to increased risk for diseases directly or indirectly linked to sexual practices, specific health care issues for transgender people, and attention to mental health, adolescent development, and violence to name a few.

In the exploration that follows, we present four interlinked inquiries. We make these inquiries with reference to the status of various sexual rights claims in the formal world of international human rights, noting particular junctures and disjunctures occasioned by the evolution of health and human rights as a growing part of the human rights movement generally. First, we are concerned with how sexuality and rights claims arise in health claims and how they function in the current political context. This global discourse contains multiple sites of contestation and surges, exclusions, and retrenchments in sexual rights work, often in the context of struggles over national sovereignty and economic power. Second, we are concerned with the operation of law vis-à-vis gender and sexuality because law is a site of power itself and is deeply implicated in these struggles, often in the guise of legal entitlements to health services. Our arguments flow from the insight that the law contributes to the creation of personages so it can attribute rights and duties to them (Lorber, 1994). Thus, we explore how, even as law comes to accept that persons can change gender, it still requires the selection of one of two genders, predicated on a biologic regime in which one can find male and female bodies.

Finally, we connect concerns for law, rights, and sexuality with an inquiry into health as a site of justice. We believe that the health systems into which sexually marginalized individuals and groups demand inclusion are often unevenly accessible because of race, gender, ethnicity, migrancy, poverty, or geographic/rural status as well as uneven distribution of resources nationally and globally (Freedman et al., 2005). Thus, if health systems are a core piece of global health, rights, and justice work today, how do health practitioners working with diverse sexualities, genders, and practices fit into this movement?

Because law as a tool of rights often plays a central gate-keeping role, our chapter seeks to explore contradictory aspects of the law that may simultaneously protect rights and undercut them. We explore the ways in which some legal successes, modeled on culturally limited terms of identity, are either exclusionary or simply insufficient. In particular, we look at specific sites, one trans-European and the other India-specific, regarding transsexuality and criminal regulation of (same sex) sexual practice, respectively, as two key issue areas that have entered many health policy debates to create new categories of people—trans-gendered persons and homosexuals.

We turn first to the connections between health and rights, and the places that sexual rights claims have arisen in health. We also highlight key principles that underlie rights-based approaches, such as account-ability, nondiscrimination, and participation. We then explore the congeries of legal rights as well as some critical fault lines through both theoretical and grounded inquiry in case studies: on the global, geopolitical engines and architecture of sexual rights claims, and on regional (Europe) and national (India) examples of sexual- and gender-linked rights claims. We close our case studies with a return to health as a site of potential justice and injustice in regard to the forces affecting health systems, in which health policy makers and practitioners work. Our conclusion notes the paradoxes of an unstable and contested rights system as the source of local work but argues that this is the best way forward to ensure that the local effects contribute to a greater system of justice and equity in health and in the society as a whole.

Our goal throughout, however, is to build the case for arguing that neither *human rights*, its sometimes handmaiden/sometimes tyrant law, nor *health*, so beneficently appearing, should be employed without examining the ways in which each concept functions to divide, rank, or make invisible the very diversity of persons and their sexuality that we seek to enable and celebrate when we use human rights claims.

2 Health and Human Rights Engage: What Is the Global Context? What Are the Principles? With What Effects on Sexual Rights?

2.1 Health and Human Rights: Tools of Accountability

Although "health and human rights are both powerful, modern approaches to defining and advancing human well being," the field of their intersection still grows slowly (Mann et al., 1999). Recent global work to develop the concepts of health and human rights includes at least four approaches to their connection: the health effects of human rights violations, the human rights effect of health policies, the syner-gistic connections between rights promotion and health promotion, and the claim to the right to health itself.

Table 1. Selected United Nations Human Rights Treaties and Their Monitoring Committees

CEDAW: Convention on the Elimination of all Forms of Discrimination against Women (adopted by U.N. General Assembly in 1979)
   CEDAW: Committee on the Elimination of Discrimination against Women

CRC: Convention on the Rights of the Child (adopted by U.N. General Assembly in 1989)
   CRC: Convention on the Rights of the Child

ICCPR: International Covenant on Civil and Political Rights (adopted by U.N. General Assembly in 1966)
   HRC: Human Rights Committee

ICERD: International Convention on the Elimination of Racial Discrimination (adopted by U.N. General Assembly in 1965)
   CERD: Convention on the Elimination of Racial Discrimination

ICESCR: International Covenant on Economic Social and Cultural Rights (adopted by U.N. General Assembly in 1966)
   CESCR: Committee on Economic Social and Cultural Rights

UDHR: Universal Declaration of Human Rights (adopted by U.N. General Assembly in 1948)

When exploring human rights, we not only call on the international system of rights-standard setting and monitoring (the United Nations) but also look to and draw from regional and national experiences. In the discussion that follows, we use the standards, reports, and determinations of a range of actors created through the United Nations' human rights system. There are rights systems at local, national, and regional levels as well, but here we concentrate on the international standards created by national governments (often through tools called treaties and conventions) that are debated publicly international and are of global reach. (See the list of major human rights treaties and committees and their commonly used abbreviations in Table 1.)

Diverse forms of engagement between rights and health evolved in part because of different doctrinal, political, and methodologic foci in human rights as it looked to health. For example, during the Cold War the prioritization of such civil and political rights as freedom from torture in the West led to a link to health through the need for health responses to torture (the health effects of human rights' violations); the end of the Cold War dissipated this privileging, opening up the discussion to the broader obligations of the right to health. Later, in Section 3, we speak to the challenges currently facing human rights claims, especially sexual rights, in part through the specific actions of the United States, and other actors globally. Before we deal with the politics of rights, including sexual rights, though, we explore the doctrinal claim of rights and its relation to the modern state.

The political assumptions of the doctrine must be held in mind. Human rights as a system is doctrinally predicated on a vision of the modern state that is, at face value, a neo-Keynesian welfare state (Sen, 2005). Politically, this state model is under attack in the current globalizing world. Critics of rights proponents' too-easy remit with status quo geopolitical state arrangements have argued that this vision of the modern state was always partial, biased, and hiding a set of interests that perpetuated regimes of control and empire (An-Na'im, 2004). We return to this critique at our conclusion, but here we engage with the doctrine on its own terms.

The foundational claim of rights is that states are legally accountable for the well-being of all the people under their jurisdiction and control. Moreover, to evaluate state accountability for rights, including health, the doctrine has evolved to use a tripartite structure that sets out the scope and nature of this accountability, using the language of *respect*, *protect*, and *fulfill*.

Governments are required to *respect* rights (the state and its agents must not through their own actions violate rights). This principle was demonstrated when an independent expert for the U.N. Commission on Human Rights, the Special Rapporteur against Torture, in 2001 reported that persons in detention were beaten or otherwise abused because of their sexual orientation or gender identity (Special Rapporteur of the Commission on Human Rights, 2001) or when in 2002 both the Committee on Economic Social and Cultural Rights (CESCR), which monitors the Covenant by the same name, and the Committee on the Elimination of Discrimination Against Women (CEDAW), which monitors the Convention of that name, criticized Kyrgyzstan for its criminalization of lesbianism as a form of violence against women (Committee on the Elimination of all forms of Discrimination against Women, 1999; Committee on Economic Social and Cultural Rights, 2000).

States are required to *protect* rights (the state must organize all branches to ensure that no other entity—private person, corporation—abuses human rights with impunity), as when the Human Rights Committee, which monitors the International Covenant on Civil and Political Rights (ICCPR), criticized the United States in 1994 not only for its then same-sex sodomy laws but also because such laws gave rise to stigma leading to discrimination and violence against persons by other private actors (Human Rights Committee, 1994). This principle is also at work when the European Court of Human Rights (a regional court, see later) found Bulgaria in violation of its obligations to protect, through failure by local police officers' investigating a rape by private persons, because their actions failed to meet the standard of due diligence—a standard of review for the obligation to investigate, prosecute, remedy, or prevent violations of rights, in this case rights that redound to promoting sexual and bodily integrity and decision-making (X, Y, and Z v. the United Kingdom, 1997).

Finally, the state must *fulfill* rights (sometimes called *promote*), meaning that the state must also ensure that its actions, at all levels, through administrative, legislative, judicial, fiscal, budgetary, or other means, make the enjoyment of rights possible. In the case of (sexual) health, this obligation could be met by taking steps to ensure that nondiscriminatory and effective mechanisms are in place to respond to epidemic diseases such as HIV/AIDS or by facilitating the infrastructure for an open and diverse society by ensuring, inter alia, that gay and lesbian advocacy groups can carry out health advocacy without legal strictures or fear of violence, as noted by the Special Rapporteurs on the Rights to Health and Human Rights Defenders (Special Rapporteur on the Right to Health, 2004).

This tripartite ordering of obligations applies to all rights and puts an end to the false dichotomization of rights between affirmative and negative, although it leaves open the actual content of each intervention. It thus puts the gender, race, and sexual ideology of the state front and center in regard to sexual rights. For example, the Committee on the Rights of the Child (overseeing the Convention on the Rights of the Child) interprets the right to information as a right for adolescents to have access to the sexual health information necessary for them to protect their health and lives, regardless of their sexual orientation—information the state must either provide or facilitate easy access to (Committee on the Rights of the Child, 2003a,b). One could imagine both wanting the state not to censor information provided by diverse sexual advocacy groups as well as needing to ensure that the information affirmatively provide by the state is free of gender and sexual stereotypes. A review of the Indian state-supported "life education" course "Learning for Life" for students in grades 9 to 11 reveals that the state-mandated education is replete with gender stereotypes for (modest) heterosexual girls and (sexually adventurous) heterosexual boys (Badrinath, 2005). As Freedman (1995a) cautioned, "the very notion of an IEC (information, education, and communication) strategy designed by government officials for the explicit purpose of changing the [sexual and reproductive] behavior and attitudes of a selected group of people, should give human rights advocates pause."

As the post-Cold War rhetoric that "all rights are universal, interdependent, and interrelated" becomes more accepted, the fact that individual nations/states are not sufficient to guarantee rights has garnered more attention. Health increasingly figures in the human rights discourse (and a competing/overlapping global public goods discourse) as an example of a right that is not within the control of any one state (Smith et al., 2003; Barrett, 2004). In the original 1940s framework for rights, there is good evidence that states were not meant to be solely responsible for the all the conditions necessary for rights, viz. the Universal Declaration of Human Rights, article 28: "Everyone is entitled to a social and international order in which the rights and freedoms set forth in this Declaration can be fully realized" (Universal Declaration of Human Rights, 1948).

Later human rights treaties are increasingly interpreted to explain the importance of state contributions to international enabling conditions and the ways that reporting states' actions affect the enjoyment of rights in entirely separate nations (Limburg Principles, 1987; Maastricht Guidelines, 1998). The Committee that monitors the CESCR has begun a practice of quizzing states' reports, based on the idea that states have accountability for the extranational health effects of their policies (Limburg Principles, 1987; Maastricht Guidelines, 1998; Yamin,

2002) The Special Rapporteur on the Right to Health has said that nations can be evaluated on the health effects of the policies they put into place through such multilateral processes as Trade-Related Aspects of Intellectual Property Rights (TRIPS). He, along with many advocates globally, has focused on rights-related questions of intellectual property (specifically patents) in regard to the inequities of cost and availability of life-saving pharmaceuticals in the context of the global HIV/AIDS pandemic (Special Rapporteur on the Right to Health, 2004).

2.2 Principles of Rights Applicable to Sexuality (and Some Examples of Their Application in Law)

The formal system of rights is comprised in part as a set of legal obligations of states, and thus a tool for certain kinds of accountability. Here, in this chapter, we are focusing on the formal tools of rights: U.N. standards, national laws and practices, health systems and their policies. Before we turn to the role of law, however, we wish to reaffirm that human rights work comes in many guises, locally and transnationally, such that the strength of human rights work derives not from treaty doctrine but from its resonance with grassroots activism and critiques of power, "the legitimate territory of those who make political demands about basic justice. . . ." (Freedman, 1995a). There is a vast, sometimes contradictory interplay between the creation and claiming of sexual rights through the action of many players, nongovernmental organizations (NGOs), and social movements and their engagement—or dismissal of law and formal rights. Although not addressed in this chapter, we hope our discussion of laws and principles is always read against this reality and not in opposition or ignorance of it.

2.2.1 Law and Principles: How Do They Relate?
As we problematize the legal paradigms around health and sexuality, a first step is noting a key aspect of law itself: Even the concept of law is not "univocal." This is probably easier to figure out in continental jurisprudence, where the notion of law is expressed by two words: *legge* and *diritto* in Italian, *loi* and *droit* in French, *ley* and *derecho* in Spanish, *Gesetz* and *Recht* in German (this distinction originates with Roman law, as expressed by the words *lex* and *jus*). In English, we would distinguish between the words *law* and *right*. Hobbes wrote that "Right, consisteth in liberty to do, or to forbear: whereas Law, determineth, and bindeth to one of them: so that law, and right, differ as much, as obligation, and liberty" (Hobbes, 1950) His words express the idea of law as linked to a positive or statutory standard (associated with *rule*), as opposed to the notion of *right*, which is seen to be an expression of a "larger body of principles."[1]

Laws and rights, rules and principles, play different roles in the understanding of health and sexuality at every level of a legal system, from the sharp divisions at the national level to the more blended

---

[1] See G. Fletcher, *Three Nearly Sacred Books in Western Law*, in 54 Arkansas Law Review 1 (2001). Fletcher underlines this distinction between statutory law and the "larger body of principles" affirming that "every European language makes this clear linguistic distinction between the code and the law based on the code."

framework of regional (such as the European and Inter-American systems of protection of human rights) or international (United Nations level) systems, in which principles create rights for individuals and duties for states. For health professionals, knowing the principles is thus a different kind of tool than knowing law: Indeed, principles can be used to challenge unjust laws. Knowing principles, such as the meaning and contents of the fundamental right to health allows health professionals set objectives and goals with reference to sexual health in their capacity as health providers. Knowing and understanding the content (and the limits) of the rules by which they operate enables them to use the system, not merely for services, but to work within it for the most effective means to provide sexual health services that conform to both the laws and the rights.

No legal system, national or international, guarantees an autonomous, fundamental right to sexuality. Therefore, the work to develop sexual rights has grown by analogy and incorporation of key principles of the right to the different aspects of sexuality. Sexual rights has particularly drawn power from the notion of *health as a fundamental right* through, at times, the discussion of reproductive health and rights (Chapman, 1995 & Hendriks, 1995) or HIV/AIDS and rights (Miller, 2000; Saiz, 2004). The recognition of principles of *equality, nondiscrimination*, and *right to privacy* (especially as formulated in evolving claims around LGBT) also contributed to this growth. For example, the promotion of equal treatment and nondiscrimination as general principles of the law is applied to eliminate discriminatory practices in public health policies as well as the access to health care services for sexual- and gender-nonconforming individuals and communities (Mann et al., 1999). Other key principles include a focus on *the dignity of the person*, the understanding that all *rights are interconnected and interdependent* in their realization, and the participation *of individuals and groups in the determination of issues* affecting them.

Nondiscrimination is a principle that encourages the realization that equality is a core value within rights—"All human beings are born free and equal in dignity and rights" (Universal Declaration of Human Rights, 1948)—yet its application is notoriously unclear. Are like things being compared, so any difference in treatment or result is unfair? Or are the things so unlike that there is no injustice in treating them differently? There are legal systems that address only formal nondiscrimination, which is to say that when the law is neutral on its face it is acceptable, regardless of the real-life barriers to equality. Human rights doctrine moves beyond formal discrimination and addresses both intentional and unintentional discrimination, but this move still leaves human rights doctrine work troubled by comparability as well as the incomprehension of one particular aspect of comparison: What aspects of sexuality can be validly compared?

Regarding discrimination in the treatment of sexual behavior, including the impact of the gender of the sexually active persons, on the one hand, many of the treaty bodies have condemned the discriminatory effect of criminal laws penalizing only same sex behavior (see Toonen, below) or penalizing only women in extramarital sexual activity (Human Rights Committee, 2002). The Committee on the Rights of the

Child has, with some hiccups, evolved a relatively robust approach to nondiscrimination, criticizing different/higher ages of consent for same sex relations (Committee on the Rights of the Child, 2000). On the other hand, as Saiz (2004) notes, "because human rights doctrine allows considerable leeway for subjective interpretation regarding what circumstances may justify unequal treatment . . . the treaty bodies have shown themselves willing to tolerate discrimination in partnership rights in the name of protection of the family." For example, the Human Rights Committee (not quite 10 years after Toonen) determined in Joslin v. New Zealand that "the right to marry" could be applied only to the union between a man and a woman (Human Rights Committee, 1999), but 3 years later, in Young v. Australia, the same committee distinguished that case and held that the denial of veteran pension benefits to the survivor of a same-sex partnership breached equal protection of the law benefits, particularly when unmarried heterosexuals could claim those benefits (Human Rights Committee, 2000).

Nondiscrimination is a potent challenge, as shown by the explosive political resistance to the Brazilian draft resolution in the Commission on Human Rights, expressing "deep concern" over human rights violations on the basis of sexual orientation and noting the Universal Declaration of Human Rights' (UDHR's) statement that all persons were entitled to all human rights without discrimination (Saiz, 2004). This simple statement called all social arrangements into question as discriminatory, thereby engendering massive political opposition. At this time, simple application of the principle of nondiscrimination to social and economic entitlements (Saiz, 2004) does not have the political engine to breach core social institutions, such as marriage, that encompass sexual relationships.

Another key value in human rights work is that of the *limit to limits* on rights: Although rights are almost never absolute, the limitations imposed on their exercise (e.g., rights limited in the interest of public health) must be strictly scrutinized for overbreadth, arbitrariness, and effectiveness. Rather stunningly, in 1994 an authoritative opinion was issued by the Human Rights Committee, the group of U.N. experts that reviews implementation of the International Covenant on Civil and Political Rights. This opinion stated that the "criminalization of homosexual practices cannot be considered a reasonable means or proportionate measure to achieve the aim of preventing the spread of HIV/AIDS" (Human Rights Committee, 1992). They stated that the invasion of privacy and the discriminatory impact of Tasmania's sodomy laws could not be justified by reference to public health needs, especially as evidence indicated that such measures were in fact counterproductive to the spread of HIV/AIDS. The Committee also found that the States' assertion of strong moral beliefs did not overcome respect for the values of privacy and nondiscrimination.

The role of *participation* in human rights has gained increasing attention in the "globalizing" debate over rights: In what way can the content of rights develop to become more truly universal (rather than being declared universal)? Whether by arguing that rights have more cultural resonance and thereby greater likelihood of being effective in diverse settings globally (An-Na'im, 1995) through greater partici-pation, or arguing that the very content of rights can be effectively addressed only through the involvement of multiple voices, including sexually minoritized persons in the Third World (Narrain, 2001), advo-cates for human rights increasingly promote participation as a core value. This value aspires to more involvement in making policies and laws, for example, such that the participation of HIV-positive persons in policy and law settings would be facilitated, or persons in sex work would be consulted when laws and policies against the trafficking of prostitution are being written (Saunders, 2004).

When considering meaningful participation, it is notable that the silence about disability in the field of sexual rights on the one hand and about sexuality in disability rights advocacy on the other is ending, with disability rights activists "taking on sexuality" (Shakespeare et al., 1996). Disability intersects with sexuality in ways that shake up easy assump-tions about embodiment, roles, and agency (Shakespeare, 2000). Notably, at the time of this writing, a draft Convention on the Rights of Persons with Disabilities is making its way through the United Nations. However, the original, relatively progressive language of the draft (people with disabilities must have "equal opportunity to experience their sexuality, have sexual and other intimate relationships, and experi-ence parenthood") has been revised to proposals qualifying the right to "experience [one's] sexuality" and "have sexual and other intimate relationships" "within a legitimate marriage," "in accordance with the national laws, customs, and traditions in each country" (Long, 2005). Dis-abled people are participating in this drafting process, but they have not yet been joined by sexual rights advocates. Participation as a value, then, must include the possibility of transformative collective action arising because of interactions across participating groups and not the mere presence of persons of the most affected identity (Shakespeare, 2000).

2.3 Health, Sexuality, and Human Rights in Action: Abuses, Remedies, and the Question of Law

Earlier, when setting out the political context of human rights' engage-ment with health, we noted that there are four frames for this engage-ment: the effect of human rights violations on health; the effect of health policies on human rights; the synergistic connections between rights promotion and health promotion; and the claim to the right to health itself. Armed with the notion of key rights principles and the political context of where and how sexual rights language arises, we now look at the practice of applying rights to sexuality in the context of health and then close with reference to law and principles.

2.3.1 Effect of Human Rights Abuses on Health
The effects of human rights abuse on health is a cornerstone of the most traditional work in human rights; yet it faces potentially radical chal-lenges. Traditional human rights work has focused on the abuse of a person by a state agent and has addressed abuses of the body or denials of such civil and political freedoms as the right of expression, freedom from arbitrary detention, and freedom from torture. Many of the

advances in sexual rights appeared first within this framework: egregious violations, such as torture and extrajudicial killing, which cannot be justified on any grounds. This became a good entry place to raise the question of killing because of homosexuality or torture because of one's gender expression or sexual behavior (Miller, 2000; Saiz, 2004). Traditional human rights work against torture fairly quickly began to look at the role of mental and physical health professionals in responding. By the mid-1980s, torture treatment centers were being founded to both treat and advocate against torture and on behalf of services for survivors (Scarry, 1985; Miller, 2004).

Since 2001, a number of the thematic mechanisms (expert/rapporteurs and working groups mandated by the U.N. Commission on Human Rights to study and report on key themes in human rights) have called for information on human rights violations against what they termed "sexual minorities."[2] Their focus was on embodied rights, often violated by violence—sometimes death. They look at arbitrary detention, freedom of expression, violence against women, and religious freedom, among others. The flow of information on sexuality-related aspects of these issues has affected human rights standard settings (e.g., since 1999), and the Special Rapporteur on Extra-Judicial Executions' reports have detailed the execution and killing of persons based on their sexual identity, same-sex sexual conduct, sexual conduct outside marriage (covering both heterosexual and homosexual sex and both capital punishment and family and community level murder tolerated by the state). The Special Rapporteur proposed as a matter of rights principles that capital punishment cannot be legitimately imposed for morals offenses.

Based in information submitted to him, the Special Rapporteur on Torture has focused not only on the extent to which persons are targeted for torture because of their gender identity and sexual identity (which he used to incorporate both orientation and behavior) but also the extent to which this harm extends into the health realm.

> While no relevant statistics are available to the Special Rapporteur, it appears that members of sexual minorities are disproportionately subjected to torture and other forms of ill-treatment, because they fail to conform to socially constructed gender expectations. Indeed, discrimination on grounds of sexual orientation or gender identity may often contribute to the process of the dehumanization of the victim, which is often a necessary condition for torture and ill-treatment to take place. . . . The Special Rapporteur further notes that members of sexual minorities are a particularly vulnerable group with respect to torture in various contexts and that their status may *also affect the consequences of their ill-treatment in terms of their access to complaint procedures or medical treatment in state hospitals, where they may fear further victimization,* [italics added] as well as in terms of legal consequences. . . .
> —Special Rapporteur of the Commission on Human Rights, 2001

---

[2]See "Sexual Minorities: Call for submissions" at http://www.pfc.org.uk/legal/uncall.htm (last checked 5/30/05).

Within this framework, health professionals have a dual concern: to advocate with the tool of rights against the laws and practices that lead to negative health effects (whether because of gender, sexual identity, sexual orientation, sexual behavior, or the use of sexualized violence) and to develop responses adequate to the after-effects of torture, regardless of its political or social predicate. As Lewin and Meyer suggested, however, responsive, respectful, and effective treatment for persons with nonheternormative sexual and gender practices or identities is not yet a norm in health structures globally or enshrined in law, although (as a matter of rights principles) it follows from the pronouncements of many rights and health experts (Lewin & Meyer, 2002).

2.3.2 Human Rights Impact of Health Practices, or Policies

As the above discussion suggests, persons in health structures may violate rights. This concern has historic roots: The International Covenant on Civil and Political Rights' (ICCPR's) article 7 prohibition against torture contains a correlate prohibition: against cruel, inhuman, or degrading treatment, including that "no one shall be subjected without his free consent to medical or scientific experimentation" (International Covenant on Civil and Political Rights, 1966). Although this principle originates in the exposure of the practices of Nazi doctors, it has modern resonance regarding unproven therapies of conversion, forensic practices "proving homosexuality" or loss of virginity (Long, 2004), drug testing, or other practices of scientific research (Meier, 2004). Rothschild pointed out that although many NGO reports increasingly highlight the need for effective health responses and "while the abuse by health care personnel has been intermittently attended to, the overall role of the health system in perpetuating the marginalization of these populations" has not been well theorized or analyzed (Rothschild, 2004), although some health-based policies, such as identity-based quarantine, travel restriction, and mandatory and coercive testing, have been addressed.

2.3.3 Potential Synergistic Effects Between Health and Human Rights

The third approach to health and human rights postulates that "promoting and protecting health requires explicit and concrete efforts to promote and protect human rights and dignity" (Mann et al., 1999). This framework examines how enjoyment of various rights must affirmatively work together in concrete contexts to make any right real. For example, if "the human rights of women include their right to have control over and decide freely and responsibly on matters related to their sexuality, including sexual and reproductive health, free of coercion, discrimination and violence" (Platform for Action of the Fourth World Conference on Women, 1995), a range of rights is needed. They include rights such as nondiscrimination, freedom of information, protection of physical integrity (freedom from torture; liberty and security of the person), the right to enjoy the benefits of scientific progress, the right of individuals and groups to participate in issues affecting them, the right to equal protection of the law.

This approach can take on the many complicated ways that discrimination on the basis of sex, race, sexual orientation, HIV status, marital status, age, and disability, for example, affect health status. It scrutinizies intersecting discriminations, as with sexualized forms of race discrimination, that affect health. Through strategies of documenting interconnected rights claims, advocates have transformed bundles of existing legal obligations into claims for sexual rights across many differently gendered or sexually identified persons. An example is determining if and how single unmarried women, including lesbians, are excluded from reproductive health technologies. At the same time, this approach, especially in regard to public health (protecting persons from discrimination, such as through combating stigma or coercive practices in the HIV/AIDS pandemic leads to better health for individuals and the community), has been an inconsistent incorporation of the fact that many rights are in tension and must be appropriately balanced and evaluated (Oppenheimer et al., 2002).

To revisit *Toonen*, then, one can see that part of the decision rests on this *principle* of interrelationship, leading to a specific critique of a *law*, as the Human Rights Committee noted that criminalizing homosexual activity tends to impede public health programs "by driving underground many of the people at the risk of infection." Criminalization of homosexual activity runs counter to the implementation of effective education programs in respect of the HIV/AIDS prevention (Human Rights Committee, 1992). Thus, rights principles can be used to evaluate the exclusionary or discriminatory effect of specific laws and to allow health policy makers to see which restrictions are justified and which are not in the light of a fuller context of rights, groups, and interventions.

Considering the operation of specific laws as *rules* makes visible the way that criminalization of same-sex sexual conducts may have indirect effects on prevention and treatment of sexually transmitted diseases as well as on measures aimed to protect the sexual health of targeted individuals who undertake the proscribed conducts. Family law and administrative regulations often contain provisions that have negative impacts on de facto couples, such as the way many spousal benefits are couched: the right to visit a partner in a health facility or other state institution or the right to make medical decisions on behalf of the incapable partner. Normative regulations may have significant consequences on equal access to health care for people in same-sex/gender couples. In those cases, the role of the health professional as mediator/rights promoter between the ideal principles, the discrimination through administration, and the patient, is essential.

Keeping in mind the move from the principle of equality to the rules of nondiscrimination (in health law or more generally), one quickly sees that country-level laws are uneven vis-à-vis the question of discrimination and the interconnectedness of rights concerning sexuality. Only Costa Rica (Costa Rica Ley General Sobre el VIH-SIDA,

1998) and South Africa (South Africa Aged Persons Amendment Act, 1998; South Africa Medical Schemes Act, 1998) have national laws prohibiting discrimination on grounds of sexual orientation that have specific applicability to health care. However, several countries in Europe, as well as states (or provinces or territories) and local governments in the United States, Australia, Canada, have enacted antidiscrimination laws that prohibit discrimination on grounds of sexual orientation (rarely, gender expression is included) in the provision of services, which may include healthcare services. Discrimination can be also a *consequence of exclusion* for LGBT people from health practices as set up by specific legal regimes, as noted in the discussions on access to fertilization techniques). As far as same-sex couples are concerned, the possibility of extending either private healthcare insurance or public healthcare benefits to the partner of the same sex has serious consequences at the level of healthcare provision, especially for low-income couples.

2.3.4 Sexual Rights and the Right to Health
The formal system of rights establishes "health" itself as a human right. The International Covenant on Economic, Social and Cultural Rights states in Article 12 that "States Parties . . . recognize the rights of everyone to the highest attainable standard of physical and mental health" (International Covenant on Economic Social and Cultural rights, 1966). The World Health Organization (WHO), pointing out that health is "a state of complete physical, mental and social well-being" that takes into account the individual's biologic and socioeconomic preconditions, rather than the mere absence of disease or infirmity, makes it clear that the notion of right to health as a principle is something very different from the right to be healthy (Chapman, 1998; Gonzalez, 2000; Kinney, 2001). Several other human rights instruments have provisions dealing with the right to health: article 11 of the ICESCR, article 25 of the UDHR, articles 23 and 24 of the Convention of the Rights of the Child (CRC), article 12(2) of CEDAW, article 5 of Committee on the Elimination of Racial Discrimination (CERD), and humanitarian law instruments, as well as article 11 of the European Social Charter, article 33 of the American Declaration of the Rights and Duties of Man, and article 16 of the African Charter of Human and Peoples' Rights. This obligation is to create conditions for health functions as any other rights claim, not as a magic grant of health but as a tool for demands. The content of the specific, useful actions to build health must be developed locally whereas the right to make the claim is global.

The 2004 Report of the Special Rapporteur on the Right to Health, Paul Hunt, squarely rooted key sexual rights in international law and then argued for their specific relevance to the right to health. In this report—which the United States and the Holy See fought to diminish in impact and validity (Williamson, 2004)—the Rapporteur noted that although sexual and reproductive rights may be controversial they are central to fundamental human rights. He also noted the lesser stage of development of sexual rights (in contrast to reproductive rights) and clarified that some aspects of sexual rights fall within "health" and others outside it (Special Rapporteur on the Right to Health, 2004). He opined that it was established that sexuality is an important characteristic of all human beings and that the full panoply of rights principles and norms (equality, privacy, and the integrity, autonomy, and well-being of the individual) must apply. He wrote that "sexual rights are human rights" and that they "include the right of all persons to express their sexual orientation, with due regard for the well-being and rights of others, without fear of persecution, denial of liberty or social interference" (Special Rapporteur on the Right to Health, 2004). He closed by linking the protection of sexual and reproductive health rights to the struggle against intolerance, gender inequality, HIV/AIDS, and global poverty.

Hunt's report—which does not make new international law but is evidence of what the status of that law is—triggered a hailstorm of attack. He synthesized a wide range of standards and attempted to keep visible the diverse concepts of inequality (age, gender, citizenship, sexual orientation, poverty, reproductive capacity). Hunt linked, but did not subsume, sexual rights to health and sexuality to reproduction. He connected them to established norms and standards of accountability using not only the tripartite framework of respect, protect, and fulfill but also the regime of evaluating health actions in terms of accessibility, *availability*, *acceptability*, and *quality* (Special Rapporteur on the Right to Health, 2004). Health seemed to be the safe site for this highly visible and political step forward for sexual rights, but the attacks by the United States and others also revealed "health" to be vulnerable, in part because of the extent to which health rights also mean affirmative state action and call forth distributive justice questions.

Moving from the international principle to national law, many national constitutions explicitly guarantee a fundamental right to health. National provisions recognizing a right to health provide different definitions, obligations, and contents (Littell, 2002) to respond to the formal set of obligations (respect, protect, fulfill). In common law systems, national courts acknowledge and define its content; in civil law systems, the law expresses the will of the parliament, which ordinary courts must apply and interpret. The impact of this claim can be broad. For instance, although the right to health falls under a section of the Indian Constitution that is more of a policy framework (article 47 of the Directive Principle of State Policy of the Indian Constitution, which establishes the duty of the state to improve public health), the Indian Supreme Court in 1981 made the right to health (as provided by article 12 of ICESCR) directly enforceable as part of the fundamental right to life protected by article 21 of the Constitution. In Francis Coralie Mullin v. The Administrator. Article 70D of the Hungarian Constitution establishes that "[e]veryone living in the territory of the Republic of Hungary has the right to the highest possible level of physical and mental health." The fundamental right to health as protected by article 32 of the Italian Constitution has been interpreted widely in the sense of including psychological and social well-being.

3 Exploring Health, Law, Rights, and Sexuality Interplay Globally and Locally: Three Case Studies

3.1 Specific Challenge for Health Policy Makers and Service Providers

When applying a rights framework to their work, can health care policy makers and practitioners recognize practices of exclusion produced by the desire for "normalization," the impulse to use professional skills resulting in the medicalization of political problems (Kleinman & Kleinman, 1997), or more general exclusions such as geographic inaccessibility or fee structures? Can we see the role of forensic medicine as an accessible tool that should be used respectfully to ensure effective responses to violence in ways that make the law more democratic? For health professionals and policy makers, their practice embodies the application of laws, and their practice reveals the limits of the law in "doing justice."

Because a whole range of material—health and rights—benefits are inherent to the application of these categories, here we explore the possibility that legal categories work as "instruments of regulatory regimes" with invidious effects (Butler, 1993). We consider the direct effects of regulatory regimes as inclusion/exclusion processes, as we believe health professionals must be aware of the possible impact on rights and health deriving from these legal categories. They are factors that determine their work—categories constructed around such ideas as sexual orientation, gender identity, sex, or the reference to LGBT issues in health policies and regulation.

3.2 European Case: The Right to Either A or B as the Basis of Rights and Gender

What follows "materializes" the arguments outlined above on how the language of law administers labels. In other words, the "language of rigid identities" ultimately implies and strengthens the "language of fixed categories" in the realm of law, disempowering the claims of sexually and gender nonnormative persons at their essence.

The shape of rights claims and standards on *gender identity* emerging in Europe provide a paradigmatic example of the vital and contradictory roles that health approaches (here, health regulation) play in the definition of sexual and gender rights. Ironically, what is indeed praiseworthy as progressive rights protection for transsexual people succeeds in part through enforcement of the rigid binary conception of identities as linked to reductive approaches to gender, sexuality, marriage, and reproduction. The cases briefly reviewed below demonstrate how this impact is constituted, as we consider the (regional) case law of the European Court of Human Rights (the Court) as well as the national legislation of some contracting (member) states.

Today, the European Court plays a fundamental role in recognizing the rights of transsexuals in Europe, although it has had a checkered history, first restricting and then often punting cases on technicalities.

The first cases arose during the early 1980s (Van Oosterwijck v. Belgium, 1980; Rees v. United Kingdom, 1986), but claimants made no progress either using claims based on right to private life issues (because of the failures of birth registers to record a male-to-female transition) or asserting their right to marry (abridged by failure to recognize their new sex). Stating that denying transgendered persons their right to marry was not a violation because marriage "refers to the traditional marriage between persons of opposite biological sex" (Rees v. United Kingdom, 1986). These early cases have been seen to betray the real motive behind the rigidly dichotomous legal conception of gender: the "concern to insulate marriage against homosexual incursion" (Rigaux, 1998; Sharpe, 2002). Sharpe (2002) writes that "homophobia of law is a feature of transgender jurisprudence," such that marriage becomes the fulcrum of the heteronormative construction of dichotomous gender, gender roles, and sex between (not within) genders, and therefore must be preserved as is, as an end itself, since it is the institution that preserves that "order of genders."

The Court followed a circuitous route on transgendered rights through the 1990s (Cossey v. United Kingdom, 1990; Sheffield & Horsham v. United Kingdom, 1998), on the one hand accepting in 1992 that there was a violation of privacy rights when French law denied new documents to a male-to-female person because official documentation played such a far-reaching role in daily life within the French civil system (B. v. France, 1992). On the other hand, in 1997 the Court found no violation of privacy rights in the denial of parental rights to nonbiologic, transsexual parents, where the "father" would have been legally a woman (X, Y, and Z v. the United Kingdom, 1997). One can see the clear imprint of the protection of the traditional gender regime even in the disparate results of the two cases. In the first case, the Court seemed more intent on "normalizing" persons within the dichotomous gender paradigm than creating rights to gender identity, as individuals who had "completed" (surgical and hormonal) transition from one gender to the other could undermine the social construction of genders in everyday life through public display as transsexuals. In the later case, the Court was primarily *extending to parental relationships* the biologic gender/sex paradigm.

The most recent and important developments of the European Court of Human Rights are the "twin" 2002 cases of Goodwin v. United Kingdom and I. v. United Kingdom. The applicants, two male-to-female postoperative transsexuals, successfully challenged British law, alleging violation of articles 8 (private life), 12 (right to marry), and 14 (nondiscrimination). The judges argued from a need to resolve the contradiction between supporting irreversible surgery and maintaining a "situation in which postoperative transsexuals live in an intermediate zone as not quite one gender" (Goodwin v. United Kingdom, 2002). The Court asserted that biologic elements do not alone determine a person's sex in life; and by recognizing the violation of the right to marry, they pointed out the need to avoid the paradoxical situation in which a transsexual, legally able to marry, can marry—under heterosexual marriage laws—only a person of the *original* opposite sex (i.e., the same current sex) and not a person of the new opposite sex.

Goodwin is a landmark decision because of its new (nonfixed/biologic) approach to the notion of legal sex and the effects of this approach on marriage, the idea of family, and procreation. In it, the judges also acknowledged rights to dignity, sexual identity, and personal development. *Goodwin* is certainly a step toward recognizing the right to gender expression, but it is limited to individuals who complete the transition from one gender to another. By means of the hormonal–surgical–legal path, these persons "disappear" within the binary sex/gender model: Thus, although *Goodwin* offers legal recognition of a new social status corresponding to a sexual and personal identity (i.e., the condition of the postoperative transsexual person), it cannot address the looming question of gendering (but not one gender) as an aspect of identity if one does not presuppose surgical intervention and absolute transition. Moreover, the underlying ideology that supports the legal recognition of persons who have transitioned from one gender to another remains governed by a heteronormative binary (often also expressed in reproductive norms) and a deep anxiety about disturbing this structure.

National laws reveal most clearly the threads of this underlying ideology. The persistence of filiation and marriage as core social institutions is underscored by the constructive requirement of *sterilization* in many national laws on transexuality. A person desirous of changing sex must render themselves unable to procreate, even as European regional and national law grows to accept same-sex couples and adoption. For example, Sweden's law, the first legal framework on transsexualism enacted in 1972 (Lag om faststallande av konstillhorighet, 1972), simultaneously advances and restricts its subjects, as conditions for certification of the new identity, to two requirements: The person must be unmarried and *unable to procreate*. Surgery is not a requirement but may be authorized (Patti & Will, 1981; Lore & Martini, 1986; Fabeni, 2002).

The most interesting legal framework on transsexualism is found in the German *Transsexuallengesetz* (Gesetz uber die Anderung der Vornamen und die Feststellung der Geschlechtszugehorigkeit in besonderen Fallen-Transsexuellengesetz, 1980). The so-called Transsexual Act, more than any other national law, responds to the individual's desire to express his or her gender identity (Fabeni, 2000). It provides two options, which may be applied either successively or independently of each other.

The first option is the *kleine Lösung* or "minor solution," according to which the judge may authorize a change of name for an applicant who, for 3 years, does not feel that she/he belongs to her/his biologic sex. This solution does not require surgical intervention and can be reversed on the applicant's request. However, the decision of the judge is annulled *if the applicant becomes a parent* after the decision is taken.

In the second option, the so-called major solution in German law, after surgical intervention the judge may authorize gender reassignment and changing the legal sex. The act also requires that the applicant is *not married* and is *not able to procreate*. Although the procedure for a change of name, or "minor solution," seems to be an optimal way to give full recognition to gender identity. Still, as Sciancalepore and Stanzione (2002) note, the German law remains within the binary system of genders.

The Dutch framework is based on the German one: according to article 29 of the Dutch Civil Code, gender reassignment is possible provided the person cannot procreate, and a change of name is possible separately and at an earlier stage without surgical reassignment (Fabeni, 2000). Thus, national solutions oscillate within a male/female paradigm tightly bound to nontransferable capacities of procreation (for both solutions) and marriage (for the major solution). Moreover, because irreversible surgical intervention—including sterilization—is required to obtain the change of legal sex, full recognition of gender identity is conditioned on "forcible surgery(ies)" (Patti & Will, 1981).

Italian national law and policy reveals another aspect of the construction of dichotomous gender in the conceptual framework on transsexualism: an anxiety about nonconforming bodies (bodies with specific gender identity and conforming sexual characteristics—in Italian *caratteri sessuali*) and the anxiety about having the wrong bodies as parents. Italian law (Italy Legge n. 164, 1982) established that the gender reassignment (change of legal sex and name on civil status records and papers) is disposed of by a decision of the Tribunal aided by experts verifying the psychophysical conditions of the individual. In principle, the gender reassignment would be possible without surgical intervention (Patti & Will, 1981). However, because the law sets out that the change of legal name and sex shall be provided if *sexual characteristics* have been modified, courts have had to interpret what is meant by the words "sexual characteristics": genitals or secondary sexual characters. Italian courts have unanimously chosen the most restrictive interpretation, considering only genitals as sexual characteristics, and therefore *surgery is always a requirement* (Sciancalepore & Stanzione, 2002). Even more tellingly about what truly counts as sexual characteristics most linked to gender identity: In cases of female-to-male transition, *sterilization* is sufficient; in the case of male-to-female transition, modification of primary sexual characteristics (i.e., external male genitals) is required (Sciancalepore & Stanzione, 2002).[3]

Ironically, although in practice the Italian situation appears to be one of the most reductively coercive, a 1985 decision of Constitutional Court no. 161 of 1985 opened the way to another understanding of fundamental *rights to gender identity*. Acknowledging the "contrast between psychological and biologic sex" in transsexual persons, it admitted that the 1982 law, by its terms, accepts a new concept of sexual identity based not only on a person's sexual/physiological attributes but also on psychological and social factors. The Constitutional Court thereby conceived of "sex as a complex feature of an individual's personality, determined by a set of factors; those factors must be balanced

---

[3]In a few isolated cases, the change of legal sex and name has been authorized even without surgical intervention, generally because of the health conditions of the patient.

in order to find and give priority to the dominant factor" (Decision no. 161, 1985). In this context, it recognized a broad notion of the "right to health" under the Constitution, including not only physical health but also mental well-being and health. Thus, any changes to one's body, if made with a view to ensuring mental well-being, are perfectly legal. Furthermore, the Court stated that the affirmation of one's sexual identity is an inviolable right of the individual, in pursuance of article 2 of the Constitution, because it allows transsexual persons the full development of their personality, both intimately and psychologically, and in their relationships with others.

How do we understand sterilization and surgery as a condition for exercising a right? The right to gender expression becomes the "right to have the opposite gender identity" and thus the right to transition from one gender to another. Sterilization erases a biologic capacity and thus eradicates a social right (reproduction) of the person; surgery acts to build a new appropriately sexed gender. In this, gender identity becomes the resexualization of bodies (Sharpe, 2002). Is this the right to gender identity that is being developed in Europe at a national level and that after *Goodwin* constitutes the minimum core standard for the 44 European countries? Is the right to gender identity in Europe a highly conditioned entitlement trapped in the apparently immutable paradigm of dichotomous male/female genders?

Here the contradictory use of the notion of health is made visible. On the one hand, the content of the right to health evolved to support transition to a new identity, with personal development as the achievement of psychological and "social" health. On the other hand, the regulatory use of health law—health services conditioned on choosing either/or; health experts as gate-keepers, benefits limited to those fitting within social norms—enforces the binary model of genders and reduces the idea of fundamental right to gender identity to a narrow field. Following the *Goodwin* case, the British Parliament approved the Gender Recognition Act 2004, according to which the person who has had gender dysphoria (certified by medical evidence), has lived in the new gender for at least 2 years, and intends to continue to live in the acquired gender for the rest of his or her life may obtain a gender recognition certificate, whose consequence is complete acquisition of the new gender, with the full range of marital and parenting rights (Conway, 2004). It is not clear how in practice the requirements will be interpreted (by doctors? by courts?), but for the first time a law allows transition without requiring surgery or the inability to procreate. This seems to be a real step toward recognition of a right to (trans)gender identity.

The problematic relationship between law and health (and health practices) with regard to gender identity is also evident in the case of persons born "intersex" where "gender attribution is essentially genital attribution" (Kessler & McKenna, 2000). More precisely, gender identity has been attributed according to the presence or absence of a penis. There is no room for "ambiguity." The experiences of intersexed persons in modern medical history reveals that even when biology/"nature" is not dichotomous social norms require that the person be classified according to dichotomous genders. Health practices and policies are required to contribute to this definition (Karzakis, 2005). The fact that the law requires determining the sex of the infant together with the (social) expectations of the parents has often been the excuse for early interventions on intersex children's genitals. Advocates for intersex persons are increasingly calling such interventions premature. Although often done out of motives of concern and protection, to the advocates, nonetheless, they are a human rights abuse (Human Rights Commission of the City and County of San Francisco, 2005). We are in a highly tentative stage of rights recognition for intersex persons' rights to self-determination, but it is perhaps necessarily still a partial self-determination: One cannot claim the right to be without a clear, exclusive male or female identity and still be human in most modern social contexts (Cabral, 2005).

Health professionals therefore *play a key role* in the legal context for transgender and often intersex persons: They are the ones who "diagnose" gender dysphoria or genital nonconformity; and they then ordain and carry out the psychological, endocrinologic, surgical paths of the transgender or intersex person. Awareness of the complexity of the sociolegal construction would allow them to act in the best interest of the person and might be a strategic tool to stimulate legal reforms that broaden the reach of sexual and gender rights. Health practice in this case mediates between national legislation and the enjoyment of rights. In transgender cases, health professionals would engage with principles deemed as rights in the European Court. With the emerging claims of intersex, new arguments navigate regional and international instruments but with only a few rules.

Health practice in this case is thus also part of the answer to the question: Is the right to health a point of celebration of the fundamental value of identities, or is health the regulatory instrument producing only certain identities? What mix of autonomy, nondiscrimination, the right to form a family, or the right to privacy among others will result in the fairest application of the rules?

3.3 When There Is No Safe Site for Sexual Rights Claiming: At the Intersection of Health, Gender, Sexuality, Age, and Class in Modern India

Examining the kaleidoscopic debates and challenges to a set of laws in the Indian Penal Code that penalize "bad sex" (the rape law and the "unnatural offenses" act, IPC Sec. 375, 376, and 377, respectively) reveals the way that sexuality's regulation by law is often configured in ways that frustrate broader rights claims unless advocates unpack the range of interests and ideologies that operate through the law.

In this case, health-oriented groups, gay identity groups, queer sexualities groups, women's groups, and child rights groups have formed and dissolved alliances and amended tactics in more than a decade's worth of attempts to reform sex and gender crime aspects of the Indian Penal Code. The struggle in India at time of this writing is unresolved. Thus, like all the law/rights/sex debates we present in this chapter, we only partially capture the many issues in the register of rights, law, and history, especially linkages to colonial and postcolonial politics (Kapur, 2002; Sukthankar, 2002).

Many commentators on the challenge to Sec. 377 ("unnatural offenses" law) draw attention to the complex engagements of local advocates vis-à-vis locally and globally defined meanings implicated in sex law reform, including concerns over law reform in isolation of social movement support (Katyal, 2004; Narrain, 2005). We, however, follow the lead of other commentators who draw on the efforts to reform the rape law and the position of children (Sec. 375/376) to press the point of how laws regulating sex often simultaneously patrol the boundaries of heterosexuality as they create the deviance of "homosexuality" and constrain acceptable gender roles simultaneously (Sukthankar, 2002; Ghosh, 1999). Paying attention to this multidirectional aspect of the law's border-patrolling function is key to understanding the complexity of reforming law regarding sex, as the reform has variously pitted queer, child rights, and women's rights advocates if not against each other then not closely allied.

Criminal law performs its border-drawing function through its paradoxical capacity to protect sexual rights for some (remedying sexual harms, as in protecting persons from coerced sexual activity) while violating sexual rights for others (through penalizing same-sex sexual activity or sex outside marriage). Differently situated groups in every country are in varied positions to command the law's protection versus being subject to its penalties for their sexual action (e.g., women seeking the right to assert the power to say yes or no in marriage, persons seeking the right to say yes to same-sex activity, children/child rights activists seeking rights for those under 18 years of age to have a say in how or when their bodies are used sexually) (Kapur, 2002; Sukthankar, 2002; Miller, 2004). Modern Indian (currently, Hindu–Right-wing driven) politics have successfully converted the sex and gender ideologies still embodied in the Code, drawn up by British Colonial rulers, into norms of gender modesty and appropriate (hetero)sexuality for contemporary Indian society (Narrain, 2004). The modern crime of rape in Section 376 is gender and procreative act-specific: vaginal intercourse forced upon a woman by a man not her husband (Indian Penal Code, 1860). Because of the gender/penetration limits of the law, when child rights advocates seek prosecution of persons suspected of sexual abuse of boys or nonpenile/vaginal abuse of girls/women, they turn to Section 377, which criminalizes "whoever voluntarily has carnal intercourse against the order of nature with any man, woman or animal shall be punished . . . penetration is sufficient to constitute the carnal intercourse necessary" (Indian Penal Code, 1860).

Thus, when advocates (operating variously from health/prevention of HIV/AIDS, gay identity, or nondiscrimination on sexual behavior rubrics) have sought to remove Section 377, they have confronted the argument that it is necessary to "protect boys and women." Although Section 377 has rarely been used to prosecute consensual adult sex between men (Katyal, 2004; Narrain, 2004) its existence has been used to justify various rights-violation practices. For example, the National

Human Rights Commission, in the face of HIV/AIDS groups' petitions, considered its unchallenged existence a reason to uphold the prohibition on condom distribution in Indian prisons (Narrain, 2004), as well as for preventing interventions focusing on men who have sex with men (People's Union for Civil Liberties Karnataka, 2003). Conversely, gay, self-identified sexual and gender minority groups, and health-oriented groups (mostly HIV/AIDS-associated) have agreed that the existence of Section 377 provides the authorizing backdrop against which blackmail, police harassment, and abuse and torture, as well as community and family abuse, is justified (Katyal, 2004; Narrain, 2004).

Advocates during the late 1990s deployed concerns for "health" in legal challenges, specifically calling for judicial reinterpretation of Section 377 in light of evidence of criminality proving to be a barrier to effective outreach efforts aimed at men having sex with men in the context of the increasing rates of HIV/AIDS in India. As Narrain (2004) and Sukthankar (2002) noted, however, this health-oriented effort proved impossible to maintain in light of a vicious police raid of two AIDS outreach and education groups in 2001 in Luknow. The men who have sex with men (MSM) outreach/health-and-harm reduction model had been crafted to fly underneath the radar of law enforcement and avoid the contemporary, politicized, exclusionary struggle over authentic Indian identities (Sukthankar, 2002; Narrain, 2004). After the raid, however, in local authorities' speeches and the media, the outreach and safer-sex materials were depicted as pornographic, and the workers were depicted as purveyors of porn or gay predators. Troublingly, some gay identity groups maintained a prolonged (now broken) silence over the arrests and abuses against the outreach workers, revealing other fault lines in addition to those discussed above. In addition to the gender/sex and age issues raised above, a multiplicity of practices of male–male eroticism arises across urban and rural areas and different regions of India, as poor, working class, and middle class men arrange their sexual and erotic lives differently across heterosexual marriages and community structure; and they are affected in radically different ways by the police powers of surveillance, bribery, and abuse tied to the crimes noted in Section 377 (Katyal, 2004).

Ironically, the raids in Lucknow and the government's response to the legal challenge to Section 377 have, Narrain (2004) notes, had the effect of a public alchemy. They have resulted in the conversion of advocates' initial MSM/health approach into promotion of a gay identity claim. This process has intensified in the glare of global conversations using gay-identity terms and has resulted in being pulled and pushed into national debates by supporters and detractors. Here, the law of Section 377 becomes a tool producing a new gay—and, in contradistinction, a new heterosexual—Indian identity; but these new gay identities are simultaneously produced and condemned by opponents of sexual diversity, a process that has been documented in other nationalizing debates in eastern Europe and southern Africa (Human Rights Watch and the International Gay and Lesbian Human Rights Commission, 1998, 2003).

Thus, health approaches to divergent sexualities have some purchase in gaining rights; but at the same time, in head-on encounters with criminal law, health as the basis of sexual rights absent additional claims may not have sufficient capacity to resist a dominant ideology intent on excluding and stigmatizing the perverse as unhealthy. A recent, more multivalent campaign in India called Voices Against 377 is striving to keep the sexuality, gender, age, caste, class, and health regulatory issues in view. This movement runs concurrent with the legal challenge to Section 377 (still at times criticized for moving too quickly and arguing with terms that were either "too gay" or not gay enough in the Indian context). While waiting for a judgment, Voices seeks to build coalitions across child rights, women's rights, and gay identified, queer-identified, nonidentified but marginalized communities (Voices against Section 377, 2004). Yet this advocacy still struggles with the triangulation of the law: If Section 377 is struck down (in contrast to being "read down," or reduced, in its reach only to consensual sex in privacy) and other aspects of the Indian Penal Code are left intact, there would be no remedy for rape of boys available in the law. Conversely, because women's groups are divided on the virtues of a gender-neutral rape (and also because a proposed reform failed to reform the marital rape exception), there is no movement on reforming the section of the law that might make it possible to prosecute equally the rape of men and women, boys and girls, regardless of orientation, gender identity, or marital status (Indian Penal Code, 1860; Sukthankar, 2002).

Engagement with the law through a legal petition on "unnatural offenses" has forced a certain politics of sexual rights to the sur face. Rooted in a movement based on rights principles of participation, nondiscrimination, and the conditions for realizing rights, the expanded campaign could become a vehicle to challenge repressive, regulatory ideologies in the broader structures of power and injustice.

3.4 Reflecting on Health as a Site for Claiming Justice

Countries with strong public health care systems would seem to be good models for the more equitable use and distribution of resources. However, our European case study revealed that although such a system may enable social inclusion through access to state-driven interventions and services it may also exclude because of its strong potential for tracking services along social (and sexual) hierarchies. Entitlement to certain rights can be subjected to close patroling, as when access to reproductive health technologies (e.g., fertilization techniques) can be controlled according to dominant ideologies of the good reproductive citizen. For example, Article 5 of the Italian Act on medically assisted insemination (Act No. 40, 2004) perpetuates inequality through providing services conditioned on a heterosexual marital model: Neither individuals nor same-sex couples can undergo the procedures. Lesbians are doubly excluded.

Finally, although global access to resources may not always be visible as an issue for sexuality, resources not only condition the realization of rights but economic development may drive a focus on health, as in the case of developing countries. The tensions in this discussion are evident: Is sexuality accepted as only "one of the key elements of human capital" and a "means to a productive life" by its service to social development through good health as determined by dominant social norms, as in the India case?

4 Conclusion: Imperilled Rights, New Rights Defenders

4.1 Sex as Geopolitics: How Does the Current Global Struggle over the Meaning of Human Rights and Health Link to Sexuality?

Health has been put at the center of global security, as when the U.N. Security Council convened a special session on HIV/AIDS as a threat to global security or as a precondition as well as a goal of development (UN Secretary General, 2004). *Sexual rights*, in the guise of a highly visible and fought-over draft resolution on nondiscrimination on sexual orientation at the U.N. Commission on Human Rights (Obanda, 2004; Phan, 2004), as well as an aspect of the right to health, has occasioned impassioned speeches by diplomats, roll call votes at the Commission, and letter writing campaigns from the Christian right wing at the international level. Thus, sexuality, health, and human rights have been politicized in new and hypervisible ways globally at the same time that movements to support diverse rights claiming struggle locally with disparate issues, resources, and strategies.

The United States increasingly seeks to turn back the positive international developments in sexual rights and the right to health (Williamson, 2004). Despite the fact that there is a limited right in the United States to engage in consensual, noncommercial sexual behavior outside marriage without penalty and the right to determine if and when sexual activity becomes reproductive, the United States currently advocates internationally with a goal of ensuring that no comparable or greater sexual rights be established elsewhere. In this globalization of the U.S. administration's domestic political/cultural struggle over sexual rights, the United States has joined unusual, issue-specific, powerful North–South alliances. In regard to sexual rights (and a panoply of reproductive rights), the United States works in tandem with the Holy See, a quasi-state player in the United Nations (Butler, 2003; Obanda, 2004; Saiz, 2004) and the Organization of the Islamic Conference (OIC). Although both the Holy See and the OIC are critical of the United States on other issues, each has muted its differences in service of their headline allegiance against expanding sexual rights (Obanda, 2004; Saiz, 2004; Saurbrey, 2004).

Sexual rights, like all human rights, have developed in a complex dynamic between national, regional, and international struggles; between court decisions (law) and diplomatic posturing; between the reasoned enunciation of principles and the manifestos of policies. Understanding sexual rights requires a lens capable of capturing the multivariate intersection of domestic, regional, and international forces and interests (Wilson, 2002; Miller, 2004; Obanda, 2004; Saiz, 2004). Local contestations over diverse sexuality and gender challenges often emerge in debates over national identity, sovereignty, and citizenship in nations buffeted by internal and international pressures. As an example, banners in Warsaw at a political rally against European Union accession hosted by the populist Catholic radio show "Radio Maria" in 2003, read (translated): "No to the EU: No Jews, No Masons, and No Sodomites." Displacing attention from economic crises and anxiety over modernization through crusades on behalf of authentic, pure national subjects—and thus against changing generational, gender, or sexual practices (Heng & Devan, 1997; Chanock, 2000)—is a common move.

If one understands the term globalization at its most general sense— "the stretching, deepening, and speeding up of global interconnectedness, i.e., the multiplicity of networks, flows, transactions and relations which transcend states" (McGrew, 1998)—it is clear that globalization operates in ways that challenge many of the traditional claims (however incompletely filled) of the contemporary state system. At the same time, other aspects of globalization offer opportunities for transnational organizing and solidarity. Thus, we arrive at some final paradoxes for rights as a tool for health actors. Human rights both needs a state and threatens forms of that state; health operates transnationally through globalization, and globalization itself threatens the state. Yet health is a fundamental right. We are thus talking about claiming a right that requires attention to the local and the global, even as our work may seem resolutely local (this body, this clinic, this community, this national law on nondiscrimination in health services).

4.2 Health Systems as Sites of Inclusion or Exclusion

Health systems can be seen as sites of citizenship affirmation at its most embodied—for all persons but especially for those of diverse sexuality and gender expression. Yet equality and adequacy of health care for any individual as a point of justice are sustainable only if we understand and support the steps needed for more just and accessible health systems for all (Freedman et al., 2005). If we conceive of health systems as relational, as "a vital part of the social fabric of any society," we see advocacy in health systems as among the tools of citizenship in society (Freedman et al., 2005). This framing reinforces the idea behind using human rights claims as a possible tool for sexually excluded persons in the context of health.

However, it also highlights that removal of the state from its legitimate role in monitoring and responding to the ways in which persons are included in or excluded from quality health care is one of the results of the dominant market-driven approaches to health care. Building accountability—formally through the law and informally through collective action among persons most affected, across differently gendered, racialized, or otherwise marginalized persons and groups— emerges as a key function of rights-based approaches in health. Such action reframes people as "citizens" in the broadest sense because rights-worthy persons are included, and it is also "how to create a system that encourages, supports, and sustains increasing inclusion, that is redistribution" (Freedman et al., 2005).

4.3 Concluding Thoughts

This chapter has tried to demonstrate the crucial role of health practitioners and policy makers in the conversation focused on rights in the context of sexual health and the health of gender and sexually non-conforming individuals. It seems to us that such a discussion is not possible without "troubling" the notions themselves of the law, sexuality, and health precisely because of their lack of uniform meaning and the complicated forms of interaction among those three "basic" elements.

We have tried to underline in our analysis the different, sometimes contradictory levels on which the legal discourse operates: as a regulatory tool and as a tool of principle. In regard to sexuality principles, both international and national systems have been moving slowly in two essential frameworks for the protection of nonnormative sexualities: within the broad notion of a right to health and as a specific discussion on sexual rights. On the other hand, in the field of law as legislative and regulatory processes, the protection of such rights for nonconforming sexualities is complicated by the "physiologic" limits of the law itself (so long as legal categories do not match with personal identities) and by the "pathologic" restrictive interpretations or applications of the law. The enforcement of legislative provisions by themselves often clash with the idea of rights, a state of well-being, and evolving protection of nonnormative sexuality.

The role of health practitioners and policy makers seems to us of great relevance in both of these domains. The daily practice of health care provision (and the consequent negotiation around rights claims and rights denials) as well as the elaboration of health policies by practitioners and policy makers should make them as the *trait d'union* between the various discourses of the law. This should configure a "triangular" situation in which practitioners and policy makers can make use of the discourse on rights and principles in the most appropriate way to broaden the interpretation of legal rules and the implementation of health practices and policies in the local and national context within the structure of the law itself. This, we argue, better responds to the needs of rights protection of sexual- and gender-nonconforming identities.

In this sense, to better mediate (and ameliorate) the negative impact of administrative regimes in health requires dismantling the rigid conceptions of two mutually constituting binaries: one built around an axis of male-female identity and one built around a heterosexual-homosexual split. For this purpose, Feinberg's depiction (Feinberg, 2001) of contemporary medical professionals refusing treatment to transgender people constitutes the tip of an iceberg of health-undermining and rights undercutting practices and policies derived from ignorance and/or animus toward a population whose gender defies traditional (and often legal) norms. Other examples of "category errors" linked to simplistic understanding of identity include the failure of health professionals to identify HIV/AIDS in women's bodies during the early stages of the epidemic in the United States (they could only "see" AIDS in male bodies) as well as the failures to address the spread of HIV in men who have sex with men but do not identify themselves as gay (Gilson & Thomas, 2003). Also, health practice operates within regulatory and administrative provisions that work through a system of rigid categorization that may frustrate the principles of justice. In Italy, for instance, a computer-based system of national health care service automatically excludes postoperative (legally) female transsexuals from reimbursable prostate tests, as the tests are considered sex-specific. How can such as system facilitate the well-being of marginalized persons?

This engagement of health practitioners' and policy makers' roles would be particularly valuable for a second reason: Specifically to consider implementing the law in terms of the critical difference between *prevention* and *remedy*. Making use of legal rules and interpreting them in a way that is favorable to sexually different people at the level of health practices and policies may be useful as a *remedial approach*. This approach, though, often limited to individual cases, is self-limiting, as it does not deal with the more general questions of troubling or changing the structural causes of stigmatization, sexual hierarchies, and exclusion. For this reason, health practitioners and policy makers should take seriously a different perspective of legal principles: seeing them as a way to implement a *preventive approach*. Attending to principles then becomes a foundation for avoiding violations of rights rather than "merely" providing remedies. Health practitioners and policy makers should look at principles as a source of ideas for developing preventive tools through the use of structure and power-aware policies and practices built on the bases of sexuality and sexual health. This fits with social history and public health histories of reform, identifying not just evidence but the causes of inequality (Oppenheimer et al., 2002). Of course, the preventive approach must take awareness of its limits, such as relying on multiple steps for implementation, a lack of effective and immediate remedies, and a need to build accountability for reform into the institutional structures.

Therefore, to develop *fair* health systems and policies, practitioners and policy makers should consider both the preventive and remedial approaches and the goals they serve to avoid engaging with the law as a tool of exclusion, as seen in the case studies. Understanding the interrelationships and the potentials arising from contemporary efforts to apply human rights to sexuality in the context of health demands a different concept of the framework of rights, sexuality, and health. More importantly, it requires an explicit understanding of the roles of the various intersectional kinds of power in meaning-making and ordering our societies, as well as around axes of difference in regard to race, citizenship, and nation and the structures of law and the market. We seek a form of inclusion that can transform the systems so they provide justice for all and are capable of incorporating discriminated-against groups into those systems.

We close, therefore, expressing the need for new coalitions and strategies to achieve health for all. We must modify our understanding of global health structures to move attention to sexual and gender identity as an instrument of value in our larger movement for social justice.

Acknowledgments: We thank Ilan Meyer for his dedicated help. We also are grateful for the wonderfully careful research assistance of Chrystal Stone and Jennifer Friedman.

References

Act No. 40 (2004) Italy: Legge n. 40. Norme in material di procreazione medicalmente assistita (February 19, 2004).

An-Na'im, A. (1995) Toward a cross-cultural approach to defining international standards of human rights: the meaning of cruel, inhuman or degrading treatment of punishment. In: An-Na'im, A. (ed), *Human rights in cross-cultural perspective: a quest for consensus.* University of Pennsylvania Press, Philadelphia, pp. 19–43.

An-Na'im, A.A. (2004) Islam and international law: toward a positive mutual engagement to realize shared ideals. In: *ASIL: Proceedings of the 98th Annual Meeting,* pp. 159–168.

B. v. France (1992) Case no. 13343/87, European Court of Human Rights.

Badrinath, S. (2005) Learning for life: sex education in India and the social construction of sexuality. Unpublished manuscript.

Barrett, S. (2004) Summary of remarks. Paper presented at the 98th annual meeting of the American Society of International Law.

Butler, J. (1993) Imitation and gender insubordination. In: Abelove, H. Barale, M.A., and Halperin, D.M. (eds) *The lesbian and gay studies reader.* Routledge, New York.

Butler, J. (2003) "New sheriff in town": the Christian right nears major victory at the United Nations. *Public Eye Magazine* 16(2).

Cabral, M.I. (2005) Organizing around transgender and inter-sex issues in Latin America: the social and political meaning for gender, sex and concepts of justice. Program for the Study of Sexuality, Gender, Health, and Human Rights, Columbia University, Mailman School of Public Health, New York (May 10, 2005).

Chanock, M. (2000) "Culture" and human rights: orientalising, occidentalising, and authenticity. In: Mamdani, M. (ed) *Beyond rights and culture talk.* St. Martin's Press, New York, pp. 15–36.

Chapman, A.R. (1995) Monitoring women's right to health under the international covenant on economic, social and cultural rights. *American University Law Review* 44(4):1157–1176.

Chapman, A.R. (1998) Conceptualizing the right to health: a violations approach. *Tennessee Law Review* 65:389–418.

Committee on Economic Social and Cultural Rights. (2000) *Concluding Comments, E/C.12/1/Add.49.*

Committee on the Elimination of all forms of Discrimination against Women. (1999) *Concluding observations, A/54/38, August 20.*

Committee on the Rights of the Child. (2000) Concluding observations of the Committee on the Rights of the Child: United Kingdom, CRC/C/15/ Add.134, paras 22 and 23.

Committee on the Rights of the Child. (2003a) *General comment no. 3: HIV/AIDS and the rights of the child, CRC/GC/2003/3.*

Committee on the Rights of the Child. (2003b) *General comment no. 4: adolescent health and development in the context of the Convention on the Rights of the Child,* CRC/GC/2003/4.

Conway, H.L. (2004) In practice—the Gender Recognition Bill—a turning point. *Family Law Journal* 34(140).

Cossey v. United Kingdom (1990) Case no.10843/84, European Court of Human Rights.

Costa Rica Ley General Sobre el VIH-SIDA (1998) No. 7771, de 28 abril de 1998.

Crenshaw, K. (1991) Mapping the margins: intersectionality, identity politics and violence against women of color. *Stanford Law Review* 43(6).

Decision no. 161 (1985) Corte Costituzionale, Italy.

Fabeni, S. (2000) *Nota all'applicazione degli artt. 158ss. Ord. St. Civ. ai casi di trans-essualismo.* http://www.cgil.it/org.diritti/transex/parere%20.htm.

Fabeni, S. (2002) *The rights of transsexual and transgender persons: the Italian legal framework and new national and European challenges.* Paper presented at the Workers Out! 2nd World Conference of Lesbian and Gay Trade Unionists, Sydney, Australia.

Farmer, P. (1999) Pathologies of power: rethinking health and human rights. *American Journal of Public Health* 89(10).

Feinberg, L. (2001) Trans health crisis: for us it's life or death. *American Journal of Public Health* 91(6):897–900.

Freedman, L. (1995a) Censorship and manipulation of reproductive health information: an issue of human rights and women's health. In: Coliver, S. (ed) *The right to know: human rights and access to reproductive health information.* University of Pennsylvania Press, Philadelphia.

Freedman, L. (1995b) Reflections on emerging frameworks of health and human rights. *Health and Human Rights* 1:314–349.

Freedman, L.P., Waldman, R.J., de Pinho, H., and Wirth, M.E. (2005) *Who's got the power? Transforming health systems for women and children. Final Report of the UN Millennium Project Task Force on Child Health and Maternal Health.* United Nations Development Programme, New York.

Fried, S., and Landsberg-Lewis, I. (2000) Sexual rights: an emerging concept in women's human rights. In: Askin, K.D. and Koenig, D.M. (eds) *Women and international human rights law.* Transnational, Ardsley.

Gesetz uber die Anderung der Vornamen und die Feststellung der Geschlecht-szugehorigkeit in besonderen Fallen-Transsexuellengesetz (1980) TSG BGB1, I, 1654.

Ghosh, S. (1999) The troubled existence of sex and sexuality: feminists engage with censorship. In: Brosius, C. and Butcher, M. (eds) *Image journeys: audio visual media and cultural change in India.* Sage, Delhi.

Gilson, L. (2003) Trust and development of health care as a social institution. *Social Science and Medicine* 56:1453–1468.

Gilson, L., and Thomas, S. (2003) Introduction: intervening in the public/private mix: the strategy of policy action. In: Söderlund, N., Mendoza-Arana, P., and Goudge, J. (eds) *The new public/private mix in health: exploring the changing landscape.* Alliance for Health Policy and Systems Research, Geneva.

Gonzalez, E. (2000) The right to health. In: *Circle of rights: economic, social and cultural rights activism: a training resource.* https://www1.umn.edu/human-rts/edumat/IHRIP/circle/modules/module14.htm.

Goodwin v. United Kingdom. (2002) Case no. 29857/95 European Court of Human Rights.

Hendriks, A. (1995) Promotion and protection of women's right to sexual and reproductive health under international law: the economic covenant and the women's convention. *American University Law Review* 44(4):1123–1144.

Heng, G., and Devan, J. (1997) State fatherhood: the politics of nationalism, sexuality and race in Singapore. In: Lancaster, R.N., and di Leonardo, M. (eds) *The gender/sexuality reader: culture, history, political economy*. Routledge, New York, pp. 107–121.

Hobbes, T. (1950) *Leviathan*. Dutton, New York.

Human Rights Commission of the City and County of San Francisco. (2005) *A human rights investigation into the medical "normalization" of intersex people*. http://www.sfgov.org/site/sfhumanrights_index.asp.

Human Rights Committee. (1992) *Toonen v. Australia, CCPR/C/50/D/488/1992*.

Human Rights Committee. (1994) General comment no. 24. General comment on issues relating to reservations made upon ratification or accession to the covenant or the optional protocols thereto, or in relation to declarations under article 41 of the Covenant.

Human Rights Committee. (1999) *Juliet Joslin et al. v. New Zealand*. Communication no. 902/1999. New Zealand, CCPR/C/75/D/902/1999.

Human Rights Committee. (2000) *Young v. Australia*. Communication no. 941/2000. Australia, CCPR/C/78/D/941/2000.

Human Rights Committee. (2002) Concluding observations: Egypt, CCPR/CO/76/EGY.

Human Rights Watch and the International Gay and Lesbian Human Rights Commission. (1998) *Public scandals: sexual orientation and criminal law in Romania*.

Human Rights Watch and the International Gay and Lesbian Human Rights Commission. (2003) *More than a name: state-sponsored homophobia and its consequences in southern Africa*.

I. v. United Kingdom (2002) Case no. 25680/94, European Court of Human Rights.

Indian Penal Code (1860) Act no. 45, 375, 376, 377.

International Covenant on Civil and Political Rights (1966) G.A. res. 2200A (XXI).

International Covenant on Economic Social and Cultural rights. (1966) GA Res. 2200A (XXI), UN G.A.O.R., Supp (No.16) 49, UN Doc. A (6316).

Italy: Legge n. 164, (1982) Norme in materia di rettificazione di attribuzione di sesso (April 14, 1982).

Kapur, R. (2002) The tragedy of victimization rhetoric: resurrecting the "native". Subject in international/post-colonial feminist legal politics. *Harvard Human Rights Journal* 15:1–37.

Karzakis, K. (2005) Science, sexuality, and human rights. Program for the Study of Sexuality, Gender, Health, and Human Rights, Columbia University, Mailman School of Public Health, New York (February 16, 2005).

Katyal, S. (2004) Exporting identity. *The Dukeminier Awards* 2(1):173–252.

Kessler, S., and McKenna, W. (2000) Who put the "trans" in transgender? Gender theory and everyday life. *The International Journal of Transgenderism* 4(3).

Kinney, E. (2001) The international human right to health: what does this mean for our nation and world? *Indiana Law Review* 34(4):1457–1476.

Kleinman, A., and Kleinman, J. (1997) The appeal of experience, the dismay of images: the cultural appropriation of suffering in our times. *Daedalus* 25(1).

Lag om faststallande av konstillhorighet (1972).

Lewin, S., and Meyer, I. (2002) Torture and ill-treatment based on sexual identity: the roles and responsibilities of health professionals and their institutions. *Health and Human Rights* 6:161–176.

Limburg Principles on the implementation of the international covenant on economic, social, and cultural rights. (1987) *Human Rights Quarterly* 9(2):122–135.

Littell, A. (2002) Can a constitutional right to health guarantee universal health care coverage or improved health outcomes? A survey of selected states. *Connecticut Law Review* 35(1):289–318.

Long, S. (2004) When doctors torture: the anus and the state in Egypt and beyond. *Health and Human Rights* 7(2):114–141.

Long, S. (2005) Personal communication to Alice Miller and Margaret Satterthwaite, May 3, 2005, on file with author.

Lorber, J. (1994) *The paradoxes of gender*. Yale University Press, New Haven.

Lore, C., and Martini, P. (1986) *Aspetti e problemi medico-legali del transessualismo*. Giuffre', Milan.

Maastricht guidelines on violations of economic, social, and cultural rights. (1998) *Human Rights Quarterly* 20(3):691–704.

Mackintosh, M. (2001) Do health care systems contribute to inequalities? In: Leon, D.A., and Walt, G. (eds) *Poverty, inequality and health: an international perspective*. Oxford University Press, Oxford.

Mann, J.M., Gruskin, S., Grodin, M., and Annas, G. (eds) (1999) *Health and human rights: a reader*. Routledge, New York.

McGrew, A. (1998) Human rights in a global age: coming to terms with globalization. In: Evans, T. (ed) *Human rights 50 years on: a reappraisal*. Manchester University Press, New York, pp. 188–210.

Meier, B.M. (2004) International criminal prosecution of physicians: a critique of Professors Annas and Grodin's proposed international medical tribunal. *American Journal of Law and Medicine* 30(4):419–452.

Meyer, I. (2001) Why lesbian, gay, bisexual, and transgender public health? *American Journal of Public Health* 91(6):856–858.

Miller, A. (2000) Sexual but not reproductive: exploring the junction and disjunction of sexual and reproductive rights. *Health and Human Rights: An International Journal* 4(2):68–109.

Miller, A. (2001) Uneasy promises; sexuality, health and human rights. *American Journal of Public Health* 91(6):861–864.

Miller, A. (2004) Sexuality, violence against women, and human rights: women make demands and ladies get protection. *Health and Human Rights* 7(2):16–47.

Miller, A., and Vance, C. (2004) Sexuality, human rights, and health. *Health and Human Rights* 7(2):5–15.

Narrain, A. (2001) Human rights and sexual minorities: global and local contexts. *Law Social Justice and Human Development* 2.

Narrain, A. (2004) The articulation of rights around sexuality and health: subaltern queer cultures in India in the era of Hindutva. *Health and Human Rights* 7(2):142–164.

Narrain, A. (2005) Presentation at the Sexuality & Rights Institute, Pune, India.

Obanda, A.E. (2004) *Sexual rights and the Commission on Human Rights*. http://www.whrnet.org/docs/issue-sexualrightscommission.html.

Oppenheimer, G., Bayer, R., and Colgrove, J. (2002) Health and human rights: old wine in new bottles? *The Journal of Law Medicine and Ethics* 30(4):522–532.

Patti, S., and Will, M. (1981) La giurisprudenza italiana e . . . l'Europa (a proposito delle rettificazioni nei registri dello stato civile). *Diritto di famiglia e delle persone* 422.

People's Union for Civil Liberties Karnataka. (2003) *Human rights violations against the transgender community: a study of kothi and hijra sex workers in Bangalore, India.* PUCL-K, Bangalore.

Phan, K. (2004) UN rejects sexual orientation as human rights. *Christian Today* (April 2, 2004).

Platform for Action of the Fourth World Conference on Women. (1995) UN Doc.A/CONF.177/20, para 96.

Rees v. United Kingdom, (1986) Case no. 9532/81, European Court of Human Rights.

Rigaux, F. (1998) Les transsexuels devant la cour europeenne des droits de l'homme: une suite d'occasions manquees. *Revue Trimestrielle des Droits de l'Homme* 33.

Rothschild, C. (2004) Not your average sex story: critical issues in recent reporting on human rights and sexuality. *Health and Human Rights* 7(2):165–178.

Rubin, G. (1984) Thinking sex: notes for a radical theory of the politics of sexuality. In: Vance, C.S. (ed) *Pleasure and danger: exploring female sexuality.* Routledge, Boston, pp. 267–319.

Saiz, I. (2004) Bracketing sexuality: human rights and sexual orientation—a decade of development and denial at the UN. *Health and Human Rights* 7(2):48–81.

Saunders, P. (2004) Prohibiting sex work projects, restricting women's rights: the international impact of the 2003 US Global AIDS Act. *Health and Human Rights* 7(2):179–192.

Saurbrey, E. (2004) US Representative to the UN Commission on the Status of Women. Remarks to the World Congress of Families III, Mexico City.

Scarry, E. (1985) *The body in pain.* Oxford University Press, New York.

Sciancalepore, P., and Stanzione, P. (2002) *Transessualismo e tutela della persona.* IPSOA, Milano.

Sen, G. (2005) Presentation at the Sexuality & Rights Institute, Pune, India.

Shakespeare, T. (2000) Disabled sexuality: toward rights and recognition. *Sexuality and Disability* 18(3):159–166.

Shakespeare, T., Davies, D., and Gillepsie-Sells, K. (1996) *The sexual politics of disability.* Casell, London.

Sharpe, A. (2002) *Transgender jurisprudence: dysphoric bodies of law.* Cavendish Publishing, London.

Sheffield & Horsham v. United Kingdom. (1998) Case no. 22985/93 and 22390/94, European Court of Human Rights.

Smith, R., Beaglehole, R., Woodward, D., and Drager, N. (eds). (2003) *Global public goods for health: health, economic, and public health perspectives.* Oxford University Press, New York.

South Africa Aged Persons Amendment Act (1998) No. 19514.

South Africa Medical Schemes Act (1998) No.131.

Special Rapporteur of the Commission on Human Rights. (2001) Report on the question of torture and other cruel inhuman or degrading treatment or punishment. UN Document A/56/156.

Special Rapporteur on the Right to Health. (2004) Report to the Secretary General of the United Nations on the right of everyone to the enjoyment of the highest attainable standard of physical and mental health, E/CN.4/2004/49/Add.1.

Sukthankar, A. (2002) The dangers of dignity and the hazards of health: sexuality, law and the language of reform in India. Unpublished manuscript.

Universal Declaration of Human Rights. (1948) G.A. res.217A (III), UN Doc A/810.

UN Secretary General. (2004) *A more secure world: our shared responsibility, a report of the high-level panel on threats, challenges, and change.* United Nations, New York.

Vance, C.S. (1999) Anthropology rediscovers sexuality: a theoretical comment. In: Parker, R., and Aggleton, P. (eds) *Culture, society and sexuality: a reader.* UCL Press, Philadelphia, pp. 39–54.

Van Oosterwijck v. Belgium. (1980) Case no. 7654/76, European Court of Human Rights.

Voices against Section 377. (2004) *Rights for all: ending discrimination under Section 377.* Voices against Section 377, New Delhi.

Williamson, R.S. (2004) Statement by the US Representative to the Commission on Human Rights, March 30, 2004.

Wilson, A. (2002) The transnational geography of sexual rights. In: Petro, P. (ed) *Truth claims: representation and human rights.* Rutgers University Press, New Brunswick, NJ, pp. 253–267.

X, Y, and Z v. the United Kingdom. (1997) Case no. 21830/93, European Court of Human Rights.

Yamin, A.E. (2002) Challenges and possibilities for the innovative praxis in health and human rights: reflections from Peru. *Health and Human Rights* 6:35–64.

6

Ethical, Legal, Social, and Political Implications of Scientific Research on Sexual Orientation

Edward Stein

1 Introduction

Scientific research on the causes of sexual orientation has captured the attention of many Americans. Some researchers, citing evidence from neuroscience, genetics, and psychology, claim that sexual orientation is either inborn or fixed at an early age. Many lesbians, gay men, bisexuals, and their allies have welcomed this claim, finding in it confirmation of their sense that they did not choose to be attracted to people of the same sex. Some parents of lesbians and gay men have also found solace in such research, finding in it assurance that nothing they did made their children homosexual. Furthermore, some lawyers, activists, politicians, religious leaders, scientists, and psychologists have tried to parlay this research into good news for lesbian and gay rights. Their main argument, which I call the "born that way" argument, goes as follows: If sexual orientations are innate, genetic, firmly rooted in biology, and/or not chosen, it is wrong to criminalize the sexual behavior of lesbians, gay men, and bisexuals, to discriminate against them, and to withhold from them benefits that heterosexuals take for granted. This argument has intuitive appeal and is deployed with increasing frequency.

This chapter concerns the social, political, legal, ethical, bioethical, and pragmatic implications of the thesis that sexual orientations are inborn or not chosen. Specifically, this chapter argues that the "born that way" argument is deeply problematic: It provides little political traction, its empirical premises are weak, and most importantly it is ethically impotent. Although I briefly discuss the empirical bases for the "born that way" argument, this chapter is not primarily concerned with the truth of scientific claims about how sexual orientations develop in humans. (For such discussions, see Byne, this volume, and Stein, 1999).

Since the later part of the nineteenth century, scientists, physicians, and mental health specialists have been interested in how people develop sexual orientations. When pursuing this interest, such researchers have typically studied gay men, occasionally studied lesbians, to an even lesser extent studied bisexuals, and to an even lesser extent studied heterosexuals. Researchers have entertained a vast range of theories to explain the differences among people's sexual orientations (Robinson, 1989; Irvine, 1990; Bullough, 1994; Minton, 2002). Until recently, a central goal of this research program was to cure or eliminate what were seen as sexual perversions. Most theories of how sexual orientations develop were articulated hand-in-hand with attempts to cure homosexuality. These attempts to cure homosexuality included hormonal injection, genital manipulation, brain surgery, hypnosis, and shock therapy (Katz, 1992, pp. 129–407). Most current research on sexual orientation is no longer motivated by a desire to cure a perceived illness. Rather, an explicit goal of such research often is to improve the legal and social landscape for lesbians, gay men, bisexuals, and transgendered people (Bailey & Pillard, 1991; Hamer & Copeland, 1994; LeVay, 1996). My conclusion is that this well intentioned goal is misguided.

This chapter proceeds as follows. After explaining the "born that way" argument in greater detail, I offer various criticisms of it. In particular, I discuss empirical, ethical, legal, bioethical, political, and pragmatic problems for this argument. I conclude that the "born that way" argument is both impotent and problematic. Although there are various reasons for doing research on sexual orientation, the reasons must be balanced against concerns about the social, political, and legal impact of such research.

2 The "Born That Way" Argument

Every version of the "born that way" argument for lesbian and gay rights begins with some sort of empirical premise—either the biological or genetic claim that sexual orientations are innate or the psychological claim that sexual orientations are immutable, that is, that they cannot be changed. The crucial step for all versions of the "born that way" argument is a bridge claim linking the empirical premise to the desired legal or ethical conclusion. Consider the following version of the "born that way" argument:

1. Sexual orientations are innate or immutable.
2. Therefore gay people do not choose their sexual orientations.
3. It is wrong to punish people or otherwise discriminate against them for something they did not choose.
4. Therefore it is wrong to punish or otherwise discriminate against gay people.

In this version of the "born that way" argument, the bridge claim is claim 3. Some simpler versions of the "born that way" argument go from a premise such as claim 1 directly to a conclusion such as claim 4. In such simpler versions of the "born that way" argument, the bridge claim is implicit in the direct inference from claim 1 to claim 4.

3 Empirical Problems

Although the empirical problems with this argument are not the main focus of this chapter, I briefly survey the empirical concerns about the "born that way" argument. First, it is far from established that sexual orientations are innate or inborn (Byne, this volume). Most current scientific research on sexual orientation faces serious methodological objections and is based on a set of unjustified assumptions about sexual orientations generally and sexual attraction to people of the same sex in particular. For example, such research typically assumes that in some biological way gay men are like women and that lesbians are like men (Stein, 1999).

Second, that a characteristic is "not chosen" does not necessarily entail that it is biologically determined. The fact that we do not choose our native language does not mean that it is innate even though the *capacity for learning* human language is innate (Pinker, 1994). Furthermore, at least some characteristics that are socially acquired are nonetheless immutable. Sexual orientations do not need to be biologically determined to be immutable. They could be impervious to change even if they are caused by social experiences (Stein, 1999, ch. 9). Moreover, biological evidence is not needed to demonstrate that a person's sexual orientation is resistant to change. Psychological research has clearly demonstrated that "reorientation therapies," that is, therapies to "convert" homosexuals to heterosexuality, are ineffective. Few, if any, of even the most highly motivated individuals have been able to change their sexual orientations despite subjecting themselves to dehumanizing aversion therapies or investing tremendous emotional and financial resources in years of more conventional psychotherapy (Haldeman, 1991, 1994; Silverstein, 1991). Spitzer (2003) claimed to show that some highly motivated gay and bisexual men could "become" heterosexual, but numerous commentators have raised serious objections to Spitzer's methodology and conclusions (Drescher & Zucker, 2006).

Third, although it is clear that people do not choose their sexual orientations in the way that they, for example, choose how to vote in an election, it is not clear that choices play no role in the development of sexual orientations. Various scholars have argued that, especially among women, choices do indeed play a significant role in the development of sexual orientations (Card, 1995; Whisman, 1996). Others have distinguished a direct choice, that is, choosing to X with the conscious intention of doing X (for example, when I flip the light switch up to turn on the light, I made a direct choice to turn on the light), from an indirect choice, that is, choosing to do something that has the effect of doing X but without having the conscious intention of doing X (for example, when I flip the light switch up and, as a result, blow a fuse and cause the entire building to lose power, I made an indirect choice to turn off the lights in the entire building). A person's sexual orientation clearly is not the result of a direct choice to have that sexual orientation; however, having a particular sexual orientation could well be the result of some other choice, or in other words, an indirect choice (Stein, 1999, ch. 9).

For these and other reasons (Byne, this volume; Stein, 1999), the empirical premises of the "born that way" argument—that lesbians, gay men, and bisexuals are born with their sexual orientations or that sexual orientations are immutable—are at best dubious.

4 Moral and Ethical Problems

The strength of its empirical premises aside, the "born that way" argument faces serious moral and ethical objections. The most important of these objections is that even if sexual orientation is innate and/or not a choice, much of what is ethically relevant about being a lesbian or a gay man is not innate and not determined; thus, these aspects of homosexuality would not be reached by the "born that way" argument. Even if sexual orientations are genetically based, actually *engaging* in sexual acts with a person of the same sex, publicly or privately *identifying* as a bisexual, a lesbian, or a gay man, and deciding to *establish* a household with a person of the same sex are *choices*—choices that one might not make, that is, one can decide to be celibate, closeted, and companion-less. On any plausible view of human nature, deciding to do these things goes beyond the characteristics with which one is born. To put the point another way, someone who was convinced that lesbians and gay men deserve rights only because sexual orientations are innate or immutable could consistently accept that people can be treated differently on the basis of choices relating to their sexual orientation. One who thinks that gay men and lesbians are born with their sexual orientations might, because of the "born that way" argument, accept that gay men and lesbians should not be discriminated against on the basis of their sexual attraction to people of the same sex. They could still, however, hold the view that people who engage in sexual acts with people of the same sex *are* appropriate targets of discrimination and that people who have their primary domestic relationship with a person of the same sex should not get recognition for their relationships.

Consider, for example, the attitudes of some religious conservatives toward homosexuality. Such people claim that *being homosexual*—desiring sex with people of the same sex—is not a sin, is not immoral, and does not warrant prejudice, discrimination, or differential treatment. The very same people claim that acting on this desire by engaging in sex with someone of the same sex, having a romantic relationship with a person of the same sex, or advocating homosexuality are morally problematic. This view of homosexuality—which is surely *not* compatible with any robust version of lesbian and gay rights—is quite compatible with the "born that way" argument. The "born that way" argument has the potential to protect a person from being discriminated on the basis of having a desire to have sex with people of the same sex, but this is a highly specific, quite limited protection.

Even assuming that sexual orientations are inborn and immutable, lesbians and gay men deserve protection against discrimination and recognition for their relationships and institutions with respect to their *actions* and *decisions* rather than for their mere orientations. Lesbians, gay men, and bisexuals need their rights protected precisely when they engage in same-sex sexual acts, when they identify as bisexuals, gay men, and lesbians, and when they create lesbian and gay families. The "born that way" argument is unable to deliver these basic ethical needs. Simply, this argument cannot provide support for claims related to rights based on choices even if these choices are related to desires that are innate (Stein, 2002b, responding to Nussbaum, 2002).

This problem with the "born that way" argument can be seen, for example, as part of the contentious issue of whether lesbians and gay men can openly serve in the U.S. Armed Forces. Under existing law (10 U.S.C. § 654) and the Department of Defense directives that implement it—together known as the "Don't Ask, Don't Tell" policy—a service member may be discharged from the Armed Forces for stating that "he or she is homosexual or bisexual," for holding hands or engaging in any other bodily contact with a person of the same sex that "demonstrates a propensity or intent to engage in sexual contact," or for "attempt[ing] to marry a person known to be of the same biological sex." Even though this policy, charitably interpreted, protects lesbians and gay men from being discriminated against for their *sexual desires*, a service member can be discharged for any public expression of homosexuality, any evidence of romantic or sexual relationships with people of the same sex, and any form of remotely intimate physical contact with people of the same sex. The "Don't Ask, Don't Tell" policy, as implemented and enforced, fails to protect lesbians and gay men. Protecting service members against discharge on the basis of the mere having of a nonheterosexual sexual orientation—and in practice, that this policy fails to provide even this limited protection (Servicemembers Legal Defense Network, 2004)—in no way prevents adverse treatment or discharge due to any behavior that might be even remotely related to such sexual orientations (Halley, 1999). The situation for lesbians and gay men in the military under the "Don't Ask, Don't Tell" policy exemplifies the sort of laws that are likely to be implemented in the face of the "born that way" argument.

Even if sexual orientations are inborn, lesbians, gay men, and bisexuals require protection and deserve recognition in virtue of their decisions and behaviors, not just their desires. Choices are clearly involved when people participate in sexual behavior, when they publicly acknowledge their homosexuality, and when they build their primary emotional and familial relationships with people of the same sex. Lesbian and gay rights concern protecting people who decide to engage in same-sex sexual acts, to identify as gay men and lesbians, and to create gay families. No plausible scientific theory can justify the ethical conclusion that such decisions demand legal and social protection. Proof that sexual orientations are genetically determined or not chosen would not preclude legislating against all conscious expressions of homosexuality. The "born that way" argument cannot bridge the gap between its empirical premises (even granting they are true) and its desired ethical conclusions.

5 Legal Problems

Another way of construing the "born that way" argument is as a legal argument rather than as an ethical one. Some ethical wrongs are not illegal (for example, it may be wrong to not keep a promise to a friend, but in most cases it is not illegal), and some legal rules are not primarily justified by ethical considerations (for example, the legal rule that a plaintiff must provide sufficient evidence to get to trial is not primarily justified by ethical principles). Even if the "born that way" argument fails as an ethical argument, it might succeed as a legal argument. In other words, it might not be ethically wrong to discriminate on the basis of sexual orientation in virtue of the (alleged) innateness of sexual orientation, but there might be legal problems with such discrimination in virtue of the origins of sexual orientation.

Although the "born that way" argument can be made in various jurisdictions (Wintemute, 1995), I focus on the United States. A primary source of civil rights in the United States is the Equal Protection Clause of the Fourteenth Amendment of the U.S. Constitution, which says, "No State shall . . . deny to any person within its jurisdiction the equal protection of the laws." The Supreme Court has interpreted this clause as requiring great skepticism (in technical legal terms, as requiring *heightened* or *strict* judicial review) toward laws that make use of racial classifications (Slaughter House Cases, 1872), ethnic classifications (Yick Wo v. Hopkins, 1886), classifications concerning national origin (Hernandez v. Texas, 1954), legitimacy (Levy v. Louisiana, 1968), and sex (Mississippi University for Women v. Hogan, 1982).[1] Classifications toward which great skepticism is not required need only pass the much weaker "rational review" test, under which laws are held constitutional so long as there exists rational justification for the classifications they use. So, for example, there are rational reasons why a firefighter might be subject to certain height and weight restrictions; such body attributes constitute, in the context of firefighting, rational classifications and would thus survive rational review.

The Supreme Court has not directly ruled on the question of whether sexual-orientation classifications warrant heightened scrutiny. In the case of *Romer v. Evans* (1996), the Court held unconstitutional a Colorado state constitutional amendment that made use of sexual-orientation classifications. (Specifically, the amendment *precluded* state and local legislative, executive, and judicial actions protecting homosexual and bisexual orientation, conduct, practices, and relationships.) The Supreme Court found the Colorado amendment unconstitutional *without* invoking heightened scrutiny, finding that the classification at issue did not satisfy the very weak rational review test.

---

[1]More precisely, sex classifications, in contrast to race classifications, receive *intermediate* scrutiny rather than *strict* scrutiny. In *United States v. Virginia* (1996), the Supreme Court somewhat blurred the boundaries between strict and intermediate scrutiny, but *Nguyen v. INS* (2001) seems to show that there remains a distinction between strict and intermediate scrutiny.

Of those courts in the United States that have directly considered the question, most have held that sexual-orientation classifications do not received heightened review (Ben-Shalom v. Marsh, 1989; Thomasson v. Perry, 1996). Of the two most noteworthy exceptions—*Tanner v. Oregon Health Sciences University* (1998) and *Watkins v. United States Army* (1988)—only *Tanner*, in which an Oregon state court decided as a matter of state law that sexual orientations deserve heightened scrutiny, remains good law.

Advocates of the "born that way" argument in the United States legal context hope to argue successfully for heightened scrutiny for sexual-orientation classifications by focusing primarily on one of the factors that the Supreme Court has, in some contexts, considered when determining the level of scrutiny required to evaluate the constitutionality of a statute under the Equal Protection Clause. Generally, the Supreme Court has said it would consider whether a classification has historically been used to discriminate intentionally against a particular group (Frontiero v. Richardson 1973), whether the use of this classification is related to ability to contribute to society (Frontiero v. Richardson, 1973), whether any group demarcated by this classification lacks the political power to combat discrimination against it (City of Cleburne v. Cleburne Living Center, 1985), and whether any group demarcated by this classification exhibits obvious, immutable, or distinguishing characteristics that defines it as a discrete and insular group (Bowen v. Gilliard, 1987). Specifically, advocates of the "born that way" argument focus on the Supreme Court's occasional consideration of whether a characteristic is immutable as part of the determination of whether a classification warrants heightened scrutiny. The Supreme Court's interest in immutability is seen as creating an opening for the immutability of sexual orientations to be relevant to lesbian and gay rights (Green, 1987; Marcosson, 2001).

The importance of immutability when determining whether a classification is suspect, however, is unclear. The Supreme Court has, on some occasions, discussed heightened scrutiny without mentioning immutability (Massachusetts Board of Retirement v. Murgia, 1976; Plyler v. Doe, 1982; City of Cleburne v. Cleburne Living Center, 1985). Various legal scholars have persuasively argued that immutability is not and should not be important when determining whether a classification is suspect (Halley, 1994; Richards, 1994; Yoshino, 1998; Stein, 2002a). More specifically, as noted above in the discussion of *Romer v. Evans* (1996), when the Supreme Court has discussed lesbian and gay rights specifically, they have not discussed immutability at all.

The most recent Supreme Court case relating to sexual orientation did not consider immutability as a factor. In the landmark case of *Lawrence v. Texas* (2003), the Supreme Court held that a Texas sodomy law was unconstitutional because it violated the Due Process Clause of the Fourteenth Amendment. Of the six justices who held the Texas sodomy law unconstitutional, only Justice Sandra Day O'Connor held that the sodomy law violated the Equal Protection Clause. When reaching the conclusion that the Texas law made use of a classification that did not bear any rational relation to a legitimate state interest,

O'Connor, following the Court's approach in *Romer*, applied what she called a "more searching form of rational . . . review" but in so doing said nothing about immutability. The other five justices who found the Texas sodomy law unconstitutional did not join O'Conner's concurring opinion, but they did say that her equal protection analysis was "tenable." The upshot of *Lawrence v. Texas* for present purposes is that even when *Lawrence* is viewed through the lens of equal protection jurisprudence (as Justice O'Connor viewed it), it is not necessary to consider the immutability of sexual orientations to reach a decision about the rights of lesbians and gay men. This provides just one recent and salient example of a court ruling in favor of lesbian and gay rights without relying on whether lesbians and gay men are "born that way."[2]

Some legal scholars have suggested, in light of *Romer v. Evans* and *Lawrence v. Texas*, that the Supreme Court has dispensed with the traditional approach (sketched out above) to assessing whether laws violate equal protection (Goldberg, 2004). Even assuming the continued vitality of the heightened scrutiny versus rational review approach to equal protection, the role of immutability in determining the level of scrutiny to which a law is subject is, at best, uncertain. More specifically, in the context of sexual orientation, there is no reason to think that U.S. federal courts will ever look at immutability as a factor to determine whether the use of sexual-orientation classifications violates equal protection. The "born that way" argument provides little or no traction for lesbian and gay rights in the U.S. legal context.

6 Political and Pragmatic Problems

In the previous sections, I argued that the connection between scientific research on sexual orientation, on the one hand, and ethical and legal claims relating to the rights of lesbians and gay men, on the other, is weak at best. Some advocates of lesbian and gay rights, aware of problems with the "born that way" argument, claim that this argument should still be embraced because it persuades many people. This political and pragmatic strategy does not focus on the validity of the "born that way" argument but, instead, focuses on the extent to which it persuades people to support lesbian and gay rights. This pragmatic approach draws support from the various opinion polls showing that people who think homosexuality is biologically based or that sexual orientations are not chosen are more likely to favor lesbian and gay rights than those who do not (Aguero et al., 1984; Ernulf et al., 1989; Whitley, 1990; Piskur & Delegman, 1992; Button et al., 1997, p. 61; Wilcox & Wolpert, 2000).

Unfortunately, this pragmatic approach is not promising. Linking lesbian and gay rights to biology is a bad strategy even in the political context. To begin, there is historical evidence for doubting the efficacy

---

[2]For an interesting discussion of a case in which immutability arguments were made in federal court, see Keen and Goldberg (1998), discussing *Evans v. Romer* (1993).

of such an argument. In early twentieth century Germany, Magnus Hirschfeld attempted to gain legal protections for homosexuals on the grounds that they constituted a third biological sex. An early version of the "born that way" argument was a centerpiece of Hirschfeld's lobbying effort for lesbian and gay rights. It is, however, suggestive to note that his belief in a biological basis for sexual orientation led Hirshfeld to refer at least some homosexual men for surgery to reduce their "homosexual inclinations" (Herrn, 1995). Prior to his death, Hirshfeld conceded that not only had he failed to prove his biological thesis, but his use of the "born that way" argument unwittingly contributed to the persecution of homosexuals by stigmatizing them as biologically defective. He presumably had in mind the fact that in Nazi Germany lesbians, gay men, and other sexual minorities were imprisoned, castrated, mutilated in other ways, and sent to death camps to remove them from the breeding stock (Plant, 1986). The example of Nazi Germany shows how claims that sexual orientation is biologically based do not guarantee a positive result for lesbians and gay men.

More generally, arguments of this form have not proven politically effective. It is widely believed—despite significant evidence to the contrary (Lewontin et al., 1984; Appiah, 1996; Gould, 1996)—that race is a biologically category and is innate. The popularity of this belief has not, however, had a mitigating influence on racism.

Focusing more specifically on empirical evidence about the pragmatic effects of arguing that lesbians and gay men are "born that way," if such an argument were politically efficacious one would expect that advocates of lesbian and gay rights would make this argument in political contexts. An interesting study by Mucciaroni and Killian (2004) reviewed 10 legislative debates at various levels of government about issues relating the rights of lesbians, gay men, and bisexuals. They found that scientific research on sexual orientation had little or no impact on the debates. In fact, they found that opponents of lesbian and gay rights were slightly more likely to assert that sexual orientations are chosen *after* the publication of scientific research that was widely believed to suggest that sexual orientations are innate. That advocates of lesbian and gay rights do not make the "born that way" argument in political contexts suggests that the argument might not be as politically expedient as some think it is.

Even granting that the belief in a biological basis for homosexuality would persuade people to favor lesbian and gay rights in the short run, the belief that a characteristic is biologically based does not in anyway guarantee that people will view this characteristic in a positive light. Many characteristics that are coded for by genes (for example, Down's syndrome, Tay Sach's syndrome, and to some extent alcoholism) are viewed as undesirable, shameful, and so on. People might believe that sexual orientations are innate but still have negative views about homosexuality.

More generally, it is a risky strategy to link lesbian and gay rights to the ups and downs of scientific research, especially because such research is, at best, in its early stages. Biological research into sexual orientation has a poor track record when it comes to reliability; what appear to be valid results today could turn out to be mistaken (Byne, 1995). Making lesbian and gay rights contingent on a particular scientific finding is simply too risky. That people are persuaded by the "born that way" argument suggests a successful short-term public relations strategy, but it does not suggest a political strategy suited to grounding a set of rights that are deeply important and that profoundly affect the lives of many people.

As an example of the risks of connecting particular scientific and/or empirical theories with lesbian and gay politics, consider the relationship of the lesbian and gay movement in America to psychiatry (Bayer, 1987). In the "pre-Stonewall" stage of the gay rights movement (from World War II to the late 1960s), many lesbian and gay rights activists embraced psychiatry and its language, partly on political grounds. The idea was that psychiatry could help legitimate lesbians and gay men, their organizations, and their quest for acceptance and civil rights (D'Emilio, 1983, pp. 116–117). But as the gay movement grew, it began to question psychiatry, ultimately protesting against the American Psychiatric Association's classification of homosexuality as a psychological disorder. This example shows that science, medicine, and psychology are tricky ethical and political weapons; at best, they are double-edged swords.

Additionally, it is worth noting that the very terminology of the biologically theories may contribute to the stigmatization of homosexuality. In some neurological and psychiatric literature, these theories are often couched in pejorative terms such as hormonal abnormality, deficiency, aberration, and "gene-controlled disarrangement of psychosexual maturation patterns" (Sedgwick, 1990, pp. 40–44; Byne & Parsons, 1993). Traits that are perceived as both innate and undesirable are frequently assumed to be amenable to medical remedy or prevention. This might harm the cause of lesbian and gay rights more than it helps it.

There is another, more limited, pragmatic version of the "born that way" argument that warrants consideration. Some have argued that establishing that sexual orientations are innate or immutable would at least discourage psychiatrists, psychologists, and therapists from trying to "cure" homosexuality (Stein, 1993, 1998). Although I have argued that scientific research on sexual orientation is not relevant to legal, ethical, and political questions concerning sexual orientation, such research may have some impact (at least in the short term) on how the mental health profession views homosexuality. The strength of this impact can, however, easily be overemphasized. First, the distinction between sexual orientations and the choices related to them is again relevant. Even if a therapist is convinced that his patient cannot change her sexual orientation, he might encourage the patient to change her behaviors, her sexual and emotional relationships, and her public sexual identity. Second, even if a therapist does not try to cure a patient's homosexuality, he might still view homosexuality as less desirable than heterosexuality and/or continue to accept a variety of mistaken and potentially harmful stereotypes about lesbians and gay men. This could adversely affect the therapeutic goals set for lesbian and gay patients. Third, the impact of the "born that way" argument would be limited because those who think homosexuality is undesirable will, in the face of credible scientific research, simply switch their support away from psychological "conversion" therapies to medical or genetic therapies. Finally and most importantly, strong arguments against conversion therapy can be made independent of any biological evidence about the origins of sexual orientation. One can argue that there is no good reason to "convert" homosexuals by arguing that there is nothing morally wrong with homosexuality (Mohr, 1990; Ball, 2003). Some have argued that there are strong ethical arguments against trying to change the sexual orientation of an individual with the strong desire to do so. For example, Suppe (1984) argued that the availability of conversion therapies may have the effect of labeling homosexuality as an inferior condition, thereby increasing prejudice and discrimination toward lesbians and gay men.

The various versions of the pragmatic form of the "born that way" argument are quite problematic. Attempts to link scientific research on sexual orientation to the political case for lesbian and gay rights are misguided. In the next section, I build on this argument to show how this attempted linkage is dangerous.

7 Bioethical Problems

The "born that way" argument has a potential negative consequence that I mentioned briefly above to which I turn to now. Using the "born that way" argument, because it emphasizes the claim that sexual orientations are innate and immutable, increases the likelihood that people will use reproductive technologies to produce heterosexual children. This result of making the "born that way" argument has potentially deleterious effects on the situation of lesbians and gay men.

Suppose that it is widely believed that sexual orientations are genetic. If scientists isolate, as some claim to have done (Hamer et al., 1993; Hamer & Copeland, 1994) a particular gene sequence associated with homosexuality, it would be relatively easy to develop a technique to determine whether a fetus has genes that code for homosexuality. If prospective parents believe that the future sexual orientation of a fetus can be determined through a prenatal screening procedure, they might make use of such a procedure or in some other way try to prevent the birth of a fetus deemed to be "at risk" of becoming homosexual.

That parents would probably make use of techniques for selecting the sexual orientation of children, what I call *orientation-selection procedures*, is not implausible for two reasons. First, parents worldwide sometimes chose to abort a fetus if it is not of the *sex* they desire. Many prospective parents throughout the world have preferences with respect to the sex of their future children; many often have preferences for sons over daughters. The preference for sons can take various forms, including preferring to have one's firstborn child be a boy, preferring to having more sons than daughters, preferring to have only boys, or preferring to have only one child and for that child to be a boy. Son preference is stronger in some cultures than others. Even in countries such as the United States where the most common preference is for having two children, one of each sex, there is still a preference for sons in the form of a preference for having a son first (Warren, 1985, pp. 12–19; Raymond, 1993, pp. 21–25; Kolker & Burke, 1994, pp. 142–150).

Second, there is widespread prejudice and discrimination against lesbians, gay men, and bisexuals. Although it is difficult to compare attitudes toward women to attitudes toward sexual minorities, it does seem that if parents sometimes chose to abort a fetus that is not of the sex they desire, some parents would also make use of orientation-selection procedures to select for heterosexual children. For this reason and others, it seems quite likely that, if technology permits, prospective parents would seek abortions and use other procedures to prevent the birth of nonheterosexual children (Stein, 1998; 1999, ch. 11). Even supportive parents of lesbians, gay men, and bisexuals admit that they would have tried to ensure that their children would be heterosexual (Savin-Williams & Dube, 1998). For example, Louise Coburn, one-time program director of Parents and Friends of Lesbians and Gays, a group active in supporting parents of lesbians, gay men, and bisexuals and working for lesbian and gay rights, acknowledged that, in the face of homophobia and heterosexism in our society, no one would want their children to be gay because "[n]o parent would chose to have a child born with any factor that would make life difficult for him or her" (Gelman, 1992). On a similar note, Judge Richard Posner (1992, p. 308)—in a book sympathetic to some claims relating to lesbian and gay rights—confidently asserted that if there was a procedure that would ensure that a child would be heterosexual, "you can be sure that the child's parents would administer it to him, believing, probably correctly, that he would be better off." The point is that most people, particularly most heterosexuals and even some lesbians and gay men, have a strong preference for having heterosexual children. The "born that way" argument, by emphasizing the claim that sexual orientations are innate and not chosen, increases the likelihood that people will want to make use of orientation-selection procedures.

Because there is no strong evidence that sexual orientations are genetically determined (Byne, this volume; Stein, 1999), it seems unlikely that any orientation-selection procedures will be successful. Regardless of whether this is correct, there remain important bioethical questions surrounding such procedures because people might make use of them even if they did not work. This is partly because it will be difficult for people who are considering making use of orientation-selection procedures to determine whether such procedures work. Most children turn out to be heterosexual even without the use of such procedures. Because of this, many parents who attempt to select for the sexual orientation of a child will believe that their interventions have been successful even though their child would have been heterosexual without the use of orientation-selection procedures. Furthermore, most people take a while to come to grips with their sexual orientation. Parents who make use of an orientation-selection procedure might think their intervention has been successful only because their child has not yet figured out his or her sexual orientation. Also, because many lesbians, gay men, and bisexuals hide their sexual orientation even once they have figured it out, many parents will think that their attempt at orientation selection has worked when in fact it has not. If a lesbian, gay man, or bisexual knows that his or her parents used an orientation-selection procedure to ensure that he or she would be heterosexual, this would just increase the likelihood that a person would hide his or her sexual orientation from his or her parents. For these reasons, even if available orientation-selection procedures fail to work, such procedures will still *appear* to work.

That orientation-selection procedures will be used even if they do not work fits with a historical pattern of gay men and lesbians being subjected to various forms of medical and psychological interventions for which no evidence of effectiveness exists (Irvine, 1990; Haldeman, 1991, 1994; Silverstein, 1991; Murphy, 1992; Katz, 1992; Somerville, 1994). For example, gay men were injected with testosterone with the aim of turning them into heterosexuals despite studies showing no correlation between sexual orientation and testosterone levels (Meyer-Bahlburg, 1984).

The general point is that even if doubts about the evidence supporting the view that sexual orientations are innate or not chosen are well founded, people will almost certainly believe studies that support such a view anyway.[3] The result could be the widespread use of techniques to avoid the birth of children thought to be carrying genes for homosexuality or bisexuality.

Perhaps the most charitable explanation for strong preference for heterosexual children versus homosexual and bisexual ones is that parents, even those not completely intolerant of homosexuality, do not want their children to experience the disapprobation, discrimination, and violence faced by lesbians and gay men. This charitable interpretation does not, in many cases, ring true. Some people find homosexuality immoral, unnatural, and/or disgusting. These people are likely to make use of orientation-selection procedures if they are available because they dislike homosexuality, not simply to protect their children from social disapprobation. The claim that a parent is simply trying to protect a child from the wrath of society's prejudice often is a rationalization for homophobia and heterosexism; it is similar to a parent who reacts to a son or daughter who is dating (or marrying) a person of a different race by saying, "What will the neighbors think?" and "Just imagine how much trouble this will cause you (and your future

---

[3]Berke (1998) compared various opinion polls and found that the percentage of people who think that sexual orientation is something a person is born with has more than doubled between 1977 and 1998.

children)!" The relevant point is that behind the preferences for heterosexual children are various negative attitudes toward homosexuality. Even if parents desire heterosexual children because they do not want their children to face homophobia and heterosexism, what matters are the *effects* of making use of orientation-selection procedures. Regardless of whether orientation-selection procedures work, their availability, the acceptability of their use, and the knowledge that they are used shape attitudes toward lesbians, gay men, and bisexuals. Specifically, the emergence of orientation-selection procedures would likely reinforce the preference for heterosexual over homosexual children and encourage the view that homosexuals and bisexuals are diseased.

Until quite recently, most people viewed homosexuality as a disease. Although some people, among them some doctors and psychologists, still see homosexuality as a mental illness, there has been a shift away from this view. One indication of this shift was the American Psychiatric Association's 1973 decision to declassify homosexuality as a mental disorder (Bayer, 1987). The effects of such a shift from seeing homosexuality as a disease have been significant: Some of the stigma associated with homosexuality has lifted, and more lesbians and gay men have become comfortable and open about their sexual orientation. The availability and use of orientation-selection procedures would suggest that screening for homosexuality is a reasonable and sanctioned medical procedure; this could potentially tip the scales of public and professional opinion back toward seeing homosexuality as a physical or mental disorder. Furthermore, the availability and use of orientation-selection procedures would increase the pressure to hide one's homosexuality and decrease the collective power of lesbians and gay men. By strengthening the disease view of homosexuality and increasing pressure to keep one's homosexuality secret, the use of orientation-selection procedures to select against nonheterosexuals would likely engender and perpetuate attitudes that lesbians and gay men are undesirable and not valuable, policies that discriminate against lesbians and gay men, violence against lesbians and gay men, and the very conditions that give rise to the preference for heterosexuals rather than nonheterosexuals (Suppe, 1984; Stein, 1998, 1999). These are serious risks that demand careful ethical consideration. The availability of orientation-selection procedures poses a serious threat to lesbians, gay men, and bisexuals in a society that is generally unfriendly to lesbians and gay men and in which most people have a strong preference for heterosexual children.[4]

---

[4]Similar sorts of ethical problems arise if it is possible—or if people think that it is possible—to use psychological procedures to change the sexual orientation of a child after he or she is born. In fact, many parents currently attempt to use psychological treatments, religious counseling, and other procedures to change the sexual orientation of children they believe might not be heterosexual.

8 Conclusions

I have argued that the "born that way" argument for lesbian and gay rights faces several problems. To review, I have argued that its empirical premises are weak, that even if true its empirical premises cannot support its ethical conclusions, that the legal interpretation of the "born that way" argument is unlikely to have any traction, that this argument is very risky in the political realm, and, in particular, there are serious bioethical risks associated with trying to convince people to believe that sexual orientations are innate.

The question remains why lesbians and gay men, in contrast to other groups arguing for civil rights, should have to appeal to the "born that way" argument. The issues of innateness and immutability seem to be selectively applied to homosexuals and not to other marginalized groups. Members of religious minorities are not asked to demonstrate that either their religious affiliation or their religious practices are innate or immutable. Despite the fact that religious affiliation is not genetic and people can and do convert from one religion to another, most modern democracies protect religious liberty. In fact, it has been argued that the basic principles that underlie the U.S. Constitution's protection of religious liberty (namely, freedom of conscience, freedom of association, and the rights to free speech and free assembly) also provide a robust defense for lesbian and gay rights that is much stronger than the lack of choice argument possibly could (Richards, 1994; Stein, 1994).

My conclusion is not, however, that scientific research on sexual orientation should cease.[5] Rather, my two main conclusions are as follows. First, research on sexual orientation should be justified on its likely scientific merits, not on its perceived legal, ethical, or political benefits. Second, advocates of lesbian and gay rights should avoid making the "born that way" argument or any other argument based on a scientific theory of how sexual orientations develop because any theory of the origins of sexual orientation may be turned against lesbians and gay men. To be strong, arguments for the rights of gay men and lesbians should be cast in terms of justice, privacy, equality, and liberty. Arguments such as this are responsible for the legal strides that have been made in the quest for lesbian and gay rights (Romer v. Evans, 1996; Baker v. Vermont, 1999; Goodridge v. Department of Public Health, 2003; Lawrence v. Texas, 2003).

---

[5]This is a much more difficult claim to make, and it is one about which my own views have changed, as can be seen by comparing Stein, et al. (1997) and Schüklenk et al. (1997) with Stein (1999, ch 12).

References

Aguero, J.E., Bloch, L., and Byrne, D. (1984) The relationship among beliefs, attitudes, experience and homophobia. *Journal of Homosexuality* 10:95–107.

Appiah, K.A. (1996) Race, culture, identity: misunderstood connections. In: Appiah, K.A., and Guttman A. (eds) *Color conscious: the political morality of race*. Princeton University Press, Princeton, pp. 30–105.

Bailey, J.M., and Pillard, R.C. (1991) Are some people born gay? *New York Times* December 17, 1991, p. A19.

Baker v. Vermont (1999) 744 A.2d 864 (Vermont).

Ball, C.A. (2003) *The morality of gay rights*. Routledge, New York.

Bayer, R. (1987) *Homosexuality and American psychiatry*, 2nd ed. Princeton University Press, Princeton.

Ben-Shalom v. Marsh (1989) 881 F.2d 454 (7th Cir).

Berke, R. (1998) Chasing the polls on gay rights. *New York Times*, August 2, 1998. Week in Review, p. 3.

Bowen v. Gilliard (1987) 483 U.S. 587.

Bullough, V. (1994) *Science in the bedroom: a history of sex research*. Basic Books, New York.

Button, J.W., Rienzo, B.A., and Wald, K.D. (1997) *Private lives, public choices: battles over gay rights in American communities*. Congressional Quarterly, Washington, DC.

Byne, W. (1995) Science and belief: psychobiological research on sexual orientation. *Journal of Homosexuality* 28:303–344.

Byne, W., and Parsons, B. (1993) Human sexual orientation: the biologic theories reappraised. *Archives of General Psychiatry* 50:228–239.

Card, C. (1995) *Lesbian choices*. Columbia University Press, New York.

City of Cleburne v. Cleburne Living Center (1985) 473 U.S. 432.

D'Emilio, J. (1983) *Sexual politics, sexual communities: the making of a homosexual minority in the United States, 1940–1970*. University of Chicago Press, Chicago.

Drescher, J., and Zucker, K.J. (2006) *Ex-gay research: analyzing the Spitzer study and its relation to science, religion, politics, and culture*. Harrington Park Press, New York.

Ernulf, K., Innala, S., and Whitam, F. (1989) Biological explanation, psychological explanation and tolerance of homosexuals: a cross-national analysis of beliefs and attitudes. *Psychological Reports* 65:1003–1010.

Evans v. Romer (1993) No. Civ. A-92-CV-7223, 1993 WL 518586 (Colo. Dist. Ct. Dec. 14, 1993).

Frontiero v. Richardson (1973) 411 U.S. 677.

Gelman, D. (1992) Born or bred? *Newsweek*, February 24, pp. 46–53.

Goldberg, S. (2004) Equality without tiers. *Southern California Law Review* 77:481–582.

Goodridge v. Department of Public Health (2003) 798 N.E.2d 941 (Mass.).

Gould, S.J. (1996) *The mismeasure of man*, rev. ed. Norton, New York.

Green, R. (1987) The immutability of (homo)sexual orientation: behavioral science implications for a constitutional (legal) analysis. *Journal of Psychiatry and Law* 16:537–575.

Haldeman, D.C. (1991) Sexual orientation conversion therapy for gay men and lesbians: a scientific examination. In: Gonsiorek, J.C., and Weinrich, J. (eds) *Homosexuality: research implications for public policy*. Sage Publications, Newbury Park, CA, pp. 149–160.

Haldeman, D.C. (1994) The practice and ethics of sexual orientation conversion therapy. *Journal of Consulting and Clinical Psychology* 62:221–227.

Halley, J. (1994) Sexual orientation and the politics of biology: a critique of the new argument from immutability. *Stanford Law Review* 46:503–568.

Halley, J. (1999) *Don't: a reader's guide to the military's anti-gay policy*. Duke University Press, Durham, NC.

Hamer, D., and Copeland, P. (1994) *The science of desire: the search for the gay gene and the biology of behavior*. Simon & Schuster, New York.

Hamer, D., Hu, S., Magnuson, V., Hu, N., and Pattatucci, A. (1993) A linkage between DNA markers on the X chromosome and male sexual orientation. *Science* 261:321–327.

Hernandez v. Texas (1954) 347 U.S. 475.

Herrn, R. (1995) On the history of biological theories of homosexuality. *Journal of Homosexuality* 28:31–56.

Irvine, J. (1990) *Disorders of desire: sex and gender in modern sexology*. Temple University Press, Philadelphia.

Katz, J.N. (1992) *Gay American history: lesbians and gay men in the U.S.A.*, rev. ed. Meridian, New York.

Keen, L., and Goldberg, S. (1998) *Strangers to the law: gay people on trial*. University of Michigan Press, Ann Arbor.

Kolker, A., and Burke, B.M. (1994) *Prenatal testing: a sociological perspective*. Bergin & Garvey, Westport, CT.

Lawrence v. Texas (2003) 539 U.S. 558.

LeVay, S. (1996) *Queer science: the use and abuse of research into homosexuality*. MIT Press, Cambridge, MA.

Levy v. Louisiana (1968) 391 U.S. 68.

Lewontin, R.C., Kamin, L.J., and Rose, S. (1984) *Not in our genes: biology, ideology, and human nature*. Pantheon, New York.

Marcosson, S. (2001) Constructive immutability. *University of Pennsylvania Journal of Constitutional Law* 3:646–721.

Massachusetts Board of Retirement v. Murgia (1976) 427 U.S. 307.

Meyer-Bahlburg, H. (1984) Psychoendocrine research on sexual orientation: current status and future options. *Progress in Brain Research* 61:375–398.

Minton, H. (2002) *Departing from deviance: a history of homosexual rights and emancipatory science in America*. University of Chicago Press, Chicago.

Mississippi University for Women v. Hogan (1982) 458 U.S. 718.

Mohr, R. (1990) *Gays/justice: a study in society, ethics and law*. Columbia University Press, New York.

Mucciaroni, G., and Killian, M.L. (2004) Immutability, science, and the legislative debate over gay, lesbian and bisexual rights. *Journal of Homosexuality* 47:53–77.

Murphy, T. (1992) Redirecting sexual orientation: techniques and justifications. *Journal of Sex Research* 29:501–523.

Nguyen v. INS (2001) 533 U.S. 53.

Nussbaum, M.C. (2002) Millean liberty and sexual orientation: a discussion of Edward Stein's The Mismeasure of Desire. *Law and Philosophy* 21:317–334.

Pinker, S. (1994) *The language instinct: how the mind creates language*. Morrow, New York.

Piskur, J., and Delegman, D. (1992) Effect of reading a summary of research about biological bases of homosexual orientation on attitudes towards homosexuals. *Psychological Reports* 71:1219–1225.

Plant, R. (1986) *The pink triangle: the Nazi war against homosexuals*. Henry Holt, New York.

Plyler v. Doe (1982) 457 U.S. 202.

Posner, R. (1992) *Sex and reason*. Harvard University Press, Cambridge, MA.

Raymond, J. (1993) *Women as wombs: reproductive technologies and the battle over women's freedom.* Harper Collins, New York.

Richards, D. (1994) Sexual preference as a suspect (religious) classification: an alternative perspective on the unconstitutionality of anti lesbian/gay initiatives. *Ohio State Law Journal* 55:491–553.

Robinson, P. (1989) *The modernization of sex: Havelock Ellis, Alfred Kinsey, William Masters and Virginia Johnson.* Cornell University Press, New York.

Romer v. Evans (1996) 517 U.S. 620.

Savin-Williams, R., and Dube, E. (1998) Parental reactions to their child's disclosure of gay/lesbian identity. *Family Relations* 47:1–7.

Schüklenk, U., Stein, E.D., Kerin, J., and Byne, W. (1997) The ethics of genetic research on sexual orientation. *Hastings Center Report* 27:6–13.

Sedgwick, E.K. (1990) *Epistemology of the closet.* University of California Press, Berkeley.

Servicemembers Legal Defense Network (2004) Conduct unbecoming: the tenth annual report on "Don't Ask, Don't Tell, Don't Pursue, Don't Harass." http://www.sldn.org/binary-data/SLDN_ARTICLES/pdf_file/2063.pdf.

Silverstein, C. (1991) Psychological and medical treatments of homosexuality. In: Gonsiorek, J.C., and Weinrich, J. (eds) *Homosexuality: research implications for public policy.* Sage Publications, Newbury Park, CA, pp. 101–114.

Slaughter House Cases (1872) 83 U.S. 36.

Somerville, S. (1994) Scientific racism and the emergence of the homosexual body. *Journal of the History of Sexuality* 5:243–266.

Spitzer, R.L. (2003) Can some gay men and lesbians change their sexual orientation? 200 participants reporting a change from homosexual to heterosexual orientation. *Archives of Sexual Behavior* 32:403–417.

Stein, E.D. (1993) Evidence for queer genes: an interview with Richard Pillard. *GLQ: A Journal of Lesbian and Gay Studies* 1:93–110.

Stein, E.D. (1994) The relevance of scientific research concerning sexual orientation to lesbian and gay rights. *Journal of Homosexuality* 27:269–308.

Stein, E.D. (1998) Choosing the sexual orientation of children. *Bioethics* 12:1–24.

Stein, E.D. (1999) *The mismeasure of desire: the science, theory and ethics of sexual orientation.* Oxford University Press, New York.

Stein, E.D. (2002a) Law, sexual orientation and gender. In: Coleman, J., and Shapiro, S. (eds) *Handbook of jurisprudence and legal philosophy.* Oxford University Press, Oxford, pp. 990–1039.

Stein, E.D. (2002b) Reply to Martha Nussbaum and Ian Hacking. *Law and Philosophy* 21:349–353.

Stein, E.D., Schüklenk, U., and Kerin, J. (1997) Scientific research on sexual orientation. In: Chadwick, R. (ed) *Encyclopedia of applied ethics*, Vol. 4. Academic Press, San Diego, pp. 101–108.

Suppe, F. (1984) Curing homosexuality. In: Baker, R., and Elliston, F. (eds) *Philosophy and sex*, rev. ed. Prometheus, Buffalo, N.Y., pp. 391–420.

Tanner v. Oregon Health Sciences University (1998) 971 P.2d 435 (Ore. App.), *review denied* 994 P.2d 129 (Ore. 1999).

Thomasson v. Perry (1996) 80 F.3d 915 (4th Cir.) (en banc).

United States v. Virginia (1996) 518 U.S. 515.

Warren, M.A. (1985) *Gendercide: the implications of sex research.* Rowman & Allenheld, Totowa, N.J.

Watkins v. United States Army (1988) 847 F.2d 1329 (9th Cir.), *vacated and affirmed on other grounds* 875 F.2d 699 (9th Cir. 1989) (en banc).

Whisman, V. (1996) *Queer by choice: lesbians, gay men and the politics of identity.* Routledge, New York.

Whitley, B.E. (1990) The relationship of heterosexuals' attributions for the causes of homosexuality to attitudes towards lesbians and gay men. *Personality and Social Psychology Bulletin* 16:369–377.

Wilcox, C., and Wolpert, R. (2000) Gay rights in the public sphere: public opinion on lesbian and gay equality. In: Rimmerman, C.A., Wald, K.A., and Wilcox, C. (eds) *The politics of gay rights*. University of Chicago Press, Chicago, pp. 409–432.

Wintemute, R. (1995) *Sexual orientation and human rights: the United States Constitution, the European Convention, and the Canadian Charter*. Oxford University Press, Oxford.

Yick Wo v. Hopkins (1886) 118 U.S. 356.

Yoshino, K. (1998) Assimilationist bias in equal protection: the visibility presumption and the case of "Don't Ask, Don't Tell." *Yale Law Journal* 108:485–571.

Targeting the State: Risks, Benefits, and Strategic Dilemmas of Recent LGBT Health Advocacy

Steven Epstein

1 Introduction

During the 1990s in the United States, lesbian, gay, bisexual, and trans-gender (LGBT) health advocates undertook a significant strategic experiment that was fraught with some peril: They turned to the state in an attempt to institutionalize a broad-based health agenda. What I call here "state-centered" LGBT health politics involves concerted efforts by activists and researchers to make demands on the state for inclusion and incorporation—demands to institutionalize LGBT (or, more often, just lesbian and gay) health as a formal concern of public health and health research bureaucracies. At the crux of state-centered advocacy is the claim that lesbians, gay men, bisexuals, and transgen-dered persons have distinctive health concerns and would benefit from research that finds them, counts them, studies them, and compares them with others. Thus the state-centered approach takes fixed cate-gories of sexual identity as the foundation of a health promotion and biomedical research strategy. Although state-centered politics has been conducted in relation to the federal, state, and local government levels in the United States, I emphasize what I take to be the most significant recent target: the U.S. Department of Health and Human Services (DHHS) and its key, health-related component agencies, such as the National Institutes of Health (NIH).

State-centered LGBT health advocacy has not been without success. There have been a number of milestones: the publication in 1999, with DHHS funding, of a landmark report (Solarz 1999) on lesbian health by the influential Institute of Medicine of the National Academy of Sci-ences; the inclusion of some discussion of sexual orientation in *Healthy People 2010*, a key federal health policy document; establishment at the DHHS of an Interagency Steering Committee on Health Disparities Related to Sexual Orientation that, among other things, bruited the issue of whether the DHHS should establish an Office of Lesbian and Gay Health; and the release by the NIH in May 2001 of a "program announcement" calling for the submission of grant proposals for research on LGBT populations. The replacement of Bill Clinton's administration by that of George W. Bush in 2000 mostly put a halt to this forward march. Yet in many respects the Bush administration's hostility toward gay rights and sexual freedoms has served only to heighten tensions built into the state-centered approach from the very outset.

Indeed, my claim is that the rise of state-centered LGBT health politics raises crucial questions about the politics of sexuality, health, identity, and belonging. When addressing these questions, I believe it is important to note the very real, practical benefits to LGBT people that may accrue from pursuing this approach to health and health research. More generally, it is also necessary to underscore the potentially emancipatory role of science in advancing the interests of sexual liberation movements (Minton, 2002). At the same time, I maintain that certain tendencies associated with the state-centered paradigm pose significant risks for the health and well-being of LGBT communities. Specifically (and consistent with some of the recent critiques of the biomedicalization of sexuality offered by Terry (1999a,b) and Scarce (1999, 2000), I suggest that state-centered LGBT health politics tends toward the reification of sexual identities, the conflation of behavior and identity in the determination of health risks, the conceptualization of difference as pathology, the playing down of sexual topics and sidestepping of nonnormative sexual practices, and the valorization of professionals and simultaneous inhibition of community participation in research design and interpretation. Avoiding these risks does not necessarily presume abandoning the state-centered approach, but it does require a careful analysis of how these risks become manifested.

2 Histories

2.1 Trajectories of Reform

The rise of state-centered LGBT health advocacy presupposes a complicated set of historical developments, including two decades of preexisting activism, the details of which are too complex to recount here. These developments include the rise of lesbian and gay health advocacy during the 1970s; the advent of radical acquired immunodeficiency syndrome (AIDS) activism during the 1980s, which spotlighted federal health agencies such as the NIH, the Food and Drug Administration (FDA), and the Centers for Disease Control and Prevention (CDC); and the attention by lesbian activists to the issue of breast cancer (Deyton & Lear, 1988; Epstein, 1996, 1997, 2003b; Terry, 1999a; Wilcox, 2000). As activist attention turned to state agencies and "big science," a small pioneering group of academic researchers began seeking to fill in the vacuum of knowledge about lesbian and gay, particularly lesbian, health concerns (Stevens & Hall, 1991; Stevens, 1992; Mays & Cochran, 1993). Operating on shoestring budgets, researchers set out to survey the state of lesbian health and found that lesbians were "underserved . . . and at greater risk than heterosexual women for a variety of health problems" (Goldstein, 1997, p. 97; see also Bowen et al., 1997). The most well known such study, the National Lesbian Health Care Survey conducted by Caitlin Ryan and Judith Bradford during the early 1980s, gathered completed health questionnaires from 1925 women (Ryan & Bradford, 1988).

In response to the complex reshaping of gay and lesbian politics that resulted from the AIDS epidemic, and on the basis of evidence generated by academic researchers on lesbian and gay health, LGBT health activism during the 1990s took increasingly diverse forms. For example, lesbians began pushing the major national lesbian and gay rights organizations, such as the National Lesbian and Gay Task Force, to devote resources and energy to health politics (Radecic & Plumb, 1993; Denenberg, 1994). Lesbian activists became increasingly involved in the burgeoning breast cancer advocacy movement, which was enjoying remarkable success in increasing the federal funding for breast cancer research. Moreover, breast cancer itself was being framed as a lesbian issue. In 1992, Dr. Suzanne Haynes of the National Cancer Institute (one of the institutes that comprise the NIH) caused a stir by suggesting at a conference that lesbians were two to three times more likely than their heterosexual female counterparts to develop breast cancer based on their profile of risk factors, as suggested by studies (including having fewer children, drinking more, and being heavier) (Haynes interview). Reporters and activists who took up a statistic popular at the time that one of nine women would develop breast cancer in their lifetimes concluded that the lifetime risk for a lesbian was therefore one in three. As breast cancer became defined as a lesbian health emergency, many gay media outlets and advocacy groups found it strategic to balance their coverage of AIDS and breast cancer as a way of giving equal time to what were sometimes conceived of as "men's" and "women's" issues (Wilcox, 2000).

At the same time, as gay men began to perceive that new antiretroviral drug regimens held out the possibility of an extended life span for those who had access to the drugs, this sense of partial progress created the breathing space for some to focus on health issues *other than* human immunodeficiency virus (HIV)/AIDS. A new, grassroots gay men's health movement took shape in the late 1990s that drew on the lessons of previous gay and AIDS-related activism—the importance of defending sexual freedom, the refusal to defer to credentialed expertise—but sought a comprehensive approach to the health issues affecting gay men (Rofes, 1999, 2000; Scarce, 1999, 2000; Mayer, 2000). To promote a new vision of gay men's health, activist and writer Eric Rofes and other organizers convened a Gay Men's Health Summit that brought together more than 300 individuals in Boulder, Colorado during the summer of 1999 to discuss such topics as health promotion in cyberspace; anal sex, anorectal disorders, and sexually transmitted diseases (STDs); drug use at circuit parties; and domestic violence as a gay men's health issue. By the following year, attendance at the summit was up to 458 participants from 37 states plus Australia, Canada, and Switzerland, and several regional meetings on gay men's health were also held. In 2002, the summit was expanded into a broader "LGBTI Health Summit," with the expectation of alternating in future years between a specific focus on gay men and an inclusive focus on lesbians, gay men, bisexuals, transgenders, and intersexuals. As I suggest later, the grassroots character and "sex-positive" ideology of this new gay men's health movement place it some critical distance from emergent "state-centered" advocacy.

Other activists during this time period sought to reform medical institutions from within. During the early 1980s a group of California doctors asked the American Medical Association (AMA) if they could establish a gay caucus within the association. When the AMA refused to recognize such a caucus, the doctors formed a separate organization called the American Association of Physicians for Human Rights (Schneider & Levin 1999). In 1994 the organization renamed itself the Gay and Lesbian Medical Association (GLMA), and 2 years later the health concerns of bisexual and transgendered patients were formally added to GLMA's charge. By the late 1990s, GLMA had become a national organization of 2000 medical professionals. As I describe later, it has played a central role in state-centered LGBT health advocacy.

2.2 A Window of Opportunity

If the turn toward state-centered advocacy presupposed a whole history of health activism, it also took advantage of a unique space of political opportunity. Beginning in the 1980s and over the course of the 1990s, a diverse assortment of health advocates (including activists, researchers, health professionals, and state employees) complained that women, racial and ethnic minorities, children, and the elderly had been systematically underrepresented as subjects in federally funded clinical research and in new drug development in the United States. Decrying a "one size fits all" approach to medicine that was believed to take heterosexual, adult white men as the standard human, these actors insisted that health research institutions attend to the particularities of distinct identities. In response, new legislation and federal policies sought specifically to include these groups in research populations and to study differences across groups. Between 1986 and 2003, more than a dozen such policies were implemented by federal health agencies within the DHHS, including the NIH, the FDA, and the CDC. In my work studying these developments, I refer to these changes in ideas and practices as the consolidation of a new "biopolitical paradigm," which I call the "inclusion-and-difference paradigm" (Epstein 2003a,b, 2004, 2006b, 2007). The key point here is that once this new paradigm was cemented in place as a way for the DHHS to respond to what it terms "special populations," it then became easier for other disenfranchised constituencies, such as lesbians, gay men, bisexuals, and transgendered persons, to call for an extension of the paradigm to cover them as well.

However, throughout the 1980s and much of the 1990s, LGBT communities were not typically considered "special populations" covered under the rubric of the inclusion-and-difference paradigm. Substantial amounts of NIH funding went to grants that listed homosexuality as a primary or secondary focus; but as one analysis of funding patterns has revealed, most of these funds (totaling about $20 million a year on average from 1982 to 1992) were directed at the HIV epidemic, with only about $532,000 per year devoted to all other health issues affecting gay men and lesbians (Silvestre, 1999; Boehmer, 2002). During the 1990s, activists sought to change this. Having learned from AIDS and breast cancer activism that they could successfully transform biomedical research practices through direct engagement with the state, activists proceeded to make the argument to DHHS officials that sexual orientation was a distinct form of difference to which researchers and physicians needed to adjust, just like sex and gender, race and ethnicity, and age. Furthermore and, I believe, crucially, proponents of lesbian health research were able to benefit from positioning themselves as a specific subgroup of women to which the new DHHS infrastructure devoted to women's health ought reasonably to attend; that is, women's health provided a strategic wedge for lesbian health advocates. The capacity of lesbians to make use of this wedge was not foreordained; in fact, the 1985 task force report on women's health that had helped to kick off the inclusion-and-difference paradigm had made no explicit mention of lesbians (PHS, 1985). However, many DHHS employees in the newly established offices promoting women's health were sympathetic to "domain expansion."

That lesbian health activists appreciated the opening provided to them by the emphasis on women's health at the DHHS is made clear in the National Gay and Lesbian Task Force's (NGLTF) 1993 report on lesbian health. Noting that federal health policy documents had called for consideration by DHHS agencies of the unique health conditions affecting women or "some subgroups of women," the authors, Peri Jude Radecic and Marj Plumb, argued that lesbians constituted one such distinct subgroup of women. They proposed, therefore, that lesbians be included "as subjects, reviewers, and principal researchers in all women's health and mental health research initiatives"; that future and ongoing longitudinal health studies funded by NIH be stratified according to sexual orientation; and that the DHHS create a "fully funded office on Lesbian Health Care" (Radecic & Plumb, 1993, pp. 1, 12, 15). In conjunction with the 1993 March on Washington in support of lesbian and gay rights, NGLTF also organized a meeting between advocates for lesbian, gay, and bisexual health and DHHS Secretary Donna Shalala, who appointed one of her assistants, Patsy Fleming (who became President Clinton's "AIDS czar" the following year) as the lesbian and gay health liaison (Plumb, 1997, p. 366). At this and subsequent meetings with DHHS officials, Dr. Vivian Pinn, the director of NIH's Office of Research on Women's Health, by all accounts played an especially supportive role, encouraging the notion that lesbian health should be included in the agenda of her office (Haynes interview; Plumb 2001, p. 873).

Building gradually over the course of the 1990s, momentum in support of lesbian health research accelerated sharply with the decision by the Institute of Medicine (IOM) of the National Academy of Sciences to prepare a report on the state of lesbian health. The report "piggybacked" on DHHS's interest in women's health in several senses. First, an earlier IOM report on the inclusion of women in biomedical research (Mastroianni et al., 1994) had been pivotal in directing attention to women's health issues, and it therefore seemed logical to advocates of lesbian health to try to replicate that success. Second, funding for the report was provided by Pinn's Office of Research on Women's Health at the NIH, as well as by the CDC's Office of Women's Health (Haynes interview; Solarz, 1999).

Published in 1999 by the National Academy Press (Solarz, 1999), the book-length report, *Lesbian Health: Current Assessment and Directions for the Future*, notably went to some pains to clarify what might be meant by a "lesbian health issue." On the basis of the data available, the report concluded, there were no grounds to maintain that lesbians were at higher risk for any health problem than heterosexual women "simply because they have a lesbian sexual orientation." It was not that being a lesbian was somehow intrinsically unhealthy; rather, certain specific health risks, such as nulliparity (not giving birth), stress effects of homophobia, and avoidance of health care, apparently were overrepresented among lesbian women (Solarz, 1999, p. 6). Precisely whether these greater risks were resulting in worse health for lesbians was a question that required additional research, and the call for such research was one of the chief thrusts of the report. Advocates for lesbian health research seized on this conclusion, referring to the report's publication as "a landmark day in the history of lesbian health" (1st U.S., 1999) and proposing that researchers take full advantage of the "window of opportunity" it had opened by launching new investigations (Bradford, 1999, p. 116). Moreover, the achievement of obtaining an IOM report propelled LGBT health advocates to train their gaze even more closely on the DHHS.

3 Projects

3.1 "Healthy People"

Perhaps the defining example of the new state-centered politics was the struggle for inclusion in *Healthy People 2010*. Running more than 800 pages, this planning document prepared by the DHHS (U.S. Department of Health and Human Services, 2000) was intended to establish the nation's health priorities for the first decade of the new century. *Healthy People* had two overarching goals: to increase the quality and length of healthy life and to eliminate health disparities between groups. More specifically, *Healthy People* consisted of 28 focus areas (listed alphabetically from "Access to Quality Health Services" to "Vision and Hearing") which were then subdivided into 467 discrete health objectives. Notwithstanding its dry and bureaucratic tone, this once-a-decade "road map" to better health is considered enormously important in setting the health agenda both nationally and for state-level and local health departments, and it has substantial implications for funding for research and service provision and for evaluating health departments' efforts.

Initially, LGBT groups were not included in the consortium of advocacy groups convened by the DHHS to participate in the *Healthy People 2010* planning process. Nevertheless, early drafts of the document did name sexual orientation up front as one dimension of health disparity: Along with "disability," sexual orientation was added to the list of forms of disparity that had been used in *Healthy People 2000* ten years before (i.e., gender, race and ethnicity, income and education, and geography). As one DHHS employee commented, this sets a nearly irreversible precedent: It is difficult to imagine that sexual orientation would get deleted from *Healthy People 2020* or *Healthy People 2030*.[1] An early draft of the document also included sexual orientation as a demographic item to be tracked in 20 of the tables corresponding to specific health objectives in the document. However, when the near-final "conference edition" of *Healthy People 2010* was released in January 2000, these specific mentions of sexual orientation mysteriously had been deleted (LGBT Nixed in Fed Plan 2000, p. 1), and only a paragraph in the introduction to the draft of *Healthy People 2010* about sexual orientation remained: There was then no mention of sexual orientation in relation to any of the 467 health objectives (Roehr, 2000; Smith, 2000a). From a practical standpoint, this absence rendered meaningless the token mention of sexual orientation in the introduction.

As GLMA and other groups mobilized, the DHHS received hundreds of letters commenting angrily on this exclusion, and an article appeared in the *Washington Blade*, a lesbian and gay newsweekly based in the capital, that criticized the Clinton administration for its omission of LGBT people from the document (Smith, 2000a). After several openly gay employees in Secretary Shalala's office became concerned about the issue (Rouse and Dunn interviews), representatives of GLMA, along with university-based lesbian and gay health researchers, were invited into the planning process (Roehr, 2000; Smith, 2000b). Shalala also designated her appointment secretary, Martin Rouse, a gay man who had been distressed to read the *Blade* article, to serve as liaison to the LGBT community in relation to *Healthy People*; and Rouse traveled around the country giving presentations to LGBT groups about the *Healthy People* process. In the end, the final version of the document incorporated sexual orientation into the "data templates" for 29 of the 467 objectives. In addition, words such as "gay," "lesbian," "bisexual," "men who have sex with men," and particularly "sexual orientation" appear in the text of the report at a number of places along the way (as revealed by a text search conducted by GLMA).

The inclusion of sexual orientation in 29 of the *Healthy People 2010* objectives highlighted an important issue: How would progress in improving the health of gay men and lesbians be tracked in relation to each objective? For tracking purposes, *Healthy People 2010* is tied to 26 different federal health surveys, but in the past few of these surveys

---

[1]Martin Rouse made this observation at the Gay Men's Health Summit in Boulder, Colorado, July 19–23, 2000 (author's field notes).

collected data about sexual identity or sexual behavior. In *Healthy People*, for all 29 data templates that include sexual orientation, the cells in the data tables contain the letters "DNC" (data not collected). As one activist characterized the situation: "It's like somebody inviting you to a wedding but there's no seat, no table, and no food for you"(Allen, 2001). In response to this absence, advocates have called for the addition of sexual orientation as a demographic item on national health surveys (Sell & Becker, 2001). For example, at the request of GLMA, the National Center for Health Statistics (part of the CDC) agreed that in 2000 it would add a question about sexual orientation to the National Health and Nutrition Examination Survey, an important and comprehensive federal health survey of 5000 individuals (Dunn interview; Brogan, 2001). Thus the successful push to include sexual orientation in *Healthy People* is giving momentum to the project of treating sexual orientation as a standard demographic item in health research.

3.2 End of an Era?

Even more so than the IOM report, the debate over *Healthy People* inspired LGBT health advocates to enter the arena of federal health policymaking. In the wake of the experience with *Healthy People*, state-centered advocates have created a new umbrella organization, the National Coalition for LGBT Health. This coalition, which represents more than 40 individual agencies and groups, was established in October 2000 at a meeting in Washington, DC. The National Coalition set a number of goals for itself, including to "increase knowledge regarding LGBT populations' health status, access to and utilization of health care, and other health-related information," "increase LGBT participation in the formation of public and private sector policy regarding health and related issues," and "eliminate disparities in health outcomes of LGBT populations" (http://www.lgbthealth.net). The group publishes a weekly newsletter that provides updates on research findings, current events, and ongoing policy debates. In effect, the coalition is positioning itself to be the chief voice of state-centered advocacy.

At the same time, advocates of LGBT health sought additional formal mechanisms for institutionalizing their concerns within the DHHS bureaucracy. Most significantly, in 2000, advocates attempted to convince DHHS officials to establish an Office of Lesbian and Gay Health that would parallel the Office on Women's Health and the Office on Minority Health. Painfully aware that if the Republican candidate won the presidential election in November the prospects for such an office would dim considerably—and hopeful that during an election year the Democratic administration would be anxious to curry favor with LGBT voters—advocates pressed hard for the DHHS to take action quickly (Dunn interview). Responding cautiously, Assistant Secretary for Health David Satcher appointed a "steering Committee on Health Disparities Related to Sexual Orientation." Consisting of representatives from each major DHHS agency, the Steering Committee took an inventory of how lesbian and gay issues were treated within DHSS and drafted a strategic plan (Bates, Dunn, Haynes, and Rouse interviews).

However, with the change in administration in 2000, these efforts effectively were put on hold. During the fall of 2002, in response to pressure from the National Coalition for LGBT Health, 19 members of Congress wrote a letter to DHHS Secretary Tommy Thompson asking the DHHS to "identify the actions that have been taken or will be taken across the department to ensure that health disparities due to sexual orientation and gender identity are being addressed and reduced" (Wolfe, 2002). In fact, the progress of LGBT state-centered advocacy in the Bush administration has been minimal. By October 2002, after DHHS withdrew $75,000 in funding previously earmarked for a lesbian health conference, researcher Judy Bradford was complaining that LGBT health concerns were moving "off the radar screen" at DHHS (Wolfe, 2002). Politically motivated crackdowns on federally funded AIDS education efforts also struck a worrisome note: In 2001 the CDC reported that it was auditing a community-based AIDS prevention organization in San Francisco (the STOP AIDS Project) that appeared to be violating federal law by using federal HIV prevention funds in ways that "encourage" sexual activity (Heredia, 2001). Audits of 14 other AIDS organizations followed. With conservative members of Congress threatening to defund NIH grants on sexual topics, researchers have been forced to adopt practices of self-censorship, such as omitting words such as "gay" from the titles and abstracts of grant proposals (Kristof, 2003; Leshner, 2003; Kaiser, 2004; Kaplan, 2004; Malakoff, 2004; Epstein, 2006a).

In modest ways, however, the incorporation of LGBT concerns in the inclusion-and-difference paradigm has continued within DHHS. In May 2001, the NIH issued a "program announcement" entitled "Behavioral, Social, Mental Health, and Substance Abuse Research with Diverse Populations" (NIH, 2001). Sponsored by a series of DHHS agencies, the program announcement invited principal investigators to apply for up to 5 years of grant support (amounts of up to $250,000 per year in direct costs) for research on "lesbian, gay, bisexual, transgendered, and related populations." However, the program announcement developed out of a workshop that took place prior to the change in administration, and the fact that words such as "gay" and "lesbian" do not actually appear in the title are indicative of caution in a changed political environment. Although skillful career civil service employees enjoy a certain amount of room in which to maneuver when promoting policies they favor, it remains unclear just how many such victories LGBT health advocates can achieve during the Bush administration. To the degree that the success of state-centered advocacy has depended on the accidental presence of LGBT persons employed in "the belly of the beast" who have been willing to take stands on LGBT health issues, it remains to be seen whether any such employees feel sufficiently emboldened to speak up.

4 Implications

The partial and limited institutionalization of LGBT health concerns in the programs, policies, interests, and rhetoric of the DHHS would have been difficult to foresee until recently. These developments are impressive and should not be underestimated. However, even if LGBT people do become more explicitly integrated according to the logic of the inclusion-and-difference paradigm (despite resistance from a conservative administration), it is important to examine just what such "success" might entail. Moreover, because state-centered advocacy inevitably places certain kinds of issues in the foreground and sidesteps others, it makes sense to analyze the explicit and implicit tensions between state-centered LGBT health advocacy and other forms of health activism of a more grassroots character. I approach these questions by suggesting some of the potential consequences of adopting a state-centered, inclusionary approach. I do so in a necessarily speculative fashion, with the goal not of making firm predictions or asserting a hard-line view but, rather, of sounding a series of cautionary notes.

4.1 State Focus

As activism is aligned to the inclusion-and-difference paradigm, the state increasingly may become the focus of political energies, and state actors and institutions may become perceived as the ultimate guarantors of equal treatment in the domain of health. Such moves may ignore what Wendy Brown has described as the "dangers in surrendering control . . . to the state, as well as in looking to the state as provider, equalizer, protector, or liberator" (Brown, 1995, p. 196). In this environment, advocacy organizations such as GLMA, which emphasize Washington, DC-based lobbying as a primary tactic and that have a close familiarity with state institutions, rise to prominence. Groups with a more critical approach to the state, such as those represented by the recent Gay Men's Health Summits, then find themselves walking a careful line, seeking to avoid both marginalization and cooptation. Thus, for example, the 2001 Gay Men's Health Summit included a plenary session on *Healthy People 2010* featuring presentations by Martin Rouse and other DHHS employees; but in the discussion that followed, both attendees and organizers voiced skepticism of relying on the government and on experts (author's field notes).

4.2 Professionalization

Adopting a state-centered approach also increases the group's dependence on professionals, including credentialed researchers, policy makers, and professional lobbyists, who may not always define the best interests of all sectors of the community in the same ways as other political actors (Mayer, 2000). "Be careful what you ask for," Vickie Mays, a UCLA health researcher, warned the audience at the Gay Men's Health Summit in 2001. Mays pointed to the growing number of researchers studying racial and ethnic minorities without any genuine knowledge of or commitment to those communities: "This does not need to be repeated in the gay men's health movement" (author's field notes). It also seems unlikely that academic health researchers are as prone to value the kinds of experiential, community-based knowledge about health, illness, and sexuality that are cultivated in grassroots activists' circles. As Marj Plumb warned in the special issue of the

American Journal of Public Health: "What is knowable about a population and its health conditions cannot be found solely through quantitative science. Community knowledge, particularly in the case of
populations that are difficult to find or to categorize, plays an increasingly important role in attempts to study these populations" (Plumb,
2001, p. 874).

In the context of state-centered politics, advocacy groups such as
GLMA that consist of a professional membership tend naturally to
move to center stage. The professional orientation of such groups then
attracts criticism from grassroots activists: When GLMA was mentioned at the Gay Men's Health Summit, audience members blasted the
organization as "white," professionalized, and insufficiently accountable to the community (author's field notes).

4.3 Visions of Health

Radical health activists frequently have challenged the mainstream biomedical presumption that the goal of health can be equated simply
with the elimination of disease. For example, in his remarks at the
opening session of the Gay Men's Health Summit in 2000, Eric Rofes
addressed the issue of what constitutes a healthy gay man, suggesting
that health meant more than just the absence of disease and criticizing
the association of health with normative cultural behavior. State-
centered efforts, by contrast, tend to adopt the DHHS goal of reducing
disparities in disease rates between groups—a worthy goal, to be sure,
but one that can bypass more fundamental questions about the
meaning of health to a community.

4.4 From Health Care to Health Research: Framing and Collective Identity

As adoption of the inclusion-and-difference paradigm directs attention
to the state and its definitions of health, the political agenda of challenging groups tends at least partially to shift away from focusing on
health care provision and toward focusing on health *research*. If in the
past the quintessential criticism concerned the insensitivity or hostility
of health care providers and the consequent limits on access to care,
the new hot issue becomes the problem of unjustified extrapolation in
research—that is, the tendency of researchers and physicians to assume
that findings from data collected through studies of straight white male
adults can be extrapolated to other groups.

This strategic shift from the conduct of health care provision to the
conduct of health care research has important implications for how
health issues are framed by LGBT movements. On one hand, the
domain of research is less accessible and more intimidating to lay
people, and it can be more difficult for nonexperts to find a voice
in such arenas. Drawing people into social movements that focus on
technical issues and mobilizing them in relation to abstruse goals can
be a challenging task (Epstein, 1996). On the other hand, the focus
on research may present activists with a relatively more achievable
set of goals. After all, compared with including LGBT people in

biomedical research, it would be much more challenging to imagine eliminating the homophobia of the health care delivery system, which is so much more decentralized and involves so many more individuals.

In addition to altering how issues are framed, the emphasis on questions of research has implications for the collective identity of a social movement, as it can change the definition of what unites the group. When a group challenges its stigmatizing treatment at the hands of health care providers, what unites them is the common experience of discrimination and oppression. However, when the focus shifts to ensuring that a categorical identity is tabulated on surveys and in clinical studies, the basis of group identity changes to one of epidemiologic similarity—sharing the same diseases, risks, and health disparities vis-à-vis the mainstream. In the former case, the group faces common external conditions but need not be internally similar: we are the same only insofar as we are treated the same by others. In the latter case, the group lays claim to internal similarity as well: what unites us is that we share a distinct, specifiable health profile. These are two quite different ways of conceiving of collective identity, and they may promote different kinds of analysis and political action.[2] For example, insofar as the group sees itself as having a distinct health profile, group members may overemphasize the threat posed by conditions that are seen as group-specific, but fail to attend to health risks (e.g., cardiovascular disease) that may be a substantially larger threat for many individuals in the group but that are not restricted to the group. In addition, group members may assume that what the group has in common (a sexual identity) is necessarily more consequential for the health of group members than the ways in which they differ (by social class, race, ethnicity, nationality, region, religion, and so on).

Indeed, insofar as the group is conceived of as internally similar, the interests of subgroups, such as gay men of color or working-class lesbians, may be systematically ignored. To be sure, the notion that LGBT communities are internally diverse is voiced repeatedly in documents such as *Healthy People 2010* and the IOM report, and commentators have warned about the risk of the "elision of important differences among populations and individuals" (Meyer, 2001, p. 858). Nevertheless, the emphasis on, for example, "gay men" as a categorical identity may inevitably tend to privilege (in the domain of health just as elsewhere in gay politics) the particular interests of middle-class gay white men.

4.5 Operationalizing the Categories: Identities and Practices

With the emphasis on "special populations," representatives of groups come to recognize that for a group to count in the polity it must

---

[2]I am grateful to Sarah Wilcox for suggesting these points. As Wilcox has argued in her analysis of lesbian health politics, strategic debates about the health politics of groups are inevitably debates about the very identities of those groups (Wilcox, 2000).

properly be counted (e.g., measured, included in surveys). With this realization comes the practical problem of how to transform social identities into categorical identities that can be "operationalized" and measured. Inevitably, researchers and advocates must then devote considerable attention to questions of definition and measurement (Solarz, 1999; Sell & Bradford 2000). For example, the index to the IOM report lists 15 page references for "definition of a lesbian." A possible consequence is that the research agenda becomes defined around precisely those questions that are amenable to quantification and measurement, which may or may not be perceived by members of the community as the questions that most crucially require answers. A possible effect is not only to privilege quantitative over qualitative data but more generally to enhance the authority of academic researchers and the kinds of knowledge they produce at the expense of the local and sometimes anecdotal knowledge about health and illness that is generated at the community level (Escoffier, 1999).

To be sure, the absence of a prior history of the institutionalization of sexual orientation categories in the federal bureaucracy means that LGBT demands for inclusion are a bit trickier than those of other groups. By contrast, when racial and ethnic minorities pressed for inclusion as subjects in biomedical research during the 1990s, the fact that race and ethnicity categories were already in long use on the U.S. census and on health surveys (however much the official list of these categories may shift every decade or so) meant that it was easier to operationalize inclusion of these groups. Government officials are far less used to thinking about categories of sexual orientation—and categories such as "transgender" are considered simply too "out there" by federal officials (Dunn interview), who are hardly prepared at present to replace the standard "male/female" demographic item with one that includes a third option (Haynes interview). (Indeed, it is not at all clear that state-centered advocacy can promote genuine inclusion of transgender health issues or if it would, instead, emphasize the variable of sexual orientation.)

By comparison with transgender, sexual orientation categories such as "homosexual" (and "heterosexual") might seem to lend themselves to straightforward operationalization. (Perhaps "bisexual" does as well, though some view this as a suspect category because of its apparent "in between" status.) These categories are also pose difficulties for a different reason: the lack of clear correspondence between identity and behavior. Surveys that ask respondents to name their sexual orientation produce one set of mappings of individuals into categories. Surveys that ask respondents who they have sex with would produce a different set of mappings, and questions about the object of desire would produce a third. As we know from empirical research (Laumann et al., 1994), these mappings would overlap but not coincide. This disjuncture between identity, practice, and desire necessarily complicates the operationalization of sexual orientation.

Although advocates of lesbian and gay health research are sensitive to these definitional difficulties, they tend not to emphasize the tangled relation between identity, practice, and desire because it brings scrutiny that may be unwelcome to a crucial underlying question in the politics of lesbian and gay health research: *What really counts as a gay or lesbian health issue?* Whereas some risks, such as higher rates of teen suicide, may indeed accrue to gays and lesbians as a consequence of their social identity, many other "gay and lesbian" health risks fundamentally reflect the propensity of gay men and lesbians to engage in specific behaviors at higher rates. If it does turn out that lesbians, as a group, are at greater risk of breast cancer, it may have little to do with their social identity as lesbians—except insofar as lesbians bypass mammography screening to avoid homophobic treatment by medical professionals—but instead may perhaps be due to the fact that lesbians are more likely not to have children. If gay men, overall, are at greater risk of anal cancer, this may be a consequence of engaging in the practice of anal sex, an activity that is neither universal among gay men nor restricted to them. The potential problem with calling these diseases "gay and lesbian health risks" is that (1) it incorrectly suggests that all members of the group are equally at risk, ignoring, for example, that many lesbians do bear children; and (2) it ignores individuals who engage in the same practices but who do not accept the group identity, such as heterosexual women who are childless, or men who have sex with men but who do not call themselves gay. Arguably, if risk is linked to practices, health promotion and health research ought to address those practices; but because the inclusion-and-difference paradigm presumes political organizing around social categories, claims about risk are more likely to be framed in terms of categorical identities. Indeed, whereas AIDS activists during the 1980s demanded that behavior and identity be disentangled, declaring that it's "what you do" and not "who you are" that puts the individual at risk for HIV infection, state-centered lesbian and gay health activists during the 1990s and beyond appear relatively unconcerned when behavior and identity are conflated.

4.6 Reification and Medicalization

The likely consequence of the association of health risk with identity categories (rather than with shared practices or shared oppression) is the reification and medicalization of those identities. This might not be so worrisome were it not for the long history, in medicine, of conceptualizing difference as pathology (Gilman, 1985; Schiebinger, 1987; Proctor, 1988; Jordanova, 1989; Terry & Urla, 1995; Waldby, 1996). Especially given the urge in many quarters to conceptualize sexual identities as biologic essences and to attribute such essences to "gay genes" or "gay brains," such reification may tend toward a presumption that LGBT individuals are actually biologically distinct from other humans. (Many advocates of lesbian and gay rights have endorsed such moves based on the belief that if sexual orientation is seen as an "immutable characteristic" conservatives cannot successfully characterize it as a sinful choice (Epstein, 1998). To be sure, some state-centered researchers appear to be skeptical of the notion that sexual orientation is a biologic classification (Sell & Becker, 2001, p. 878); and many discussions of LGBT health research emphasize mental health and substance abuse issues that do not necessarily lend themselves to a biologic framing, especially when linked to claims about the social oppression to which LGBT people are subjected. Often, however, the reification of identity tends to support the idea that certain groups are either susceptible to illness as a result of their biologic differences or prone to illness as a result of "bad habits" and customs that are intrinsic to the group (Ong, 1995; Shah, 2001; Briggs & Mantini-Briggs, 2003).

4.7 Politics of Sexuality

There may be another reason why advocates of state-centered health tend to emphasize identity rather than behavior. Although an emphasis on behaviors might often be a more precise way of talking about health risk in the case of lesbian, gay, and bisexual health, speaking of identity tends to keep the focus on personhood, whereas emphasizing behavior inevitably would mean talking explicitly about sexuality. It can be argued, in fact, that the limited political viability of state-centered LGBT health politics has depended substantially on the avoidance of explicit discussion of sexuality. In the corridors of Washington, it is far less threatening to speak of "sexual orientation as a demographic variable" than it is to speak of fellatio or fisting. In recent decades, Republicans in Congress have torpedoed the funding even for survey research related to sexuality (such as the National Health and Social Life Survey) (Laumann et al., 1994), and federal agencies have shown a distinct disinterest in health research that seems "too gay," such as research on anal condoms or rectal microbicides. Indeed, the explanation for why lesbian health research seemed to take off ahead of (non-HIV-related) gay men's health research may be, in part, that in the popular imagination gay men are more "sexualized" than lesbians. As Pat Dunn, the former policy director for GLMA, observed: "I have heard political analysis that lesbians are easier to talk about: it's not as politically or socially unacceptable to talk about lesbian health issues, [whereas the perception is that] gay men's health issues have a lot to do with anal intercourse and that kind of thing" (Dunn interview).

Although state-centered LGBT health advocates and researchers may themselves be quite open-minded on sexual matters, the inevitable need to play down issues of sexuality to pursue their agenda may place them at odds with significant strands of the LGBT movement, which historically has defended a liberated sexuality. Indeed, the new, grassroots gay men's health movement (like the AIDS activist movement before it) has adopted a strong "sex-positive" stance that is reflected in the blunt, unapologetic language used at their conferences and in their printed materials. (The cover of the conference program for the 2000 Gay Men's Health Summit displayed a collage of session titles, including "The Dick—A User's Guide" and "Perceptions of Semen.")

The historical linkage of LGBT politics with a sex-positive stance may give the LGBT health agenda a specific kind of critical "edge" that distinguishes it from that of other social groups that have been folded into the inclusion-and-difference paradigm. The inability of agencies of the state to incorporate this sexual politics may lead to a clearer articulation of an alternative, non-state-centered, LGBT health politics. For example, at a panel discussing *Healthy People* at the 2000 Gay Men's Health Summit, Daniel Wolfe, a New York City-based activist and writer, asked rhetorically: "When will we see research on how prostate cancer treatments diminish pleasure during anal sex? Never, from *Healthy People 2010!*" (author's field notes). Such questioning and the implicit call for a broader agenda for research, prevention, and treatment potentially put grassroots activists on a collision course with the requirements of state-centered advocacy.

5 Conclusions

As writing by Terry (1999a) and Scarce (2000) in different ways suggest, the rise of a state-centered health agenda poses important strategic choices for LGBT communities—especially so if the political climate for LGBT health advocacy improves. The partial institutionalization of LGBT health concerns in the federal health bureaucracy may result in substantial amounts of funding for research on health issues that affect lesbian and gay (and perhaps, to a lesser degree, bisexual and transgendered) people. Researchers committed to improving the health of those communities may in practice find few constraints on their use of government funds and may be able to "take the money and run"—or they may find that funding is available only to the degree that research conforms to government prescriptions about health, sexuality, and identity. As Ilan Meyer warned in a special issue of the *American Journal of Public Health*, "we may see that for every sensitive effort to include the target population in decision making, there may be another program that seeks to restore health by eliminating practices essential to self-expression and identity, leading to alienation and damage" (Meyer 2001, p. 858).

How can the risks of cooptation by state bureaucracies best be avoided? What does it mean for LGBT people to become subjects and objects of biomedical scrutiny in these new ways and to themselves adopt biomedical modes of understanding their identities and communities? Is the focusing of medical attention on sex/gender subjectivities a good thing in the sense that it attracts people and resources to the study of previously underserved communities? Or is it a dangerous thing in the sense that it encourages us to treat sexual and gender identities as fixed biologic or cultural types and as an illness category?

Engagement with the state and with biomedical expertise and modes of understanding appears inevitable and probably crucial, but the risks that accompany this engagement are not insignificant. In the present era, as more and more social groups demand inclusion in biomedical research, calls for such incorporation are, in effect, calls to be treated as citizens. Historically, however, "biomedical citizenship" (Ong, 1995; Shah, 2001; Briggs & Mantini-Briggs, 2003) has been closely linked to the policing of social groups and demarcation of the boundaries of normality. Analyses of "sexual citizenship" and its limitations (Duggan, 1994; Berlant, 1997; Richardson, 1998; Weeks, 1998; Bell & Binnie 2000; Plummer, 2003) may prove instructive here. As Diane Richardson has observed, the extension of citizenship on the basis of sexual identity has encountered stiff resistance and has been "based on a politics of tolerance and assimilation" (Richardson, 1998, p. 89). There is no reason to assume that "biomedical citizenship" for LGBT people will be any less begrudgingly bestowed or any less riddled with contradictions than citizenship for such people generally.

Acknowledgments: Much of the material presented here has been adapted from Epstein, 2003b. Some of the work on which this chapter was based was supported by an Investigator Award in Health Policy Research from the Robert Wood Johnson Foundation. In addition, portions of this material are based on work supported by the National Science Foundation under grant SRB-9710423. Any opinions, findings, and conclusions or recommendations expressed in this material are those of the author and do not necessarily reflect the views of the National Science Foundation.

References

Cited Interviews (affiliations were current at the time of the interview)

Bates, C. (2000) Office of HIV/AIDS Policy, Department of Health and Human Services. Interviewed in Washington, DC, August 7.

Dunn, P. (2000) Director of Public Policy for the Gay and Lesbian Medical Association. Interviewed in San Francisco, July 28.

Haynes, S. (2000) Office of Women's Health, Department of Health and Human Services. Interviewed in Washington, DC, August 7.

Rouse, M. (2000) Scheduling assistant in Department of Health and Human Services. Interviewed in Boulder, CO, July 21.

Text References

1st U.S. lesbian health report. (1999). Planet Out News Planet. http://www.planetout.com/newsplanet/article.html?1999/01/14/1.

Allen, J.E. (2001) Health agenda focuses attention on gay's needs. *Los Angeles Times* April 30.

Bell, D., and Binnie, J. (2000) *The sexual citizen: queer politics and beyond*. Polity, Cambridge, UK.

Berlant, L. (1997) *The queen of America goes to Washington city: essays on sex and citizenship*. Duke University Press, Durham, NC.

Boehmer, U. (2002) Twenty years of public health research: inclusion of lesbian, gay, bisexual, and transgender populations. *American Journal of Public Health* 92:1125–1130.

Bowen, D., Powers, D., and Greenlee, H. (1997) Lesbian health research: perspectives from a research team. In: White, J., and Martínez, M.C. (eds) *The lesbian health book: caring for ourselves*. Seal Press, Seattle, pp. 299–320.

Bradford, J. (1999) Emergence of an infrastructure for lesbian health research [editorial]. *Journal of the Gay and Lesbian Medical Association* 3:115–117.

Briggs, C.L., and Mantini-Briggs, C. (2003) *Stories in times of cholera: racial profiling during a medical nightmare*. University of California Press, Berkeley.

Brogan, D.J. (2001) Implementing the institute of medicine report on lesbian health. *Journal of the American Medical Women's Association* 56:24–26.

Brown, W. (1995) *States of injury: power and freedom in late modernity*. Princeton University Press, Princeton, NJ.

Denenberg, R. (1994) *Report on lesbian health*. National Gay and Lesbian Task Force Policy Institute, Washington DC.

Deyton, B., and Lear, W. (1988) A brief history of the gay/lesbian health movement in the USA. In: Shernoff, M., Scott, W.A. (eds) *The sourcebook on lesbian/gay health care*. National Lesbian and Gay Health Foundation, Washington, DC, pp. 15–19.

Duggan, L. (1994) Queering the state. *Social Text*: 1–14.

Epstein, S. (1996) *Impure science: AIDS, activism, and the politics of knowledge*. University of California Press, Berkeley.

Epstein, S. (1997) AIDS activism and the retreat from the genocide frame. *Social Identities* 3:415–438.

Epstein, S. (1998) Gay and lesbian movements in the United States: dilemmas of identity, diversity, and political strategy. In: Adam, B., Duyvendak, J.W., and Krouwel, A. (eds) *The global emergence of gay and lesbian politics: national imprints of a worldwide movement*. Temple University Press, Philadelphia, pp. 30–90.

Epstein, S. (2003a) Inclusion, diversity, and biomedical knowledge making: the multiple politics of representation. In: Oudshoorn, N., and Pinch, P. (eds) *How users matter: the co-construction of users and technology*. MIT Press, Cambridge, MA, pp. 173–190.

Epstein, S. (2003b) Sexualizing governance and medicalizing identities: the emergence of "state-centered" LGBT health politics in the United States. *Sexualities* 6:131–171.

Epstein, S. (2004) Bodily differences and collective identities: representation, generalizability, and the politics of gender and race in biomedical research in the United States. *Body and Society* 10:183–203.

Epstein, S. (2006a) The new attack on sexuality research: morality and the politics of knowledge production. *Sexuality Research and Social Policy* 3:1–12.

Epstein, S. (2006b) Institutionalizing the new politics of difference in U.S. biomedical research: thinking across the science/state/society divides. In: Frickel, S., and Moore, K. (eds) *The new political sociology of science: institutions, networks and power*. University of Wisconsin Press, Madison, pp. 327–350.

Epstein, S. (2007, in press) *Inclusion: gender, race, and the politics of difference in medical research*. University of Chicago Press, Chicago.

Escoffier, J. (1999) The invention of safer sex: vernacular knowledge, gay politics, and HIV prevention. *Berkeley Journal of Sociology* 43:1–30.

Gilman, S.L. (1985) *Difference and pathology: stereotypes of sexuality, race and madness*. Cornell University Press, Ithaca.

Goldstein, N. (1997) Lesbians and the medical profession: HIV/AIDS and the pursuit of visibility. In: Goldstein, N., and Manlowe, J. (eds) *The gender politics of HIV/AIDS in women*. New York University Press, New York, pp. 86–110.

Heredia, C. (2001) S.F.'S HIV fight may be too sexy. *San Francisco Chronicle*, November 16, A-25.

Jordanova, L. (1989) *Sexual visions: images of gender in science and medicine between the eighteenth and twentieth centuries*. University of Wisconsin Press, Madison.

Kaiser, J. (2004) Biomedical politics: Democrats blast a sunny-side look at U.S. health disparities. *Science* 303:451.

Kaplan, E. (2004) Follow the money. *The Nation*, November 1, pp. 20–23.

Kristof, N.D. (2003) The secret war on condoms [Op-Ed]. *New York Times*, January 10, A25.

Laumann, E.O., Gagnon, J.H., Michael, R.T., and Michaels, S. (1994) *The social organization of sexuality: sexual practices in the United States.* University of Chicago Press, Chicago.

Leshner, A.I. (2003) Don't let ideology trump science. *Science* 302:1479.

LGBT Nixed in Fed Plan. (2000) *GLMA Report*, Spring, p. 10.

Malakoff, D. (2004) White House rebuts charges it has politicized science. *Science* 304:184–185.

Mastroianni, A.C., Faden, R., and Federman, D. (eds) (1994) *Women and health research: ethical and legal issues of including women in clinical studies.* National Academy Press, Washington, DC.

Mayer, K. (2000) Beyond Boulder: a glance back and the road ahead. *Journal of the Gay and Lesbian Medical Association* 4:1–2.

Mays, V.M., and Cochran, S.D. (1993) The impact of perceived discrimination on the intimate relationships of black lesbians. *Journal of Homosexuality* 25:1–14.

Meyer, I.H. (2001) Why lesbian, gay, bisexual, and transgender public health? *American Journal of Public Health* 91:856–859.

Minton, H.L. (2002) *Departing from deviance: a history of homosexual rights and emancipatory science in America.* University of Chicago Press, Chicago.

NIH. (2001) Behavioral, social, mental health, and substance abuse research with diverse populations. NIH Program Announcement PA-01-096. National Institutes of Health, Bethesda, MD, May 21.

Ong, A. (1995) Making the biopolitical subject: Cambodian immigrants, refugee Medicine and cultural citizenship in California. *Social Science and Medicine* 40:1243–1257.

PHS (1985) Women's health: report of the Public Health Service Task Force on Women's Health Issues: Volume 1. *Public Health Reports* 100:73–106.

Plumb, M. (1997) Blueprint for the future: the lesbian health advocacy movement. In: White, J., and Martínez, M.C. (eds) *The lesbian health book: caring for ourselves.* Seal Press, Seattle, pp. 362–377.

Plumb, M. (2001) Undercounts and overstatements: will the IOM report on lesbian health improve research? *American Journal of Public Health* 91:873–875.

Plummer, K. (2003) *Intimate citizenship.* University of Washington Press, Seattle.

Proctor, R.N. (1988). *Racial hygiene: medicine under the nazis.* Harvard University Press, Cambridge, MA.

Radecic, P.J., and Plumb, M. (1993) Lesbian health issues & recommendations. National Gay and Lesbian Task Force Policy Institute, Washington, DC, April 1.

Richardson, D. (1998) Sexuality and citizenship. *Sociology* 32:83–100.

Roehr, B. (2000) Master plan for US health now includes gays. *San Francisco Gay & Lesbian Times*, January 27, p. 27.

Rofes, E. (1999) Foreword to smearing the queer: medical bias in the health care of gay men, by Michael Scarce. Harrington Park, New York, pp. xi–xiv.

Rofes, E. (2000) Resuscitating the body politic: creating a gay men's health movement. *Baltimore Alternative*, August 8, p. 21.

Ryan, C., and Bradford, J. (1988) The National Lesbian Health Care Survey: an overview. In: Shernoff, M., and Scott, W.A. (eds) *The sourcebook on lesbian/gay health care.* National Lesbian and Gay Health Foundation, Washington, DC, pp. 30–40.

Scarce, M. (1999) *Smearing the queer: medical bias in the health care of gay men.* Harrington Park, New York.

Scarce, M. (2000) The second wave of the gay men's health movement: medicalization and cooptation as pitfalls of progress [editorial]. *Journal of the Gay and Lesbian Medical Association* 4:3–4.

Schiebinger, L. (1987) Skeletons in the closet: the first illustrations of the female skeleton in eighteenth century anatomy. In: Gallagher, C., and Lacquer, T. (eds) *The making of the modern body: sexuality and society in the nineteenth century.* University of California Press, Berkeley, pp. 42–82.

Schneider, J., and Levin, S. (1999) Uneasy partners: the lesbian and gay health care community and the AMA. *JAMA* 282:1287–1288.

Sell, R.L., and Becker, J.B. (2001) Sexual orientation data collection and progress toward healthy people 2010. *American Journal of Public Health* 91:876–882.

Sell, R.L, and Bradford, J. (2000) Elimination of health disparities based upon sexual orientation: inclusion of sexual orientation as a demographic variable in healthy people 2010 objectives. Unpublished observations.

Shah, N. (2001) *Contagious divides: epidemics and race in San Francisco's Chinatown.* University of California Press, Berkeley.

Silvestre, A.J. (1999) Gay male, lesbian and bisexual health-related research funded by the national institutes of health between 1974 and 1992. *Journal of Homosexuality* 37:81–94.

Smith, R. (2000a) Healthy criticism: activists complain report omits gays. *Washington Blade*, February 25, pp. 1, 21, 23.

Smith, R. (2000b) Healthy people 2010 document may be changed. *Washington Blade*, June 2, p. 23.

Solarz, A.L. (ed) (1999) *Lesbian health: current assessment and directions for the future.* National Academy Press, Washington, DC.

Stevens, P.E. (1992) Lesbian health care research: a review of the literature from 1970 to 1990. *Health Care for Women International* 13:91–120.

Stevens, P.E., and Hall, J.M. (1991) A critical historical analysis of the medical construction of lesbianism. *International Journal of Health Services* 21:291–307.

Terry, J. (1999a) Agendas for lesbian health: countering the ills of homophobia. In: Clarke, A.E., and Olesen, V.L. (eds) *Revisioning women, health, and healing: feminist, cultural, and technoscience perspectives.* Routledge, New York, pp. 324–342.

Terry, J. (1999b) *An American obsession: science, medicine, and homosexuality in modern society.* University of Chicago Press, Chicago.

Terry, J., and Urla, J. (eds) (1995) *Deviant bodies: critical perspectives on difference in science and popular culture.* Indiana University Press, Bloomington.

U.S. Department of Health and Human Services. (2000) *Healthy people 2010: understanding and improving health.* U.S. Government Printing Office, Washington, DC.

Waldby, C. (1996) *AIDS and the body politic: biomedicine and sexual difference.* Routledge, London.

Weeks, J. (1998) The sexual citizen. *Theory Culture & Society* 15:35–52.

Wilcox, S. (2000) Framing AIDS and breast cancer as lesbian health issues: social movements and the alternative press. Department of Sociology, University of Pennsylvania.

Wolfe, K. (2002) Gay health off radar screen of Bush HHS. *Washington Blade*, October 11.

Part III

Prejudice and Pride in Health

Sexual Stigma: Putting Sexual Minority Health Issues in Context

Gregory M. Herek, Regina Chopp, and Darryl Strohl

1 Introduction

In the United States today, lesbians, gay men, bisexual women, and bisexual men are stigmatized. They are subjected to explicit and subtle discrimination, marginalized or made virtually invisible by many of society's institutions, and often vilified. To understand the health-related experiences and behaviors of sexual minorities, it is necessary to examine this stigma and prejudice, including its sources and dimensions, how it is enacted, and how it is experienced. Such an examination is the goal of the present chapter.

2 Definitions and Conceptual Framework

To begin, we propose a conceptual framework for understanding stigma and prejudice directed at sexual minorities. Building on an earlier discussion of these topics (Herek, 2004), this framework integrates the sociological construct of *stigma* with the psychological construct of *prejudice*. Although these terms are often used interchangeably, differentiating them permits a more refined social psychological analysis of hostility toward sexual minorities. Drawing on insights from multiple theoretical perspectives (e.g., Allport, 1954; Goffman, 1963; Scambler & Hopkins, 1986; Meyer, 2003), the proposed framework incorporates institutional and individual levels of analysis and, within the latter, addresses the experiences of members of both the nonstigmatized majority and the stigmatized minority group.

In brief, we conceptualize *sexual stigma* as society's shared belief system through which homosexuality is denigrated, discredited, and constructed as invalid relative to heterosexuality. Society's institutions incorporate this belief system into an ideology that reinforces stigma and the power differentials associated with it, a phenomenon we label *heterosexism*. Virtually all members of society are aware that gay, lesbian, and bisexual people are stigmatized, regardless of whether they personally endorse society's negative views. This awareness affects social interactions. For heterosexuals, sexual stigma tends to be salient only when sexual orientation becomes personally relevant (e.g., when they knowingly encounter a gay, lesbian, or bisexual person). For sexual minority individuals, by contrast, stigma awareness is chronic. It results in *felt stigma*, which translates into ongoing appraisals of social situations for possible enactments of stigma (e.g., discrimination, mistreatment). As a result of these appraisals, the minority individual may employ proactive or reactive coping strategies, including various stigma management strategies. When gay, lesbian, and bisexual individuals internalize society's negative ideology about sexual minorities, the result is *internalized homophobia*. When heterosexuals internalize it, the result is *sexual prejudice*. In the remainder of this section, we elaborate on this framework and its central components.

Stigma historically has referred to a condition or attribute that discredits the individual who manifests it (e.g., Goffman, 1963; Jones et al., 1984). This discrediting can be specific to a particular social situation, or it can endure across social settings. In any social interaction, the roles of the stigmatized and the "normal" (as Goffman, 1963, labeled the non-stigmatized) are defined such that the former has a relatively inferior status and, consequently, generally less power and access to resources than the latter. As the determinant of a social role, stigma has a social reality independent of individual actors. It is a part of culture, a knowledge shared among society's members that is rationalized and justified by society's ideological systems. (We use *ideology* here in its social structural sense, not to describe any particular individual's belief system but, rather, to refer to a set of hierarchical social relations that are both expressed through and perpetuated by various practices.)

Sexual stigma is stigma based on sexual orientation. We define it here as society's negative regard for any nonheterosexual behavior, identity, relationship, or community (Herek, 2004). Like other stigmas, sexual stigma creates social roles and expectations that are widely shared by the members of society. Regardless of their own sexual orientation or personal attitudes, people living in the United States generally know that homosexual acts and desires—as well as people whose personal identities are based on same-sex attractions, behaviors, and relationships, or on membership in the gay community—are widely considered bad, sick, and inferior to heterosexuality. Like other types of stigma, sexual stigma is rationalized and justified by the ideological systems of society, including ideologies of gender, morality, and citizenship that define homosexuality and sexual minorities as deviant, sinful, and outside the law.

Because conceptualizations of human sexuality have changed over time, sexual stigma must be understood in its historical context. Whereas homosexual and heterosexual behaviors are ubiquitous among human societies (e.g., Murray, 2000), the idea that individuals are defined in terms of their sexual attractions and behaviors is of relatively recent origin. Exactly how individuals in other times and cultures subjectively experienced their sexuality and exactly when various constructs related to sexual orientation entered the dominant world view in Western societies are topics of lively debate whose resolution is beyond the scope of the present chapter (for discussions, see, for example, Foucault, 1978; Chauncey, 1982–1983; Trumbach, 1989; Van der Meer, 1997). Nevertheless, historians now widely agree that modern notions of homosexuality and heterosexuality, and indeed the very concept of sexual orientation, are relatively new and that the latter nineteenth century witnessed significant changes in how sexuality was understood.

Similarly, whereas homosexual acts have been stigmatized to varying degrees throughout history, the stigma attached to homosexual and bisexual identities is mainly a phenomenon of the nineteenth and twentieth centuries. When discussing sexual stigma, therefore, it is useful to differentiate the stigma attached to homosexual desires and behaviors from that directed at individuals who, as a result of their lesbian, gay, or bisexual identity, are regarded as embodying homosexuality.

Sexual stigma has been an integral part of many of society's institutions, including religion, the law, and medicine. We refer here to institutionalized sexual stigma as heterosexism. Heterosexism comprises the organizing rules whereby the institutions of society make gay and bisexual people invisible in most social situations or, when they become visible, designate them as appropriate targets for hostility, discrimination, and attack (Herek, 2004). Consequently, lesbian, gay, and bisexual people have less access than heterosexuals to the benefits afforded by those institutions. In many cases, they are directly targeted for punishment. Thus, heterosexism perpetuates the power differential at the heart of sexual stigma.

Shifting from a sociological to a psychological frame, we distinguish among individuals' awareness that sexual stigma exists, their perception that they may be the target of enactments of stigma (which, borrowing from Scambler and Hopkins, 1986, we refer to as *felt stigma*), and their personal embrace or rejection of it (which we refer to as *internalized stigma*). Heterosexuals and lesbian, gay, and bisexual people alike recognize the existence of sexual stigma to varying degrees. Most sexual minority individuals and many heterosexuals experience felt stigma. However, not everyone considers such stigma legitimate. As discussed below, the proportion of the U.S. population that embraces sexual stigma has declined dramatically in recent decades. We refer to heterosexuals' internalization of sexual stigma as *sexual prejudice*. Among lesbian, gay, and bisexual people, we refer to it as *internalized homophobia*. In the present chapter, we use these constructs—sexual stigma, heterosexism, stigma awareness, felt stigma, and internalized stigma (both sexual prejudice and internalized homophobia)—to discuss the context in which lesbian, gay, and bisexual people encounter and respond to health concerns and challenges.[1]

---

[1]Contemporary discourse about sexuality often attempts to address lesbian, gay, bisexual, and transgender issues simultaneously. This practice is exemplified by the widespread use of the "LGBT" acronym and its variations. Although we recognize the value of such a combination in cultural and political contexts, we nevertheless believe it warrants critical scrutiny in scientific discourse. Unpacking the LGBT acronym is important both for theoretical and

3 Heterosexism: Institutional Enactment of Sexual Stigma

Throughout much of the twentieth century, sexual stigma kept homosexual and bisexual people largely hidden. Their experiences were negated by society's major institutions and most social interaction proceeded on the premise that all participants were heterosexual. When gay and bisexual people became visible, they usually were condemned, pathologized, ridiculed, or attacked. Thus sexual stigma has functioned both to render sexual minorities invisible and to legitimize their ostracism and abuse.

At the same time, the targets of sexual stigma have repeatedly contested it during the past half century. Resistance to the stigmatized status of homosexuality was nascent at the end of World War II, and burgeoned during the 1970s after the Stonewall riots. Although sexual stigma remains widespread today, it is continually challenged; and as explained below, some of its institutional manifestations have largely disappeared. In the discussion that follows, we note how sexual stigma has been successfully challenged as well as the ways in which it remains hegemonic.

In this section, we briefly review the operation of heterosexism through the law, religion, and psychiatry. Each of these institutions has articulated its own rationales for denigrating homosexual behavior and people. Within each of them, sexual minorities and sympathetic heterosexuals have challenged heterosexism with varying success. Our discussion begins with the institution in which such resistance has, to date, had the least impact (religion). We then move to an institution in which it has led to significant changes (law) and conclude with the institution in which heterosexism has been largely negated, so much so that the institution now devotes considerable energy to eradicating the stigma it once promulgated (psychiatry and psychology).

3.1 Heterosexism in Religion

Christianity has always been the dominant religious faith in the United States, and Christian condemnation of homosexual behavior predates

---

empirical purposes. Combining lesbians and gay men (the "L" and "G") under a single rubric obscures gender differences in the experiences of homosexual people. Bisexuality (the "B" component) is seriously underconceptualized and understudied. Moreover, collapsing the experiences of bisexual women and men further obscures gender differences. For all the problems associated with the "LGB" combination, at least its components are all part of the broader phenomenon commonly called sexual orientation. By contrast, transgender issues (a wide variety of phenomena collapsed under "T" in the acronym) implicate an analysis based mainly on gender rather than sexuality. Although these two aspects of human experience are closely related, they are conceptually and empirically distinct. We believe that societal and individual reactions to transgender individuals warrant a separate treatment that fully explores the unique theoretical and empirical issues specific to stigma based on gender identity and gender-related behavior. We do not presume to offer such an analysis in the present chapter.

the founding of the American colonies. Historically, antipathy toward homosexual acts was part of a broader condemnation of an entire class of behaviors that included nonprocreative sexual conduct (e.g., masturbation, bestiality), sex not sanctioned by marriage (fornication, adultery), and marital sex that focused on sensual gratification (e.g., intercourse in positions other than the man lying on top of the woman). This array of sexual activities was collected under the rubric of "sodomy" around the eleventh century. Condemnation of sodomy—including homosexual acts—as "unnatural" received official expression in the writings of Thomas Aquinas and other theologians (Jordan, 1997). By the latter twelfth century, hostility toward "sins against nature" had taken root and eventually spread throughout European religious and secular institutions (Boswell, 1980). Whereas historians disagree about the extent of religious hostility toward homosexual behavior before this time, they generally concur that such moral condemnation subsequently was the rule. Some acts that once were considered sodomy are now widely condoned. Homosexuality, however, remains a focus of intense religious hostility.

Christian teachings distinguish between homosexual acts and individuals with a homosexual orientation. Being homosexual is not, in itself, considered a sin by most religions. Acting on one's homosexual feelings by having a sexual encounter or relationship with someone of the same sex, however, constitutes a sin. Homosexuals are encouraged to become heterosexual, but those who cannot do so are welcomed in the church so long as they remain celibate. However, "practicing" homosexuals—including those who wish to pursue a lifelong monogamous relationship with a same-sex partner—are not officially accepted.

For example, the Roman Catholic church has long maintained that "homosexual acts are intrinsically disordered and can in no case be approved of" while counseling that persons with a homosexual orientation "must certainly be treated with understanding and sustained in the hope of overcoming their personal difficulties and their inability to fit into society" (Congregation for the Doctrine of the Faith, 1975, Section VIII, ¶4). Similarly, although the Presbyterian Church (USA) General Assembly has acknowledged that "The church should be sensitive to the difficulty of rejecting a person's sexual orientation without rejecting the person" (Presbyterian Church USA, 2001, ¶5), it regards homosexual acts as sinful and has declared that "self-affirming, practicing homosexual persons may not be ordained as ministers of the Word and Sacrament, elders, or deacons" (Presbyterian Church USA, 2001, "The Ordination of Homosexuals" section, ¶4). The United Methodist Church (UMC) asserts that, "Homosexual persons no less than heterosexual persons are individuals of sacred worth" but also that "we do not condone the practice of homosexuality and consider this practice incompatible with Christian teaching" (United Methodist Church, 2004a, ¶5). The UMC Book of Discipline also directs that "[s]ince the practice of homosexuality is incompatible with Christian teaching, self-avowed practicing homosexuals are not to be accepted as candidates, ordained as ministers, or appointed to serve in The United

Methodist Church" (United Methodist Church, 2004b, "Regarding the Ministry of the Ordained" section).

This distinction between acts and actors is often expressed by conservative Christians in the maxim, "Love the sinner but hate the sin," an admonition probably derived from Augustine of Hippo's *cum dilectione hominum et odio vitiorum*, which is usually translated as "with love of mankind and hatred of sins" (Knowles, 1997, p. 191). Although characterized by its adherents as embodying compassion and tolerance, this philosophy clearly conveys sexual stigma. Unlike heterosexual conduct, homosexual behavior is regarded unequivocally as evil, with the circumstances in which it occurs (e.g., whether it is practiced in the context of a committed, loving relationship) considered irrelevant to its status as a sin. To the extent that being a gay or lesbian person is fundamentally about one's sexual and romantic relationships, the validity of distinguishing behavior from identity for purposes of stigma is highly questionable. Indeed, the problematic nature of this distinction is readily evident in Christian discourse.

For example, in a 1986 document authored by Cardinal Joseph Ratzinger (now Pope Benedict XVI), the Catholic Church declared that although being homosexual is not itself a sin "it is a more or less strong tendency ordered toward an intrinsic moral evil; and thus the inclination itself must be seen as an objective disorder" (Congregation for the Doctrine of the Faith, 1986, Point 3, ¶2). Similarly, whereas the Evangelical Lutheran Church, the Presbyterian Church, and other Protestant denominations admit gay men and lesbians as congregants and permit the ordination of gay and lesbian clergy, most require those individuals to abstain from homosexual acts. Thus, religious condemnation of homosexual behavior inevitably stigmatizes people who are homosexual.

Some denominations have made this equation explicit by translating their doctrinal condemnation of homosexual behavior into active political opposition to gay rights. In 1992, for example, the Catholic Church explained its opposition to laws prohibiting discrimination based on sexual orientation, stating that "such initiatives, even where they seem more directed toward support of basic civil rights than condonement of homosexual activity or a homosexual life-style, may in fact have a negative impact on the family and society" (Congregation for the Doctrine of the Faith, 1992, ¶1) and declaring that "there are areas in which it is not unjust discrimination to take sexual orientation into account, for example, in the placement of children for adoption or foster care, in employment of teachers or athletic coaches, and in military recruitment" (¶11).

White evangelical Protestantism has been the major source of antigay activism in the United States since the advent of the modern gay movement after the 1969 Stonewall riots. Prior to that time, evangelical discourse urged Christians to reduce their vilification of homosexuality and to try instead to win homosexuals over through love and compassion (Herman, 1997). By the late 1960s and early 1970s, however, evangelical publications such as *Christianity Today* evidenced a growing concern with "gay militancy" and increasingly linked homosexuality with sexual crime. The image of homosexuals shifted from one of wayward individuals to be pitied and saved to gay men and lesbians as "an anti-Christian force, promoting a heresy increasingly sanctioned by the state in the form of decriminalization and the extension of civil rights" (Herman, 1997, p. 50).

By the late 1970s, when Anita Bryant launched her crusade to repeal a Dade County (Florida) antidiscrimination ordinance, lesbians and gay men were increasingly demonized by politically active religious conservatives, who subsequently came to be known as the Religious Right or the Christian Right.[2] By the early 1990s, this animosity, coupled with the Christian Right's increasing political strength, led to attempts in several states to pass antigay laws through voter initiatives. The rallying cry of these initiatives was "no special rights" for homosexuals, a framing strategy that proved to be more effective with secular voters than the morality-based arguments that worked well within the ranks of Christian conservatives (Herman, 1997).

Historically, Black evangelical Protestants have followed a different path from their White counterparts. Like other Christian denominations, Black churches have condemned homosexuality and marginalized their gay and lesbian members, often forcing them to remain invisible although their sexual orientation was an open secret in their congregations (Fullilove & Fullilove, 1999). Although condemning homosexuality at least as much as Whites, however, Black Americans have been more supportive of civil liberties for gay people and more strongly opposed to antigay discrimination (Lewis, 2003). Since the 1990s, the overwhelmingly White Christian Right has attempted to recruit Black Evangelicals with only limited success (Herman, 1997). The national debate about marriage rights for same-sex couples has provided another opportunity in this regard, and some Black clergy publicly supported George Bush in the 2004 election, applauding his support for a Constitutional amendment to block marriage rights for gay couples (Kirkpatrick, 2004).

Some religious denominations have welcomed lesbian and gay members, and some of the most liberal—Unitarians, the United Church of Christ, and Reform Judaism, for example—have accepted gay people into their ministry and blessed same-sex marriages or same-sex "holy unions" (e.g., Dewan, 2005). In several Protestant denominations, specific congregations have declared themselves to be "welcoming" or "affirming" of gay men and lesbians (Sanders, 2001; Trevison, 2005). In other denominations, resistance to established teachings about homosexuality was evidenced by the formation during the late twentieth

---

[2]The Christian Right is a social movement that attempts to mobilize evangelical Protestants and other orthodox Christians into political action with the goal of embodying conservative values in public policy (Wilcox, 1996; Green, 2000). It is important to note that the political movement known as the Christian Right does not include all white Evangelicals and Fundamentalists. Evangelicals comprise a diverse group; and although most generally agree that homosexual behavior is a sin, they do not all endorse the antigay agenda of the Christian Right.

century of groups whose central purpose was to promote a positive theological stance toward homosexuality. In 1969, for example, gay Catholics formed Dignity, an organization whose goals are to provide a gay- and lesbian-affirmative Catholic ministry (Dignity USA, 2005). Other groups include Integrity (in the Episcopal Church), Affirmation (Methodist and Mormon Churches), Lutherans Concerned, and More Light Presbyterians.

In summary, although it is contested in individual congregations, heterosexism currently pervades organized religion. Most denominations define romantic love, committed relationships, and families solely in heterosexual terms and condemn homosexuality as sinful. Through these doctrines, religion simultaneously negates homosexuality in the realms of relationships and families while providing a rationale for marginalizing and attacking people who are gay, lesbian, or bisexual.

3.2 Heterosexism in the Law

Historically, the U.S. legal system built upon religious heterosexism by defining homosexuality mainly in terms of criminality, omitting consideration of same-sex relationships from family law and policy and condoning or encouraging discrimination against sexual minorities. Legal prohibitions that codify stigma have taken at least three forms: (1) laws that prohibit or restrict private sexual *acts* between consenting adults; (2) laws that specifically deny basic civil liberties to gay and lesbian *individuals*; and (3) laws that reinforce the *power differential* at the heart of stigma.

Continuing the religious traditions, laws criminalized sodomy in France and Spain during the early thirteenth century, in Italian cities such as Florence, Siena, and Venice during the fourteenth century, in the Holy Roman Empire and England during the sixteenth century, and in Prussia and Denmark during the seventeenth century (Fone, 2000). Approximately 350 men were prosecuted for sodomy in The Netherlands between 1730 and 1732 following the discovery of "a nationwide network of sodomites, including men from all social strata" (Van der Meer, 1993, p. 141). At least 75 of those men were executed. By the late eighteenth century, women also were prosecuted solely because they had sex with other women (Van der Meer, 1993).

Many of the American colonies enacted stiff criminal penalties for sodomy (which the statutes often described only in Latin or with oblique phrases such as "the unmentionable vice" or "wickedness not to be named"), and the purview of these laws included homosexual conduct. Men were executed for sodomy in colonial Virginia in 1624 and in New Haven and New Netherland in 1646 (Katz, 1976). Except for a brief period when the New Haven colony penalized "women lying with women," sodomy laws in the American colonies applied exclusively to acts initiated by men—whether with another man, a woman, a girl, a boy, or an animal (Chauncey, 2004). The colonial laws gave rise to state sodomy statutes during the 1700s and 1800s, some of which survived until the U.S. Supreme Court ruled them unconstitutional in 2003 (Lawrence et al. v. Texas, 2003).

During the early twentieth century, legal persecution began to extend beyond sexual behaviors to encompass gay and lesbian individuals and their communities. Solidification of the modern categories of homosexuality and heterosexuality, and the stigma attached to the former, were accelerated by events surrounding World War II. Prior to the declaration of war, civilian and military courts classified homosexual behavior as a criminal offense and subjected it to sanction, but homosexual individuals were not officially barred from military service (Haggerty, 2003). As the country mobilized and psychiatric screening became part of the induction process, however, psychiatry's then-dominant view of homosexuality as a psychopathology was introduced into the military. For the first time, the military sought to exclude homosexual persons from its ranks based on a medical rationale (Bérubé, 1990). During the War's early years, when the armed services' need for personnel was great, many homosexual individuals were inducted, allowed to enlist, or retained in the service, even after their sexual orientation became known to peers and superior officers. As personnel needs declined during the War's waning years, however, antihomosexual policies were enforced with increasing vigilance, and many gay and lesbian service members were involuntarily discharged as sexual psychopaths (Bérubé, 1990).

Around this time, stigma directed at people who assumed a homosexual identity intensified dramatically in civilian society, fueled by a series of sex crime panics and, in the postwar years, the McCarthy witch hunts (Johnson, 2004). Although law enforcement records do not indicate a rise in the number of sexual crimes during this era, the news media gave sensationalized coverage to several brutal sexual murders of children before and after the War. In response, the public called for government action against sexual deviants in what historians now refer to as sex crime panics (Freedman, 1989; Chauncey, 1993). In the public mind and in criminal statutes, homosexuals often were not differentiated from child molesters, rapists, and sexual murderers. All were officially labeled "sexual psychopaths." In the rising hysteria about sex crimes, gay people—whose fledgling urban communities made them visible to police and the public—were often targets of civic morality campaigns. Once arrested, they were subjected to the sexual psychopath statutes, which allowed indeterminate imprisonment until the individual was judged to be "cured" of her or his sexual deviance. Even those who escaped arrest often had their homosexuality publicly revealed, which could mean loss of employment, ostracism by friends and family, and public shame. Some committed suicide in response to (or in fear of) such stigma (Freedman, 1989; Chauncey, 1993).

The postwar sex crime panics had lasting effects on society. Most U.S. laws that specifically denied basic civil liberties to gay and lesbian individuals were passed during this period. They included laws denying licenses to "sexual deviates" in a variety of professions, ranging from cosmetology to law, as well as laws that forbade the sale of liquor to homosexuals and prohibited people from dancing in public with someone of the same sex; they even barred commercial establishments from creating settings in which homosexuals could congregate

(D'Emilio, 1983). It was also during this era that gay men came to be widely regarded as child molesters, a stereotype that antigay activists continue to promote (e.g., Cameron, 1994).

Sodomy laws had important effects that extended well beyond criminalizing specific sexual acts. They were used to justify discrimination against gay men and lesbians in employment, housing, services, and child custody. The threat of a felony conviction made many gay men and lesbians reluctant to act on their same-sex desires or acknowledge their identity. Thus, sodomy laws played an important role in keeping gay men and lesbians invisible (Leslie, 2000).

Today the U.S. legal system continues to reinforce the power differential at the heart of stigma through discriminatory statutes and the absence of laws protecting sexual minorities from discrimination in employment, housing, and services. Federal law does not prohibit antigay discrimination, but it expressly prohibits military personnel from engaging in sex with another person of the same sex, being involved in a homosexual relationship, or seeking to be married to a person of the same sex (U.S. Code 654, 1993). As of July, 2005, a total of 17 states had enacted antidiscrimination laws, most of which cover employment but not housing or services. Approximately 285 municipalities had passed local ordinances. Consequently, about half of the U.S. population was protected by some form of antidiscrimination law (National Gay and Lesbian Task Force, 2005c,d).

As of July 2005, two adults of the same sex were allowed to marry only in Massachusetts. At the federal level, the 1996 Defense of Marriage Act expressly defines marriage to exclude same-sex couples from federal benefits and stipulates that the states are not obligated to recognize same-sex marriages performed in other states. Most states have passed their own statutes banning marriage for same-sex couples or have amended their constitutions to define marriage as a heterosexual union. Several of these statutes and amendments prohibit domestic partnerships and civil unions as well. The U.S. Congress considered such an amendment in 2004, strongly supported by President Bush, but failed to pass it (Hulse, 2004; Peterson, 2004; National Gay and Lesbian Task Force, 2005a).

In the realm of parenting, same-sex couples are prohibited from adopting children in Utah and Mississippi, and gay and lesbian individuals are expressly forbidden by statute from any form of adoption in Florida. In roughly half of the states, a member of a same-sex couple can establish a parental relationship with a partner's biological or adoptive child through a procedure called second-parent adoption. However, courts in several states (including Nebraska, Colorado, Ohio, and Wisconsin) have ruled that second-parent adoption is not permissible under current statute, and adoption law in most other states is unclear about the permissibility of second-parent adoption (Patterson et al., 2002; National Gay and Lesbian Task Force, 2005e).

To the extent that the law creates barriers to same-sex couples creating a life together, grants fewer rights and privileges to same-sex couples than to their heterosexual counterparts, and discriminates against families headed by same-sex couples, it stigmatizes individuals in committed same-sex relationships. Legal prohibitions against marriage by same-sex couples effectively declare that homosexual relationships are considered inferior to heterosexual relationships and that individuals in same-sex relationships are inherently less deserving of society's recognition than heterosexual couples. They single out gay people for special ostracism, marginalizing their relationships and providing a justification for the overall stigma that society directs against them. Thus, the legal system is an important institution through which stigma is expressed and reinforced. Laws are enacted and enforced to systematically deny stigmatized outgroups access to resources and benefits that the ingroup enjoys. In addition to controlling access to valuable resources, laws that advantage one group over another also send a message to society about the relative status of the ingroup and outgroup. Moreover, they provide a justification for the unequal status of the outgroup.

3.3 Heterosexism in Psychiatry and Psychology

During the nineteenth century, medicine and psychiatry began to compete successfully with religion and the law for jurisdiction over sexuality. As a consequence, discourse about homosexuality expanded beyond the realms of sin and crime to include pathology. The expansion of discourse about homosexuality from the realms of sin and crime to that of pathology was generally considered progressive at the time because a sick person was less blameful than a sinner or criminal (e.g., Chauncey, 1982–1983; D'Emilio & Freedman, 1988; Duberman et al., 1989). It was also around this time that the idea that individuals could be defined in terms of their sexual attractions and behaviors—that is, the modern notions of "the homosexual" and "the heterosexual"— began to emerge in medical discourse.

From the outset, homosexuality was defined in opposition to normalcy. Karl Maria Benkert, the Hungarian writer widely credited with coining the term *homosexual* in 1869, originally contrasted it to *normalsexual*. *Heterosexual* did not emerge until later as the preferred term for describing sexual attraction to and behavior with the other sex (Dynes, 1985). Even within medicine and psychiatry, however, homosexuality was not universally viewed as pathology during the early twentieth century. Richard von Krafft-Ebing described it as a degenerative sickness in his *Psychopathia Sexualis*, but Havelock Ellis urged that homosexuality be considered a normal variant of human behavior, like left-handedness (Krafft-Ebing, 1900; Ellis, 1901). Sigmund Freud (1953) believed that homosexuality represented a less than optimal outcome for psychosexual development but nevertheless asserted in a now-famous 1935 letter that "it is nothing to be ashamed of, no vice, no degradation, it cannot be classified as an illness" (Freud, 1951, p. 786).

"Sexual inversion" preceded "homosexuality" as a topic of medical and scientific scrutiny. During the 1860s, Karl Ulrichs, a German activist and himself a homosexual, was the first writer to discuss inversion in a public forum outside the medical profession. He proposed that male inverts, or "Urnings," should be understood as "individuals who are born with the sexual drive of women and who have male bodies" (Ulrichs, 1994, vol. 1, p. 35). Ulrichs' theory was adopted by the next generation of "homosexual" activists, including his countryman Magnus Hirschfeld. The latter argued that inverts represented an intermediate sex, combining the psychic qualities of both male and female (Hirschfeld, 2000).

As Chauncey (1982–1983) explained, sexual inversion originally described the totality of the individual including but not limited to her or his sexual conduct. Male inverts were believed to be passive, effeminate, and weak. Their sexual attraction to "masculine" males followed naturally from these characteristics, but they were also assumed to be attracted in many cases to dominant ("masculine") females. Female inverts were believed to be active, in contrast to what was considered normal feminine passivity. Because women were regarded as lacking sexual passion, female inverts were considered abnormal simply because they manifested any sexual attractions. Whether these attractions were to men or to women was less important than the fact that they displayed an active sexuality (Chauncey, 1982–1983).

Freud's (1953) conceptualization of homosexuality, articulated in 1905 in the first of his *Three Essays on the Theory of Sexuality*, dramatically changed thinking about inversion and sexual orientation. Freud introduced a distinction between preferences for particular types of sexual activity (sexual aim) and the kind of person or thing toward whom (or which) the sexual aim was directed (sexual object). Whereas the notion of the sexual invert focused on the individual's sexual aim (passive sexuality among male inverts, active sexuality among females), Freud's focus on the sexual object eventually prevailed. "Homosexuals" came to be understood entirely in terms of their sexual object choice (i.e., a person of the same sex), and the construct of the invert fell into disuse (Freud, 1953; Chauncey, 1982–1983).

The view of homosexuality as pathology became entrenched in the period between World Wars I and II. It was around this time that many American psychoanalysts began to reject Freud's beliefs about the inherent bisexuality of humans. They argued instead that homosexuality is a pathological departure from the natural state of heterosexuality that resulted from pathological family relationships, and that it represents a phobic response to members of the other sex. This position soon became dominant in American psychoanalysis (Bayer, 1987; Silverstein, 1991). As noted above, it also became part of official U.S. military policies concerning homosexuality. By 1942, revised army mobilization regulations included a paragraph defining both the homosexual and the "normal" person and clarifying procedures for rejecting gay draftees (Bérubé, 1990). In 1952, the first edition of the *Diagnostic and Statistical Manual of Mental Disorders* (DSM) presented a systematic approach to psychiatric diagnosis. Reflecting then-prevalent assumptions, homosexuality was included under the category of sociopathic personality disturbances (American Psychiatric Association, 1952).

If homosexuality was a pathology, the logical response was to cure or prevent it. Large numbers of homosexual men and women spent countless hours in psychotherapy in what proved to be, for most, a vain attempt to change their sexual orientation (Haldeman, 1991). When psychotherapy did not work, many tried more drastic methods, including hypnosis, administration of hormones, aversive conditioning with electric shock or nausea-inducing drugs, lobotomy, electroshock, and castration (Katz, 1976).

Just as the sodomy laws had widespread effects that did not depend on their actual enforcement, the classification of homosexuality as a mental illness played an important role in rationalizing sexual stigma and creating specific ways in which it could be enacted. The pathologization of homosexuality provided an important justification for barring homosexual individuals from many occupations, denying them child custody, and generally treating them as inferior to heterosexuals. Individual homosexuals who did not seek cure or who refused to conceal their sexuality were seen as deserving little sympathy.

Although the assumption that homosexuality was a sickness enjoyed widespread acceptance during the 1950s, challenges to the psychiatric orthodoxy soon emerged. One of the first and most famous of these came in the empirical research of psychologist Evelyn Hooker. Her landmark study (Hooker, 1957) was innovative in several important respects. First, rather than simply accepting the predominant view of homosexuality as pathology, she posed the question of whether homosexuals and heterosexuals actually differed in their psychological adjustment. Second, rather than studying psychiatric patients, she recruited a sample of homosexual men who were functioning normally in society. Third, she employed a procedure whereby disinterested experts rated the adjustment of her research participants without prior knowledge of their sexual orientation. This method addressed an important source of bias that was common in previous studies of homosexuality.

Hooker administered three projective tests—Rorschach, Thematic Apperception Test (TAT), and Make-A-Picture-Story (MAPS) Test—to 30 homosexual males and 30 heterosexual males recruited through community organizations and matched for age, intelligence quotient (IQ), and education. None of the men was in therapy at the time of the study. Unaware of each subject's sexual orientation, two independent Rorschach experts evaluated the men's overall adjustment using a 5-point scale and ultimately classified two-thirds of the heterosexuals and two-thirds of the homosexuals in the three highest categories of adjustment. When asked to identify which Rorschach protocols were obtained from homosexuals, the experts could not distinguish respondents' sexual orientation at a level better than chance. A third expert used the TAT and MAPS protocols to evaluate the men's psychological adjustment. As with the Rorschach responses, the adjustment ratings of the homosexuals and heterosexuals did not differ significantly. Hooker concluded from her data that homosexuality as a clinical entity does not exist, and that it is not inherently associated with psychopathology.

Hooker's basic findings were subsequently replicated by other investigators using a variety of research methods. Freedman (1971), for example, adapted Hooker's design to study lesbian and heterosexual women. Instead of projective tests, he administered objectively scored personality tests to the women. His conclusions were similar to those of Hooker (Freedman, 1971). Today, a large body of published empirical research clearly refutes the notion that homosexuality per se is indicative of psychopathology (Hart et al., 1978; Riess, 1980; Gonsiorek, 1991).

Confronted with the overwhelming empirical evidence and changing cultural views of homosexuality, psychiatrists and psychologists radically altered their stance during the latter decades of the twentieth century. In 1973, the Board of Directors of the American Psychiatric Association voted to remove homosexuality from the DSM. In response to this action, a faction of psychiatrists who opposed the change instigated a vote of the Association's entire membership in 1974. That vote, however, supported the Board's decision.

Subsequently, a new diagnosis, ego-dystonic homosexuality, was created for the DSM's third edition in 1980. Ego dystonic homosexuality was said to be indicated by: (1) persistent lack of heterosexual arousal, which the patient experienced as interfering with initiation or maintenance of wanted heterosexual relationships; and (2) persistent distress from a sustained pattern of unwanted homosexual arousal. The new diagnostic category, however, was criticized professionally on numerous grounds. It was viewed by many as a political compromise to appease the psychiatrists—mainly psychoanalysts—who still considered homosexuality a pathology. Others questioned the appropriateness of having a separate diagnosis that described the content of an individual's dysphoria. They argued that the psychological problems related to ego-dystonic homosexuality could be addressed just as well by other general diagnostic categories, and that the existence of the diagnosis perpetuated sexual stigma. Moreover, widespread prejudice against homosexuality in the United States meant that "almost all people who are homosexual first go through a phase in which their homosexuality is ego dystonic," according to the American Psychiatric Association (1987, p. 426). In 1986, the diagnosis was removed entirely from the DSM. The only vestige of ego-dystonic homosexuality in the revised DSM-III occurred under Sexual Disorders Not Otherwise Specified, which included persistent and marked distress about one's sexual orientation (American Psychiatric Association, 1987; see Bayer, 1987, for an account of the events leading up to the 1973 and 1986 decisions). The American Psychological Association (APA) promptly endorsed the psychiatrists' actions and has since worked intensively to eradicate the stigma historically associated with a homosexual orientation (Conger, 1975; Morin & Rothblum, 1991).

Thus, the medical and scientific institutions that provided much of the ideological rationale for stigmatizing homosexuality during the first half of the twentieth century displayed a remarkable reversal in the latter third of the century. Although some religiously oriented therapists still dissent, the dominant position among contemporary clinicians and researchers is that homosexuality is a normal variant of human sexual expression that is no more inherently associated with psychopathology than is heterosexuality. This shift has played an important role in influencing societal attitudes and in providing a basis for reversing many of the antigay policies and laws that were enacted earlier in the twentieth century (e.g., Zaller, 1992).

4 Experience of Sexual Stigma Among Sexual Minority Individuals

Recognition that sexual stigma impinges on the lives of sexual minority individuals has led to the development of theoretical models for understanding minority stress, that is, the stress uniquely experienced by minority group members as a result of their stigmatized status (Brooks, 1981; Meyer, 1995, 2003; DiPlacido, 1998). Meyer (1995) proposed three key minority stressors for gay, lesbian, and bisexual people: (1) external, objective stressful events and conditions; (2) the minority individual's expectations of such events and the vigilance this expectation requires; and (3) the minority individual's internalization of negative societal attitudes. These sources of stress correspond to the present chapter's constructs of (1) sexual stigma, (2) stigma awareness and felt stigma, and (3) internalized homophobia. With the previous section's discussion of sexual stigma as a backdrop, we address the latter two processes of minority stress in the present section.

4.1 Stigma Awareness and Felt Stigma

Felt stigma refers to an individual's subjective experience of stigma, including her or his awareness of its prevalence and manifestations (Scambler & Hopkins, 1986; Scambler, 1989). Scambler (1989) offered the insight that for some members of stigmatized groups the consequences of felt stigma can be even more profound than those of enacted stigma (e.g., employment discrimination, physical attack). This is because felt stigma often motivates individuals with a stigmatized condition to engage in preemptive, protective behaviors to avoid enactments of stigma. For example, they may avoid contact with the nonstigmatized majority or may attempt to pass as members of that majority. Such strategies can reduce the likelihood of experiencing overt enactments of stigma but can also significantly disrupt the lives of the stigmatized, narrow their options, and increase their psychological distress.

Writing about epilepsy, Scambler and Hopkins (1986) proposed that "felt stigma refers principally to the fear of enacted stigma, but also encompasses a feeling of shame associated with being epileptic." This conceptualization implies three components for felt stigma, which have counterparts in the psychological literature.

First, the underlying basis of felt stigma is knowledge about a stigma's existence and the forms in which it is enacted as well as the beliefs and expectancies about the likelihood of stigma enactments in various circumstances. Those expectancies, as Scambler explained, can be more or less accurate among both the stigmatized and the nonstigmatized. We have referred to this knowledge in the present chapter as stigma awareness.

Second, felt stigma involves stigmatized individuals' desire to avoid enactments of stigma, which is the motivational basis for modifying their behavior. Scambler and Hopkins (1986) characterized this desire in terms of fear. Whereas the emotion of fear may indeed be a response to the anticipation of enacted stigma, this need not always be so. Instead of fear, we propose that the expectation of an enactment of stigma can better be considered a potential stressor that can elicit different emotional responses in different individuals.

Conceptualized as a potential stressor, felt stigma can be considered in terms of psychological theories of stress and coping (Lazarus & Folkman, 1984; Miller & Major, 2000; Meyer, 2003). Within this framework, stigma can be seen as leading an individual to appraise both the threat posed by a social situation and her or his options and resources for avoiding harm. If a situation is evaluated as stressful—that is, if the threat exceeds the individual's available resources for responding to it—the individual engages in some form of coping behavior. Coping can be problem-focused or emotion-focused, and it can be prospective or reactive.

Scambler's model posits that felt stigma motivates an individual to avoid situations in which enactments of stigma are possible, that is, to employ a strategy of proactive coping (Aspinwall & Taylor, 1997). These self-protective behaviors are often in tune with social realities. To the extent that the individual accurately assesses the risks for enactments of stigma in her or his social environment, this appraisal process can minimize her or his risks for discrimination and attack and thus can be highly adaptive.

In the most influential theoretical account of stigma, Goffman (1963) discussed a variety of stigma management strategies. He observed that the primary challenge in social interactions faced by persons with a concealable stigma is to control who knows about their stigmatized status. He referred to persons with a concealable stigma as the *discreditable* to highlight the importance of such information management. As the term discreditable suggests, having one's stigma revealed to others often carries negative consequences, ranging from having social stereotypes inaccurately applied to oneself, to social ostracism and discrimination, to outright physical attack. Once an individual's stigma is revealed, according to Goffman (1963), he or she becomes one of the *discredited*, and her or his primary task in social interaction shifts from managing personal information to attempting to influence how others use that information in forming impressions about her or him.

Gay men and lesbians frequently find this task complicated by the widespread perception that acknowledging one's homosexual orientation to others is a highly intimate disclosure, unlike routine acknowledgments of heterosexuality (e.g., mentioning or introducing one's spouse to others). When they self-disclose, gay people are likely to be regarded as inappropriately flaunting their sexuality. By contrast, heterosexuals' self-disclosures about their sexual orientation occur routinely, even during casual interactions with strangers; and they are usually not considered noteworthy because everyone is presumed to be heterosexual. This asymmetry creates difficulties in maintaining reciprocal levels of self-disclosure in social interactions between heterosexuals and homosexuals (Herek, 1996).

Moreover, once a person is known to be homosexual, that fact is regarded by others as the most (or one of the most) important pieces of information they possess about her or him. It establishes this individual as a member of the outgroup, relative to heterosexuals, and colors all other information about her or him, even information totally unrelated to sexual orientation. The individual's uniqueness is likely to be ignored or minimized, and she or he is likely to be perceived as highly similar to all other gay, lesbian, or bisexual people.

Consequently, stereotypes about homosexuals are likely to be applied to the individual. A *stereotype* is a fixed belief that all or most members of a particular group share a characteristic that is unrelated to their group membership (e.g., that Blacks are lazy or Jews are greedy). Some stereotypes of gay men and lesbians also are commonly applied to other disliked minority groups in this and other cultures. They include the stereotypes that members of the minority are hypersexual; a threat to society's most vulnerable members (e.g., children); secretive, clannish, and untrustworthy; and physically or mentally sick (Adam, 1978; Gilman, 1985; Herek, 2002a). Other stereotypes are more specific to homosexuality, such as the beliefs that gay men are effeminate, and lesbians are masculine (e.g., Kite & Deaux, 1987; Herek, 2002a).

Stereotypes foster distortions in how majority group members process information about minority individuals. Heterosexuals who hold stereotypes about sexual minorities tend to perceive and remember information about gay, lesbian, and bisexual individuals that is consistent with their stereotypes. They tend to selectively notice behaviors and characteristics that fit with their preconceived beliefs about gay men or lesbians while failing to notice behaviors and characteristics that are inconsistent with those beliefs (a phenomenon labeled *selective perception*). When they are trying to remember information about a gay person, their recollections and guesses about that individual tend to fit with their preconceived beliefs (*selective recall*). (See, for example, Snyder & Uranowitz, 1978; Gross et al., 1980; and Herek, 1991).

The foregoing discussion might be read as suggesting that hiding their stigmatized status is the safest strategy for gay men and lesbians. Passing as a nonstigmatized person, however, requires considerable effort, constant vigilance, and effective deployment of a variety of strategies. These strategies can include *discretion* (i.e., simply refraining from disclosing personal information to others), *concealment* (actively preventing others from acquiring information about oneself), and *fabrication* (deliberately providing false information about oneself to others) (Zerubavel, 1982). Whichever strategies are used, "passing" requires the individual to lead a kind of double life (e.g., Ponse, 1976). It interferes with normal social interaction, creates a multitude of practical problems, and requires psychological and physical work.

Moreover, attempts to pass are not always successful. Lesbians and gay men often find that others have acquired information about their homosexuality through astute observation, from a third party, or simply by guessing (Herek & Capitanio, 1996). Even when they can pass, many gay people find the process personally objectionable. Thus, they reveal their status to others to facilitate honest relationships, to make their lives simpler, to avoid the stress associated with passing, to enhance their own self-esteem while overcoming the negative psychological effects of stigmatization, and to change societal attitudes and help others who share their stigma (for further discussion of the reasons for coming out, see Herek, 1996).

4.2 Internalized Stigma and "Internalized Homophobia"

Stigma management strategies can afford protection from enactments of stigma. However, internalizing society's negative attitudes toward sexual minorities, accepting them as deserved, and consequently feeling negative attitudes toward the self (e.g., shame) are likely to be maladaptive. Weinberg (1972), who coined the term homophobia, originally defined it to encompass the self-hatred that homosexuals themselves sometimes manifest, which he labeled "internalized homophobia" (p. 83). According to Weinberg (1972), "the person who from early life has loathed himself for homosexual urges arrives at this attitude by a process exactly like the one occurring in heterosexuals who hold the prejudice against homosexuals" (p. 74). This process, he explained, involves forming impressions about homosexuality in a cultural context that is "almost wholly derogatory" (p. 74). Especially for boys, those impressions become the basis for actions, such as ridiculing suspected homosexuals (Kimmel, 1997).

Using a psychodynamic perspective, Malyon (1981–1982) described the development and operation of internalized homophobia in gay men. According to his analysis, internalized homophobia is based on "the mythology and opprobrium which characterize current social attitudes toward homosexuality" (*exogenous homophobia*) which are internalized by "the incipient homosexual individual" during the course of socialization (Malyon, 1981–1982, p. 60). Malyon argued that internalized homophobia exists in the form of conscious antigay attitudes, which he believed could be modified fairly easily in the course of psychotherapy, and more pernicious unconscious introjections. The latter give rise to "low self-esteem, lack of psychological congruity and integration, overly embellished and ossified defenses, problems with intimacy, and a particular vulnerability to depression" (Malyon, 1981–1982, p. 65).

The notion that members of a stigmatized group experience psychological difficulties as a consequence of accepting society's negative evaluation of them is not unique to sexual minorities. Allport (1954) observed that racial, ethnic, and religious minority group members often develop defenses for coping with prejudice, noting that "since no one can be indifferent to the abuse and expectations of others we must anticipate that ego defensiveness will frequently be found among members of groups that are set off for ridicule, disparagement, and discrimination. It could not be otherwise" (Allport, 1954, p. 143). Allport distinguished defenses directed at the source of discrimination (*extropunitive*) from those that are inwardly focused (*intropunitive*). Relevant to internalized homophobia, the latter category includes the defense of identification with the dominant group, leading to self-hate, which can involve "one's sense of shame for possessing the despised qualities of one's group" as well as "repugnance for other members of one's group because they 'possess' these qualities" (Allport, 1954, p. 152).

In contrast to the hostility that heterosexuals direct at homosexuals (i.e., exogenous homophobia), internalized homophobia necessarily involves an intrapsychic conflict between what people think they should be (i.e., heterosexual) and how they experience their own sexuality (i.e., as homosexual or bisexual). Weinberg (1972) prescribed multiple strategies for addressing this conflict, all based on a model of acting in accordance with the attitude one wants to adopt toward the self.

Internalized homophobia has also been labeled *internalized heterosexism* (Szymanski & Chung, 2003) or *internalized homonegativity* (Mayfield, 2001; Currie et al., 2004; Tozer & Hayes, 2004). Whatever it is called, mental health practitioners and researchers generally agree that negative feelings about one's own homosexual desires lie at the core of this phenomenon (Williamson, 2000) but they vary widely in how they conceptualize and operationalize it (Shidlo, 1994; Herek et al., 1998). Based on Malyon's (1981–1982) formulation, we might expect the principal manifestations of internalized homophobia to be negative affect directed at the self and a desire to be heterosexual. In practice, however, internalized homophobia has been operationally defined not only as dislike of one's own homosexual feelings and behaviors but also as hostile and rejecting attitudes toward other gay people, unwillingness to disclose one's homosexuality to others, perceptions of stigma associated with being homosexual, and acceptance of societal stereotypes about homosexuality (Wolcott et al., 1986; Nicholson & Long, 1990; Lima et al., 1993; Ross & Rosser, 1996; Wagner et al., 1996; Szymanski & Chung, 2001; Currie et al., 2004). Many of these constructs might more appropriately be considered correlates or consequences rather than manifestations of internalized homophobia (Shidlo, 1994). Despite the lack of consensus about the definition, the operationalization, and even the labeling of internalized homophobia, negative attitudes toward oneself that are rooted in sexual stigma are likely to have important consequences for physical and psychological well-being (for reviews, see Williamson, 2000; Meyer, 2003).

5 Internalization of Sexual Stigma Among Heterosexuals: Sexual Prejudice

Sexual prejudice is the internalization of sexual stigma by heterosexuals resulting in hostility and negative attitudes toward sexual minorities (Herek, 2004). Although sexual prejudice remains widespread in the

United States, heterosexuals' attitudes toward lesbians and gay men have become somewhat more accepting in recent years, especially in the realms of civil rights and the right to freedom from employment discrimination. Most adult Americans still regard homosexual behavior as immoral, but the trend appears to be in the direction of less condemnation. In the next section, we briefly review public opinion data about the nature and prevalence of sexual prejudice.[3]

5.1 Extent and Manifestations of Sexual Prejudice

5.1.1 Homosexual Behavior

Since the early 1970s, the National Opinion Research Center (NORC) at the University of Chicago has included questions about homosexuality in its General Social Survey (GSS), an ongoing, face-to-face national poll. One item asks whether sexual relations between two adults of the same sex are "always wrong, almost always wrong, wrong only sometimes, or not wrong at all." Between 1973 and 1993, more than two-thirds of the public considered homosexuality to be "always wrong." The proportion responding "never" or "only sometimes" wrong ranged around 20%. During the early 1990s, however, a shift occurred in responses to this item. The proportion saying homosexual behavior is "always wrong" began to decline in 1993, dropping to 54% in 1998, and has remained fairly stable since then. Although most still regard homosexual behavior as wrong, the trend clearly has been in the direction of less condemnation.

This question's phrasing may bias responses because it frames homosexual relations as wrong to at least some extent. Nevertheless, data from other surveys with differently worded items assessing the morality of homosexual behavior have yielded similar findings. In national Gallup polls between 2001 and 2005, for example, 52% to 55% of respondents believed that homosexual behavior is morally wrong, whereas 38% to 44% believed it is not morally wrong (Saad, 2005).

Gallup polls have also assessed opinions about whether homosexuality should be considered an acceptable alternative life-style. Responses to this item between 1982 and 1992 indicated a roughly 3:2 ratio of no/yes responses. By a margin of 17 points (51–34%), respondents did not consider homosexuality an acceptable life-style in 1982. In 1992, the margin was 19 points (57–38%). By May 2003, however, 54% considered homosexuality an acceptable life-style compared to 43% who regarded it as unacceptable. Except for a brief fluctuation immediately after the U.S. Supreme Court's 2003 Lawrence v. Texas ruling (when 49% of those surveyed thought that homosexuality was unacceptable compared to 46% who thought it acceptable), this pattern has held. In May 2005, a total of 51% of respondents considered homosexuality an acceptable life-style, whereas 45% regarded it unacceptable.

---

[3]Unless otherwise indicated, public opinion data reported here were obtained from the Public Opinion On-Line database at the Roper Center (http://roperweb.ropercenter.uconn.edu/).

The Gallup poll also has asked whether homosexual relations between consenting adults should or should not be legal. This issue has displayed greater volatility than any of those considered above. In 1977, respondents were evenly split, with 43% favoring legalization and 43% opposing it. By 1982, a plurality favored legalization (45–39% opposed). During the mid-1980s, however, the trend sharply reversed, probably due in part to public concerns about the acquired immune deficiency syndrome (AIDS) epidemic, which in the United States disproportionately affected gay and bisexual men. In 1986, for example, only 32% supported legalizing homosexual relations, whereas 57% opposed it. That was also the year in which the U.S. Supreme Court upheld the right of states to enact sodomy laws (Bowers v. Hardwick, 1986). During the 1990s, public opinion about consensual same-sex relations fluctuated, with a plurality of Americans favoring legalization in 1992 (48–44%) but a similar plurality opposing it in 1996 (47–44%). In 1999, half (50%) of the Gallup respondents favored legalization, compared to 43% who opposed it. By 2001, there were 54% who favored legalization, and 42% who opposed it.

At the time of the Supreme Court's 2003 Lawrence v. Texas ruling, 60% favored legalization of same-sex relations compared to 35% who opposed legalization. In the wake of that ruling, however, responses indicated increased opposition to legalizing same-sex relations. Interpreting these data is made more difficult by the fact that the national debate about same-sex marriage grew in intensity during this period. Interpretation of terms such as "same-sex relations" and "homosexual relations" may have been influenced by this debate. Some poll respondents may have equated these terms with same-sex relationships rather than private, consensual sexual activity. At the beginning of 2004, the public was closely divided as to whether homosexual relations between consenting adults should or should not be legal. By May of that year, however, legalization was again favored by most (52%), a finding that held in another survey conducted in May 2005.

5.1.2 Sexual Prejudice Targeting Lesbians and Gay Men
The GSS regularly includes three items concerning respondents' willingness to grant basic free speech rights to "a man who admits that he is a homosexual." Respondents are asked if they would allow such a man to "make a speech in your community" or "teach in a college or university" and if they would favor removing "a book he wrote in favor of homosexuality" from the public library. Even in 1973, responses to these items showed fairly strong support for First Amendment rights in connection with homosexuality. That year, 61% would have allowed a homosexual man to speak, 47% would have allowed him to teach in a college, and 54% would have opposed censoring a book that he wrote in favor of homosexuality. By 2002, the proportions endorsing First Amendment rights regarding homosexuality had grown to 84% for speech, 78% for teaching, and 75% against library censorship. The percentage of respondents opposing rights for a male homosexual showed a corresponding decrease.

The Gallup poll also assessed attitudes toward equal employment opportunities. Support for equal rights in job opportunities generally has increased steadily and dramatically: from 56% in 1977 to 87% in 2005. The proportion opposing employment rights was initially in the minority (33% in 1977) and decreased even further over time to 11% in 2005. The public's support for employment equality has been somewhat less enthusiastic when questions are asked about specific occupations. Nevertheless, the trend over the past quarter century still has been toward steadily increasing support. One of the most remarkable changes has been in the proportion of Americans who believe homosexuals should be hired as elementary school teachers: It grew from 27% in 1977 to 54% in 2005. This trend has also been documented by the Pew Research Center for the People and the Press. Their national polls show that the proportion of U.S. adults who believe that school boards should be able to fire "teachers who are known homosexuals" dropped from 51% in 1987 to 33% in 2003. The proportion who disagreed rose from 42% to 62% during that period.

In contrast to the public's generally strong support for employment rights, opposition to marriage equality for same-sex couples has been widespread. Gallup polls conducted between 2000 and 2005 found that between 55% and 68% (median 61%) of respondents believed "marriages between homosexuals" should not be "recognized by the law as valid, with the same rights as traditional marriages," whereas 28% to 42% (median 34%) believed such marriages should be valid (Saad, 2005). Similarly, a July 2005 poll by the Pew Research Center found that 53% of respondents opposed "allowing gays and lesbians to marry legally" compared to 36% who supported marriage rights (Pew Research Center, 2005). Interestingly, the greatest support for marriage equality (42%) was recorded in a 2004 Gallup survey in which the marriage question was asked after a series of questions on gay rights, suggesting that attitudes toward marriage may be affected by the broader frame in which the issue is considered.

5.2 Correlates of Sexual Prejudice Targeting Gay Men and Lesbians

Empirical research shows that heterosexuals' attitudes toward gay men and lesbians are consistently correlated with various demographic, psychological, and social variables. In contrast to heterosexuals with favorable attitudes toward gay people, those with negative attitudes are more likely to be men, older, less well educated, and residing in geographic areas where negative attitudes represent the norm (e.g., rural areas or the midwestern or southern United States). They are more likely to attend religious services frequently, more likely to endorse orthodox religious beliefs such as the literal truth of the Bible, more likely to be Republican than Democrat or Independent, and more likely to describe themselves as politically conservative rather than liberal or moderate. They tend to display higher levels of psychological authoritarianism, are less sexually permissive, and are more supportive of traditional gender roles. They are more likely to believe that a homosexual orientation is freely chosen and less likely to have had close personal friends or family members who are openly lesbian or gay (e.g., Herek, 1984, 1994).

Interpretation of these patterns requires caution because the data are correlational. For example, the belief that homosexuality is freely chosen is consistently associated with higher levels of sexual prejudice. This relationship may mean that believing homosexuality is a choice causes a heterosexual person to hold negative attitudes toward gay men and lesbians, consistent with the tenets of attribution theory (e.g., Weiner, 1995). Alternatively, it may mean that people who hold negative attitudes are more receptive to beliefs that seem to attach blame to gay men and lesbians. Yet a third factor may be involved. In the United States, for example, White heterosexuals who believe that sexual orientation is not a matter of personal choice are substantially more likely than those who believe homosexuality is chosen to have one or more close gay or lesbian friends (Herek & Capitanio, 1995). This pattern suggests that the relationship between attributions of choice and attitudes toward gay people may result mainly from a third variable— personal contact with openly gay men and lesbians.

5.3 Sexual Prejudice Targeting Bisexual Men and Women

Sexual prejudice targeting bisexuals overlaps in many ways with antigay prejudice (e.g., Ochs, 1996). Bisexuals have commented that heterosexuals appear to regard them as homosexuals, which suggests that expressions of hostility toward bisexuals are often rooted in antigay attitudes (e.g., Weinberg et al., 1994; Rust, 2000). It is not surprising, therefore, that the few published studies in this area have found significant correlations between heterosexuals' attitudes toward bisexuals and their attitudes toward lesbians and gay men (Eliason, 1997; Mohr & Rochlen, 1999). Among the possible reasons for this pattern are that many heterosexuals may equate bisexuality with sexual promiscuity or nonmonogamy; bisexual men and women might be regarded as vectors of human immunodeficiency virus (HIV) infection or other sexually transmitted diseases (STDs); and bisexuals might be a source of anxiety or discomfort because they are perceived as challenging the widely accepted heterosexual-homosexual dichotomy of sexuality (Herek, 2002b; for discussion of these and other reasons, see Paul & Nichols, 1988; Ochs & Deihl, 1992; Ochs, 1996; Paul, 1996; Rust, 1996).

In a national telephone survey, Herek (2002b) found that bisexual men and women were rated more negatively than gay men and lesbians (see also Eliason, 1997; Spalding & Peplau, 1997). In the same survey, more negative attitudes toward bisexuals were associated with higher age, less education, lower annual income, residence in the South and rural areas, higher religiosity, political conservatism, traditional values concerning gender and sexual behavior, authoritarianism, and lack of contact with gay men or lesbians. White heterosexual women expressed significantly more favorable attitudes than other women and all men. A gender difference was observed in attitudes toward bisexuals and homosexuals: Heterosexual women rated bisexuals significantly less favorably than they rated homosexuals, regardless of gender, whereas heterosexual men rated sexual minority males less favorably than sexual minority females, regardless of whether the target was bisexual or homosexual.

6 Consequences of Sexual Stigma: Two Examples

Sexual stigma—acting through heterosexism at the institutional level and sexual prejudice at the individual level—affects the lives of gay, lesbian, and bisexual people in a variety of ways. We conclude this chapter by considering two examples of such impact: economic discrimination and antigay violence.

6.1 Economic Discrimination

A stereotype widely disseminated by both the Christian Right and marketing professionals is that gay men and lesbians are more affluent than heterosexuals and have larger disposable incomes that can be spent on luxury consumer goods and services (DeLozier & Rodrigue, 1996; Herman, 1997). This claim has been used, on the one hand, to foster resentment against gay people and buttress the claim that antidiscrimination laws amount to special rights (Herman, 1997) and, on the other hand, to urge corporations to market their products to the gay and lesbian community (Badgett, 1997). To the extent that it is based on empirical evidence, the claim of gay affluence is derived mainly from marketing surveys conducted with convenience samples of gay men and lesbians drawn from magazine subscriber lists, organizational memberships, and similar sources. Such samples are highly problematic because they overrepresent the affluent (Badgett, 1997; Baker, 1997).

Moreover, a variety of factors might affect the earnings of gay men and lesbians. Marital status is reliably associated with income: Married men have higher average incomes than unmarried men, and married couples generally have more household income than singles or cohabiting adults (e.g., Loh, 1996; Stack & Eshleman, 1998). Because people of the same sex are barred from marrying in all states except Massachusetts, gay and lesbian couples would not be expected to benefit from this marriage premium. Income also is affected by education, location of residence, and occupation. Compared to heterosexuals, gay men and lesbians might attain a higher level of formal education (e.g., Rothblum & Factor, 2001) and might be more likely to reside in areas where incomes are higher, such as large urban centers (e.g., Laumann et al., 1994). At the same time, they might sacrifice financial rewards for careers in lower-paying occupations where tolerance of sexual minorities is high (Badgett & King, 1997). Finally, because men generally earn more than women, any discussion of the earnings of sexual minorities must consider the incomes of gay men separately from those of lesbians (for further discussion of these issues, see: Klawitter & Flatt, 1998; Badgett, 2001).

Thus, comparing the incomes of lesbians and gay men with their heterosexual counterparts is a complex task, one made even more difficult by the lack of extensive data on respondents' sexual orientation and income from probability samples. To address this problem, economists and demographers have used a variety of available data sets. They include data on sexual behavior from ongoing national surveys with large cumulative samples (mainly the GSS) and U.S. Census data, which included questions about cohabitation with a same-sex partner in 1990 and 2000. Both types of data have limitations. Inferring a person's identity as gay, lesbian, or bisexual from their self-reported sexual behavior inevitably leads to misclassifications (because, for example, some self-identified heterosexuals have engaged in homosexual behavior and some self-identified gay people are celibate). The census data do not identify gay, lesbian, and bisexual people not residing with a same-sex partner. Even cohabiting couples are not detected by the census if one member is not the head of the household. Moreover, both types of sample are affected by underreporting. Given the pervasiveness of sexual stigma, many people who are in a same-sex relationship or who self-identify as gay, lesbian, or bisexual are simply unwilling to disclose their status to researchers. Nevertheless, with appropriate recognition of the data's limitations and controls for other relevant variables, findings from high-quality probability samples can be validly generalized to the population. By contrast, the validity of generalizations from data obtained from convenience samples cannot be known.

Because the patterns of findings differ for men and women, it is appropriate to discuss them separately. The data obtained from probability samples and the census alike indicate that, contrary to the stereotype, gay men earn disproportionately less than their heterosexual counterparts. In the first study of its kind, Badgett (1995) compared GSS respondents reporting any same-sex sexual activity to respondents reporting only heterosexual activity. Defining the sexual orientation variable in several ways and controlling for age, education, and other relevant variables, she found that men who reported same-sex behavior earned 11% to 27% less than behaviorally heterosexual men. A follow-up study that added data from the 1992 National Health and Social Life Survey (NHSLS) (Laumann et al., 1994) yielded similar findings (Badgett, 2001). Using GSS data from 1989 to 1996, Blandford (2003) found that gay and bisexual men experienced a 30% to 32% income disadvantage compared to heterosexual men (see also Berg & Lien, 2002; Black et al., 2003).

Using a subset of the 1990 Census data, Allegretto and Arthur (2001) found that gay men earned 14% less than married heterosexual men with comparable levels of education, controlling for age, race, location, and occupation. To assess whether this difference could be explained by marital status, they compared members of male cohabiting couples to unmarried men who were cohabiting with a female partner. They found that men in a same-sex cohabiting relationship earned 2% less. Thus, although the marriage premium substantially contributed to the earnings differential in this sample, it did not explain it entirely

(Allegretto & Arthur, 2001; see also Carpenter, 2004). Klawitter and Flatt (1998) replicated these findings.

The findings for lesbians are less clear-cut but suggest that lesbians' earnings, although considerably lower than those of men, are similar to or greater than those for comparable heterosexual women. Badgett's studies yielded mixed findings, with lesbians appearing to earn less than heterosexual women in one study (Badgett, 1995) and more in the other (Badgett, 2001). Neither difference, however, was statistically significant. In their analysis of census data, focusing on full-time, year-round workers, Klawitter and Flatt (1998) found that the earnings of women in same-sex couples did not differ significantly from those of married women and unmarried women with a cohabiting male partner (see also Carpenter, 2004). Using GSS data, however, other studies have found that lesbians and bisexual women earn significantly more than comparable heterosexual women (Berg & Lien, 2002; Black et al., 2003; Blandford, 2003).

Apart from income differentials, other research has documented direct employment discrimination based on sexual orientation, that is, overt and intentional differential treatment of sexual minorities in hiring, promotion, and other aspects of employment (Levine, 1979; Levine & Leonard, 1984; Croteau, 1996; Thompson & Nored, 2002). Adam (1981), for example, found that a law student whose résumé included membership in a gay organization was offered fewer interviews for internships than a student with an otherwise identical résumé. In a field experiment, Hebl and her colleagues found that gay-identified job applicants were not treated differently in overt ways but did evoke more negative nonverbal behaviors from job interviewers; these nonverbal biases, in turn, affected how the applicants responded to the interviewer (Hebl et al., 2002).

In addition to direct discrimination, the earnings differential may result from other factors. As noted above, a significant portion of the income gap appears to result from the fact that gay people are not allowed to marry and thus are denied the so-called marriage premium in earnings. In addition, many gay men and lesbians might opt for self-employment or choose occupations in which they expect sexual prejudice to be minimal. The price for a more tolerant workplace may be lower income (Badgett & King, 1997).

Alternatively, lesbian and gay workers who perceive that their workplace is hostile to their sexual orientation (i.e., workers with a high degree of felt stigma) might keep their sexual orientation secret to avoid enactments of stigma. In a questionnaire study with a gay and lesbian community sample, Waldo (1999) found that outness in the workplace was associated with experiences of overt sexual orientation-based harassment or discrimination, which in turn were associated with greater psychological distress and job dissatisfaction (see also Croteau, 1996; Ragins & Cornwell, 2001). Woods and Lucas (1993) described several strategies for avoiding antigay prejudice in the workplace. Some workers "play it straight," making sure that they do not conform to gay stereotypes and even inventing a heterosexual love life when their coworkers try to set them up with a date. Others dodge the issue by putting on an asexual facade. They become skilled at avoiding conversations and situations in which any discussion of personal life might arise. Still others rigidly segregate their lives so their work life and their life as a gay person do not overlap, sometimes even traveling to other cities to socialize with other gay people where the danger of running into a coworker is minimal (Woods & Lucas, 1993).

These strategies may avoid discrimination, but they also require considerable psychic (and sometimes physical) energy. Moreover, they all involve some degree of dishonesty and secretiveness, which may make it difficult for a worker to develop close ties with coworkers or supervisors through informal interactions, attendance at company parties, and the like. This lack of social integration, in turn, might reduce a worker's chances of receiving promotions and pay raises, an effect that Badgett (2001) termed *indirect discrimination*. Having to conceal one's sexuality in the workplace is also correlated with reduced job satisfaction and performance (Day & Schoenrade, 1997; Griffith & Hebl, 2002).

6.2 Violence Based on Sexual Orientation

Criminal victimization of sexual minorities has a long history. For years, violence was widely considered a normal response to gay people, and the perpetrators of antigay violence were rarely arrested or prosecuted (Herek & Berrill, 1992). During the 1980s, however, the gay community began to challenge this view successfully, arguing that antigay attacks should be considered *hate crimes*. For the present discussion, hate crimes are defined as actions intended to inflict physical injury, emotional suffering, or property damage to a person because of her or his race, sexual orientation, religion, or other comparable group identification (Herek, 1989; Levin & McDevitt, 1993). Because the targets of such acts are selected primarily on the basis of their group membership, hate crimes represent an attack not only upon an individual's physical self or property but also on her or his identity and on the other members of her or his community. Antigay hate crimes convey a message not only to the victim but also to the entire community. Each such crime is, in effect, both a punishment for stepping outside culturally accepted boundaries and a warning to all gay, lesbian, and bisexual people to remain invisible.

Throughout the 1980s, community antiviolence projects were organized to prevent and respond to antigay hate crimes in cities such as San Francisco and New York (Herek, 1992; Wertheimer, 1992). At the national level, lesbian and gay groups—mainly under the leadership of Kevin Berrill, director of the National Gay and Lesbian Task Force's Violence Project—successfully forged coalitions with law enforcement officials, victim advocacy groups, professional associations, and other minority community groups in a campaign to redefine antigay violence as a significant social and legal problem that warranted a serious response at all levels of society (e.g., Berrill, 1992b; Berrill & Herek, 1992). As a result of this activism, society's policy makers began to redefine antigay violence, recognizing it as a problem requiring their response. Congressional hearings on antigay victimization were first held in 1986 (United States Congress House Committee on the Judiciary, 1987) and eventually led to enactment of the Hate Crimes Statistics Act (Public Law 101–275, 104 Stat. 140) in 1990. The Act directed the federal government to collect statistics on hate crimes based on race, ethnicity, religion, and sexual orientation. When it was signed by President George H.W. Bush on April 23, 1990, it became the first federal law ever to include recognition of problems experienced by individuals because of their sexual orientation.

Thousands of crimes based on the victim's sexual orientation have been reported to the Federal Bureau of Investigation (FBI) since it began tabulating statistics in 1991. In the first set of statistics compiled under the Act, 4558 hate crimes were tallied in 1991, of which 422 (9%) were related to sexual orientation (Skorneck, 1993). In 2003, the most recent year for which data were available at the time of this writing, 1239 (17%) of the 7489 reported hate crime incidents were based on the victim's sexual orientation (Federal Bureau of Investigation, 2004). These figures only roughly indicate national trends because reporting hate crimes by law enforcement agencies is voluntary, and the quality of data varies widely from one jurisdiction to another. Some police departments extensively train their personnel to identify and report hate crimes, and some have special staff to deal with crimes that might be bias-motivated. These agencies are in the minority, however, and many (perhaps most) police departments do not devote special resources to hate crimes. In addition, many victims never report their experiences to the police, fearing further harassment or simply believing that the police will never be able to apprehend their assailants (Herek et al., 2002). Consequently, many hate crimes go uncounted.

The official response to antigay crimes lags far behind the response to crimes based on the victim's racial, ethnic, or religious group membership. By the end of 2004, for example, 44 states and the District of Columbia had enacted laws that either monitor crimes motivated by prejudice or enhance the penalties attached to them, but such laws specifically addressed antigay violence in only 30 of those jurisdictions (29 states and the District of Columbia). Fourteen other states had hate crime laws on the books, but the laws did not include sexual orientation (National Gay and Lesbian Task Force, 2005b). In several of those states, the exclusion of sexual orientation was not merely an oversight. Their hate crime legislation has been blocked, defeated, or amended to delete sexual orientation because legislators objected to any form of statutory recognition or protection for lesbian and gay male citizens.

Official criminal justice statistics represent only one strategy for tracking the prevalence of antigay hate crimes. Another way to assess the extent of hate crime victimization is through surveys conducted with community samples of lesbians, gay men, and bisexuals. In those surveys, respondents are recruited through various methods and are asked to complete a self-administered questionnaire that includes items about criminal victimization and harassment based on one's sexual orientation. Data from such surveys suggest that a substantial proportion (perhaps as many as one in five) have experienced some type of criminal victimization because of their sexual orientation since age 16. This includes assaults, rapes, robberies, and acts of vandalism directed at people because they are perceived to be gay, lesbian, or bisexual.

Based on a 1992 comprehensive review of 24 separate questionnaire studies with convenience samples of gay men and lesbians, Berrill reported that a median of 9% of respondents had been assaulted with a weapon because of their sexual orientation; 17% reported simple physical assault, and 19% reported vandalism of property (Berrill, 1992a). In a survey of more than 2200 lesbian, gay, and bisexual residents of the greater Sacramento (California) area, 19% of lesbians and 28% of gay men had experienced some type of criminal victimization because of their sexual orientation since age 16 (Herek et al., 1999). Among bisexual women and men, the figures were, respectively, 15% and 27%.[4] Many of those victimizations had occurred in the recent past. Altogether, 13% of the lesbians, 18% of the gay men, 10% of the bisexual women, and 16% of the bisexual men reported criminal victimization because of their sexual orientation during the previous 5 years (Herek et al., 1999). Because none of these surveys utilized probability samples, the percentages cannot be generalized to the entire U.S. gay and lesbian population. Although we do not know exactly how many people have been targeted for criminal victimization because of their presumed sexual orientation (and heterosexuals are sometimes mistaken for homosexuals in antigay attacks), it is clear that an alarming number of attacks based on sexual orientation have occurred in the past and continue to occur today.

In addition to the violence, lesbians and gay men routinely face harassment, threats, intimidation, and hostility because of their sexual orientation. In Berrill's (1992a) review of 24 community studies, a median of 44% of respondents had been threatened with violence because of their sexual orientation; 33% had been chased or followed; 25% had had objects thrown at them; and 13% had been spat upon. Verbal harassment was an almost universal experience: across studies, a median of 80% of respondents had experienced it. In the Sacramento study, more than half of the respondents (56%) said they had been verbally harassed because of their sexual orientation during the previous year. In that same time period, 19% of the sample had been threatened with violence, 17% had been chased or followed, 12% had an object thrown at them, and 5% had been spat upon because of their sexual orientation (Herek et al., 1999).

Hate crime victimization takes a serious toll. In addition to the physical harm hate crimes inflict on victims, they appear to create greater psychological trauma than other kinds of violent crime. One study found that gay men and lesbians who had experienced a crime against their person based on their sexual orientation manifested significantly higher levels of depressive symptoms, traumatic stress symptoms, anxiety, and anger compared to lesbians and gay men

---

[4]Percentages are based on 2259 responses: 980 from lesbians, 898 from gay men, 190 from bisexual women, and 191 from bisexual men.

who had experienced comparable crimes during the same time period that were unrelated to their sexual orientation (Herek et al., 1999). Although difficult to measure empirically, such crimes probably also function as a form of terrorism, creating generalized anxiety among members of sexual minority communities where they occur (e.g., Noelle, 2002).

7 Conclusions

Homosexuality continues to be stigmatized in the United States. Lesbians, gay men, and bisexual people are confronted with heterosexism in the institutions of society while also encountering sexual prejudice from many heterosexuals. Some of them have internalized societal stigma, which creates an additional threat to their psychological well-being. At the same time, sexual minorities continue to contest stigma, heterosexism, and sexual prejudice. Although efforts to transform society's institutions have achieved mixed success, sexual prejudice has declined significantly during the past three decades. It is against this backdrop that the health-related experiences and behaviors of sexual minority individuals must be understood.

References

Adam, B.D. (1978) Inferiorization and self-esteem. *Social Psychology* 41:47–53.

Adam, B.D. (1981) Stigma and employability: discrimination by sex and sexual orientation in the Ontario legal profession. *Canadian Review of Sociology & Anthropology* 18:216–221.

Allegretto, S.A., and Arthur, M.M. (2001) An empirical analysis of homosexual/heterosexual male earnings differentials: unmarried and unequal? *Industrial & Labor Relations Review* 54:631–646.

Allport, G.W. (1954) *The nature of prejudice.* Doubleday, Garden City, NY.

American Psychiatric Association. (1952) *Mental disorders: diagnostic and statistical manual,* 1st ed. APA, Washington, DC.

American Psychiatric Association. (1987) *Diagnostic and statistical manual of mental disorders,* 3rd, ed. APA, Washington, DC.

Aspinwall, L.G., and Taylor, S.E. (1997) A stitch in time: self-regulation and proactive coping. *Psychological Bulletin* 121:417–436.

Badgett, M.V.L. (1995) The wage effects of sexual orientation discrimination. *Industrial & Labor Relations Review* 48:726–739.

Badgett, M.V.L. (1997) Beyond biased samples: challenging the myths on the economic status of lesbians and gay men. In: Gluckman, A., and Reed, B. (eds) *Homo economics: capitalism, community, and lesbian and gay life.* Routledge, New York, pp. 65–71.

Badgett, M.V.L. (2001) *Money, myths, and change: the economic lives of lesbians and gay men.* University of Chicago Press, Chicago.

Badgett, M.V.L., and King, M.C. (1997) Lesbian and gay occupational strategies. In: Gluckman, A., and Reed, B. (eds) *Homo economics: capitalism, community, and lesbian and gay life.* Routledge, New York, pp. 73–86.

Baker, D. (1997) A history in ads: the growth of the gay and lesbian market. In: Gluckman, A., and Reed, B. (eds) *Homo economics: capitalism, community and lesbian and gay life*. Routledge, New York, pp. 11–20.

Bayer, R. (1987) *Homosexuality and American psychiatry: the politics of diagnosis*, rev. ed. Princeton University Press, Princeton, NJ.

Berg, N., and Lien, D. (2002) Measuring the effect of sexual orientation on income: evidence of discrimination? *Contemporary Economic Policy* 20:394–414.

Berrill, K.T. (1992a) Antigay violence and victimization in the United States: an overview. In: Herek, G.M., and Berrill, K.T. (eds) *Hate crimes: confronting violence Against lesbians and gay men*. Sage, Thousand Oaks, CA, pp. 19–45.

Berrill, K.T. (1992b) Organizing against hate on campus: strategies for activists. In: Herek, G.M., and Berrill, K.T. (eds) *Hate crimes: confronting violence against lesbians and gay men*. Sage, Thousand Oaks, CA, pp. 259–269.

Berrill, K.T., and Herek, G.M. (1992) Primary and secondary victimization in anti-gay hate crimes: official response and public policy. In: Herek, G.M., and Berrill, K.T. (eds) *Hate crimes: confronting violence against lesbians and gay men*. Sage, Thousand Oaks, CA, pp. 289–305.

Bérubé, A. (1990) *Coming out under fire: the history of gay men and women in World War two*. Free Press, New York.

Black, D.A., Makar, H.R., Sanders, S.G., and Taylor, L.J. (2003) The earnings effects of sexual orientation. *Industrial & Labor Relations Review* 56:449–469.

Blandford, J.M. (2003) The nexus of sexual orientation and gender in the determination of earnings. *Industrial & Labor Relations Review* 56:622–642.

Boswell, J. (1980) *Christianity, social tolerance, and homosexuality: gay people in western Europe from the beginning of the Christian era to the fourteenth century*. University of Chicago Press, Chicago.

Bowers v. Hardwick (1986) 478 U.S. 186.

Brooks, V.R. (1981) *Minority stress and lesbian women*. Lexington Books, Lexington, MA.

Cameron, P. (1994) *The gay 90s: what the empirical evidence reveals about homosexuality*. Adroit Press, Franklin, TN.

Carpenter, C. (2004) New evidence on gay and lesbian household incomes. *Contemporary Economic Policy* 22:78–94.

Chauncey, G. (2004) "What gay studies taught the court": the historians' amicus brief in Lawrence v Texas. *GLQ: A Journal of Lesbian & Gay Studies* 10:509–538.

Chauncey, G., Jr. (1982–1983) From sexual inversion to homosexuality: medicine and the changing conceptualization of female deviance. *Salmagundi* 58–59:114–146.

Chauncey, G., Jr. (1993) The postwar sex crime panic. In: Graebner, W. (ed) *True stories from the American past*. McGraw-Hill, New York, pp. 160–178.

Conger, J.J. (1975) Proceedings of the American Psychological Association, Incorporated, for the year 1974: minutes of the annual meeting of the Council of Representatives. *American Psychologist* 30:620, 632–633.

Congregation for the Doctrine of the Faith. (1975) *Declaration on certain questions concerning sexual ethics*. March 18, 2005; http://www.vatican.va/roman_curia/congregations/cfaith/documents/rc_con_cfaith_doc_19751229_persona-humana_en.html.

Congregation for the Doctrine of the Faith. (1986) *Letter to the Bishops of the Catholic Church on the pastoral care of homosexual persons*. July 8, 2003; http://www.vatican.va/roman_curia/congregations/cfaith/documents/rc_con_cfaith_doc_19861001_homosexual-persons_en.html.

Congregation for the Doctrine of the Faith. (1992) *Some considerations concerning the response to legislative proposals on non-discrimination of homosexual persons*. July 8, 2003; http://www.ewtn.com/library/CURIA/CDFHOMOL. HTM.

Croteau, J.M. (1996) Research on the work experiences of lesbian, gay, and bisexual people: an integrative review of methodology and findings. *Journal of Vocational Behavior* 48:195–209.

Currie, M.R., Cunningham, E.G., and Findlay, B.M. (2004) The short internalized homonegativity scale: examination of the factorial structure of a new measure of internalized homophobia. *Educational & Psychological Measurement* 64:1053–1067.

Day, N.E., and Schoenrade, P. (1997) Staying in the closet versus coming out: relationships between communication about sexual orientation and work attitudes. *Personnel Psychology* 50:147–163.

DeLozier, M.W., and Rodrigue, J. (1996) Marketing to the homosexual (gay) market: a profile and strategy implications. *Journal of Homosexuality* 31(1–2): 203–212.

D'Emilio, J. (1983) *Sexual politics, sexual communities: the making of a homosexual minority in the United States 1940–1970*. University of Chicago Press, Chicago.

D'Emilio, J., and Freedman, E.B. (1988) *Intimate matters: a history of sexuality in America*. Harper & Row, New York.

Dewan, S. (2005) United Church of Christ backs same-sex marriage. *New York Times*, July 5, p. A10.

Dignity, USA. (2005) *What is dignity?* March 22 ,2005; http://www.dignityusa.org/whatis.html.

DiPlacido, J. (1998) Minority stress among lesbians, gay men, and bisexuals: a consequence of heterosexism, homophobia, and stigmatization. In: Herek, G.M. (ed) *Stigma and sexual orientation: understanding prejudice against lesbians, gay men, and bisexuals*. Sage, Thousand Oaks, CA, pp. 138–159.

Duberman, M.B., Vicinus, M., and Chauncey, G., Jr. (1989) *Hidden from history: reclaiming the gay and lesbian past*. New American Library, New York.

Dynes, W. (1985) *Homolexis: a historical and cultural lexicon of homosexuality*. Gay Academic Union, New York.

Eliason, M.J. (1997) The prevalence and nature of biphobia in heterosexual undergraduate students. *Archives of Sexual Behavior* 26:317–326.

Ellis, H. (1901) *Sexual inversion*. F.A. Davis, Philadelphia.

Federal Bureau of Investigation. (2004) *Hate crime statistics 2003*. U.S. Department of Justice, Washington, DC.

Fone, B.R. (2000) *Homophobia: a history*. Metropolitan, New York.

Foucault, M. (1978) In: Hurley, R. (trans.) *The history of sexuality*. Vol. 1. *An introduction*. Pantheon, New York.

Freedman, E. (1989) "Uncontrolled desires": the response to the sexual psychopath, 1920–1960. In: Peiss, K., and Simmons, C. (eds) *Passion and power: sexuality in history*. Temple University Press, Philadelphia.

Freedman, M. (1971) *Homosexuality and psychological functioning*. Wadsworth, Belmont, CA.

Freud, S. (1951) A letter from Freud. *American Journal of Psychiatry* 107:786–787.

Freud, S. (1953) Three essays on the theory of sexuality. In: Strachey, J. (ed. and trans.) *The standard edition of the complete psychological works of Sigmund Freud*, Vol. 7. Hogarth Press, London, pp. 123–243. (original work published in 1905).

Fullilove, M.T., and Fullilove, R.E.I. (1999) Stigma as an obstacle to AIDS action. *American Behavioral Scientist* 42:1117–1129.

Gilman, S.L. (1985) *Difference and pathology: stereotypes of sexuality, race, and madness*. Cornell University Press, Ithaca, NY.

Goffman, E. (1963) *Stigma: notes on the management of spoiled identity*. Prentice-Hall, Englewood Cliffs, NJ.

Gonsiorek, J.C. (1991) The empirical basis for the demise of the illness model of homosexuality. In: Gonsiorek, J.C., and Weinrich, J.D. (eds) *Homosexuality: research implications for public policy*. Sage, Thousand Oaks, CA, pp. 115–136.

Green, J.C. (2000) Antigay: varieties of opposition to gay rights. In: Rimmerman, C.A., Wald, K.D., and Wilcox, C. (eds) *The politics of gay rights*. University of Chicago Press, Chicago, pp. 121–138.

Griffith, K.H., and Hebl, M.R. (2002) The disclosure dilemma for gay men and lesbians: "coming out" at work. *Journal of Applied Psychology* 87:1191–1199.

Gross, A.E., Green, S.K., Storck, J.T., and Vanyur, J.M. (1980) Disclosure of sexual orientation and impressions of male and female homosexuals. *Personality & Social Psychology Bulletin* 6:307–314.

Haggerty, T. (2003) History repeating itself: a historical overview of gay men and lesbians in the military before "don't ask, don't tell." In: Belkin, A., and Bateman, G. (eds) *Don't ask, don't tell: debating the gay ban in the military*. Lynne Rienner Publishers, Boulder, CO, pp. 9–49.

Haldeman, D.C. (1991) Sexual orientation conversion therapy for gay men and lesbians: a scientific examination. In: Gonsiorek, J.C., and Weinrich, J.D. (eds) *Homosexuality: research implications for public policy*. Sage, Thousand Oaks, CA, pp. 149–160.

Hart, M., Roback, H., Tittler, B., Weitz, L., Walston, B., and McKee, E. (1978) Psychological adjustment of nonpatient homosexuals: critical review of the research literature. *Journal of Clinical Psychiatry* 39:604–608.

Hebl, M.R., Foster, J.B., Mannix, L.M., and Dovidio, J.F. (2002) Formal and interpersonal discrimination: a field study of bias toward homosexual applicants. *Personality & Social Psychology Bulletin* 28:815–825.

Herek, G.M. (1984) Beyond "homophobia": a social psychological perspective on attitudes toward lesbians and gay men. *Journal of Homosexuality* 10:1–21.

Herek, G.M. (1989) Hate crimes against lesbians and gay men: issues for research and policy. *American Psychologist* 44:948–955.

Herek, G.M. (1991) Stigma, prejudice, and violence against lesbians and gay men. In: Gonsiorek, J.C., and Weinrich, J.D. (eds) *Homosexuality: research implications for public policy*. Sage, Thousand Oaks, CA, pp. 60–80.

Herek, G.M. (1992) The community response to violence in San Francisco: an interview with Wenny Kusuma, Lester Olmstead-Rose, and Jill Tregor. In: Herek, G.M., and Berrill, K.T. (eds) *Hate crimes: confronting violence against lesbians and gay men*. Sage, Thousand Oaks, CA, pp. 241–258.

Herek, G.M. (1994) Assessing heterosexuals' attitudes toward lesbians and gay men: a review of empirical research with the ATLG scale. In: Greene, B., and Herek, G.M. (eds) *Lesbian and gay psychology: theory, research, and clinical applications*. Sage, Thousand Oaks, CA, pp. 206–228.

Herek, G.M. (1996) Why tell if you're not asked? Self-disclosure, intergroup contact, and heterosexuals' attitudes toward lesbians and gay men. In: Herek, G.M., Jobe, J., and Carney, R. (eds) *Out in force: sexual orientation and the military*. University of Chicago Press, Chicago, pp. 197–225.

Herek, G.M. (2002a) Gender gaps in public opinion about lesbians and gay men. *Public Opinion Quarterly* 66:40–66.

Herek, G.M. (2002b) Heterosexuals' attitudes toward bisexual men and women in the United States. *Journal of Sex Research* 39:264–274.

Herek, G.M. (2004) Beyond "homophobia": thinking about sexual stigma and prejudice in the twenty-first century. *Sexuality Research and Social Policy* 1(2):6–24.

Herek, G.M., and Berrill, K.T. (1992) *Hate crimes: confronting violence against lesbians and gay men*. Sage, Thousand Oaks, CA.

Herek, G.M., and Capitanio, J.P. (1995) Black heterosexuals' attitudes toward lesbians and gay men in the United States. *Journal of Sex Research* 32:95–105.

Herek, G.M., and Capitanio, J.P. (1996) "Some of my best friends": intergroup contact, concealable stigma, and heterosexuals' attitudes toward gay men and lesbians. *Personality & Social Psychology Bulletin* 22:412–424.

Herek, G.M., Cogan, J.C., Gillis, J.R., and Glunt, E.K. (1998) Correlates of internalized homophobia in a community sample of lesbians and gay men. *Journal of the Gay & Lesbian Medical Association* 2:17–25.

Herek, G.M., Gillis, J.R., and Cogan, J.C. (1999) Psychological sequelae of hate crime victimization among lesbian, gay, and bisexual adults. *Journal of Consulting & Clinical Psychology* 67:945–951.

Herek, G.M., Cogan, J.C., and Gillis, J.R. (2002) Victim experiences in hate crimes based on sexual orientation. *Journal of Social Issues* 58:319–339.

Herman, D. (1997) *The antigay agenda: orthodox vision and the Christian right*. University of Chicago Press, Chicago.

Hirschfeld, M. (2000) In: Lombardi-Nash, M.A. (trans.) *The homosexuality of men and women*, 2nd ed. Prometheus Books, Buffalo, NY.

Hooker, E. (1957) The adjustment of the male overt homosexual. *Journal of Projective Techniques* 21:18–31.

Hulse, C. (2004) Senators block initiative to ban same-sex unions. *New York Times*. July 15, p. A1.

Johnson, D.K. (2004) *The lavender scare: the cold war persecution of gays and lesbians in the federal government*. University of Chicago Press, Chicago.

Jones, E.E., Farina, A., Hastorf, A.H., Markus, H., Miller, D.T., and Scott, R.A. (1984) *Social stigma: the psychology of marked relationships*. W.H. Freeman, New York.

Jordan, M.D. (1997) *The invention of sodomy in Christian theology*. University of Chicago Press, Chicago.

Katz, J.N. (1976) *Gay American history: lesbians and gay men in the U.S.A.* Thomas Y. Crowell Company, New York.

Kimmel, M.S. (1997) Masculinity as homophobia: fear, shame and silence in the construction of gender identity. In: Gergen, M.M., and Davis, S.N. (eds) *Toward a new psychology of gender*. Routledge, New York, pp. 223–242.

Kirkpatrick, D.D. (2004) Black pastors backing Bush are rarities, but not alone. *New York Times*. October 5, p. A15.

Kite, M.E., and Deaux, K. (1987) Gender belief systems: homosexuality and the implicit inversion theory. *Psychology of Women Quarterly* 11:83–96.

Klawitter, M.M., and Flatt, V. (1998) The effects of state and local antidiscrimination policies on earnings for gays and lesbians. *Journal of Policy Analysis & Management* 17:658–686.

Knowles, E. (1997) *The Oxford dictionary of phrase, saying, and quotation*. Oxford University Press, New York.

Krafft-Ebing, R.V. (1900) *Psychopathia sexualis with especial reference to antipathetic sexual instinct: a medico-forensic study*. W.T. Keener, Chicago.

Laumann, E.O., Gagnon, J.H., Michael, R.T., and Michaels, S. (1994) *The social organization of sexuality: sexual practices in the United States*. University of Chicago Press, Chicago.

Lawrence et al. v. Texas, 539 U.S. 558 (2003).

Lazarus, R.S., and Folkman, S. (1984) *Stress, appraisal, and coping*. Springer, New York.

Leslie, C. (2000) Creating criminals: the injuries inflicted by "unenforced" sodomy laws. *Harvard Civil Rights-Civil Liberties Law Review* 35(1):103–181.

Levin, J., and McDevitt, J. (1993) *Hate crimes: the rising tide of bigotry and bloodshed.* Plenum, New York.

Levine, M.P. (1979) Employment discrimination against gay men. *International Review of Modern Sociology* 9:151–163.

Levine, M.P., and Leonard, R. (1984) Discrimination against lesbians in the work force. *Signs: Journal of Women in Culture & Society* 9:700–710.

Lewis, G.B. (2003) Black-white differences in attitudes toward homosexuality and gay rights. *Public Opinion Quarterly* 67:59–78.

Lima, G., Lo Presto, C.T., Sherman, M.F., and Sobelman, S.A. (1993) The relationship between homophobia and self-esteem in gay males with AIDS. *Journal of Homosexuality* 25(4):69–76.

Loh, E.S. (1996) Productivity differences and the marriage wage premium for white males. *Journal of Human Resources* 31:566–589.

Malyon, A.K. (1981–1982) Psychotherapeutic implications of internalized homophobia in gay men. *Journal of Homosexuality* 7(2–3):59–69.

Mayfield, W. (2001) The development of an internalized homonegativity inventory for gay men. *Journal of Homosexuality* 41(2):53–76.

Meyer, I.H. (1995) Minority stress and mental health in gay men. *Journal of Health & Social Behavior* 36:38–56.

Meyer, I.H. (2003) Prejudice, social stress, and mental health in lesbian, gay, and bisexual populations: conceptual issues and research evidence. *Psychological Bulletin* 129:674–697.

Miller, C.T., and Major, B. (2000) Coping with stigma and prejudice. In: Heatherton, T.F., Kleck, R.E., Hebl, M.R., and Hull, J.G. (eds) *The social psychology of stigma.* Guilford, New York, pp. 243–272.

Mohr, J.J., and Rochlen, A.B. (1999) Measuring attitudes regarding bisexuality in lesbian, gay male, and heterosexual populations. *Journal of Counseling Psychology* 46:353–369.

Morin, S.F., and Rothblum, E.D. (1991) Removing the stigma: fifteen years of progress. *American Psychologist* 46:947–949.

Murray, S.O. (2000) *Homosexualities.* University of Chicago Press, Chicago.

National Gay and Lesbian Task Force. (2005a) Anti-gay marriage measures in the US. August 30, 2005; http://thetaskforce.org/downloads/marriagemap.pdf.

National Gay and Lesbian Task Force. (2005b) Hate crime laws in the U.S. August 30, 2005; http://thetaskforce.org/downloads/hatecrimesmap.pdf.

National Gay and Lesbian Task Force. (2005c) State nondiscrimination laws in the U.S. August 30, 2005; http://www.thetaskforce.org/downloads/nondiscriminationmap.pdf.

National Gay and Lesbian Task Force. (2005d) The issues: nondiscrimination. August 30, 2005; http://thetaskforce.org/theissues/issue.cfm?issueID=18.

National Gay and Lesbian Task Force. (2005e) The issues: parenting. August 30, 2005; http://thetaskforce.org/theissues/issue.cfm?issueID=30.

Nicholson, W.D., and Long, B.C. (1990) Self-esteem, social support, internalized homophobia, and coping strategies of HIV+ gay men. *Journal of Consulting & Clinical Psychology* 58:873–876.

Noelle, M. (2002) The ripple effect on the Matthew Shepard murder: impact on the assumptive worlds of members of the targeted group. *American Behavioral Scientist* 46:27–50.

Ochs, R. (1996) Biphobia: it goes more than two ways. In: Firestein, B.A. (ed) *Bisexuality: the psychology and politics of an invisible minority.* Sage, Thousand Oaks, CA, pp. 217–239.

Ochs, R., and Deihl, M. (1992) Moving beyond binary thinking. In: Blumenfeld, W.J. (ed) *Homophobia: how we all pay the price.* Beacon Press, Boston, pp. 67–75.

Patterson, C.J., Fulcher, M., and Wainright, J. (2002) Children of lesbian and gay parents: research, law, and policy. In: Bottoms, B.L., Bull Kovera, M., and McAuliff, B.D. (eds) *Children, Social Science, and the Law.* Cambridge University Press, New York, pp. 176–199.

Paul, J.P. (1996) Bisexuality: exploring/exploding the boundaries. In: Savin-Williams, R.C., and Cohen, K.M. (eds) *The lives of lesbians, gays, and bisexuals: children to adults.* Harcourt Brace College Publishers, Ft. Worth, TX, pp. 436–461.

Paul, J.P., and Nichols, M. (1988) "Biphobia" and the construction of a bisexual identity. In: Shernoff, M., and Scott, W. (eds) *The sourcebook on lesbian/gay health care.* National Lesbian and Gay Health Foundation, Washington, DC, pp. 142–147.

Peterson, K. (2004) 50-State rundown on gay marriage laws. November 13, 2004; http://www.stateline.org/stateline/?pa=story&sa=showStoryInfo&id=353058.

Pew Research Center. (2005) Abortion and rights of terror suspects top court issues. August 14, 2005; http://people-press.org/.

Ponse, B. (1976) Secrecy in the lesbian world. *Urban Life* 5:313–338.

Presbyterian Church USA. (2001) *Homosexuality.* September 3, 2005; http://www.pcusa.org/101/101-homosexual.htm.

Ragins, B.R., and Cornwell, J.M. (2001) Pink triangles: antecedents and consequences of perceived workplace discrimination against gay and lesbian employees. *Journal of Applied Psychology* 86:1244–1261.

Riess, B.F. (1980) Psychological tests in homosexuality. In: Marmor, J. (ed) *Homosexual behavior: a modern reappraisal.* Basic Books, New York, pp. 296–311.

Ross, M.W., and Rosser, B.R.S. (1996) Measurement and correlates of internalized homophobia: a factor analytic study. *Journal of Clinical Psychology* 52:15–21.

Rothblum, E.D., and Factor, R. (2001) Lesbians and their sisters as a control group: demographic and mental health factors. *Psychological Science* 12:63–69.

Rust, P.C. (1996) Monogamy and polyamory: relationship issues for bisexuals. In: Firestein, B.A. (ed) *Bisexuality: the psychology and politics of an invisible minority.* Sage, Thousand Oaks, CA, pp. 127–148.

Rust, P.C. (2000) Bisexuality: a contemporary paradox for women. *Journal of Social Issues* 56(2):205–221.

Saad, L. (2005) Gay rights attitudes a mixed bag. *The Gallup Report.* May 20, 2005; http://www.gallup.com

Sanders, E. (2001) Methodist clergy create activist alliance: group will fight discrimination against gays in the church. *Seattle Times.* July 28, p. B1.

Scambler, G. (1989) *Epilepsy.* Routledge, London.

Scambler, G., and Hopkins, A. (1986) Being epileptic: coming to terms with stigma. *Sociology of Health & Illness* 8:26–43.

Shidlo, A. (1994) Internalized homophobia: conceptual and empirical issues in measurement. In: Greene, B., and Herek, G.M. (eds) *Lesbian and gay psychology: theory, research, and clinical applications.* Sage, Thousand Oaks, CA, pp. 176–205.

Silverstein, C. (1991) Psychological and medical treatments of homosexuality. In: Gonsiorek, J.C., and Weinrich, J.D. (eds) *Homosexuality: research implications for public policy.* Sage, Thousand Oaks, CA, pp. 101–114.

Skorneck, C. (1993) FBI's first report on hate crimes. *San Francisco Examiner.* January 5, p. A-5.

Snyder, M., and Uranowitz, S.W. (1978) Reconstructing the past: some cognitive consequences of person perception. *Journal of Personality & Social Psychology* 36:941–950.

Spalding, L.R., and Peplau, L.A. (1997) The unfaithful lover: heterosexuals' perceptions of bisexuals and their relationships. *Psychology of Women Quarterly* 21:611–625.

Stack, S., and Eshleman, J.R. (1998) Marital status and happiness: a 17-nation study. *Journal of Marriage & the Family* 60:527–536.

Szymanski, D.M., and Chung, Y.B. (2001) The lesbian internalized homophobia scale: a rational/theoretical approach. *Journal of Homosexuality* 41(2): 37–52.

Szymanski, D.M., and Chung, Y.B. (2003) Feminist attitudes and coping resources as correlates of lesbian internalized heterosexism. *Feminism & Psychology* 13:369–389.

Thompson, R.A., and Nored, L.S. (2002) Law enforcement employment discrimination based on sexual orientation: a selective review of case law. *American Journal of Criminal Justice* 26:203–217.

Tozer, E.E., and Hayes, J.A. (2004) Why do individuals seek conversion therapy? The role of religiosity, internalized homonegativity, and identity development. *Counseling Psychologist* 32:716–740.

Trevison, C. (2005) Spiritual allies continue support of gay marriages. *The Oregonian.* May 4, p. C2.

Trumbach, R. (1989) Gender and the homosexual role in modern Western culture: the 18th and 19th centuries compared. In: Altman, D., Vance, C., Vicinus, M., Weeks, J., et al. *Homosexuality, which homosexuality?* GMP Publishers, London, pp. 149–169.

Ulrichs, K.H. (1994) In: Lombardi-Nash, M.A. (trans.) *The riddle of "man-manly" love: the pioneering work on male homosexuality.* Prometheus Books, Buffalo, NY.

United Methodist Church. (2004a) Human sexuality. August 31, 2005a; http://archives.umc.org/interior.asp?ptid=1&mid=1728.

United Methodist Church. (2004b) What is the denomination's position on homosexuality? August 31, 2005b; http://archives.umc.org/interior.asp?ptid=1&mid=1324.

United States Congress House Committee on the Judiciary. (1987) *Anti-gay violence: hearing before the subcommittee on criminal justice of the committee on the judiciary House of Representatives: ninety-ninth Congress second session on anti-gay violence.* U.S. Government Printing Office, Washington, DC.

U.S. Code 654. (1993) Pub. L. 103–160 571, 107 Stat., 1547. Government Printing Office, Washington, DC.

Van der Meer, T. (1993) Sodomy and the pursuit of a third sex in the early modern period. In: Herdt, G.H. (ed) *Third sex, third gender: beyond sexual dimorphism in culture and history.* Zone Press, New York, pp. 137–212.

Van der Meer, T. (1997) Sodom's seed in The Netherlands: the emergence of homosexuality in the early modern period. *Journal of Homosexuality* 34(1):1–16.

Wagner, G., Brondolo, E., and Rabkin, J. (1996) Internalized homophobia in a sample of HIV+ gay men, and its relationship to psychological distress, coping, and illness progression. *Journal of Homosexuality* 32(2):91–106.

Waldo, C.R. (1999) Working in a majority context: a structural model of heterosexism as minority stress in the workplace. *Journal of Counseling Psychology* 46:218–232.

Weinberg, G. (1972) *Society and the healthy homosexual.* St. Martin's, New York.

Weinberg, M.S., Williams, C.J., and Pryor, D.W. (1994) *Dual attraction: understanding bisexuality.* Oxford University Press, New York.

Weiner, B. (1995) *Judgments of responsibility: a foundation for a theory of social conduct.* Guilford Press, New York.

Wertheimer, D.M. (1992) Treatment and service interventions for lesbian and gay male crime victims. In: Herek, G.M., and Berrill, Kevin, T. (eds) *Hate crimes: confronting violence against lesbians and gay men.* Sage, Thousand Oaks, CA, pp. 227–240.

Wilcox, C. (1996) *Onward Christian soldiers? The religious right in American politics.* Westview Press, Boulder, CO.

Williamson, I.R. (2000) Internalized homophobia and health issues affecting lesbians and gay men. *Health Education Research* 15:97–107.

Wolcott, D.L., Namir, S., Fawzy, F.I., Gottlieb, M.S., and Mitsuyasu, R.T. (1986) Illness concerns, attitudes toward homosexuality, and social support in gay men with AIDS. *General Hospital Psychiatry* 8:395–403.

Woods, J.D., and Lucas, J.H. (1993) *The corporate closet: the professional lives of gay men in America.* Free Press, New York.

Zaller, J.R. (1992) *The nature and origins of mass opinion.* Cambridge University Press, New York.

Zerubavel, E. (1982) Personal information and social life. *Symbolic Interaction* 5:97–109.

Globalization, Structural Violence, and LGBT Health: A Cross-Cultural Perspective

Mark B. Padilla, Ernesto Vásquez del Aguila, and Richard G. Parker

1 Introduction

It is a daunting task to provide even a partial analysis of the health of lesbians, gays, bisexuals, and transsexuals (LGBTs) from a global perspective owing to the cross-cultural and regional variation in the social construction and expression of sexuality as well as the still incomplete scholarly literature on the topic. This chapter, however, argues that it is precisely such a global vantage point that is required to apprehend the contemporary context of health and illness among LGBT populations. Although LGBT health is shaped by local cultural meanings and practices, it is also inherently embedded in large-scale processes and the position of local LGBT populations within the global system. In the era of a highly mobile, hybrid, and fundamentally interconnected world in which material and symbolic cultures are linked across vast distances, the meanings of LGBT sexuality and their consequences for health in specific locales cannot be understood if nations are viewed in isolation (Altman, 1989). Indeed, the nature of global interconnectedness requires us to engage LGBT health as a fundamentally transnational phenomenon involving the interplay of meanings, practices, and vulnerabilities that extend beyond the purely local. For example, the acquired immune deficiency syndrome (AIDS) epidemic among gay-identified men in the United States and Europe may be intimately related to the meanings and practices that drive risky practices in Papua New Guinea, Uganda, or Bolivia. Furthermore, the flow of the discourses, meanings, persons, and practices that shape LGBT health are always multidirectional, necessitating a more complicated theoretical approach that truly engages the issue of LGBT health from the global perspective.

This chapter draws on a growing ethnographic and social scientific literature on LGBT persons to analyze LGBT health at both local and global levels. Approaching LGBT health from an anthropologic perspective, we take the position that the meanings and social consequences of socially deviant or nonnormative sexualities are subject to cross-cultural variations because LGBT persons are always situated within specific cultural systems and are also connected to larger political and economic inequalities that are expressed at a global scale. Thus, although this review is necessarily partial and is constrained by the limits of the literature currently available, particularly the relative paucity of cross-cultural studies of both lesbian and transgender health, the discussion seeks to organize the literature available within a dual conceptual framework that emphasizes two fundamental features of LGBT health: (1) the large-scale structural inequalities at work both locally and globally that influence LGBT health; and (2) the cultural variations in the meaning, expression, and practice of LGBT persons in various contexts. As other chapters in this volume examine the literature on LGBT health in developed settings, we draw primarily on ethnographic evidence in the developing world to illustrate the ways that the social and structural context (including both cultural meanings and political-economic forces) manifests in the health of LGBT persons.

We want to emphasize from the outset that although we use the designation LGBT throughout this text, readers must be mindful that this category, like others we discuss in this chapter, is not unproblematic when viewed cross-culturally. Whereas the notion of an LGBT population seeks, at one level, to emphasize diversity (clearly calling attention to the L, the G, the B, and the T as distinct subsets of this heterogeneous population), when applied cross-culturally it can itself become an ethnocentric imposition. Some activists in non-Western and developing societies have adopted it, whereas others have questioned its application. Even some who have adopted it have wished to further diversify it: In many parts of Latin America, for example, reference is made to the LGBTT population, with the second T having been added to distinguish between *transgender* and *transvestite* subgroups. In short, from a cross-cultural perspective, whenever LGBT is used in this analysis, we ask that readers remember that this is a somewhat problematic construct that must be subjected to constant critique to avoid imposing a category that fails to have a fully agreed upon (or universally shared) meaning across social and cultural boundaries.

2 Structural Violence and LGBT Health

The concept of *structural violence* provides an important point of departure for discussions of LGBT health in cross-cultural settings. Structural violence refers to the ways by which social inequalities and political-economic systems place particular persons or groups in situations of extreme vulnerability, and this vulnerability is expressed in patterns of morbidity and mortality (Farmer et al., 1996). Precisely because social inequalities such as class, race, and ethnicity intersect with sexual inequalities, the shape of LGBT health in any social or cultural setting is inextricably linked to the relations that exist between these various forms of social inequality. This highlights the importance of placing any discussion of LGBT health in a broader historical and political-economic framework to understand the range of social forces that affect the health of LGBT communities and populations around the world in an era of intense globalization.

A growing cross-cultural literature has emerged that is relevant for our discussion of the social inequalities that shape the environments in which LGBT populations live and the specific expressions of structural violence they face. In the developing world, much of this literature has focused on processes that have been stimulated by the extension of industrialization and capitalist economic restructuring in a wide range of societies—as much in Latin America, Asia, and Africa as in the more extensively researched societies of western Europe or North America (Altman, 1989; Parker, 1999; Drucker, 2000; Appadurai, 2001). These studies have demonstrated that certain expressions of global capitalism have led to the transnational spread of identities, meanings, and terms of Western notions of LGBT identity in a broad range of societies, including, for example, Argentina (Pecheny, 2001; Brown, 2002), Brazil (Parker 1999, 2002), Chile (Frasca, 1997, 2003), China (Wah-shan, 2000), the Dominican Republic (Padilla, 2007, in press), India (Reddy, 2004), Indonesia (Wieringa, 1994, 1995), Mexico (Carrier, 1995, 1999; Carrillo, 1999, 2002), Namibia (Croucher, 2002), Peru (Cáceres, 1996; Cáceres & Rosasco, 1999), Senegal (Teunis, 1998), South Africa (Gevisser & Cameron, 1995; Donham, 1998; Phillips, 2000, 2004), Taiwan (Chao, 2000), or Thailand (Jackson, 1997, 2000; Jackson & Cook, 2000). Despite this diverse literature, relatively less attention has been placed on what has been described as "dependent development and gay identity" (Parker & Caceres, 1999), in which the shape of these appropriated cultural forms and identities is analyzed within local and global systems of power and inequality. Such a framework is essential when considering the influence of structural violence on LGBT health, and it has several consequences for our understanding of the health of LGBT populations in the developing world.

First, in resource-poor areas of the world, the large-scale political-economic environment—and therefore many of the structural vulnerabilities faced by LGBT persons—is quite distinct from the structural circumstances that have been described for LGBT communities in developed, industrialized nations such as the United States (D'Emilio, 1993). For example, integration into the wage economy may have facilitated independence from natal households among some LGBT men and women in the United States, thereby allowing them financial independence from the what D'Emilio (1993) describes as the "imperative to procreate." In contrast, the formal wage economy in the developing world is often highly constrained and precarious, functionally precluding large numbers of LGBT persons from achieving material independence. Murray (1992) has discussed this phenomenon as the "underdevelopment of gay communities," a somewhat problematic term intended to draw attention to the ways LGBT communities in the developing world may be constrained by structural factors characteristic of the larger conditions of underdevelopment, such as economic dependence on family and kin networks, lack of housing, low literacy, low access to education, and high unemployment.

Indeed, a growing ethnographic literature on LGBT populations in a variety of cultural settings has begun to document the specific ways that *nonnormative sexualities*—understood as expressions of sexual identity or practice that deviate from the expectations of particular hegemonic "sexual cultures" (Parker, 1990)—may be particularly vulnerable to the structural and social inequalities routinely experienced by poor populations in many areas of the world (Farmer, 1990, 1992). This literature, although not always informed by applied public health approaches, has nevertheless described some of the ways that the inequalities confronting many poor populations in the developing world are often particularly pronounced among those who are further stigmatized by their nonnormative gender, sexuality, or sexual behavior. We believe that to understand the social epidemiology of LGBT health in the developing world we must also understand the particular structural constraints LGBT persons face, and this requires attention to the linkages between political-economic factors and the disadvantaged position of LGBTs as a marginal and stigmatized group within local systems of gender and sexuality. Furthermore, because much of this structural violence is reinforced by institutionalized and governmental policies that systematically undermine the human rights of LGBT populations, some international agencies have begun to recognize such expressions as violations of sexual rights (Ungar, 2000; Schliefer, 2004).

Various studies from Latin America of transgendered persons, for example, demonstrate that same-sex attraction or cross-gender behavior during childhood or adolescence can produce vehement retribution or violence from family and community members. In her study of effeminate *jotas*, or young men displaying cross-gender behavior in a poor section of Mexico City, Prieur's research showed that many of these persons were forced out of school—and often out of their homes—because of their effeminacy, leaving them, according to Prieur, "largely excluded from the educational system and from ordinary working life" (Prieur, 1998, p. 67). Structurally excluded from numerous domains of productive life and subject to various forms of systematic abuse, Prieur concludes that commercial sex work may actually be (somewhat paradoxically) an *upwardly mobile choice* for these adolescents, or at least one that does not contribute further to their marginal social status: "For the young jotas who have left school and not had the opportunity to enter the labor market, starting to sell sexual services does not represent further exclusion, does not mean that the distance from *straight* society increases" (Prieur, 1998, p. 72). Kulick's (1997, 1998) work on transgendered Brazilian prostitutes, or *travestís*, similarly demonstrates that once detached from extended kin networks, and after being violently expelled from home, many *travestís* were left largely without support structures when they became homeless, hungry, ill, or reached the final stages of human immunodeficiency virus (HIV) infection. He further demonstrates the ways that international sex work networks facilitate the *travestís'* trips to European cities, where many of them are made further vulnerable by restrictive policies, antiimmigrant laws, abusive authorities, drugs, and violence. Thus, although it is inappropriate to think of Mexican *jotas* or

Brazilian *travestís* as in some way bereft of autonomy or agency—because both of these ethnographic studies also demonstrate the elaborate and poignant ways that transgendered sex workers use their expert knowledge of gender and sexuality to survive—the studies exemplify the persistent and extreme structural violence that confronts transgendered persons in Latin America, shaping their vulnerability to physical and psycho-emotional risks.

The stigma and discrimination experienced by transgendered persons demonstrates, on one hand, the extreme consequences of non-normative gender and sexuality in many cultural contexts and, on the other hand, the logic behind the desire—even perhaps the *necessity*—to pass as normal for those LGBTs who are able to do so. "Passing" is a phenomenon often associated with the sociologist Erving Goffman's (1963) classic analysis of stigma management; it refers to an individual's ability to convince others, through the use of a variety of strategies and techniques, that she/he does not belong to a stigmatized social category. For instance, Carrillo described a case from his ethnographic research in Mexico involving two lesbian women who over an extended period of time "had engaged in elaborate schemes and arrangements to be able to live as a lesbian couple while also pretending that they were divorced women supporting each other as close friends" (Carrillo, 2002, p. 145). Such patterns are consistent with observations about lesbian invisibility throughout Latin America, where remaining silent about one's sexuality is a functional response to the fear of losing the privileged social status conferred by heterosexuality; it is a rational coping mechanism in the context of very real threats to lesbian women's well-being (Eiven, 2003). Indeed, an International Gay and Lesbian Human Rights Commission (IGLHRC) report on Spain suggests that owing to tradition and economic crisis most unmarried women are forced to live with their parents until their early thirties, and lesbians who reveal their sexual orientation to their family face nearly insurmountable rejection and condemnation (Hernandez, 2003).

Although the health implications of passing—often overlapping with what Carrillo refers to as *sexual silence*—is only beginning to be documented, the HIV/AIDS epidemic has spurred a number of authors to draw connections between cultural silence about homoeroticism and the spread of HIV. In an important piece on the epidemic among Latin American and Latino populations, for example, Alonso and Koreck (1993) argued that the continued transmission of the HIV virus was closely related to the deeply ingrained cultural silence about sex and sexuality, particularly same-sex behavior, despite the commonality of clandestine same-sex encounters in Latin American societies. In the case of sex between men, they argued that Latino silence was a fundamental barrier to effective prevention of HIV, an argument that has been put forward in various versions by other researchers as well (Parker, 1992, 1996, 1999, 2000; Cáceres, 1996; Díaz, 1997, 1998; Carrillo, 2002; Arend, 2003; Padilla, 2007, in press).

One of the least studied aspects of sexual silence is the way it influences LGBT health in the context of their familial and household relationships. For example, some cross-cultural literature on gender and household health suggests that in many cultural contexts relationships with family and other household members may be crucial determinants of numerous health outcomes, and relationships with adult women may be particularly important in this regard (Browner, 1989; Browner & Leslie, 1996; Clark, 1993). However, for LGBTs who may not feel capable of discussing or acknowledging their sexuality with their immediate household and family, adequate support for LGBT-related health concerns is unlikely to be forthcoming. Furthermore, even if household members become aware of one's sexuality, the rejection, reprimand, or even physical abuse that can result may further place LGBT persons in more precarious health situations or contribute to negative health outcomes. For example, Díaz's (1998) work among Latino gay men in the United States suggests that when the familial support for one's gay identity was not forthcoming many men in his study were in danger of losing access to crucial social networks they needed for survival. Díaz sees these contacts as essential for assisting individuals in an already marginalized ethnic group to cope with the structural conditions they face in the larger society. Furthermore, Carrillo argued, Díaz "has gone so far as to suggest that sexual silence creates a psychological split between sex and affection that among homosexual men results in a search for anonymous sex, loneliness, longing for a romantic relationship, problems practicing safer sex, and a deep-seated absence of affective intimacy in the context of sex" (Carrillo, 2002, p. 149). In addition to maintaining sexual silence, family members may also directly influence or manipulate sexual behaviors and practices, as dramatically illustrated by Bolt-Gonzales's (1996) analysis of lesbians in Nicaragua, which demonstrates that lesbians' relatives and significant others may play an important role in imposing reproductive decisions and forcing maternity.

Ironically, even as LGBT activism and movement politics in certain countries have led to the possibility of LGBT persons adopting children or raising their own biologic children, LGBT families continue to face social and legal restrictions that reinforce sexual marginalization. The Human Rights Watch (2004a) reported the case of a Chilean lesbian mother who was deprived custody of her children by the High Court because she refused to hide her lesbian relationship from her children. Similarly, in the relatively progressive political environment of Spain, where lesbians are legally permitted to adopt a child, a report by the International Gay and Lesbian Human Rights Commission reported in 2003 that women were not allowed to adopt as a couple, and a lesbian mother who is open about her sexuality may face serious social consequences (Hernandez, 2003). Although Spain has recently resolved legislative ambiguities that allowed continuing discrimination in marriage and adoption (McLean, 2005), these examples demonstrate the broad impact of institutionalized discrimination on the private lives and sexual rights of LGBT persons, even in presumably progressive social and political contexts.

The fact that sexual silence may be related to certain health risks may lead one to assume that open self-identification as gay or lesbian may mitigate such risks for LGBT persons. However, there is no reason to believe that this is necessarily so based on the highly limited evidence presently available. The literature on the relation between self-identification as gay and HIV risk behavior among minority men in the United States, for example, has provided ambiguous results. Whereas some scholars argue that gay identification can lead to positive health behaviors among men who have sex with men because of positive gay community norms that reinforce safer sex practices (Seibt et al., 1993; Turner et al., 1993; Kelly et al., 2002; Chng et al., 2003), other studies suggest that gay identification among Latino men may actually *increase* high-risk behavior (Marks et al., 1998). From a global perspective, part of the ambiguity involves the fact that the very notion of sexual disclosure assumes there is a fundamental LGBT essence that is either hidden or truthfully exposed, and this is not a universal understanding of sexuality or sexual identity across cultures and societies. A significant proportion of the same-sex behavior in many cultural settings may not be definitive of a homosexual identity in any way analogous to gay identity in places such as the United States or western Europe. Therefore, any attempt to understand the relation between sexual identification and health risks in the developing world, by necessity, must consider the local meanings of same-sex practices in specific cultural settings in addition to the nature of social inequalities and structural violence.

In sum, the existing cross-cultural literature on LGBT persons demonstrates that the combination of social marginality and large-scale structural inequality often leads to particularly acute manifestations of structural violence among marginalized genders and sexualities in the developing world, and this disadvantaged position of LGBTs is a crucial factor—perhaps *the* most crucial factor—in shaping LGBT health outcomes. At the same time, the ways that structural violence unfolds and its linkages to local cultural meanings and definitions of sexuality are variable and depend on the local cultural context. Understanding both of these processes is essential for conceptualizing LGBT health. Moreover, we argue, it demands greater emphasis on ethnographic and qualitative approaches to LGBT health in the developing world to better understand the local meanings of sexuality in specific cultural contexts and their connections to the structural violence faced by LGBT persons.

3 Violence, Human Rights, and LGBT Health

The literature on violence against LGBT persons, although far from comprehensive, demonstrates that the structural violence faced by LGBT persons is not limited to the impersonal domain of social, political, and economic inequalities. Indeed, such violence frequently manifests in very real expressions of physical and sexual abuse against this population. Although relatively little is known about exposure to violence and abuse from within LGBT communities (as in the case of domestic violence by sexual partners) or from individuals or groups outside these communities who perpetrate physical violence against LGBT persons, a growing international human rights literature attests to systematic and institutionalized abuses and social cleansing practices perpetrated by governments or their functionaries (police, military, paramilitary forces, death squads) against LGBT persons in many parts of the world. Furthermore, the existing literature on domestic violence in LGBT communities demonstrates the close connections between the larger social inequalities and silences faced by LGBT persons and the risk of domestic violence in LGBT communities. Here we summarize this emerging literature, drawing on the few descriptive or ethnographic studies available as well as the documentation of such human rights abuses now available through international organizations such as Amnesty International.

Whereas the practice of domestic violence among same-sex partners has been well documented in the United States (Merrill & Wolfe, 2000; Relf, 2001a,b), there is still a lack of literature about battered LGBT persons in many parts of the world. In the United States, lesbians report pushing or being pushed more frequently than gay men, a pattern that is reflected in a suggestive study from Brazil, which demonstrated that 20% of the calls to a telephone hotline involved women who were assaulted by their female partners (Eiven, 2003). Nevertheless, this may be a reflection of the underreporting of battering among men, an artifact of the fact that the authorities tend to underestimate partner abuse among gay men, or a consequence of the reduced believability of battered men in comparison to (heterosexual or lesbian) women (Poorman et al., 2003). However, because of the paucity of literature on LGBT domestic abuse in developing settings, it is unclear to what degree the patterns observed in the United States are generalizable cross-culturally. Some ethnographic studies suggest that in developing settings underreporting may be similarly pronounced because prior experiences of persecution or abuse by authorities toward sexual minorities is likely to result in the fear that admission to same-sex behaviors will result in further police abuse (Kulick, 1998; Prieur, 1998; Padilla, 2007, in press). In addition, the generalized shame and stigma surrounding nonnormative sexual behaviors and identities is likely to contribute to underreporting.

An important study of abuse in LGBT relationships in Australia, which reported that domestic violence is the third most severe health problem facing gay men today after AIDS and substance abuse, demonstrates the intimate connections between societal homophobia and the risk of domestic violence (Vickers, 1996). Describing LGBT domestic violence as "the second closet," the author argues that LGBT persons who abuse their partners often use homophobia and heterosexism as a weapon of control over the partner in a variety of ways, such as threatening to reveal the partner's sexuality to friends, family, employers, or the wider community; convincing their partner that violence is an expression of gay life; or arguing that nobody is going to help or believe the story of violence due to homophobia (Vickers, 1996). Because of the discretion about the relationship that both partners are supposed to protect, domestic violence therefore functions as a second closet for many LGBTs who do not reveal their situation owing to the institutionalized homophobia and heterosexism present in the criminal justice system, support services, and the larger society (Vickers, 1996). The lack of ability in many cases to discuss such relationships with family and other social peers creates further barriers to reporting the abuse and to seeking any support systems or programs that may be available.

The situation of domestic violence is further exacerbated by the patterns of hate crimes, abuse, and persecution of LGBT persons by those outside the community. In the 2001 global report on torture and hate crimes against LGBT person by Amnesty International, provocatively titled "Crimes of Hate, Conspiracy of Silence," LGBT populations are said to be systematically denied human rights and full citizenship throughout the world. Importantly, the report argues that this denial is often rooted in a conspiracy of silence between the state, other institutions, and society, and that such silence functions to maintain and reinforce human rights violations against LGBT persons, such as discrimination in employment, access to military or state professions, and access to social and medical services (Amnesty International, 1997). Systematic abuse and discrimination based on sexual identity are often legitimized by law, policy, and practice in many countries, and torture may even be legitimized when employed against LGBT persons. A parallel indictment of international human rights abuses published by the International Gay and Lesbian Human Rights Commission (2003) argues that torture is a widespread means for regulating sexuality and enforcing norms of gender and sexuality, and that the effects of *sodomy laws* in many parts of the world justifies detention of people based on their sexual orientation, denial of public services, and the abuse of LGBT persons by police, doctors, and health practitioners. Recently, additional human rights organizations, such as the Human Rights Watch, have released statements denouncing the systematic torture, persecution, assassination, and hate crimes against the LGBT population the world over. Their report highlights numerous tragic cases of systematic abuse, such as one recent atrocity in Sierra Leone in which a lesbian activist—the victim of constant harassment and violence from neighbors and the compliance of local police and the government—was found murdered after being repeatedly raped and stabbed (Human Rights Watch, 2004c). The graphic nature of the abuses detailed in this report emphasizes that such violence is rarely based on simple political differences that can be addressed through traditional mechanisms of legal or policy reform; rather, it is generated by deep hatred and moral outrage that is systemic and pervasive, requiring broad social and cultural transformation.

The extent of the human rights violations against LGBT persons underlines the need to consider these phenomena as an additional expression of structural violence that is expressed in the very physical risks to life and limb that are confronted by LGBT in many settings as a consequence of institutionalized discrimination. Policies and programs aimed at improving LGBT health, in addition to providing health services and programs specifically designed for LGBT persons, must therefore also address themselves to abusive policies of states or international organizations, and seek to apply political pressure through existing human rights bodies that are increasingly document-ing such human rights violations among sexual minorities.

4 HIV/AIDS and LGBT Health in Cross-Cultural Perspective

Within the broader context of structural violence and the global and local structural constraints LGBT persons face, we turn to the phe-nomenon that has become emblematic of the intersection between sex-uality and health in the contemporary world: the HIV/AIDS pandemic. As Cáceres (2005) argues in a review of LGBT health issues focusing primarily on Latin America, discussions of LGBT health urgently need to move "beyond AIDS," a sentiment with which we wholeheartedly agree. Nevertheless, in many ways HIV/AIDS provides an essential context for our discussion of LGBT health in the developing world, as so much of the social, economic, and political context of LGBT health has been irrevocably shaped by this single health problem. In this section, we argue that the impact of HIV/AIDS on LGBT health in the developing world cannot be adequately understood without consider-ing at least three factors: (1) the complex ways the development of the local HIV epidemic intersects with existing patterns of stigmatization and discrimination toward LGBT persons; (2) the general lack of emphasis placed on designing appropriate programs to meet the sexual health needs of a *diversity* of LGBT groups and identities in specific sociocultural contexts; and (3) the relations among LGBT populations, community-based organizations, and patterns of state funding and support for LGBT communities and programs. We believe it is essen-tial that this discussion be viewed within a self-consciously global context because the discourses surrounding HIV, as much as the virus itself, are highly mobile, such that scientific or popular understandings of the epidemic in Washington may have intimate connections to beliefs, practices, or policies in Bombay, Durbin, or Buenos Aires. Thus, consideration of the responses to AIDS among LGBTs in the develop-ing world can never be understood as entirely independent of the influ-ence of models and interpretations in the high-income countries from which much of the AIDS-related research, funding, media, and schol-arly literature has emanated since the beginning of the epidemic.

For a number of reasons related to global patterns in the epidemiol-ogy of HIV/AIDS, as well as the historical timing of recognizable gay and lesbian communities in the urban industrialized West, the HIV epi-demic in the United States and Western Europe became associated early in the epidemic with gay-identified men (Epstein, 1996). As argued in several critical analyses of popular interpretations of AIDS early in the epidemic (Treichler, 1988; Watney, 1988; Patton, 1990), the somewhat arbitrary historical impact of HIV infection on gay men in the urban West has led to an incautious yet persistent association between HIV and gay *identity* that tends to reinforce existing social stigma toward LGBT persons and to confirm the popular perception of their inherent perversion and pathology. This tautologic association—

what might be termed the *homosexualization of AIDS*—became a highly influential conceptual model that was rapidly globalized during the first decade of the pandemic and has continued to inform both popular and scientific interpretations of emerging epidemics in various parts of the world (Bolton, 1992a,b; Hoffman & Bolton, 1996; Treichler, 1999).

In the most general terms, there have been at least two consequences for the developing world of this particular restigmatization of LGBT persons vis-à-vis their conceptual association with HIV/AIDS. First, as HIV becomes more prevalent in a given region, LGBT persons—particularly gay-identified men or their analogous identities in a given cultural system—may be presumed to be the primary vectors of HIV infection, often regardless of the actual behavioral epidemiology of HIV transmission, and may also be blamed for the negative consequences of HIV on the wider community. That is, the tautologic association between gay identity and HIV has functioned to reinforce convenient stereotypes that exist in many societies (Human Rights Watch, 2004b), notwithstanding their inevitable cross-cultural variations in expression and intensity, while also offering a convenient explanation for the apparent cause of the epidemic. Not only has this compounded the historical discrimination and scapegoating experienced by LGBT persons in numerous locales, it has created many challenges for HIV prevention campaigns as the epidemic has evolved, as individuals who do not identify themselves with any nonnormative sexual identity or behavior may not consider themselves at risk for HIV infection and may therefore forego appropriate behavioral or preventative measures.

For example, in Farmer's ethnographic account of the emergence of the HIV/AIDS epidemic in Haiti, the initial victims—who were apparently infected through heterosexual contact—did not believe they could be HIV-infected because of their assumption that only homosexuals get AIDS (Farmer, 1992). Such notions were directly in line with reports emanating from the United States and elsewhere at the time in which gay men were configured as the prototypical (or even exclusive) victims of what was often referred to as a "gay plague." These discourses and stereotypes have emerged in many parts of the world in their various local manifestations, and the erroneous beliefs they generate about who is at risk for HIV (and by extension, who is *not* at risk) have been repeatedly identified as barriers to HIV prevention in countries as wide-ranging as India (Bhattacharya, 2004), South Africa (Toms, 1990; de Gruchy & Germond, 1997), and Mexico (Liguori et al., 1996; Liguori & Lamas, 2003). Thus, a growing amount of social science research in international contexts has now demonstrated that as the AIDS epidemic expands the stigma and fears of contagion that are associated with it—what Jonathan Mann referred to as the "Third Epidemic" in the evolution of AIDS—are often linked to the historical patterns of social inequality and hierarchy in the local setting (Mann, 1987; Parker & Aggleton, 2003). LGBT persons are typically disadvantaged in such hierarchies. This not only makes them vulnerable to further discrimination, which may in turn increase their risk for HIV infection, it also, and ironically, results in greater risk to the so-called general population, who may see AIDS as a problem exclusive to the Other and thus fail to understand that the boundaries between self and other are rarely as impermeable as social stereotypes would have us believe.

The permeability of the boundaries between LGBT persons and the general population has been a key epistemologic issue in both public health and social scientific research on HIV/AIDS since the beginning of the epidemic. Early in the epidemic, the notion of a *bisexual bridge* between what was often conceived as a relatively self-contained high risk group of homosexually behaving men and the general population was frequently invoked both as an impending threat to the larger society and as a potential epidemiologic explanation for the different male-to-female ratios of HIV infection in various areas of the world (Aggleton, 1996a). In 1987, for example, Padian (1987) pondered the marked difference between the 1:1 male/female ratio of HIV infection in Africa and the 14:1 ratio in the United States; she offered that higher levels of bisexual behavior among men could conceivably account for this contrast (Padian, 1987, pp. 951–954). Such analyses were also centrally concerned with the global transition from what was then termed *Pattern I*—the epidemiologic scenario originally emerging in the United States and western Europe in which gay men, IV-drug users, and recipients of blood products were the primary victims—to *Pattern II*, whose ideal representation is the generalized, predominantly heterosexual epidemic in sub-Saharan Africa (Patton, 1990). Aggleton (1996a) describes the concept of the bisexual bridge as follows:

[M]ale bisexuals have often been characterized as a "bridging group," enabling HIV to be transmitted from apparently discrete sub-populations of behaviourally homosexual and behaviourally heterosexual individuals. Most usually, it is suggested that bisexual men pose a special threat to their female partners through having had sex with other men, particularly exclusively homosexual men. Such accounts stereotype reality in that they posit the existence of two identifiable and discrete groups of individuals, the "homosexual" and the "heterosexual," that are capable of being "bridged" by a third type.

Early in the epidemic, bisexual behavior and the notion of a bisexual bridge therefore provided a convenient framework for conceptualizing—however crudely—an epidemiologic transition that appeared to be occurring particularly rapidly in some world regions. Yet, as implied by Aggleton's comment, the categorizations used in this framework also tended to impose definitions of sexual identity that may not correspond to social reality in other societies and cultures.

Partly as a response to these epistemologic questions and pushed by social scientific critiques (Parker, 1987, 1990, 1992; Parker & Carballo, 1990; Bolton, 1992a, b), the 1990s brought a growing awareness of the problematic dimensions of epidemiologic language, including its tendency to equate gay identity with an independent risk group or to neglect the various ways that homosexuality is understood in cross-cultural settings. This led to a shift in public health terminology toward the use of the term men who have sex with men, or MSM, in an attempt to separate sexual *identity*, which has nothing to do with HIV risk per se, and sexual risk *behavior*. Although this new terminology has been useful for addressing much of the stereotyping and stigmatization inherent in earlier risk group language and avoids the assumption that all homosexually behaving men can be glossed as *gay*, it is not a label with which individual men can identify and may therefore alienate them from HIV/AIDS interventions (Muñoz-Laboy, 2004). Perhaps more importantly, the new term has tended to perpetuate the erroneous assumption that the highly diverse groups of MSM subsumed under this label share certain broad features that would warrant their categorization as a single vulnerable population. It therefore presumes that the complex social and cultural meanings of sexual identity are universal to all those who participate in same-sex behavior, a notion that is at least partially based on the heterosexist premise that the social complexity of the LGBT experience is somehow reducible to sexual behaviors (Young & Meyer, 2005). Yet this entirely neglects the broad range of meanings, behaviors, social contexts, and identities associated with different subgroups of LGBT persons and across cultural settings, a diversity that is even more striking when placed in global perspective. For example, a growing ethnographic literature on homoeroticism—and perhaps most significantly on Latin American homoeroticism—now exists to conclude that a significant proportion of men who engage in homosexual acts do not identify themselves as *gay*, and their needs are rarely addressed by prevention approaches designed for gay-identified men (Parker, 1987, 1992, 1996, 1999; Alonso & Koreck, 1993; Carrier, 1995; Cáceres, 1996; De Moya & Garcia, 1996; Díaz, 1998; Carrillo, 2002; Cáceres & Stall, 2003; Padilla, 2007, in press).

Some analogous definitional problems have limited the creation of appropriate responses to the HIV prevention and treatment needs of what has come to be termed women who have sex with women (WSW). Partly because of the widespread assumption that lesbians face less risk of HIV infection than men, most studies and public health interventions exclude WSW who do not consider themselves lesbians, as well as the range of structural risks for HIV faced by many of the subgroups of women included in this broad category (Arend, 2005). For example, some of these women—most notably those who are marginalized because of class or race—bear much higher risks of exposure to violence, homelessness, sex work, and intravenous drug use (Arend, 2005). There is also a lack of information about other sexually transmitted diseases among lesbians, such as human papilloma virus (HPV) infection, gonorrhea, syphilis, vulvitis, vaginitis, and cervicitis, that can be transmitted among women (Eiven, 2003). Additionally, some of these women engage in sexual relations with men, realities neglected by generic categories that erase the diversity of behavioral patterns characteristic of certain subgroups of WSW (Young et al., 1992; Eiven, 2003). Lesbians are therefore invisible for many researchers, providers, and health professionals; and their rights to health are ignored or subsumed under the umbrella of reproductive health, a category of health services that is notoriously heterosexist (Eiven, 2003).

An additional complexity obscured by catch-all categories such as MSM and WSW is that transmission of HIV in these broad populations is subject to significant regional and cultural variation. For example, whereas there is now significant (and growing) evidence that MSM are an important population vulnerable to HIV infection everywhere in the world (Turner et al., 1993; McKenna, 1996; UNAIDS, 2002), prevalence levels and the behavioral epidemiology of HIV among MSM is quite variable. In Latin America, despite growing levels of heterosexual transmission in some countries, prevalence levels among MSM have ranged from 20% to 35% in major cities of large countries such as Argentina, Brazil, and Mexico and from 5% to 10% in provincial areas and in small countries such as Costa Rica (Izazola Licea, 2001). Whereas in Mexico and Brazil, the homo/bisexual category of HIV transmission accounts for 56% and 35%, respectively, of all AIDS cases reported (PAHO/WHO, 2002), official interpretations of surveillance data in the adjacent Caribbean region are quite distinct, where the epidemic is described as predominantly heterosexual (Camara, 2001). Surveillance data on cases of HIV/AIDS in the Caribbean estimate that somewhere between 76% and 80% of infections are currently due to heterosexual transmission, with homo/bisexual transmission accounting for around 12% (PAHO/WHO, 2002). The relatively low proportion of HIV infections attributed to same-sex activities in the Caribbean therefore contrasts rather sharply with some other countries in the region, despite the fact that the Caribbean is immediately adjacent to these countries and there is considerable and continuous interchange of populations between them. It is unclear to what degree these differences are reflections of true distinctions in the epidemiology of HIV in these regions and to what degree they are consequences of social or cultural distinctions in the organization of same-sex desire and behavior—differences that are not captured by epidemiological categories.

Prevalence and incidence data for MSM are less available for countries in Asia and Africa, where a clearly defined *gay* identity seems to be less common than in the United States, Europe, or even Latin America and where the widespread denial of sexual activity between men may have resulted in a lack of research attention to these hidden populations (McKenna, 1996). Throughout Asia, however, behavioral surveys of men generally have reported high levels of bisexual behavior, and male–male sex has been responsible for an important part of reported HIV infections. For example, in a study of military conscripts in Thailand, although male–male sex was reported by only 7% of the sample, it was associated with 13% of the HIV infections in this population in 1995 (UNAIDS, 2002). The diverse and dynamic nature of these behavioral patterns is further highlighted when we consider the emergence and growth of LGBT identities and sexual politics in Asia, which may have influences on hidden populations and transform the meaning of HIV-related risk practices. For example, a growing literature based on ethnographic research now exists that documents the emergence of increasingly complex LGBT communities and movements in Thailand (Jackson, 2000), Indonesia (Boellstorff & Oetomo, 1996; Oetomo, 2000; Boellstorff, 2004, 2005), India and Bangladesh (Khan, 1994, 1998; Nanda, 1999; Reddy, 2004), and the Philippines (Tan,

1993, 1995). Such movements and politics are directly applicable to the shape of vulnerability to HIV infection as well as institutional representation from which to engage in HIV prevention activities for LGBT populations in the region.

In sub-Saharan Africa, where denial of male homosexual behavior has been described as especially strong, social and behavioral studies by African researchers have increasingly begun to call this denial into question, suggesting that in many countries largely hidden homosexual practices may in fact be far more common than previously reported (Cameron & Gevisser, 1994; Gevisser & Cameron, 1995; Murray & Roscoe, 1998; Teunis, 1998; Phillips, 2000, 2004; Lorway, 2003), and that levels of male–male transmission may be hidden in the HIV prevalence estimates for supposedly uniformly heterosexual men (Murray & Roscoe, 1998; Padilla, 2007, in press). Undoubtedly, part of the problem here derives from the fact that categories such as *homosexuality* fail to describe adequately the diverse forms of traditional male–male sex in many African societies, even though closer study of the contexts within which male–male sex occurs has revealed that male same-sex practices occur throughout the world but are rarely defined as homosexual or gay (McKenna, 1996; Parker & Terto, 1998). Yet even in sub-Saharan Africa, historical and ethnographic research carried out over the course of the past decade has emphasized the existence of multiple forms of hidden same-sex interactions in traditional cultures (Murray & Roscoe, 1998; Lorway, 2003), in the institutions and economies of colonial and early postcolonial societies, such as the mines of southern Africa (Moodie & Ndatshe, 1994; Morrell, 1998; Niehaus, 2002; Phillips, 2004), and most recently in the rapidly changing societies of contemporary Africa (Preston-Whyte et al., 2000; Lorway, 2003; Phillips, 2004).

The emerging literature on homosexuality in such settings suggests that lack of available data on HIV/AIDS and MSM in some regions is itself probably a result of official denial feeding into the limitation of HIV/AIDS research agendas. These limitations have almost certainly masked important forms of vulnerability to HIV infection that have been hidden or even mystified in epidemiologic reports on the epidemic. Recent work coming out of sub-Saharan Africa, for example, suggests that homosexual transmission among men is often incorrectly interpreted as heterosexual transmission due to the inability of researchers, physicians, and public health officials to recognize hidden homosexual relations (Teunis, 1998; Lorway, 2003; Phillips, 2004; Padilla, 2007, in press). Equally perverse, studies now suggest that some women in sub-Saharan African societies who are primarily active in sexual relations with other women (and often self-identified as lesbians) may also be at high risk of infection due to social pressure to be heterosexually active, and may even experience male violence and rape employed in the service of compulsory heterosexuality (Lorway, 2003).

As Parker and colleagues have argued, the result of denial and neglect in HIV/AIDS research has been the reproduction of denial and neglect in the development of AIDS-related programs and services for LGBT populations: "Virtually no official governmental or intergovernmental programs have prioritized men who have sex with men, even in regions where homosexual transmission has been pronounced, such as in Latin America and parts of Asia" (Parker et al., 2000, p. 529). This persistent neglect, related to the stigmatization of LGBT more generally, has been clearly documented in a study carried out by the Panos Institute in association with the Norwegian Red Cross (McKenna, 1996). A targeted survey was conducted with national AIDS programs, AIDS-service organizations (ASOs), nongovernmental organizations (NGOs) involved in AIDS-related work, and gay groups and individuals in countries around the world to document both the extent of same-sex behavior and the kinds of programmatic and prevention responses that had been generated in response to HIV among MSM in the developing world. Data were collected from more than 40 national AIDS programs, more than 100 ASOs and NGOs, and more than 50 gay organizations in countries throughout Africa, Asia, and Latin America. Only 25% of national AIDS programs listed MSM as a target group for AIDS prevention, and only 9% reported programs for male sex workers (in contrast to 84% targeting heterosexual adults, 78% targeting adolescents, and 69% targeting female sex workers) (McKenna, 1996). These results were confirmed when national AIDS programs were asked if any AIDS-related services were available to MSM in their countries: again, a large number, 74%, stated that no such services were available; only 24% reported some services available. When asked what kinds of services, 23% reported counseling services, 18% information and education programs, 16% condom distribution, 12% outreach work, and 9% HIV testing or treatment for MSM (McKenna, 1996).

Throughout the developing world, in the absence of meaningful governmental programs, primary responsibility for HIV prevention has depended on community-based NGOs (McKenna, 1996; Parker et al., 1998). Thus far, the most limited efforts for MSM still characterize sub-Saharan Africa (Gevisser & Cameron, 1995; McKenna, 1996; Murray & Roscoe, 1997, 1998; Parker et al., 1998; Lorway, 2003). In a number of southern and southeastern Asian countries, important programs oriented toward MSM and to the newly emerging gay communities found in many countries have now been initiated (WHO, 1993; Boellstorff & Oetomo, 1996; Kahn, 2003), as is the case in Latin America where gay and AIDS activist organizations have taken the lead in developing programs largely aimed at community mobilization and HIV prevention (Schifter & Madrigal, 1992; Parker et al., 2001). Given their limited scale, however, it is no surprise that such programs have had a relatively small impact on slowing the epidemic, which is exacerbated by the fact that these programs have almost never been systematically evaluated through the use of rigorous research designs; nor have they provided the kind of empirical information base that would ideally be available to programmers and policy makers seeking models to replicate in developing prevention programs for homosexually and bisexually active men (Parker et al., 1998). Indeed, one of the clearest conclusions from the available literature is the urgent need for rigorous intervention and evaluation research on the structure, process, and outcomes of prevention programs designed for MSM in developing countries.

The fact that most governments have generally failed to address adequately the nuances and local realities of the HIV/AIDS epidemic among LGBTs is a clear illustration of the ways that social stigma is expressed in political institutions and economic structures. Where government policies and programs should have sought to reduce the social inequalities that fuel the HIV/AIDS epidemic, they have often chosen to ignore the record of research and programs demonstrating the importance of reaching out to marginalized groups, building communities capable of providing supportive structures, empowering LGBTs to take action on their own behalf, and ensuring their human rights and dignity in the face of persistent stigma and discrimination in the wider society (Parker et al., 1998). Ironically, institutionalized discrimination in the form of the systematic neglect of such programmatic needs only contributes to the cycle of stigma and vulnerability that fuels the epidemic. As shown in a growing number of studies in the developed world, experiences of stigma and discrimination among LGBT persons may in fact be primary factors contributing to high risk behavior. Understanding the precise structural, social, and psychological bases for these connections is a crucial area of future research for LGBT health (Lang, 1990, 1991; Savin-Williams, 1994; Meyer, 1995; Díaz, 1997, 1998; Diaz et al., 2000). Nevertheless, although we might suspect that this synergistic relation between social stigma and HIV/AIDS vulnerability will have analogous expressions in the developing world, their specific manifestations depend on local cultural definitions of nonnormative sexuality, the nature and intensity of social and institutional oppression, and the role played by the state in mitigating the negative consequences of discrimination against LGBT persons. Unfortunately, most governments are far from understanding and addressing these linkages in their specific cultural settings.

Finally, when considering the relationship between institutional and political contexts as they relate to HIV/AIDS among LGBTs, it is important to mention what we might call the epistemologic barriers that often hinder the ability of public health programs to address effectively the HIV prevention and treatment needs of LGBT populations. What is particularly clear from the international anthropological literature on AIDS is that there are vast cultural differences in definitions of what constitutes a *homosexual*, and these definitions have consequences for at least two factors that influence the delivery of appropriate HIV/AIDS services to LGBTs: (1) Such definitions affect how accurately epidemiologists and public health officials interpret patterns of morbidity and mortality among specific LGBT populations; and (2) they influence how effectively public health interventions are specifically designed to address the *broad range* of same-sex identities and practices in the local culture. Unfortunately, only in rare cases are epidemiologic or behavioral data pertaining to HIV/AIDS (or any health-related phenomenon significantly affecting LGBTs) analyzed and interpreted in reference to the local meanings and practices that define homoerotic experience in specific cultural settings. Once again, behavioral bisexuality serves as a useful example. A number of researchers have described the invisibility of bisexual behavior in many parts of the world as being due to the fact that certain homoerotic behaviors are not locally understood to be homosexual, much same-sex desire and behaviors are hidden to avoid social stigma, or private inversion of the sexual norm is considered erotic (Aggleton, 1996b). For example, in his discussion of male bisexuality and HIV in Peru, Cáceres argues that the typical epidemiologic construction of AIDS as essentially a homosexual plague with bisexuality serving as a "bridge connecting an infected (and infectious) constituency to the general population" serves to falsely essentialize sexual behaviors in a manner that has little relationship to the actual behavioral epidemiology of HIV in Peru (Cáceres, 1996, p. 137).

As has been articulated also in Parker's work in Brazil (1987, 1990, 1992, 1996, 1999), another implicit assumption behind much HIV prevention is that all or most men who engage in homosexual sex will be successfully reached by programs targeting the *gay* or *homosexual* community. This perspective—fostered in some settings by the overgeneralization and somewhat uncritical exportation of standard approaches to HIV prevention among urban, white, middle-class, gay-identified men in the United States—has therefore tended to conflate a gay sexual identity with homosexual behavior, a conflation that does not reflect the psychosocial reality for some (perhaps most) men who regularly engage in same-sex sexual behavior in many areas of the world. It is only gradually, and still in a limited number of (relatively well resourced) settings, that what might be described as emerging gay communities have begun to articulate their own hybrid (indigenous yet also globally engaged) responses and program designs for HIV/AIDS prevention and mitigation (Parker & Terto, 1998).

In sum, when viewed from the global and cross-cultural perspective, the HIV/AIDS epidemic among LGBT populations is far from a unitary phenomenon. The interpretation and analysis of local epidemics requires recognition of the mounting evidence showing that although LGBT populations are vulnerable to HIV/AIDS in all settings, the nature and expression of this vulnerability is dependent on numerous contextual factors. To be successful, future programs must recognize the diversity of both identity and behavior in LGBT populations and their distinct HIV prevention and sexual health needs. Furthermore, intervention approaches must recognize that in many cultures concepts such as homosexuality, bisexuality, or gay may have little meaning, and that even in societies in which such categories are present many men who have same-sex relations may not consider these practices to be definitive of their sexual identities. Finally, programs must recognize the importance of mobilizing communities and developing community support structures to reach LGBT persons and to provide them with both social and psychological support for adopting and sustaining safer sexual practices. Such collective empowerment, in the face of otherwise widespread stigma and discrimination, is a key element of all interventions for so-called MSM and WSW; and it is only with widespread state support for basic human rights among all LGBTs that a social climate can be created to reduce the impact of HIV/AIDS among the broad range of LGBT communities as well as the so-called general population.

5 Incarceration and LGBT Health

The fact that LGBT persons are often criminalized by institutionalized sexual discrimination has at least two consequences for considerations of LGBT health in prisons and detention centers. First, because of such discriminatory laws and policies—supported by social prejudices—LGBT persons are at very high risk of incarceration and/or persecution by the authorities. A number of studies in international settings, particularly studies focusing on HIV/AIDS prevention, have demonstrated that prisons can be harmful environments in terms of epidemics and public health (Sagarin, 1976; Moss et al., 1979; Douglas et al., 1989; Wiggs, 1989; Carbajal et al., 1991; Guerena Burgueno et al., 1992; Ducos et al., 1993; Anonymous, 1998; Odujinrin & Adebajo, 2001; Chen et al., 2003; Green et al., 2003). Thus, if LGBT persons are at high risk of exposure to prison environments, they are similarly at high risk for exposure to the various risks associated with being incarcerated. The epidemiologic significance of this is emphasized by the fact that prison environments, although often considered marginal institutions disconnected from the rest of the society, are part of a continuous flow of people between prison environments and the "outside world" that can contribute significantly to epidemiologic patterns of infectious diseases in the larger society (Wiggs, 1989). Thus, LGBT persons may be implicated in epidemiologic relationships that link incarcerated settings with outside settings, an argument that has been made frequently in the context of HIV infection and transmission to women among African American populations in the United States (Peterson, 1997; Lichtenstein, 2000; Lemelle & Battle, 2004).

The second consequence of the institutionalized discrimination faced by LGBT persons is that once they are placed in prison environments they are vulnerable to additional abuses by both fellow inmates and the prison staff. In terms of nonconsensual sex, violence in prisons is a complex phenomenon not only occurring between and among inmates but also wielded as a form of institutional violence committed by the authorities in charge of the prison (Moss et al., 1979; Aubrey & Christiaan, 1995). Many studies report high numbers of men who report having been coerced into having sex at some point during their imprisonment (Green et al., 2003), and in some cases this violence results in the victim's suicide (Wiggs, 1989).

In the case of HIV/AIDS, the situation is made worse by the fact that there is often a common cultural opposition to providing condoms in prison, often because this service would represent institutional recognition of active homosexual behavior among inmates (Anonymous, 1998). In Malawi prisons, for example, prison inmates are not allowed access to condoms because of the belief that such an intervention could encourage homosexuality, which is illegal in the country (Zachariah et al., 2002). In his analysis of South African prisons, Achmat (1993) argued that biomedical and other hegemonic discourses about sexuality seek to neutralize the subversive and destabilizing effects of same-sex sexuality in all-male environments such as compounds and prisons. In this sense, efforts to provide condoms to prisoners confront strong opposition from politicians and government officials, who frequently share the view that introducing condom in prisons is an invitation to (or an acknowledgement of) forbidden homosexual practices. An additional problem is that many programs for preventing HIV infection in prisons emphasize the idea of mandatory HIV testing as a way of preventing the spread of the disease, rather than offering voluntary programs with emphasis on education and counseling (Andrus et al., 1989). In the context of societal discrimination against HIV-positive persons, such mandatory testing programs could add another layer of discrimination and abuse, as inmates may be forcibly tested and their HIV status exposed.

As in any other homosocial environments, highly diverse sexual cultures and practices occur in incarcerated populations. Indeed, imprisonment itself creates conditions for the exchange of intimacy and sexual experiences. Several studies show not only different forms of sexual behavior but also the constitution of new forms of social and sexual identities based on the daily life experience in prison (Awofeso & Naoum, 2002; Vásquez del Aguila, 2002). There may be a reconfiguration of eroticism in such settings, such that sexual identities are more fluid and express an array of sexual practice, such as sex between inmates and their male and female visitors (which are not always conjugal visitors); consensual homosexual sex among inmates; group masturbation; various forms of prostitution; sex between prisoners and prison staff; and rape and sexual violence among prison inmates (Awofeso & Naoum, 2002; Vásquez del Aguila, 2002).

Despite the strong potential for regulations on the use of illicit substances in incarcerated populations, prison life in the developing world may involve routine use of drugs, alcohol, and other substances as part of the daily life of the inmates. For example, in a study in Tijuana, Mexico, prisoners reported high rates of drug use even in comparison with several nonincarcerated populations (Guerena Burgueno et al., 1992). As many studies demonstrate in other contexts, the use of drugs can reduce the possibility of sexual negotiation and the incorporation of safe sex behavior, including the use of condoms. In this sense, the presence of drugs in prisons reinforces the inmate's vulnerability and increases the possibilities for the spread of sexually transmitted infections.

As Arnott (2001) states, it is necessary to incorporate a human rights approach in prisons with the assumption that these institutions are not a different world in which human rights and other international conventions do not apply. From a public health perspective, human rights in prisons include preventing the spread of HIV, which requires the provision of condoms, education, counseling, and access to health services. In fact, periods of incarceration may represent a unique opportunity to convey prevention messages that focus on high-risk behaviors outside the incarcerated setting (Wohl et al., 2000). Finally, the LGBT approach to health advocacy has rarely been linked to protecting the sexual health of incarcerated populations; but given the vulnerability of LGBT persons to institutional abuse and incarceration—as well as the overlapping nature of prison homosexuality and the larger LGBT community—greater awareness of these linkages may serve to improve the health of both incarcerated populations and LGBT populations more generally.

6 Sexual Migration, Mobility, and Health

Migration is a regional or global movement of people who cross domestic and/or international boundaries for a variety of reasons, such as an economic crisis, the search for educational improvement, escape from political violence, and as may be the case for LGBT persons, the perception of greater openness to sexual diversity. Although the social scientific and demographic literature on migration and the process of acculturation has expanded significantly during the last few decades, few studies have addressed the particular issues faced by LGBT migrant populations (Carrillo, 2004). On one hand, decisions to migrate for LGBT persons may involve political and economic considerations similar to those of heterosexual persons, such as opportunities for employment, professional advancement, or escape from oppressive economic or political circumstances. On the other hand, this decision is shaped by other factors and considerations that are particular to LGBT persons, such as sexual identity, exposure to sexual stigma, and the perception of improved possibilities for sexual experiences or community building in other regions or countries (Carrillo, 2004). This problematizes traditional approaches to migration that presume that sexuality involves exchanges between male and female heterosexual partners, or that the meanings of family and kinship for migrants are necessarily the same for the wide range of genders and sexualities.

For many migrants, international migration is not a new experience but, rather, a continuum linking rural communities or small cities to urban or mega cities in their country of origin. Therefore to conceptualize migration among LGBTs as a process, it is necessary to consider the sexual and social situation of the immigrants prior to relocation, during migration, at the various migratory phrases, upon arrival in the new place of residence, and in many cases upon return to their country of origin (Carrillo, 2004). Migration from developing countries is not a homogeneous phenomenon; rather, it involves diverse patterns of separation from the homeland, transition, and so-called acculturation to the new social environment. Cultures vary enormously in how they approve or disapprove of sexual behaviors, and LGBT migrants therefore may encounter dramatic shifts in ideologies, sexual practices, social stigma, and sexual identities. Certain attitudes and behaviors that gay men perform in a new situation are not possible to imagine in their homeland owing to the stigma and discrimination these attitudes might engender, not only for themselves but also for their families and social networks (Bronfman et al., 1989; Bronfman & Minello, 1992).

As suggested by recent critiques of the concept in public health, the notion of *acculturation* has often led to analyses that stereotype reality, reducing complex social phenomena to two ideal types that are seen to interact rather simplistically and in a somewhat linear fashion (Hunt et al., 2004). The reality of contemporary migration and mobility patterns questions analyses that depict a somewhat mechanistic assimilation to the mainstream society rather than dynamic processes, always in tension, conflict, negotiation, and resistance between the various migrant groups and the (often multiethnic) receiving society. Indeed, patterns of population movement are considerably more complex than the traditional *culture contact model* implies, illustrated by phenomena such as circular migration, global media communications, and the complex transnational kin structures that are everywhere in evidence today.

Interestingly, the notion of acculturation has been applied in a number of recent studies on the LGBT population to understand the relation between assimilation to a gay model and its relation to sexual health. For example, a significant amount of HIV/AIDS research on the acculturation process among Latino MSM has sought to determine whether greater incorporation into a gay-identified sexual system leads to greater or lesser rates of sexual risk behavior. A number of studies have argued that integration into the North American gay community is protective for immigrant Latino MSM, either because these men are able to learn safe sex norms espoused by gays or because they gain access to the social support of the gay community (Seibt et al., 1993; Turner et al., 1993; Kelly et al., 1995; Chng & Geliga-Vargas, 2000). Nevertheless, the presumed positive effects of gay acculturation are not universal findings. In a study of HIV-positive gay, bisexual, and heterosexual Latinos in Los Angeles, greater levels of acculturation were associated with greater rates of sexual risk disclosure but significantly higher rates of unprotected sex (Marks et al., 1998). Similarly, other investigators have found that men with higher connectedness to gay communities and organizations were *less* likely to disclose high-risk behavior or unprotected anal intercourse (Doll et al., 1994).

As with the wider literature on acculturation, we believe that studies of LGBT health need to move beyond reductionistic or stereotyped models of culture contact to examine the lived experiences of migration and the situational contexts of health for specific migrant populations. Transnational migration, rather than simple geographic movement of people from one country to another, is a dynamic and complex phenomenon related to social networks and transnational linkages that constitute important economic, emotional, and social exchanges between people's homelands and their new place of living (Hirsch et al., 2002; Hirsch, 2003). These complexities are further magnified for LGBT migrants because, in addition to cultural differences in the normative society, they are often moving within and between dramatically different sexual communities with quite variable consequences for social stigma, same-sex behavior, and discrimination. Furthermore, because of the often stark differences in the material and structural contexts of the various places migrants traverse, there may be quite different material consequences for LGBT persons depending on where they are in their specific migration route, the legal rights (if any) for LGBT persons in each location, the willingness of the government and authorities to protect the rights of migrant LGBTs, and so on. Future research on health among migrant LGBTs should therefore seek to conceptualize not only the ways that cultural exchange occurs regarding the meanings of homoeroticism and the processes of sexual self-identification but also how structural factors are operating to influence health among LGBT migrants.

Tourism is not a form of migration but, rather, a particular combination of mobility, consumption, and leisure (MacCannell, 1976; Urry, 1995, 2002). Nevertheless, it may be closely linked to health among LGBT populations, particularly in geographic areas highly dependent on the tourism industry. Farmer, for example, pointed to the epidemiologic linkages between gay North American sex tourism and the AIDS epidemic in Haiti, arguing that despite epidemiologic data to the contrary, U.S. public health officials during the early 1980s depicted the island as an isolated reservoir of endemic HIV infection (Farmer, 1992). He argued that this rhetorical construction belies the extensive epidemiologic linkages between the United States and Haiti through the commercial sex industry, which provided the most likely route for the introduction of HIV from North America to Haiti: "Sufficient data now exist to support the assertion that economically driven male prostitution, catering to a North American clientele, played a major role in the introduction of HIV to Haiti" (Farmer, 1992, p. 145). Paralleling many aspects of Farmer's argument, a growing number of studies have emphasized the epidemiologic and historical importance of these regional nodes of international sex work in various parts of the Caribbean, such as Cuba (Leiner, 1994; Lumsden, 1996), Barbados (Press, 1978), and the Dominican Republic (De Moya et al., 1992; De Moya & Garcia, 1998; Padilla, 2007, in press). The need for interventions to improve sexual health among tourists and the locals with whom they have contact, including but not limited to sex workers, has been argued repeatedly, drawing on studies from a wide range of geographic and cultural contexts (Isaacs & McKendrick, 1992; Murray & Roscoe, 1998; McCamish et al., 2000; Visser, 2002; Padilla, 2007, in press). It remains a priority for future efforts to improve LGBT health to examine the intersection between tourism, sex work, and the health of LGBT populations and to prioritize programs to address the needs of both hosts and guests in the global tourism sector.

In addition to tourism, it should be mentioned that in the contemporary globalized world cross-cultural contact and LGBT relationships are taking increasingly complex and varied forms, including configurations such as transnational relationships, partnerships between foreign expatriates and locals in the developing world, or circular migratory arrangements. In part, these emerging expressions of LGBT sexuality and identity are the product of different kinds of cultural contact and fluidity that characterize late capitalism itself (Harvey, 1990; Appadurai, 1996). Indeed, the structures of what has been called *flexible accumulation* may lead to different types of population flow that also have implications for LGBT sexuality, identity, and health, as illustrated by the influence of multinational offshore modes of production on the sexual mixture of employees from various cultural backgrounds, or the increasing presence of expatriate aid workers in the developing world who now live for long periods in the South. Thus, the movement and flow of LGBT populations is quite complex in their contemporary capitalist expressions; and these flows, and the relationships they generate, are as important as the shorter, more clearly commodified relations typical of sex tourism. Research and interventions have only begun to address the ways that such processes influence LGBT health in specific settings, but they must be examined in future work on these issues if we are to improve patterns of morbidity and mortality in LGBT communities in the contemporary globalized world.

7 Conclusions

This chapter has sought to outline the existing ethnographic and social science literature relevant to LGBT health from a theoretical perspective that highlights both political-economic conditions and the structural violence LGBT populations confront, as well as the cross-cultural variations in the social norms and perceptions that shape LGBT vulnerability in specific locales. As described at the outset, we believe that such a dual conceptual approach is essential to the consideration of LGBT health in the contemporary world, given that both social inequality and the diverse meanings of nonnormative sexuality have an influence on the health-related vulnerabilities LGBT persons face. Unfortunately, there is a paucity of cross-cultural studies that specifically seek to examine LGBT health within such an analytical framework, requiring us to extrapolate ethnographic observations regarding the discrimination and health risks of LGBT persons from broader anthropological studies about nonnormative genders and sexualities in various developing countries. On the other hand, health-related research and public health programs targeting LGBT populations rarely consider health outcomes as the product of structural violence or social inequalities, resulting in a theoretical myopia that limits the ability of such work to address the larger social forces that shape LGBT health. We therefore advocate for the development of social science perspectives and intervention approaches that conceive of LGBT health as embedded in various social inequalities and that seek to understand the precise linkages between structural violence and sexual marginality in specific cultural settings.

In addition, we believe that the growing field of globalization studies has much to offer the examination of health issues among LGBT populations, as so many of the fundamental features of contemporary sexualities—from Guadalajara to Hong Kong—are embedded in transnational modes of production/consumption and the rapid flow of bodies, sexual identities, and sexual meanings. Although the latter aspects of globalization have been theorized in many of the cross-cultural studies of sexuality cited above, there has been relatively little work done that places LGBT health at the center of the analysis, examining how global processes relate to health circumstances in specific places. This is perhaps related to the tendency for globalization to be conceptualized as a process primarily involving the flow of the meanings and identities related to LGBT sexualities, rather than the stark social inequalities and patterns of structural violence that are central to the experiences of globalization among many LGBT populations, particularly in the developing world. To conceptualize the multifaceted connections between global processes and the health risks and vulnerabilities experienced by LGBT persons, future work must combine these perspectives, examining how processes of globalization function to create new health risks for LGBT persons as well as considering ways that public health programs, structural interventions, political activism, and policy changes might function to mitigate these risks.

References

Achmat, Z. (1993) "Apostles of civilised vice": "immoral practices" and "unnatural vice" in South African prisons and compounds, 1890–1920. *Social Dynamics* 19(2):92–110.

Aggleton, P. (1996a) Introduction. In: Aggleton, P. (ed) *Bisexualities and AIDS: international perspectives*. Taylor & Francis, London, pp. 1–2.

Aggleton, P. (ed) (1996b) *Bisexualities and AIDS: international perspectives*. Taylor & Francis, London.

Alonso, A.M., and Koreck, M.T. (1993) Silences: "Hispanics," AIDS, and sexual practices. In: Abelove, H., Barale, M.A., and Halperin, D.M. (eds) *The lesbian and gay studies reader*. Routledge, New York, pp. 110–126.

Altman, D. (1989) AIDS and the reconceptualization of homosexuality. In: Altman, D. (ed) *Homosexuality, which homosexuality?* GMP, London, pp. 35–48.

Amnesty International. (1997) *Breaking the silence: human rights violations based on sexual orientation*. Amnesty International United Kingdom, London.

Andrus, J.K., Fleming, D.W., Knox, C., McAlister, R.O., Skeels, M.R., Conrad, R.E., Horan, J.M., and Foster, L.R. (1989) HIV testing in prisoners: is mandatory testing mandatory? *American Journal of Public Health* 79:840–842.

Anonymous. (1998) AIDS in prisons—good intentions, harsh realities in Africa's penitentiaries. *AIDS Analysis in Africa* 8(3):12.

Appadurai, A. (1996) *Modernity at large*. University of Minnesota Press, Minneapolis.

Appadurai, A. (2001) Grassroot globalization and the reseach imagination. In: Appadurai, A. (ed) *Globalization*. Duke University Press, Durham, pp. 1–21.

Arend, E. (2005) The politics of invisibility: homophobia and low-income HIV-positive women who have sex with women. *Journal of Homosexuality* 49(1):97–122.

Arend, E.D. (2003) The politics of invisibility: HIV-positive women who have sex with women and their struggle for support. *Journal of the Association of Nurses in AIDS Care* 14(6):37–47.

Arnott, H. (2001) HIV/AIDS, prisons and the Human Rights Act. *European Human Rights Law Review* 1:71–77.

Aubrey, T., and Christiaan, B. (1995) *Anti-gay hate crimes: need for police involvement to curb violence committed against gays*. Centre for the Study of Violence and Reconciliation, Braamfontein.

Awofeso, N., and Naoum, R. (2002) Sex in prisons—a management guide. *Australian Health Review* 25:149–158.

Bhattacharya, G. (2004) Sociocultural and behavioral contexts of condom use in heterosexual married couples in India: challenges to the HIV prevention program. *Health Education & Behavior* 31(1):101–117.

Boellstorff, T. (2004) Zines and zones of desire: mass mediated love, national romance, and sexual citizenship in gay Indonesia. *Journal of Asian Studies* 63:367–402.

Boellstorff, T. (2005) *The gay Archipelago: sexuality and nation in Indonesia*. Princeton University Press, Princeton.

Boellstorff, T., and Oetomo, D. (1996) Community outreach in Indonesia: a practical and sustainable technique for HIV Prevention. International Conference on AIDS. 11:502 (abstract Pub. D. 1414).

Bolt-Gonzales, M. (1996) *Sencillamente diferentes: la autoestima de las mujeres lesbianas en los sectores urbanos de Nicaragua*. Fundacion Xochiquetzal, Managua.

Bolton, R. (1992a) AIDS and promiscuity: muddles in the models of HIV prevention. In: Bolton, R., and Singer, M. (eds) *Rethinking AIDS prevention: cultural approaches*. Gordon & Breach, Montreux.

Bolton, R. (1992b) Mapping terra incognita: sex research for AIDS prevention: an urgent agenda for the 1990s. In: Herdt, G., and Lindenbaum, S. (eds) *The time of AIDS: social analysis, theory, and method*. Sage, London.

Bronfman, M., and Minello, N. (1992) Sexual habits of temporary Mexican-migrants to the United States of America: risk practices for HIV infection. *International Conference on AIDS* 8(2):D423 (abstract PoD 5219).

Bronfman, M., Camposortega, S., and Medina, H. (1989) Myths and realities of the migration-AIDS relationship: the case of Mexican migration to the United States. International Conference on AIDS, Mexico City, 5:893 (abstract E.546).

Brown, S. (2002) Con discriminación y represión no hay democracia: the lesbian and gay movement in Argentina. *Latin American Perspectives* 29:119–138.

Browner, C.H. (1989) Women, household, and health in Latin America. *Social Science and Medicine* 28:461–473.

Browner, C.H., and Leslie, J. (1996) Women, work, and household health in the context of development. In: Sargent, C.F., and Brettell, C.B. (eds) *Gender and health: an international perspective*. Prentice Hall, Upper Saddle River, NJ, pp. 260–277.

Cáceres, C.F. (1996) Male bisexuality in Peru and the prevention of AIDS. In: Aggleton, P. (ed) *Bisexualities and AIDS: international perspectives*. Taylor & Francis, Bristol, PA, pp. 126–147.

Cáceres, C. (2005) Más allá del SIDA: la cuestión de la salud en las comunidades GLBT. In: Minayo, M.C.S.S., and Coimbra, C.E.A. (eds) *Criticas e atuantes: ciências sociais e humanas em saúde na América Latina*. Editoria Fiocruz, Rio de Janeiro, pp. 427–439.

Cáceres, C.F., and Rosasco, A.M. (1999) The margin has many sides: diversity among gay and homosexually active men in Lima. *Culture Health and Sexuality* 1(3):261–275.

Cáceres, C.F., and Stall, R. (2003) Commentary: the human immunodeficiency virus/AIDS epidemic among men who have sex with men in Latin America and the Caribbean: it is time to bridge the gap. *International Journal of Epidemiology* 32:740–743.

Camara, B. (2001) 20 Years of the HIV/AIDS epidemic in the Caribbean. CAREC-SPSTI, Port of Spain, Trinidad.

Cameron, E., and Gevisser, M. (1994) *Defiant desire: gay and lesbian lives in South Africa*. Ravan Press, Johannesburg.

Carbajal, C.L., Vallina, E., Arribas, J.M., Diaz, J., and Dominguez, B. (1991) Epidemiological study of prisoners at risk for AIDS in a Spanish prison. *Anales de Medicina Interna* 8:382–386.

Carrier, J. (1995) *De los otros: intimacy and homosexuality among Mexican men.* Columbia University Press, New York.

Carrier, J. (1999) Reflections on ethical problems encountered in field research on Mexican male homosexuality: 1968 to present. *Culture Health Sex* 1:207–221.

Carrillo, H. (1999) Cultural change, hybridity and male homosexuality in Mexico. *Culture Health and Sexuality* 1:223–238.

Carrillo, H. (2002) *The night is young: sexuality in Mexico in the time of AIDS.* University of Chicago Press, Chicago.

Carrillo, H. (2004) Sexual migration, cross-cultural sexual encounters, and sexual health. *Sexuality Research and Social Policy* 1(3):58–70.

Chao, A. (2000) Global metaphors and local strategies in the construction of Taiwan's lesbian identities. *Culture Health and Sexuality* 2:377–390.

Chen, J.L., Bovee, M.C., and Kerndt, P.R. (2003) Sexually transmitted diseases surveillance among incarcerated men who have sex with men—an opportunity for HIV prevention. *AIDS Education and Prevention* 15(Suppl A):117–126.

Chng, C.L., and Geliga-Vargas, J. (2000) Ethnic identity, gay identity, sexual sensation seeking and HIV risk taking among multiethnic men who have sex with men. *AIDS Education and Prevention* 12:326–339.

Chng, C.L., Wong, F.Y., Park, R.J., Edberg, M.C., and Lai, D.S. (2003) A model for understanding sexual health among Asian American/Pacific Islander men who have sex with men (MSM) in the United States. *AIDS Education and Prevention* 15:21–38.

Clark, L. (1993) Gender and generation in poor women's household health production experiences. *Medical Anthropology Quarterly* 7:386–402.

Croucher, S. (2002) South Africa's democratisation and the politics of gay liberation. *Journal of Southern African Studies* 28:315–330.

D'Emilio, J. (1993) Capitalism and gay identity. In: Abelove, H., Barale, M.A., and Halperin, D.M. (eds) *The lesbian and gay studies reader.* Routledge, New York, pp. 467–476.

De Gruchy, S., and Germond, P. (1997) *Aliens in the household of God: homosexuality and Christian faith in South Africa.* David Philip, Cape Town.

De Moya, A., and Garcia, R. (1998) Three decades of male sex work in Santo Domingo. In: Aggleton, P. (ed) *Men who sell sexuality: international perspectives on male prostitution and AIDS.* Taylor & Francis, London.

De Moya, E.A., and Garcia, R. (1996) AIDS and the enigma of bisexuality in the Dominican Republic. In: Aggleton, P. (ed) *Bisexualities and AIDS: international perspectives.* Taylor & Francis, Bristol, PA, pp. 121–135.

De Moya, E.A., Garcia, R., Fadul, R., and Herold, E. (1992) Sosua sanky-pankies and female sex workers: an exploratory study. La Universidad Autonoma, Santo Domingo.

Díaz, R.M. (1997) Latino gay men and psycho-cultural barriers to AIDS prevention. In: Levine, M.P., Nardi, P.M., and Gagnon, J.H. (eds) *In changing times: gay men and lesbians encounter HIV/AIDS.* University of Chicago Press, Chicago, pp. 221–244.

Díaz, R.M. (1998) *Latino gay men and HIV.* Routledge, New York.

Diaz, R.M., Ayala, G., and Marin, B.V. (2000) Latino gay men and HIV: risk behavior as a sign of oppression. *Focus: a Guide to AIDS Research* 15(7):1–5.

Doll, L.S., Harrison, J.S., Frey, R.L., McKirnan, D., Bartholow, B.N., Douglas, J.M., Jr., Joy, D., Bolan, G., and Doetsch, J. (1994) Failure to disclose HIV risk among gay and bisexual men attending sexually transmitted disease clinics. *American Journal of Preventive Medicine* 10:125–129.

Donham, D. (1998) Freing South Africa: the "modernization" of male male sexuality in Soweto. *Cultural Anthropology* 13(1):3–21.

Douglas, R.M., Gaughwin, M.D., Ali, R.L., Davies, L.M., Mylvaganam, A., and Liew, C.Y. (1989) Risk of transmission of the human immunodeficiency virus in the prison setting. *Medical Journal of Australia* 150:722.

Drucker, P. (ed) (2000) *Different rainbows*. Gay Men's Press, London.

Ducos, J., Ramirez, A., Perez, J., Florencio, M., and Perdomo, C. (1993) HIV and syphilis among inmates of the Dominican Republic. *International Conference in AIDS* 9:650 (abstract PO-C02-2601).

Eiven, L. (2003) Lesbians, health and human rights: a Latin American perspective: a contribution for discussion and reflection. *Women's Health Collection* 7:44–54.

Epstein, S. (1996) *Impure science: AIDS, activism, and the politics of knowledge*. University of California Press, Berkeley.

Farmer, P. (1990) *Infections and inequalities: the modern plagues*. University of California Press, Berkeley.

Farmer, P. (1992) *AIDS and accusation: Haiti and the geography of blame*. University of California Press, Berkeley.

Farmer, P., Connors, M., and Simmons, J. (eds) (1996) *Women, poverty, and AIDS: sex, drugs and structural violence*. Common Courage Press, Monroe, ME.

Frasca, T. (1997) *De amores y sombras: poblaciones y culturas homo y bisexuales en hombres de Santiago*. Corporación Chílena de Prevención de SIDA, Santiago.

Frasca, T. (2003) Men and women—still far apart on HIV/AIDS. *Reproductive Health Matters* 11(22):12–20.

Gevisser, M., and Cameron, E. (1995) *Defiant desire*. Routledge, New York.

Goffman, E. (1963) *Stigma: notes on the management of spoiled identity*. Simon & Schuster, New York.

Green, J., Strang, J., Hetherton, J., Whiteley, C., Heuston, J., and Maden, T. (2003) Same-sex sexual activity of male prisoners in England and Wales. *International Journal of STD & AIDS* 14:253–257.

Guerena Burgueno, F., Benenson, A.S., Bucardo Amaya, J., Caudillo Carreno, A., and Curiel Figueroa, J.D. (1992) Sexual behavior and drug abuse in homosexuals, prostitutes and prisoners in Tijuana, Mexico. *Revista Latinoamericana de Psicología* 24(1–2):85–96.

Harvey, D. (1990) *The condition of postmodernity*. Blackwell, Cambridge.

Hernandez, M. (2003) Unspoken rules. International Gay and Lesbian Human Rights Commission (IGLHRC), New York.

Hirsch, J. (2003) *A courtship after marriage: sexuality and love in Mexican transnational families*. University of California Press, Berkeley.

Hirsch, J., Higgins, J., Bentley, N., and Nathanson, C. (2002) The social constructions of sexuality: marital infidelity and sexually transmitted disease-HIV risk in a Mexican migrant community. *American Journal of Public Health* 92:1227–1237.

Hoffman, V., and Bolton, R. (1996) Patterns of sexual risk-taking among heterosexual men. *Medical Anthropology* 16:341–362.

Human Rights Watch. (2004a) *Chile: high court discriminates against lesbian mother*. HRW, Santiago.

Human Rights Watch. (2004b) *Hated to death: homophobia, violence and Jamaica's HIV/AIDS epidemic. Human Rights Watch* 16(6):1–79.

Human Rights Watch. (2004c) Sierra Leone: lesbian rights activist brutally murdered. HRW report online: http://www.hrw.org/english/docs/2004/10/04/sierra9440.htm.

Hunt, L.M., Schneider, S., and Comer, B. (2004) Should "acculturation" be a variable in health research? A critical review of research on US Hispanics. *Social Science & Medicine* 59:973–986.

International Gay and Lesbian Human Rights Commission. (2003) *More than a name: state-sponsored homophobia and its consequences in southern Africa.* Human Rights Watch, New York.

Isaacs, G., and McKendrick, B. (1992) *Male homosexuality in South Africa: identity formation, culture, and crisis.* Oxford University Press, Cape Town, South Africa.

Izazola Licea, J. (2001) *Políticas públicas y prevención del VIH/SIDA en América Latina y el Caribe.* Fundación Mexicana para la Salud/SIDALAC/ ONUSIDA, México, pp. 151–182.

Jackson, P. (2000) An explosion of Thai identities: global queering and re-imagining queer theory. *Culture Health and Sexuality* 2:405–424.

Jackson, P.A. (1997) Kathoey><gay><man: the historical emergence of gay male identity in Thailand. In: Manderson, L., and Jolly, M. (eds) *Sites of desire economies of pleasure: sexualities in Asia and the Pacific.* University of Chicago Press, Chicago, pp. 166–190.

Jackson, P.A., and Cook, N.M. (eds) (2000) *Genders and sexualities in modern Thailand.* Silkworm Books, Chiang Mai.

Kahn, S. (2003) Culture, sexualities, and identities: men who have sex with men in India. *Journal of Homosexuality* 40(3/4):99–115.

Kelly, J.A., Sikkema, K.J., Winett, R.A., Solomon, L.J., Roffman, R.A., Heckman, T.G., Stevenson, L.Y., Perry, M.J., Norman, A.D., and Desiderato, L.J. (1995) Factors predicting continued high-risk behavior among gay men in small cities: psychological, behavioral, and demographic characteristics related to unsafe sex. *Journal of Consulting & Clinical Psychology* 63:101–107.

Kelly, J.A., Amirkhanian, Y.A., McAuliffe, T.L., Granskaya, J.V., Borodkina, O.I., Dyatlov, R.V., Kukharsky, A., and Kozlov, A.P. (2002) HIV risk characteristics and prevention needs in a community sample of bisexual men in St. Petersburg, Russia. *AIDS Care* 14(1):63–76.

Khan, S. (1994) Cultural context of sexual behaviour and identities and their impact upon preventive models: an overview of South Asian men who have sex with men. *Indian Journal Social Work* 55:633–646.

Khan, S. (1998) Through a window darkly: men who sell sex to men in India and Bangladesh. In: Aggleton, P. (ed) *Men who sell sex: International perspectives on male prostitution and AIDS.* Temple University Press, Philadelphia, pp. 195–212.

Kulick, D. (1997) The gender of Brazilian transgendered prostitutes. *American Anthropologist* 99:574–585.

Kulick, D. (1998) *Travestí: sex, gender and culture among Brazilian transgendered prostitutes.* University of Chicago Press, Chicago.

Lang, N.G. (1990) Sex, politics, and guilt: a study of homophobia and the AIDS phenomenon. In: Feldman, D. (ed) *Culture and AIDS.* Praeger, New York, pp. 169–182.

Lang, N.G. (1991) Stigma, self-esteem and depression: psycho-social responses to risk of AIDS. *Human Organization* 50:66–72.

Leiner, M. (1994) *Sexual politics in Cuba: machismo, homosexuality, and AIDS.* Westview Press, Boulder, Co.

Lemelle, A.J., Jr., and Battle, J. (2004) Black masculinity matters in attitudes toward gay males. *Journal of Homosexuality* 47(1):39–51.

Lichtenstein, B. (2000) Secret encounters: black men, bisexuality, and AIDS in Alabama. *Medical Anthropology Quarterly* 14:374–393.

Liguori, A.L., and Lamas, M. (2003) Gender, sexual citizenship and HIV/AIDS. *Culture Health & Sexuality* 5:87–90.

Liguori, A.L., Block, M.G., and Aggleton, P. (1996) Bisexuality and HIV/AIDS in Mexico. In: Aggleton, P. (ed) *Bisexualities and AIDS: international perspectives*. Taylor & Francis, London, pp. 99–120.

Lorway, R. (2003) Inventing Namibian queer selfhood in the era of HIV/AIDS. Presented at the conference of the International Association for the Study of Sexuality, Culture and Society, Johannesburg.

Lumsden, I. (1996) *Machos, maricones, and gays: Cuba and homosexuality*. Temple University Press, Philadelphia.

MacCannell, D. (1976) *The tourist: a new theory of the leisure class*. Shocken Books, New York.

Mann, J.M. (1987) Statement at an informal briefing on AIDS to the 42nd Session of the United Nations General Assembly. United Nations, New York.

Marks, G., Cantero, P.J., and Simoni, J.M. (1998) Is acculturation associated with sexual risk behaviors? An investigation of HIV-positive Latino men and women. *AIDS Care* 10:283–295.

McCamish, M., Storer, G., and Carl, G. (2000) Refocusing HIV/AIDS interventions in Thailand: the case for male sex workers and other homosexually active men. *Culture Health and Sexuality* 2:167–182.

McKenna, N. (1996) *On the margins: MSM and HIV in the developing world*. Panos Institute, London.

McLean, R. (2005) First gay couples apply for marriage under new Spanish law. New York Times. July 5, A3.

Merrill, G.S., and Wolfe, V.A. (2000) Battered gay men: an exploration of abuse, help seeking, and why they stay. *Journal of Homosexuality* 39(2):1–30.

Meyer, I.H. (1995) Minority stress and mental health in gay men. *Journal of Health and Social Behavior* 36:38–56.

Moodie, D., and Ndatshe, V. (1994) *Going for gold: men, mines, and migration*. University of California Press, Berkeley.

Morrell, R. (1998) Of boys and men: masculinity and gender in southern African studies. *Journal of Southern African Studies* 24:605–630.

Moss, C.S., Hosford, R.E., and Anderson, W.R. (1979) Sexual assault in a prison. *Psychological Reports* 44(3 Pt 1):823–828.

Muñoz-Laboy, M. (2004) Beyond "MSM": sexual desire among bisexually-active Latino men in New York City. *Sexualities* 7(1):55–80.

Murray, S., and Roscoe, W. (1997) *Islamic homosexualities*. New York University Press, New York.

Murray, S., and Roscoe, W. (1998) Boy-wives and female husbands: studies of African homosexualities. St. Martin's Press, New York.

Murray, S.O. (1992) The "underdevelopment" of modern/gay homosexuality in Mesoamerica. In: Plummer, K. (ed) *Modern homosexualities fragments of lesbian and gay experience*. Routledge, London, pp. 29–38.

Murray, S.O., and Roscoe, W. (eds). (1998) *Boy-wives and female husbands: studies in African homosexualities*. Palgrave, New York.

Nanda, S. (1999) The Hijrasof India: cultural and individual dimensions of an institutionalized third gender role. In: Parker, R., and Aggleton, P. (eds) *Culture, society and sexuality: a reader*. University of California Press, Berkeley, pp. 226–238.

Niehaus, I. (2002) Renegotiating masculinity in the South African lowveld: narratives of male-male sex in labour compounds and in prisons. *African Studies* 61(1):77–97.

Odujinrin, M.T., and Adebajo, S.B. (2001) Social characteristics, HIV/AIDS knowledge, preventive practices and risk factors elicitation among prisoners in Lagos, Nigeria. *West African Journal of Medicine* 20:191–198.

Oetomo, D. (2000) Masculinity in Indonesia: genders, sexualities, and identities in a changing society. In: Parker, R., Barbosa, R., and Aggleton, P. (eds) *Framing the sexual subject*. University of California Press, Berkeley, pp. 46–59.

Padian, N. (1987) Heterosexual transmission of acquired immunodeficiency syndrome: international perspectives and national projections. *Reviews of Infectious Diseases* 9:947–960.

Padilla, M. (2007, in press) *Caribbean pleasure industry: tourism, sexuality, and AIDS in the Dominican Republic*. University of Chicago Press, Chicago.

PAHO/WHO. (2002) AIDS surveillance in the Americas: biannual report. Pan American Health Organization, Geneva.

Parker, R. (1987) Acquired immunodeficiency syndrome in urban Brazil. *Medical Anthropology Quarterly* 1:155–175.

Parker, R. (1992) Male prostitution, bisexual behaviour and HIV transmission in urban Brazil. In: Dyson, T. (ed) *Sexual behaviour and networking: anthropological and sociocultural studies on the transmission of HIV*. International Union for the Scientific Study of Population, Liege, Belgium, pp. 109–122.

Parker, R. (1999) *Beneath the equator: cultures of desire, male homosexuality, and emerging gay communities in Brazil*. Routledge, New York.

Parker, R. (2002) Change of sexuality: masculinity and male homosexuality in Brazil. *Alteridades* 12(23):49–62.

Parker, R., and Caceres, C. (1999) Alternative sexualities and changing sexual cultures among Latin American men. *Culture Health and Sexuality* 1:201–206.

Parker, R., and Carballo, M. (1990) Qualitative research on homosexual and bisexual behavior relevant to HIV/AIDS. *Journal of Sexuality Research* 27:497–525.

Parker, R., Khan, S., and Aggleton, P. (1998) Conspicuous by their absence? Men who have sex with men (MSM) in developing countries—implications for intervention. *Critical Public Health* 8:329–346.

Parker, R., Rios, L., and Terto, V., Jr. (2001) Intervenciones para hombres que tienen sexo con hombres: una revision de la investigación y prácticas preventivas en América Latina. In: Licea, J.I. (ed) *Políticas Públicas y Prevención del VIH/SIDA en América Latina y el Caribe*. Fundación Mexicana para la Salud/SIDALAC/ ONUSIDA, México, pp. 151–182.

Parker, R.G. (1990) Sexual culture and AIDS education in urban Brazil. In: Kulstad, R. (ed) *AIDS 1988: AAAS symposia papers*. American Association for the Advancement of Science, Washington, DC, pp. 169–173.

Parker, R.G. (1996) Bisexuality and HIV/AIDS in Brazil. In: Aggleton, P. (ed) *Bisexualities and AIDS*. Taylor & Francis, London, pp. 148–160.

Parker, R.G. (2000) AIDS prevention and gay community mobilization in Brazil. *Development* 2:49–53.

Parker, R.G., and Aggleton, P. (2003) HIV- and AIDS-related stigma and discrimination: a conceptual framework and implications for action. *Social Science & Medicine* 57:13–24.

Parker, R.G., and Terto, V., Jr. (1998) *Entre homens: homosexualidade e AIDS no Brasil*. ABIA, Rio de Janeiro.

Parker, R.G., Easton, D., and Klein, C.H. (2000) Structural barriers and facilitators in HIV prevention: a review of international research. *AIDS* 14(Suppl 1):S22–S32.

Patton, C. (1990) *Inventing AIDS*. Routledge, New York.

Pecheny, M. (2001) *De la "no discriminacion" al "reconocimiento social": un analisis de la evolucion de las demandas politicas de las minorias sexuales en America Latina*. Paper presented at the XXIII Congress of the Latin American Studies Association, Washington, DC, September 6–8, 2001.

Peterson, J.L. (1997) AIDS-related risks and same-sex behaviors among African American men. In: Levine, M.P., Nardi, P.M., and Gagnon, J.H. (eds) *In changing times: gay men and lesbians encounter HIV/AIDS*. University of Chicago Press, Chicago, pp. 283–301.

Phillips, O. (2000) Constituting the global gay: issues of individual subjectivity and sexuality in Southern Africa. In: Herman, D., C, S. (eds) *Sexuality in the legal arena*. Athlone Press, London, pp. 17–33.

Phillips, O. (2004) The invisible presence of homosexuality: implications for HIV/AIDS and rights in southern Africa. In: Kalipeni, E., Craddock, S., Oppong, J.R., and Ghosh, J. (eds) *HIV/AIDS in Africa: beyond epidemiology*. Blackwell Publishing, Malden, pp. 155–166.

Poorman, P.B., Seelau, E.P., and Seelau, S.M. (2003) Perceptions of domestic abuse in same-sex relationships and implications for criminal justice and mental health responses. *Violence and Victims* 18:659–669.

Press, C.M. (1978) Reputation and respectability reconsidered: hustling in a tourist setting. *Caribbean Issues* 4(1).

Preston-Whyte, E., Varga, C., Oosthuizen, H., Roberts, R., and Blose, F. (2000) Survival sex and HIV/AIDS in an African city. In: Parker, R., Barbosa, R., and Aggleton, P. (eds) *Framing the sexual subject*. University of California Press, Berkeley, pp. 165–190.

Prieur, A. (1998) *Mema's house, Mexico City: on transvestites, queens, and machos*. University of Chicago Press, Chicago.

Reddy, G. (2004) *With respect to sex: negotiating Hijra identity in south India*. University of Chicago Press, Chicago.

Relf, M.V. (2001a) Battering and HIV in men who have sex with men: a critique and synthesis of the literature. *Journal of the Association of Nurses in AIDS Care* 12(3):41–48.

Relf, M.V. (2001b) Childhood sexual abuse in men who have sex with men: the current state of the science. *Journal of the Association of Nurses in AIDS Care* 12(5):20–29.

Sagarin, E. (1976) Prison homosexuality and its effect on post-prison sexual behavior. *Psychiatry* 39:245–257.

Savin-Williams, R.C. (1994) Verbal and physical abuse as stressors in the lives of lesbian, gay male, and bisexual youths: associations with school problems, running away, substance abuse, prostitution, and suicide. *Journal of Consulting and Clinical Psychology* 62:261–269.

Schifter, J., and Madrigal, J. (1992) *Hombres que aman hombres*. ILEP-SIDA, San Jose.

Schliefer, R. (2004) Hated to death: homophobia, violence, and Jamaica's HIV/AIDS Epidemic. *Human Rights Watch* 16(6B).

Seibt, A., McAlister, A., Freeman, A., Krepcho, M., Hedrick, A., and Wilson, R. (1993) Condom use and sexual identity among men who have sex with men—Dallas. *MMWR Morbidity and Mortality Weekly Report* 42(6–7):12–13.

Tan, M. (1993) Socio-economic impact of HIV/AIDS in the Philippines. *AIDS Care* 5:283–288.

Tan, M. (1995) From Bakla to gay: shifting gender identities and sexual behaviors in the Philippines. In: Parker, R., and Gagnon, J.H. (eds) *Conceiving sexuality: approaches to sex Research in a postmodern world*. Routledge, New York, pp. 85–96.

Teunis, N. (1998) Same-sex sexuality in Africa: a case study from Senegal. *AIDS and Behavior* 5:173–182.

Toms, I. (1990) AIDS in South Africa: potential decimation on the eve of liberation. *Progress Report on Health Development in South Africa*:13–16.

Treichler, P. (1999) *How to have theory in an epidemic: cultural Chronicles of AIDS*. Duke University Press, Durham.

Treichler, P.A. (1988) AIDS, homophobia, and biomedical discourse: an epidemic of signification. In: Crimp, D. (ed) *AIDS: cultural analysis, cultural activism*. MIT Press, Cambridge, pp. 31–70.

Turner, H.A., Hays, R.B., and Coates, T.J. (1993) Determinants of social support among gay men: the context of AIDS. *Journal of Health & Social Behavior* 34(1):37–53.

UNAIDS. (2002) *Report on the global HIV/AIDS epidemic*. Joint United Nations Programme on AIDS, Geneva.

Ungar, M. (2000) State violence and lesbian, gay, bisexual and transgender (LGBT) rights. *New Political Science* 22(1):61–75.

Urry, J. (1995) *Consuming places*. Routledge, New York.

Urry, J. (2002) *The tourist gaze: leisure and travel in contemporary societies*. Sage, London.

Vásquez del Aguila, E. (2002) Placer y poder en un mundo de hombres: identidades sexuales e identidades de género en internos de una institución penitenciaria de Lima. In: Cáceres, C. (ed) *La salud sexual como derecho en el Peú de hoy*. REDDES Jóvenes, Lima, pp. 149–180.

Vickers, L. (1996) The second closet: domestic violence in lesbian and gay relationships: a western Australian perspective. *Murdoch University Electronic Journal of Law* 3(4).

Visser, G. (2002) Gay tourism in South Africa: issues from the Cape Town experience. *Urban Forum* 13(1):85–94.

Wah-shan. (2000) Homosexuality and the cultural politics of Tongzhi in Chinese societies. *Journal of Homosexuality* 40(3/4):27–46.

Watney, S. (1988) AIDS, "moral panic" theory and homophobia. In: Aggleton, P., and Homans, H. (eds) *Social aspects of AIDS*. 1st ed. Falmer Press, Philadelphia.

WHO. (1993) Effective approaches to AIDS prevention: report of a meeting. Geneva, May 26–29, 1992. World Health Organization, Global Programme on AIDS.

Wieringa, S. (1994) Women's interests and empowerment: gender planning reconsidered. *Development and Change* 25:829–848.

Wieringa, S. (1995) *Sub-versive women: women's movements in Africa, Asia, Latin America and the Caribbean*. ZED, London.

Wiggs, J.W. (1989) Prison rape and suicide. *Journal of the American Medical Association* 262:3403.

Wohl, A.R., Johnson, D., Jordan, W., Lu, S., Beall, G., Currier, J., and Kerndt, P.R. (2000) High-risk behaviors during incarceration in African-American men treated for HIV at three Los Angeles public medical centers. *Journal of Acquired Immune Deficiciency Syndrome* 24(4):386–392.

Young, R., and Meyer, I. (2005) The trouble with "MSM" and "WSW": erasure of the sexual-minority person in public health discourse. *American Journal of Public Health* 95:1144–1149.

Young, R.M., Weissman, G., and Cohen, J.B. (1992) Assessing risk in the absence of information: HIV risk among women injection drug users who have sex with women. *AIDS & Public Policy Journal* 7:175–183.

Zachariah, R., Harries, A.D., Chantulo, A.S., Yadidi, A.E., Nkhoma, W., and Maganga, O. (2002) Sexually transmitted infections among prison inmates in a rural district of Malawi. *Transactions of the Royal Society of Tropical Medicine and Hygiene* 96:617–619.

10

Prejudice and Discrimination as Social Stressors

Ilan H. Meyer

1 Introduction

Lesbians, gay men, and bisexuals (LGBs) vary in sociodemographic characteristics such as cultural, ethnic or racial identity, age, education, income, and place of residence as well as in the degree to which their LGB identities are central to their self-definition, their level of affiliation with other LGB people, and their rejection or acceptance of societal stereotypes about and prejudice against homosexuality. In that diversity, it is difficult to describe many common themes. Despite the many differences that separate them, LGB people share remarkably similar experiences related to prejudice, stigma, discrimination, rejection, and violence directed toward them across cultures and locales (Espin, 1993; Fullilove & Fullilove, 1999; Herek, 2000; Diaz et al., 2001). Even after a historic U.S. Supreme Court ruling that the criminalization of homosexuality is unconstitutional, gay men and lesbians continue to be subjected to legal discrimination in housing, employment, and basic civil rights—most prominent in recent years are discrimination related to family law, including marriage and adoption.

Within this social context, LGB people have responded to prejudice and discrimination with resilience and resolve, forming communities as varied and diverse as the LGB individuals that comprise them. These communities have provided safe spaces for LGBs to congregate; and within these communities LGBs have developed norms and values and created institutions where LGB identities and relationships are acknowledged, supported, and respected (D'Emilio, 1983).

The social environment plays an important role in the health of LGBs. Prejudice affects the health of LGB people in many ways. Direct routes are easily discernible: They include exposure to violence and discrimination. Indirect routes are less visible but more pervasive: They include inadequate attention to health concerns of LGB people, lack of knowledge and insensitivity regarding the cultural aspects of LGB groups, barriers to accessing health care, and poor quality of care (Garnets et al., 1990; Malebranche et al., 2004).

That social conditions characterized by prejudice, rejection, and discrimination are stressful has been suggested regarding various social categories, including groups defined by race/ethnicity, gender, and sexual orientation (Barnett & Baruch, 1987; Mirowsky & Ross, 1989; Pearlin, 1999; Swim, 2001; Meyer, 2003); heavyweight people (Miller & Myers, 1998); people with stigmatizing physical illnesses such as acquired immunodeficiency syndrome (AIDS) and cancer (Fife & Wright, 2000); and people who have taken on stigmatizing attributes, or "marks," as psychologists call the targets of stigma, such as body piercing (Jetten et al., 2001).

The U.S. Public Health Service declared its goal of eliminating disparities in health in the United States (U.S. Department of Health and Human Services, 2000). Anticipating and accompanying this work, there has been increased interest in the minority stress model for explaining causes of disparities in health outcomes, for example, and in particular as it applies to the social environment of African Americans' experience of stress related to racism (Allison, 1998; Clark, 1999). Social psychology theory has begun to explicitly incorporate these experiences into stress discourse (Allison, 1998; Miller & Major, 2000). Researchers and the Healthy People 2010 document have also identified LGBT (with the T representing transgender) populations at risk and identified disparities in health outcomes between them and the general U.S. population. Such disparities have been explained by social stressors (Dean et al., 2000; Gay and Lesbian Medical Association, 2001).

Krieger discussed the ways that discrimination becomes embodied, relating to the multiple ways that such social conditions affect the health of minority populations (Krieger, 2001). Here, I present a conceptual model that describes social conditions as stressors and describe their putative effect on mental health. The model specifies some of the stressful social processes that affect risk for mental disorders and opportunities for well-being in LGB populations but also accounts for resilience and coping, which may buffer the stress.

2 A Conceptual Model: Prejudice and Discrimination as Minority Stress

When developing the concept of minority stress, researchers' underlying assumptions are that minority stress is (1) unique—that is, minority stress is additive to general stressors that are experienced by all people, and therefore that stigmatized people require an adaptation effort above that required of similar others who are not stigmatized; (2) chronic—that is, minority stress is related to relatively stable underlying social and cultural structures; and (3) socially based—that is, it stems from social processes, institutions, and structures beyond the individual rather than individual events or conditions that characterize general stressors, or biologic, genetic, or other nonsocial characteristics of the person or the group. Applied to lesbians, gay men, and bisexuals, a minority stress model posits that sexual prejudice is stressful and may lead to adverse mental health outcomes (Brooks, 1981; Meyer, 1995, 2003; Krieger & Sidney, 1997; DiPlacido, 1998; Cochran, 2001; Mays & Cochran, 2001). A more recent contribution is the interest of stress researchers in the relation of identity with stress. Reviewing the literature on stress and identity, Thoits called the investigation of stressors related to minority identities a "crucial next step" in the study of identity and stress (Thoits, 1999, p. 361). Understanding identity may help researchers formulate hypotheses about the interaction of stress and identity—for example, whether stress in a gay-related area has more impact on a health outcome in individuals with high versus low commitment to gay identity.

2.1 Minority Stress Processes in LGB Populations

There is no consensus about specific stress processes that affect LGB people, but psychological theory, stress literature, and research on the health of LGB populations provide some ideas for articulating a minority stress model. A distal-proximal distinction can help with cataloguing minority stress processes. The distal-proximal dimension relies on stress conceptualization that seems most relevant to minority stress and its concern with the impact of external social conditions and structures on individuals. Lazarus and Folkman (1984) described social structures as "distal concepts whose effects on an individual depend on how they are manifested in the immediate context of thought, feeling, and action—the proximal social experiences of a person's life" (p. 321). Distal social attitudes gain psychological importance through cognitive appraisal and become proximal concepts with psychological importance to the individual. Crocker et al. (1998) make a similar distinction between "objective reality," which includes prejudice and discrimination, and "states of mind that the experience of stigma may create in the stigmatized." They noted that "states of mind have their grounding in the realities of stereotypes, prejudice, and discrimination," again echoing Lazarus and Folkman's (1984) conceptualization of the proximal, subjective appraisal as a manifestation of distal objective environmental conditions.

I described minority stress processes along a continuum: from distal stressors, which are typically defined as objective events and conditions, to proximal personal processes, which are by definition subjective because they rely on individual perceptions and appraisals. I have suggested that specific processes of minority stress are relevant to lesbians, gay men, and bisexuals (Meyer, 1995, 2003; Meyer & Dean, 1998). From distal to proximal they are (1) external objective stressful events and conditions (chronic and acute), (2) expectations of such events and the vigilance this expectation requires, (3) concealment of one's sexual orientation, and (4) the internalization of negative societal attitudes. It should be noted that additional processes may be added that are general to all LGB individuals or that are unique to some populations, such as women, ethnic minorities, and so on.

Distal minority stressors can be defined as *objective stressors* in that they do not depend on the person's perceptions or appraisals, although certainly their report depends on perception and attribution (Kobrynowicz & Branscombe, 1997; Operario & Fiske, 2001). As objective stressors, distal stressors can be seen as independent of personal identification with the assigned minority status (Diamond, 2000). For example, a woman may have a romantic relationship with another woman but not identify as a lesbian (Laumann et al., 1994). Nevertheless, she may be perceived as a lesbian by others and as such may suffer from stressors associated with prejudice toward LGB people (e.g., antigay violence). In contrast, the more proximal stress processes are *subjective* and are therefore more affected by one's self-identity as lesbian, gay, or bisexual. Thus, because subjective stressors are more closely related to identities, and because identities vary in the social and personal meanings that are attached to them, variability in identity could lead to variability in health outcomes in the face of stress.

2.2 Stress and Identity

There are specific characteristics of minority identity (e.g., the prominence of minority identity in the person's sense of self) that may be related to minority stress and its impact on health outcomes. Group identities are essential for individual emotional functioning as they address conflicting needs for individuation and affiliation (Brewer, 1991).

Characteristics of identity may be related to mental health both directly and in interaction with stressors. A *direct effect* mechanism suggests that identity characteristics themselves can cause distress. For example, Burke (1991) said that feedback from others that is incompatible with one's self-identity—a process he called "identity interruptions"—can cause distress. An *interactive effect* with stress suggests that characteristics of identity would modify the effect of stress on health outcomes. For example, Linville (1987) found that subjects with more complex self identities were less prone to depression in the face of stress. Another mechanism was suggested by Thoits (1999, p. 346), who explained, "Since people's self conceptions are closely linked to their psychological states, stressors that damage or threaten self concepts are likely to predict emotional problems." This suggests that a stronger commitment to a gay identity may enhance the impact of stressors in gay-related areas. The reverse is also plausible: Stronger identity may ameliorate the impact of stress. This may be the case if a stronger minority identity leads to stronger affiliations with one's community. Stronger affiliations in the minority community and social support, in turn, may aid in buffering the impact of stress (Crocker & Major, 1989; Branscombe et al., 1999b; Brown et al., 1999). I discuss below prominence, valence, and integration of identities (Rosenberg & Gara, 1985; Thoits, 1991, 1999; Deaux, 1993).

Prominence (or salience) of an identity may exacerbate stress because "the more an individual identifies with, is committed to, or has highly developed self-schemas in a particular life domain, the greater will be the emotional impact of stressors that occur in that domain" (Thoits, 1999, p. 352). In coming-out models and in some models of racial identity, there has been a tendency to see minority identity as prominent and ignore other personal and social identities (de Monteflores & Schultz, 1978; Cross, 1995; Eliason, 1996), but this is not necessarily the case. Minority identities, which may seem prominent to observers, are often not endorsed as prominent by minority group members themselves, leading to variability in identity hierarchies of minority persons (Massey & Ouellette, 1996). For example, Brooks (1981) noted that the stress process for lesbians is complex because it involves both sexual orientation and gender identities. Similarly, research on African American and Latino LGBs has shown that they often confront homophobia in their racial/ethnic communities and alienation from their racial/ethnic identity in the lesbian/gay community (Espin, 1993; Loiacano, 1993; Diaz et al., 2001). LGB members of racial/ethnic minorities thus manage diverse identities. Unlike the more simplistic picture painted by identity models, then, it is plausible that salience of minority identities—including race/ethnic, sexual orientation, and gender, among others—are dynamic. Rather than view identity as stable, researchers now view identity structures as fluid, with prominence of identity often shifting with the social context (Brewer, 1991; Deaux & Ethier, 1998; Crocker & Quinn, 2000).

Valence refers to the evaluative features of identity and is tied to self-validation. Negative valence has been described as a good predictor of mental health problems, with an inverse relation to depression (Woolfolk et al., 1995; Allen et al., 1999). Identity valence is a central characteristic of coming-out models, as internalized homophobia diminishes and self-acceptance increases. Thus, overcoming negative self-evaluation is the primary aim of the LGB person's development in coming out and is a central theme of gay-affirmative therapies (Coleman, 1982; Maylon, 1982; Troiden, 1989; Loiacano, 1993; Rotheram-Borus & Fernandez, 1995; Meyer & Dean, 1998; Diaz et al., 2001). Negative valence is most likely related to increased impact of the stressor in the relevant area. For example, Meyer and Dean (1998) found that in the face of antigay violence gay men who had more positive self-perceptions of their gay identity fared better than gay men who had more negative self-perceptions of their gay identity in terms of mental health outcomes. The authors explained that gay men with negative self-perceptions may have had fewer internal resources to cope with the antigay experience, in a sense identifying with the antigay aggression.

Distinct identities are interrelated through a hierarchal organization (Rosenberg & Gara, 1985; Linville, 1987). *Integration* of identities refers to the relationship of the minority identity and other identities of the person. In coming-out models, integration of the minority identity with the person's other identities is seen as the optimal stage of identity development. For example, Cass (1979) saw the last stage of coming out as "identity synthesis," where the gay identity becomes merely one part of this integrated total identity. During optimal identity development, various aspects of the person's self, including but not limited to other minority identities, such as those based on gender or race/ethnicity, are integrated (Eliason, 1996).

For example, Crawford et al. (2002) see in gay Black men's identities a conflict between two cultures with unique and sometimes conflicting stressors and resources. Crawford and colleagues suggested a model for understanding the experiences of African American gay and bisexual men as a dual minority. The authors described four types of potential adaptation to the challenges of the intersection of the sexual and racial identities: (1) *assimilation*, high racial/ethnic identification and low sexual orientation identification; (2) *integration*, both racial/ethnic and sexual orientation identifications are high; (3) *separation*, low racial/ethnic identification and high sexual orientation identification; and (4) *marginalization*, both racial/ethnic and sexual orientation identifications are low. Consistent with identity development models, Crawford and colleagues hypothesized that the *integration* type of identification would be associated with more positive outcomes, including self-esteem, symptoms of mental disorders, and responsiveness to human immunodeficiency virus (HIV) prevention efforts. The authors found evidence in support of this hypothesis and concluded (Crawford et al., 2002, p. 186): "The fusion of ethnic and sexual identity into an integrated whole that is characterized by holding positive attitudes toward one's ethnic group, homosexuals and homosexuality, and engaging in social participation and cultural practice in the African-American and gay subcultures appear to be key to this process."

3 LGB Minority Stress Model

Based on the distal-proximal distinction, I propose a minority stress model that incorporates the elements discussed above. When developing the model I emulated Dohrenwend's stress model to highlight minority stress processes. Dohrenwend has described the stress process within the context of strengths and vulnerabilities in the larger environment and within the individual. For the purpose of succinctness, I have included in my discussion only those elements of the stress process unique to or necessary for the description of minority stress. It is important to note, however, that the elements I omitted—including advantages and disadvantages in the wider environment, personal predispositions, biologic background, ongoing situations, appraisal and coping—are integral parts of the stress model and are essential for a comprehensive understanding of the stress process (Dohrenwend, 2000).

The model (Fig. 10.1) depicts stress and coping and their impact on mental health outcomes (box i). Minority stress is situated in general environmental circumstances (a), which may include advantages and disadvantages related to factors such as socioeconomic status. An important aspect of these circumstances in the environment is the person's minority status (e.g., gay or lesbian) (b). These are depicted as

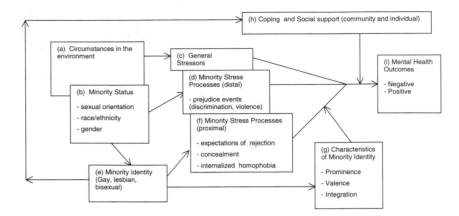

Figure 10.1 Stress, coping, and mental health in LGB populations.

overlapping boxes in the figure to indicate the close relation to other circumstances in the person's environment. For example, minority stressors for a gay man who is poor would undoubtedly be related to his poverty; together, these characteristics would determine his exposure to stress and coping resources (Diaz et al., 2001). Circumstances in the environment lead to exposure to stressors, including general stressors such as job loss or death of an intimate (c); and minority stressors unique to minority group members, such as discrimination in employment (d). Similar to their source circumstances, the stressors are depicted as overlapping as well, representing their interdependence (Pearlin, 1999). For example, an experience of antigay violence (d) is likely to increase vigilance and expectations of rejection (f). Often minority status leads to personal identification with one's minority status (e). In turn, such minority identity leads to additional stressors related to the individual's perception of self as a stigmatized and devalued minority (Miller & Major, 2000). Because they involve self-perceptions and appraisals, these minority stress processes are more proximal to the individual, including, as described above for LGB individuals, expectations of rejection, concealment, and internalized homophobia (f).

Of course, minority identity is not only a source of stress but also an important effect modifier in the stress process. First, characteristics of minority identity can augment or weaken the impact of stress (g). For example, minority stressors may have a greater impact on health outcomes when the LGB identity is prominent than when it is secondary to the person's self-definition (Thoits, 1999). Second, LGB identity may also be a source of strength (h) when it is associated with opportunities for affiliation, social support, and coping that can ameliorate the impact of stress (Crocker & Major, 1989; Branscombe et al., 1999b; Miller & Major, 2000).

3.1 Minority Stress Processes

Many researchers have studied minority stress processes—not necessarily classifying or labeling them as I do—and have often demonstrated that such stress affects the mental health of LGB individuals. These studies have typically measured mental health outcomes using psychological scales (e.g., depressive symptoms) rather than the criteria-based mental disorders (e.g., major depressive disorder). These studies concluded that minority stress processes are related to an array of mental health problems including depressive symptoms, substance use, and suicide ideation (D'Augelli & Hershberger, 1993; Cochran & Mays, 1994; Meyer, 1995; Rosario et al., 1996; Waldo, 1999; Diaz et al., 2001). Such studies have shown, for example, that stigma leads LGB persons to experience alienation, lack of integration with the community, and problems with self-acceptance (Greenberg, 1973; Maylon, 1982; Massey & Ouellette, 1996; Frable et al., 1997; Grossman & Kerner, 1998; Stokes & Peterson, 1998).

3.1.1 Prejudice Events

Researchers have described antigay violence and discrimination as core stressors affecting gay and lesbian populations (Garnets et al., 1990; Herek & Berrill, 1992; Herek et al., 1999; Kertzner, 1999). Antigay prejudice has been perpetrated throughout history: institutionalized forms of prejudice, discrimination and violence ranged from Nazi extermination of homosexuals to enforcement of sodomy laws punishable by imprisonment, castration, torture, and death (Adam, 1987). With the formation of a gay community, as LGB individuals became more visible and more readily identifiable by potential perpetrators, they increasingly became targets of antigay violence and discrimination (Herek & Berrill, 1992; Badgett, 1995; Safe Schools Coalition of Washington, 1999; Human Rights Watch, 2001). In 2001 Amnesty International reported that LGBT people are subject to widespread human rights abuses, torture, and ill-treatment ranging from loss of dignity to assault and murder. Many of these abuses are conducted with impunity—sanctioned by the state and society through formal mechanisms such as discriminatory laws and informal mechanisms, including prejudice and religious traditions (Amnesty International, 2001).

Surveys have documented that lesbians and gay men are disproportionately exposed to prejudice events, including discrimination and violence. For example, in a probability study of U.S. adults, LGB people were twice as likely as heterosexuals to have experienced a life event related to prejudice, such as being fired from a job (Mays & Cochran, 2001). In a study of LGB adults in Sacramento, California, approximately one-fifth of the women and one-fourth of the men experienced victimization (including sexual assault, physical assault, robbery, and property crime) related to their sexual orientation (Herek et al., 1999). Some research has suggested variation by ethnic background as well, although the direction of the findings is not clear. Thus, among urban adults aged 25 to 37 who reported same-sex sexual partners, Krieger and Sidney (1997) found that one-half of Whites compared with one-third of Blacks reported discrimination based on sexual orientation. On the other hand, in a study of HIV-positive gay men in New York City, Siegel and Epstein (1996) found that African American and Puerto

Rican men had significantly more gay-related minority stressors than Caucasian men.

Research has suggested that LGB youth are even more likely than adults to be victimized by antigay prejudice events, and the psychological consequences of their victimization may be more severe. Surveys of schools in several regions of the United States showed that LGB youth are exposed to more discrimination and violence events than their heterosexual peers. Several such studies, conducted on population samples of high school students, converge in their findings and show that the social environment of sexual minority youth in U.S. high schools is characterized by discrimination, rejection, and violence (Faulkner & Cranston, 1998; Garofalo et al., 1998). Compared with heterosexual youth, LGB youth are at increased risk for being threatened and assaulted, are more fearful for their safety at school, and miss school days because of this fear (Safe Schools Coalition of Washington, 1999). For example, in a random sample of Massachusetts high schools students, LGB students more often than heterosexual students had property stolen or deliberately damaged (7% vs. 1%), were threatened or injured with a weapon (6% vs. 1%), and were in a physical fight requiring medical treatment (6% vs. 2%). A national survey of LGBT youth conducted by the advocacy organization Gay, Lesbian, and Straight Education Network (GLSEN) reported that youth experienced verbal harassment (61%), sexual harassment (47%), physical harassment (28%), and physical assault (14%). Most LGBT youth (90%) sometimes or frequently heard homophobic remarks at their schools, and many (37%) reported hearing these remarks from faculty or school staff (GLSEN, 1999).

Gay men and lesbians are also discriminated against in the workplace. Waldo (1999) demonstrated a relation between employers' organizational climate and the experience of heterosexism in the workplace, which was subsequently related to adverse psychological health, and job-related outcomes in gay, lesbian, and bisexual employees. Badgett's (1995) analysis of national data showed that gay and bisexual male workers earned 11% to 27% less than heterosexual male workers with the same experience, education, occupation, marital status, and region of residence.

Garnets and colleagues (1990) described psychological mechanisms that could explain the association between victimization and psychological distress. The authors noted that victimization interferes with a person's perception of the world as meaningful and orderly. In an attempt to restore order to their perception of the world, survivors ask "Why me?" and often respond with self-recrimination and self-devaluation. More generally, experiences of victimization take away the victim's sense of security and invulnerability. Health symptoms of victimization include "sleep disturbances and nightmares, headaches, diarrhea, uncontrollable crying, agitation and restlessness, increased use of drugs, and deterioration in personal relationships" (Garnets et al., 1990, p. 367). Antigay bias crimes had a greater mental health impact on LGB persons than did similar crime's not related to bias and that bias-crime victimization may have short- or long-term consequences, including severe reactions such as posttraumatic stress disorder (Herek et al., 1999; McDevitt et al., 2001).

3.1.2 Stigma: Expectations of Rejection and Discrimination

Goffman (1963) discussed the anxiety with which the stigmatized individual approaches interactions in society. Such an individual "may perceive, usually quite correctly, that whatever others profess, they do not really 'accept' him and are not ready to make contact with him on 'equal grounds'" (p. 7). Allport (1954) described vigilance as one of the traits that targets of prejudice develop for defensive coping. This concept helps explain the stressful effect of stigma. Like other minority group members, gay men, lesbians, and bisexuals learn to anticipate—indeed expect—negative regard from members of the dominant culture. To ward off potential negative regard, discrimination, and violence, they must maintain vigilance. The greater one's perceived stigma, the greater is the need for vigilance in interactions with dominant group members. By definition, such vigilance is chronic in that it is repeatedly and continually evoked in the everyday life of the minority person. Crocker and colleagues (1998, p. 517) described this as the "need to be constantly 'on guard' . . . alert, or mindful of the possibility that the other person is prejudiced." Jones and colleagues (1984) described the effect of societal stigma on the stigmatized individual as creating a conflict between self-perceptions and others' perceptions. As a result of this conflict, self-perception is likely to be at least somewhat unstable and vulnerable. Maintaining the stability and coherence of self-concept is likely to require considerable energy and activity.

This exertion of energy in maintaining one's self-concept is stressful and would increase as the perceptions of others' stigmatization increase. Branscombe et al. (1999a) described four sources of threat relevant to the discussion of stress due to stigma: *Categorization threat* involves the threat that the person will be categorized by others as a member of a group against his or her will, especially when group membership is irrelevant in the particular context (e.g., categorization as a woman when applying for a business loan). *Distinctiveness threat* is an opposite threat, relating to denial of distinct group membership when it is relevant or significant (also Brewer, 1991). *Threats to the value of social identity* involves undermining the minority group's values, such as its competence and morality. A fourth threat, *threat to acceptance*, emerges from negative feedback from one's ingroup and the consequent threat rejection by the group. For example, Ethier and Deaux (1994) found that Hispanic American students at an Ivy League university were conflicted, divided between identification with white friends and their culture and the desire to maintain an ethnic cultural identity.

Research evidence on the impact of stigma on health, psychological, and social functioning comes from a variety of sources. Link (1987; Link et al., 1997) showed that in mentally ill individuals perceived stigma was related to adverse effects in mental health and social functioning. In a cross-cultural study of gay men, Ross (1985) found that anticipated social rejection was more predictive of psychological distress outcomes than actual negative experiences. However, research on the impact of stigma on self-esteem, a main focus of social psychological research, has not consistently supported this theoretical perspective: Such research often fails to show that members of stigmatized groups have lower self-esteem than others (Crocker & Major, 1989; Crocker et al., 1998; Crocker & Quinn, 2000). One explanation for this finding is that, along with its negative impact, stigma has self-protective properties related to group affiliation and support that ameliorate the effect of stigma (Crocker & Major, 1989). This finding is not consistent across various ethnic groups: Although African Americans have scored higher than Whites on measures of self-esteem, other ethnic minorities have scored lower (Twenge & Crocker, 2002).

Experimental social psychological research has highlighted other processes that can lead to adverse outcomes. This research may be classified as somewhat different from that related to the vigilance concept discussed above. Vigilance is related to fear of possible (even if imagined) negative events and may therefore be classified as more distal along the continuum ranging from the environment to the self. Stigma threat, as described below, relates to internal processes that are more proximal to the self. This research has shown that expectations of stigma can impair social and academic functioning of stigmatized persons by affecting their performance (Farina et al., 1968; Steele & Aronson, 1995; Steele, 1997; Crocker et al., 1998; Pinel, 2002). For example, Steele (1997, p. 614) described stereotype threat as the "social-psychological threat that arises when one is in a situation or doing something for which negative stereotype about one's group applies" and showed that the emotional reaction to this threat can interfere with intellectual performance. When situations of stereotype threat are prolonged they can lead to "disidentification," whereby a member of a stigmatized group removes a domain that is negatively stereotyped (e.g., academic success) from his or her self-definition. Such disidentification with a goal undermines the person's motivation—and therefore effort—to achieve in this domain. Unlike the concept of life events, where stress stems from some concrete offense (e.g., antigay violence), here it is not necessary that any prejudice event has actually occurred. As Crocker (1999) noted, because of the chronic exposure to a stigmatizing social environment, "[t]he consequences of stigma do not require that a stigmatizer in the situation holds negative stereotypes or discriminates" (p. 103). As Steele (1997) described it, for the stigmatized person there is "a threat in the air."

3.1.3 Concealment Versus Disclosure
Another area of research on stigma, moving more proximally to the self, concerns the effect of concealing one's stigmatizing attribute. Paradoxically, concealing one's stigma is often used as a coping strategy, aimed at avoiding negative consequences of stigma, but it is a coping strategy that can backfire and become stressful (Miller & Major, 2000). In a study of women who felt stigmatized by abortion, Major and Gramzow (1999) demonstrated that concealment was related to suppressing thoughts about the abortion, which led to intrusive

thoughts about it, and resulted in psychological distress. Smart and Wegner (2000) described the cost of hiding one's stigma in terms of the resultant cognitive burden involved in the constant preoccupation with hiding. They described complex cognitive processes, both conscious and unconscious, that are necessary to maintain secrecy regarding one's stigma, and called the inner experience of the person who is hiding a concealable stigma a "private hell" (p. 229).

Gay men, lesbians and bisexuals may conceal their sexual orientation in an effort to protect themselves from real harm (e.g., being attacked, getting fired from a job) or out of shame and guilt (D'Augelli & Grossman, 2001). Concealment of one's homosexuality is an important source of stress for gay men and lesbians (DiPlacido, 1998). Hetrick and Martin (1987) described "learning to hide" as the most common coping strategy of gay and lesbian adolescents and noted that "individuals in such a position must constantly monitor their behavior in all circumstances: How one dresses, speaks, walks, and talks become constant sources of possible discovery. One must limit one's friends, one's interests, and one's expression, for fear that one might be found guilty by association. . . . The individual who must hide of necessity learns to interact on the basis of deceit governed by fear of discovery. . . . Each successive act of deception, each moment of monitoring which is unconscious and automatic for others, serves to reinforce the belief in one's difference and inferiority" (pp. 35–36).

Hiding and fear of being identified do not end with adolescence. For example, studies of the workplace experience of lesbians, gay men, and bisexuals found that fear of discrimination and concealment of sexual orientation are prevalent (Croteau, 1996), and that they have adverse psychological, health, and job-related outcomes (Waldo, 1999). These studies showed that gay men, lesbians, and bisexuals engage in identity disclosure and concealment strategies that address fear of discrimination on one hand and a need for self-integrity on the other. These strategies range from "passing," which involves lying in order to be seen as heterosexual; covering, which involves censoring clues about one's self so the gay/lesbian identity is concealed; being implicitly "out," which involves telling the truth without using explicit language that discloses one's sexual identity; and being explicitly "out" (Griffin, 1992; in Croteau, 1996).

Another source of evidence comes from psychological research that has shown that expressing emotions and sharing important aspects of one's self with others—through confessions and disclosures involved in interpersonal or therapeutic relationships, for example—are important factors in maintaining physical and mental health (Pennebaker, 1995). Studies showed that suppression, such as hiding secrets, is related to adverse health outcomes, and that expressing and disclosing traumatic events or characteristics of the self improve health by reducing anxiety and promoting assimilation of the revealed characteristics (Bucci, 1995; Stiles, 1995). In one class of studies, investigators have shown that repression and inhibition affect immune function and health outcome, whereas expression of emotions, such as writing about traumatic experiences, produces improved immune function, fewer physician visits, and diminished symptoms for diseases such as asthma and arthritis (Petrie et al., 1995; Smyth et al., 1999). Research evidence for gay men supports these formulations. Cole and colleagues found that HIV infection advanced more rapidly among gay men who concealed their sexual orientation than those who were open about it (Cole et al., 1996b). In another study, among HIV-negative gay men, those who concealed their sexual orientation were more likely to have had health problems than those who were open about their sexual orientation (Cole et al., 1996a).

In addition to suppressed emotions, concealment prevents LGB people from identifying and affiliating with others who are gay. The psychology literature has demonstrated the positive effect of affiliation with other similarly stigmatized persons on self-esteem (Jones et al., 1984; Crocker & Major, 1989; Postmes & Branscombe, 2002). This effect has been demonstrated by Frable et al. (1998) in day-to-day interactions. The researchers assessed self-perception and well-being in the context of the immediate social environment. College students with concealable stigmas, such as homosexuality, felt better about themselves when they were in an environment with others who are like them than when they were with others who are not similarly stigmatized. In addition, if LGB people conceal their sexual orientation, they are not likely to access formal and informal support resources in the LGB community. Thus, by concealing their sexual orientation LGB people suffer from the health-impairing properties of concealment and lose the ameliorative self-protective effects of being "out."

3.1.4 Internalized Homophobia

In the most proximal position along the continuum from the environment to the self, internalized homophobia represents a form of stress that is internal and insidious. In the absence of overt negative events, and even if one's minority status is successfully concealed, lesbians and gay men may be harmed by directing negative social values toward the self. Thoits (1985, p. 22) described such a process of self-stigmatization, explaining: "[R]ole-taking abilities enable individuals to view themselves from the imagined perspective of others. One can anticipate and respond in advance to others' reactions regarding a contemplated course of action."

Clinicians use the term *internalized homophobia* to refer to the internalization of societal antigay attitudes in lesbians and gay men (e.g., Malyon, 1982). Meyer and Dean (1998) defined internalized homophobia as "the gay person's direction of negative social attitudes toward the self, leading to a devaluation of the self and resultant internal conflicts and poor self-regard" (p. 161). After they accept their stigmatized sexual orientation, gay men, lesbians, and bisexuals begin a process of coming out. Optimally, through this process they come to terms with their homosexuality and develop a healthy identity that incorporates their sexuality (Cass, 1979, 1984; Coleman, 1982; Troiden, 1989). Internalized homophobia signifies failure of the coming-out process to ward off stigma and thoroughly overcome negative self-perceptions and attitudes (Morris et al., 2001). Although it is most acute early during the coming-out process, it is unlikely that internalized homophobia completely abates even when the person has accepted his or her homosexuality. Because of the strength of early socialization experiences and continued exposure to antigay attitudes, internalized homophobia remains an important factor in the gay person's psychological adjustment throughout life. Gay people maintain varying degrees of residual antigay attitudes that are integrated into their self-perception that can lead to mental health problems (Malyon, 1982; Nungesser, 1983; Hetrick & Martin, 1984; Cabaj, 1988). Gonsiorek (1988, p. 117) termed such residual internalized homophobia "covert," and said: "Covert forms of internalized homophobia are the most common. Affected individuals appear to accept themselves, yet sabotage their own efforts in a variety of ways."

Williamson (2000) reviewed the literature on internalized homophobia and described the wide use of the term in gay and lesbian studies and gay-affirmative psychotherapeutic models. He noted the intuitive appeal of internalized homophobia to "almost all gay men and lesbians" (p. 98). Much of the literature on internalized homophobia has come from theoretical writings and clinical observations, although some research has been published. Despite significant challenges to measuring internalized homophobia and lack of consistency in its conceptualization and measurement (Shidlo, 1994; Ross & Rosser, 1996; Mayfield, 2001; Szymanski & Chung, 2001), research showed that internalized homophobia is a significant correlate of mental health, including depression and anxiety symptoms, substance use disorders, and suicide ideation (DiPlacido, 1998; Meyer & Dean, 1998; Williamson, 2000). Research has also suggested a relation between internalized homophobia and various forms of self-harm, including eating disorders (Williamson, 2000) and HIV risk-taking behaviors (Meyer & Dean, 1998), although some studies failed to show this relation (Shidlo, 1994). Nicholson and Long (1990) showed that internalized homophobia was related to self-blame and poor coping in the face of HIV infection/ AIDS. Other research showed that internalized homophobia was related to difficulty with intimate relationships and sexual functioning (Dupras, 1994; Rosser et al., 1997; Meyer & Dean, 1998).

3.1.5 Stress-Ameliorating Factors
As early as 1954, Allport suggested that minority members respond to prejudice with coping and resilience. Modern writers agree that positive coping is common and beneficial to members of minority groups (Clark et al., 1999). Therefore, minority status is associated not only with stress but with important resources such as group solidarity and cohesiveness that protect minority members from the adverse mental health effects of minority stress (Kessler et al., 1985; Crocker & Major, 1989; Shade, 1990; Branscombe et al., 1999b; Clark et al., 1999; Miller & Major, 2000; Postmes & Branscombe, 2002). Empirical evidence supports these contentions. For example, in a study of African American participants, Branscombe et al. (1999b) found that attributions of prejudice were directly related to negative well-being and hostility toward Whites but also, through the mediating role of enhanced in-group

identity, to positive well-being. In a separate study, Postmes and Branscombe (2002) found that among African Americans a segregated racial environment contributed to greater in-group acceptance and improved well-being and life satisfaction.

The importance of coping with stigma has also been asserted in LGB populations. Weinberg and Williams (1974, pp. 150–151) noted that "occupying a 'deviant identity' need not necessarily intrude upon [gay men's] day-to-day functioning" and urged scientists to "pay more attention to the human capacity for adaptation." Through coming out LGB people learn to cope with and overcome the adverse effects of stress (Morris et al., 2001). Thus, stress and resilience interact in predicting mental disorder. Gay men, lesbians, and bisexuals counteract minority stress by establishing alternative structures and values that enhance their group (D'Emilio, 1983; Crocker & Major, 1989). In a similar vein, Garnets et al. (1990, p. 367) suggested that although antigay violence creates a crisis with potential adverse mental health outcomes it also presents "opportunities for subsequent growth." Among gay men, personal acceptance of one's gay identity and talking to family members about AIDS showed the strongest positive associations with concurrent measures of support and changes in support satisfaction (Kertzner, 2001). Similarly, in a study of LGB adolescents, family support and self-acceptance ameliorated the negative effect of antigay abuse on mental health outcomes (Hershberger & D'Augelli, 1995).

A distinction between personal and group resources is often not addressed in the coping literature. It is important to distinguish between resources that operate on the individual level (e.g., personality), in which members of minority groups vary, and resources that operate on a group level and are available to all minority members (Branscombe & Ellemers, 1998). Like other individuals who cope with general stress, lesbians, gay men, and bisexuals utilize a range of personal coping mechanisms, resilience, and hardiness to withstand stressful experiences (Antonovsky, 1987; Ouellette, 1993; Masten, 2001). In addition to such personal coping, group-level social-structural factors can have mental health benefits (Peterson et al., 1996). Jones and colleagues (1984) described two functions of coping achieved through minority group affiliations: to allow stigmatized persons to experience social environments in which they are not stigmatized by others and to provide support for negative evaluation of the stigmatized minority group. Social evaluation theory suggests another plausible mechanism for minority coping (Pettigrew, 1967). Members of stigmatized groups who have a strong sense of community cohesiveness evaluate themselves in comparison with others who are like them rather than with members of the dominant culture. The group may provide a reappraisal of the stressful condition, yielding it less injurious to psychological well-being. Through reappraisal, the group validates deviant experiences and feelings of minority persons (Thoits, 1985). Indeed, reappraisal is at the core of gay-affirmative, black-affirmative, and feminist psychotherapies that aim to empower the minority person

(Smith & Siegel, 1985; Shade, 1990; Garnets & Kimmel, 1991; Hooks, 1993).

The distinction between personal and group-level coping may be somewhat complicated because even group-level resources (e.g., services of a gay-affirmative church) need to be accessed and utilized by individuals. Whether individuals can access and use group-level resources depends on many factors, including personality variables. Nevertheless, it is important to distinguish between group-level and personal resources because when group-level resources are absent even otherwise resourceful individuals have deficient coping. Group-level resources may therefore define the boundaries of individual coping efforts. Thus, "minority coping" may be conceptualized as a group-level resource, related to the group's ability to mount self-enhancing structures to counteract stigma. This formulation highlights the degree to which minority members may be able to adopt some of the group's self-enhancing attitudes, values, and structures rather than the degree to which individuals vary in their personal coping abilities. Using this distinction, it is conceivable that an individual has efficient personal coping resources but lacks minority coping resources. For example, a lesbian or gay member of the U.S. Armed Forces, where a "don't ask, don't tell" policy discourages affiliation and attachments with other LGB persons, may be unable to access and utilize group-level resources and is therefore vulnerable to adverse health outcomes regardless of his or her personal coping abilities. Finally, it is important to note that coping can also have a stressful impact (Miller & Major, 2000). For example, concealing one's stigma is a common way of coping with stigma and avoiding negative regard, yet it takes a heavy toll on the person using this coping strategy (Smart & Wegner, 2000).

4 Discussion

I have suggested a conceptual model that describes sexual prejudice as the social environmental context within which to examine the mental health of LGB individuals. The model can serve as a guide for directing research of LGB mental health by identifying areas of investigation. It can also aid in suggesting areas for intervention. The model is not meant to be finite or all-inclusive. Other stress and ameliorative processes could be added, depending on particular issues of the population studied. The model might elaborate different areas when applied to LGBs who are young versus older, White versus ethnic minorities, and men versus women. For example, when studying African American men, Crawford et al. (2002) highlighted aspects of identity and affiliation related to and conflicts among Black and sexual orientation identities. Fieland and colleagues (Chapter 11) described history and spirituality as resources with unique significance for two-spirit American Indian/Alaskan Natives.

Similarly, generational differences affect the stress process. Although oppression of LGB youth, including discrimination and violence, continues to be a serious challenge to public health and public policy, there are new opportunities for LGB youth that have never been present before and that may affect the shape of stressors and the opportunities for resilience and coping (Herdt & Boxer, 1996; Cohler & Galatzer-Levy, 2000). Individuals born during the late 1980s and 1990s, are being raised in a period where legal barriers are falling and social institutions—most remarkably, marriage—that previous generations of LGB individuals could not fathom are becoming available. Such social environmental changes should result in changes in conceptual and theoretical formulations of LGB development such as described by Eliason and Schope (see Chapter 1) and Savin-Williams and Cohen (see Chapter 2).

For example, social changes in the meaning of other minority statuses, such as race/ethnicity, have opened new possibilities, most significantly the possibility that multiple identities can complement one another rather than compete, and that identification and connections with different communities can coexist (see Chapter 1). These concepts are inconsistent with current conceptual models of LGB youth. Coming-out models typically envision a transformation where one sheds a prior identity and replaces it with an LGB identity. Postmodern conceptions of identity make it clear that this is rarely the case. Identity is now understood by theorists as multifaceted and contextual (Ashmore et al., 2004). Youth are more likely to enact various identities and confront struggles and challenges in multiple fronts; for example, they may integrate race/ethnic and sexual minority identities in ways that prior generations could not conceive. Therefore, stress processes related to sexual orientation and race/ethnicity may need to be viewed as more integrated and more contextual. This means, for example, that for Black LGBs sexual prejudice and racism are not, as older generations have described it, parallel concerns that shift with the social environment but an amalgama that travels with them everywhere they go. Such questions need to be answered as research addresses more complex LGB identities and related coping.

4.1 Intervention and Treatment

Kitzinger (1997) warned against relying on the stress model, seeing "stress" as a subjective, individually focused concept that can lead to ignoring the need for important political and structural changes: "If [psychologists'] aim is to decrease 'stress' and to increase the 'ego strength' of the victim," she asked, "do they risk forgetting that it is the perpetrator, not the victim, who is the real problem? What political choices are they making in focusing on the problems of the oppressed rather than on the problem of the oppressor?" This is an important reminder that public health should pay attention to, but it fails to take into account the full range of, and the variety of interventions implied by, the stress model. As a construct, the stress model can be useful not only for helping articulate the various components—or stress processes, as I described them—that affect health but also point out to areas of intervention. Utilizing the stress model more fully, researchers and policy makers should attend to the full spectrum of interventions implied by the model (Ouellette, 1998): The stress model points to both distal and proximal causes and should direct us to relevant interventions at both the individual and structural levels.

It is important for public health to focus on distal causes of distress by eliminating sources of stress in the social environment. For that, public health and public policy interventions are necessary that would eliminate prejudice and discrimination, reduce antigay violence, and create a supportive social environment for LGB individuals. Many initiatives address this need. Such initiatives include political action by individuals and groups and the establishment of organizations and facilities that combat sexual prejudice, homophobia, and heterosexism. For example, LGB organizations work on a national and local level to lobby legislators and mobilize the gay community to political action (e.g., the Human Rights Campaign, National Gay and Lesbian Task Force), to challenge laws that discriminate against LGBs (e.g., Lambda Legal Defense and Education Fund, National Center for Lesbian Rights), and to fight homophobia and advocate for more accepting social environments for LGBTs (Gay, Lesbian and Straight Education Network; Senior Action in Gay Environment). For example, GLSEN brings LGB and straight students and educators together in schools across the country to work toward the elimination of antigay discrimination and the incorporation of LGB issues into school curricula (GLSEN, 2004). Other efforts use scientific work to have an impact on legal battles that affect LGBT rights via *amicus curiae* (friends of the court) briefs filed in important court cases. For example, in the case before the Supreme Court that led it to strike down sodomy laws in the United States (Lawrence & Garner v. Texas, 2003), an amicus brief led by the American Public Health Association directly addressed the implication of the stress model as described above. Responding to claims that sodomy laws *promote* public health and HIV prevention, the brief not only rejected that notion but also affirmed that sodomy laws adversely affect the physical and mental health of LGB persons (American Public Health Association, 2003).

The stress model also points to individual-level interventions. Denying individual agency and resilience would ignore an impressive body of social psychological research that demonstrates the importance and utility of coping with stigma (Crocker & Major, 1989; Branscombe & Ellemers, 1998; Miller & Myers, 1998; Miller & Major, 2000). Individual-level interventions include prevention programs that would enhance LGB youth's sense of self and help them with coming out and clinical interventions that would help LGB individuals with issues related to internalized homophobia, antigay violence, and rejection and discrimination (American Psychological Association, 2000). The individual and the social environment are highlighted in the minority stress model I described, and both need to be addressed in regard to prevention and intervention (Minkler, 1999). Ignoring the social environment would erroneously place the burden on the individual, suggesting that minority stress is only a personal problem for which individuals must be treated (Hobfoll, 1998). However, neglecting individual-based interventions that enhance coping and resilience of LGB individuals and communities is also wrong. It would go against a rich history of resistance and self-reliance that has characterized the history of LGB groups in the United States (D'Emilio, 1983).

References

Adam, B.D. (1987) *The rise of a gay and lesbian movement*. Twayne Publishers, Boston.

Allen, L.A., Woolfolk, R.L., Gara, M., and Apter, J.T. (1999) Possible selves in major depression. *Journal of Nervous and Mental Disease* 184:739–745.

Allison, K.W. (1998) Stress and oppressed social category membership. In: Swim, J.K., and Stangor, C. (eds) *Prejudice: the target's perspective*. Academic Press, San Diego, pp. 145–170.

Allport, G.W. (1954) *The nature of prejudice*. Addison-Wesley, Reading, MA.

American Psychological Association. (2000) Guidelines for psychotherapy with lesbian, gay, and bisexual clients. *American Psychologist* 55:1440–1451.

American Public Health Association. (2003) Amicus brief filed in Lawrence v. Texas (date filed: January 16, 2003).

Amnesty International. (2001) *Crimes of hate, conspiracy of silence: torture and ill-treatment based on sexual identity*. Amnesty International, London.

Antonovsky, A. (1987) *Unraveling the mystery of health: how people manage stress and stay well*. Jossey-Bass, San Francisco.

Ashmore, R.D., Deaux, K., and McLaughlin-Volpe, T. (2004) An organizing framework for collective identity: articulation and significance of multi-dimensionality. *Psychological Bulletin* 130:80–114.

Badgett, L.M.V. (1995) The wage effects of sexual orientation discrimination. *Industrial and Labor Relations Review* 48:726–739.

Barnett, R.C., and Baruch, G.K. (1987) Social roles, gender, and psychological distress. In: Barnett, R.C., Biener, L., and Baruch, G.K. (eds) *Gender and stress*. Free Press, New York, pp. 122–143.

Branscombe, N.R., and Ellemers, N. (1998) Coping with group-based discrimination: individualistic versus group-level strategies. In: Swim, J.K., and Stangor, C. (eds) *Prejudice: the target's perspective*. Academic Press, San Diego, pp. 243–266.

Branscombe, N.R., Ellemers, N., Spears, R., and Doosje, B. (1999a) The context and content of social identity threats. In: Ellemers, N., Spears, R., and Doosje, B. (eds) *Social identity: context, commitment, and content* Blackwell, Oxford, pp. 35–58.

Branscombe, N.R., Schmitt, M.T., and Harvey, R.D. (1999b) Perceiving pervasive discrimination among African Americans: implications for group identification and well-being. *Journal of Personality and Social Psychology* 77:135–149.

Brewer, M.B. (1991) The social self: on being the same and different at the same time. *Personality and Social Psychology Bulletin* 17:475–482.

Brooks, V.R. (1981) *Minority stress and lesbian women*. Lexington Books Lexington, MA.

Brown, T.N., Sellers, S.L., Brown, K.T., and Jackson, J. (1999) Race, ethnicity, and culture in the sociology of mental health. In: Aneshensel, C.S., and Phelan, J.C. (eds) *Handbook of the sociology of mental health*. Kluwer Academic/Plenum Publishers, New York, pp. 167–182.

Bucci, W. (1995) The power of the narrative: a multiple code account. In: Pennebaker, J.W. (ed) *Emotion, disclosure, & health*. American Psychological Association, Washington, DC, pp. 93–122.

Burke, P. (1991) Identity processes and social stress. *American Sociological Review* 56:836–849.

Cabaj, R.P. (1988) Homosexuality and neurosis: considerations for psychotherapy. In: Ross, M.W. (ed) *The treatment of homosexuals with mental health disorders*. Harrington Park Press, New York, pp. 13–23.

Cass, V.C. (1979) Homosexual identity formation: a theoretical model. *Journal of Homosexuality* 4:219–235.

Cass, V.C. (1984) Homosexual identity formation: testing a theoretical model. *Journal of Sex Research* 20:143–167.

Clark, R., Anderson, N.B., Clark, V.R., and Williams, D.R. (1999) Racism as a stressor for African Americans: a biopsychosocial model. *American Psychologist* 54:805–816.

Cochran, S.D. (2001) Emerging issues in research on lesbians' and gay men's mental health: does sexual orientation really matter? *American Psychologist* 56:931–947.

Cochran, S.D., and Mays, V.M. (1994) Depressive distress among homosexually active African-American men and women. *American Journal of Psychiatry* 151:524–529.

Cohler, B.J., and Galatzer-Levy, R.M. (2000) *The course of gay and lesbian lives: social and psychoanalytic perspectives*. Chicago: Chicago University Press.

Cole, S.W., Kemeny, M.E., Taylor, S.E., and Visscher, B.R. (1996a) Elevated physical health risk among gay men who conceal their homosexual identity. *Health Psychology* 15:243–251.

Cole, S.W., Kemeny, M.E., Taylor, S.E., Visscher, B.R., and Fahey, J.L. (1996b) Accelerated course of human immunodeficiency virus infection in gay men who conceal their homosexual identity. *Psychosomatic Medicine* 58:219–231.

Coleman, E. (1982) Developmental stages of the coming out process. *Journal of Homosexuality* 7:31–43.

Crawford, I., Allison, K.W., Zamboni, B.D., and Soto, T. (2002) The influence of dual-identity development on the psychosocial functioning of African-American gay and bisexual men. *Journal of Sex Research* 39:179–189.

Crocker, J. (1999) Social stigma and self-esteem: situational construction of self-worth. *Journal of Experimental Social Psychology* 35:89–107.

Crocker, J., and Major, B. (1989) Social stigma and self-esteem: the self-protective properties of stigma. *Psychological Review* 96:608–630.

Crocker, J., and Quinn, D.M. (2000) Social stigma and the self: meanings, situations, and self-esteem. In: Heatherton, T.F., Kleck, R.E., Hebl, M.R., and Hull, J.G. (eds) *The social psychology of stigma*. Guilford Press, New York, pp. 153–183.

Crocker, J., Major, B., and Steele, C. (1998) Social stigma. In: Gilbert, D., Fiske, S.T., and Lindzey, G. (eds) *The handbook of social psychology*, 4th ed. McGraw-Hill, Boston, pp. 504–553.

Cross, W. (1995) The psychology of nigrescence: revising the cross model. In: Ponterotto, J.G., Casa, J.M., Suzuki, L.A., and Alexander, C.M. (eds) *Handbook of multicultural counseling*. Sage Publications, Thousand Oaks, CA, pp. 93–122.

Croteau, J.M. (1996) Research on the work experience of lesbian, gay, and bisexual people: an integrative review of methodology and findings. *Journal of Vocational Behavior* 48:195–209.

D'Augelli, A.R., and Grossman, A.H. (2001) Disclosure of sexual orientation, victimization, and mental health among lesbian, gay, and bisexual older adults. *Journal of Interpersonal Violence* 16:1008–1027.

D'Augelli, A.R., and Hershberger, S.L. (1993) Lesbian, gay, and bisexual youth in community settings: personal challenges and mental health problems. *American Journal of Community Psychology* 21:1–28.

Dean, L., Meyer, I.H., Sell, R.L., Sember, R., Silenzio, V., Bowen, D.J., et al. (2000) Lesbian, gay, bisexual, and transgender health: findings and concerns. *Journal of the Gay and Lesbian Medical Association* 4:101–151.

Deaux, K. (1993) Reconstructing social identity. *Personality and Social Psychology Bulletin* 19:4–12.

Deaux, K., and Ethier, K. (1998) Negotiating social identity. In: Swim, J.K., and Stangor, C. (eds) *Prejudice: the target's perspective*. Academic Press, San Diego, pp. 301–323.

D'Emilio, J. (1983) *Sexual politics, sexual communities: the making of a homosexual minority in the United States, 1940–1970*. University of Chicago Press, Chicago.

De Monteflores, C., and Schultz, S.J. (1978) Coming out: similarities and differences for lesbians and gay men. *Journal of Social Issues* 34:59–72.

Diamond, L.M. (2000) Sexual identity, attractions, and behavior among young sexual-minority women over a 2-year period. *Developmental Psychology* 36:241–250.

Diaz, R.M., Ayala, G., Bein, E., Jenne, J., and Marin, B.V. (2001) The impact of homophobia, poverty and racism on the mental health of Latino gay men. *American Journal of Public Health* 91:927–932.

DiPlacido, J. (1998) Minority stress among lesbians, gay men, and bisexual: a consequence of heterosexism, homophobia, and stigmatization. In: Herek, G.M. (ed) *Stigma and sexual orientation: understanding prejudice against lesbians, gay men, and bisexuals*, Vol. 4. Sage, Thousand Oaks, CA, pp. 138–159.

Dohrenwend, B.P. (2000) The role of adversity and stress in psychopathology: some evidence and its implications for theory and research. *Journal of Health and Social Behavior* 41:1–19.

Dupras, A. (1994) Internalized homophobia and psychosexual adjustment among gay men. *Psychological Reports* 75:23–28.

Eliason, M.J. (1996) Identity formation for lesbian, bisexual, and gay persons: beyond a "minoritizing" view. *Journal of Homosexuality* 30:31–58.

Espin, O.M. (1993) Issues of identity in the psychology of Latina lesbians. In: Garnets, L.D., and Kimmel, D.C. (eds) *Psychological perspectives on lesbian and gay male experiences*. Columbia University Press, New York, pp. 348–363.

Ethier, K., and Deaux, K. (1994) Negotiating social identity when contexts change. *Journal of Personality and Social Psychology* 67:243–251.

Farina, A., Allen, J.G., and Saul, B.B. (1968) The role of the stigmatized person in affecting social relationships. *Journal of Personality* 36:169–182.

Faulkner, A.H., and Cranston, K. (1998) Correlates of same-sex sexual behavior in a random sample of Massachusetts high school students. *American Journal of Public Health* 88:262–266.

Fife, B.L., and Wright, E.R. (2000) The dimensionality of stigma: a comparison of its impact on the self of persons with HIV/AIDS and cancer. *Journal of Health and Social Behavior* 41:50–67.

Frable, D.E., Wortman, C., and Joseph, J. (1997) Predicting self-esteem, well-being, and distress in a cohort of gay men: the importance of cultural stigma, personal visibility, community networks, and positive identity. *Journal of Personality* 65:599–624.

Frable, D.E.S., Platt, L., and Hoey, S. (1998) Concealable stigmas and positive self-perceptions: feeling better around similar others. *Journal of Personality and Social Psychology* 74:909–922.

Fullilove, M.T., and Fullilove, R.E. (1999) Stigma as an obstacle to AIDS action. *American Behavioral Scientist* 42:1117–1129.

Garnets, L.D., and Kimmel, D.C. (1991) Lesbian and gay male dimensions in the psychological study of human diversity. In: Garnets, L.D., Jones, J.M.,

Kimmel, D.C., Sue, S., and Tarvis, C. (eds) *Psychological perspectives on human diversity in America*. American Psychological Association, Washington, DC.

Garnets, L.D., Herek, G.M., and Levy, B. (1990) Violence and victimization of lesbians and gay men: mental health consequences. *Journal of Interpersonal Violence*, 5:366–383.

Garofalo, R., Wolf, R.C., Kessel, S., Palfrey, J., and DuRant, R.H. (1998) The association between health risk behaviors and sexual orientation among a school based sample of adolescents. *Pediatrics* 101:895–902.

Gay and Lesbian Medical Association and LGBT Health Experts. (2001) *Healthy people 2010 companion document for lesbian, gay, bisexual, and transgender (LGBT) health*. Gay and Lesbian Medical Association, San Francisco.

GLSEN. (1999) *GLSEN's national school climate survey: lesbian, gay, bisexual and transgender students and their experiences in school*. GLSEN, New York.

GLSEN. (2004) History. http://www.glsen.org/cgi-bin/iowa/all/about/index.html.

Goffman, E. (1963) *Stigma: notes on the management of spoiled identity*. Touchstone, New York.

Gonsiorek, J.C. (1988) Mental health issues of gay and lesbian adolescents. *Journal of Adolescent Health Care* 9:114–122.

Greenberg, J.S. (1973) Study of self-esteem and alienation of male homosexuals. *Journal of Psychology* 83:137–143.

Griffin, P. (1992) From hiding out to coming out: empowering lesbian and gay educators. In: Harbeck, K.M. (ed) *Coming out of the classroom closet*. Harrington Park Press, Binghamton, NY, pp. 167–196.

Grossman, A.H., and Kerner, M.S. (1998) Self-esteem and supportiveness as predictors of emotional distress in gay male and lesbian youth. *Journal of Homosexuality* 35(2):25–39.

Herdt, G., and Boxer, A. (1996) *Children of horizons*. Beacon Press, Boston.

Herek, G.M. (2000) The psychology of sexual prejudice. *Current Directions in Psychological Sciences* 9:19–22.

Herek, G.M., and Berrill, K.T. (1992) *Hate crimes: confronting violence against lesbian and gay men*. Sage, Thousand Oaks, CA.

Herek, G.M., Gillis, J.R., and Cogan, J.C. (1999) Psychological sequelae of hate-crime victimization among lesbian, gay, and bisexual adults. *Journal of Consulting and Clinical Psychology* 67:945–951.

Hershberger, S.L., and D'Augelli, A.R. (1995) The impact of victimization on the mental health and suicidality of lesbian, gay, and bisexual youth. *Developmental Psychology* 31:65–74.

Hetrick, E.S., and Martin, A.D. (1984) Ego-dystonic homosexuality: a developmental view. In: Hetrick, E.S., and Stein, T.S. (eds) *Innovations in psychotherapy with homosexuals*. American Psychiatric Association Press, Washington, DC.

Hetrick, E.S., and Martin, A.D. (1987) Developmental issues and their resolution for gay and lesbian adolescents. *Journal of Homosexuality* 14:25–43.

Hobfoll, S.E. (1998) The social and historical context of stress. In: *Stress, culture, and community: the psychology and philosophy of stress*. Plenum Press, New York, pp. 1–23.

Hooks, B. (1993) *Sisters of the yam: black woman and self-recovery*. South End Press, Boston.

Human Rights Watch. (2001) *Hatred in the hallways: violence and discrimination against lesbian, gay, bisexual, and transgender students in U.S. schools*. Human Rights Watch, New York.

Jetten, J., Branscombe, N.R., Schmitt, M.T., and Spears, R. (2001) Rebels with a cause: group identification as a response to perceived discrimination from the mainstream. *Personality and Social Psychology Bulletin* 27:1204–1213.

Jones, E.E., Farina, A., Hestrof, A.H., Markus, H., Miller, D.T., and Scott, R.A. (1984) *Social stigma: the psychology of marked relationships*. W.H. Freeman, New York.

Kertzner, R.M. (1999) Self-appraisal of life experience and psychological adjustment in midlife gay men. *Journal of Psychology and Human Sexuality* 11:43–64.

Kertzner, R.M. (2001) The adult life course and homosexual identity in midlife gay men. *Annual Review of Sex Research* 12:75–92.

Kessler, R.C., Price, R.H., and Wortman, C.B. (1985) Social factors in psychopathology: stress, social support, and coping processes. *Annual Review of Psychology* 36:572.

Kitzinger, C. (1997) Lesbian and gay psychology: a critical analysis. In: Fox, D., and Prilleltensky, I. (eds) *Critical psychology: an introduction*. Sage, Thousand Oaks, CA, pp. 202–216.

Kobrynowicz, D., and Branscombe, N.R. (1997) Who considers themselves victims of discrimination? Individual difference predictors of perceived gender discrimination in women and men. *Psychology of Women Quarterly* 21:347–363.

Krieger, N. (2001) Theories for social epidemiology in the 21st century: an ecosocial perspective. *International Journal of Epidemiology* 30:668–677.

Krieger, N., and Sidney, S. (1997) Prevalence and health implications of anti-gay discrimination: a study of black and white women and men in the CARDIA cohort. *International Journal of Health Services* 27:157–176.

Laumann, E.O., Gagnon, J.H., Michael, R.T., and Michaels, S. (1994) *The social organization of sexuality: sexual practices in the United States*. University of Chicago Press, Chicago.

Lazarus, R.S., and Folkman, S. (1984) *Stress, appraisal, and coping*. Springer, New York.

Link, B.G. (1987) Understanding labeling effects in the area of mental disorders: an assessment of the effects of expectations of rejection. *American Sociological Review* 52:96–112.

Link, B.G., Struening, E.L., Rahav, M., Phelan, J.C., and Nuttbrock, L. (1997) On stigma and its consequences: evidence from a longitudinal study of men with dual diagnoses of mental illness and substance abuse. *Journal of Health and Social Behavior* 38:177–190.

Linville, P. (1987) Self-complexity as a cognitive buffer against stress related illness and depression. *Journal of Personality and Social Psychology* 52:663–676.

Loiacano, D.K. (1993) Gay identity among black Americans: racism, homophobia, and the need for validation. In: Garnets, L.D., and Kimmel, D.C. (eds) *Psychological perspectives on lesbian and gay male experiences*. Columbia University Press, New York, pp. 364–375.

Major, B., and Gramzow, R.H. (1999) Abortion as stigma: cognitive and emotional implications of concealment. *Journal of Personality and Social Psychology* 77:735–745.

Malebranche, D.J., Peterson, J.L., Fullilove, R.E., and Stackhouse, R.W. (2004) Race and sexual identity: perceptions about medical culture and healthcare among black men who have sex with men. *Journal of the National Medical Association* 96:97–107.

Malyon, A.K. (1982) Psychotherapeutic implications of internalized homophobia in gay men. *Journal of Homosexuality* 7:59–69.

Massey, S., and Ouellette, S.C. (1996) Heterosexual bias in the identity self-portraits of gay men, lesbians, and bisexuals. *Journal of Homosexuality* 32:57–76.

Masten, A.S. (2001) Ordinary magic: resilience processes in development. *American Psychologist* 56:227–238.

Mayfield, W. (2001) The development of an internalized homonegativity inventory for gay men. *Journal of Homosexuality* 4:53–76.

Mays, V.M., and Cochran, S.D. (2001) Mental health correlates of perceived discrimination among lesbian, gay, and bisexual adults in the United States. *American Journal of Public Health* 91:1869–1876.

McDevitt, J., Balboni, J., Garcia, L., and Gu, J. (2001) Consequences for victims: a comparison of bias- and non-bias-motivated assaults. *American Behavioral Scientist* 45:697–713.

Meyer, I.H. (1995) Minority stress and mental health in gay men. *Journal of Health and Social Behavior* 36:38–56.

Meyer, I.H. (2003) Prejudice, social stress and mental health in lesbian, gay, and bisexual populations: conceptual issues and research evidence. *Psychological Bulletin* 129:674–697.

Meyer, I.H., and Dean, L. (1998) Internalized homophobia, intimacy, and sexual behavior among gay and bisexual men. In: Herek, G.M. (ed) *Stigma and sexual orientation: understanding prejudice against lesbians, gay men, and bisexuals*. Sage, Thousand Oaks, CA, pp. 160–186.

Miller, C.T., and Major, B. (2000) Coping with stigma and prejudice. In: Heatherton, T.F., Kleck, R.E., Hebl, M.R., and Hull, J.G. (eds) *The social psychology of stigma*. Guilford Press, New York, pp. 243–272.

Miller, C.T., and Myers, A.M. (1998) Compensating for prejudice: how heavyweight people (and others) control outcomes despite prejudice. In: Swim, J.K., and Stangor, C. (eds) *Prejudice: the target's perspective*. Academic Press, San Diego, pp. 191–218.

Minkler, M. (1999) Personal responsibility for health? A review of the arguments and the evidence at century's end. *Health Education & Behavior* 26:121–140.

Mirowsky, J., and Ross, C.E. (1989) *Social causes of psychological distress*. Aldine De Gruyter, Hawthorne, NY.

Morris, J.F., Waldo, C.R., and Rothblum, E.D. (2001) A model of predictors and outcomes of outness among lesbian and bisexual women. *American Journal of Orthopsychiatry* 71:61–71.

Nicholson, W.D., and Long, B.C. (1990) Self-esteem, social support, internalized homophobia, and coping strategies of HIV+ gay men. *Journal of Consulting and Clinical Psychology* 58:873–876.

Nungesser, L.G. (1983) *Homosexual acts, actors, and identities*. Praeger, New York.

Operario, D., and Fiske, S.T. (2001) Ethnic identity moderates perceptions of prejudice: judgments of personal versus group discrimination and subtle versus blatant bias. *Personality and Social Psychology Bulletin* 27:550–561.

Ouellette, S.C. (1993) Inquiries into hardiness. In: Goldbeger, L., and Breznitz, S. (eds) *Handbook of stress: theoretical and clinical aspects*, 2nd ed. Free Press, New York, pp. 77–100.

Ouellette, S.C. (1998) The value and limitations of stress models in HIV/AIDS. In: Dohrenwend, B.P. (ed) *Adversity, stress, and psychopathology*. Oxford University Press, New York, pp. 142–160.

Pearlin, L.I. (1999) The stress process revisited: reflections on concepts and their interrelationships. In: Aneshensel, C.S., and Phelan, J.C. (eds) *Handbook of the sociology of mental health*. Kluwer Academic/Plenum Publishers, New York, pp. 395–415.

Pennebaker, J.W. (1995) *Emotion, disclosure, and health*. American Psychological Association, Washington, DC.

Peterson, J.L., Folkman, S., and Bakeman, R. (1996) Stress, coping, HIV status, psychosocial resources, and depressive mood in African American gay, bisexual, and heterosexual men. *American Journal of Community Psychology* 24:461–487.

Petrie, K.J., Booth, R.J., and Davison, K.P. (1995) Repression, disclosure, and immune function: recent findings and methodological issues. In: Pennebaker, J.W. (ed) *Emotion, disclosure, & health*. American Psychological Association, Washington, DC, pp. 223–237.

Pettigrew, T.F. (1967) Social evaluation theory: convergencies and applications. In: Levine, D. (ed) *Nebraska symposium on motivation*, 15th ed. University of Nebraska Press, Lincoln, pp. 241–304.

Pinel, E.C. (2002) Stigma consciousness in intergroup contexts: the power of conviction. *Journal of Experimental Social Psychology* 38:178–185.

Postmes, T., and Branscombe, N.R. (2002) Influence of long-term racial environmental composition on subjective well-being in African Americans. *Journal of Personality and Social Psychology* 83:735–751.

Rosario, M., Rotheram-Borus, M.J., and Reid, H. (1996) Gay-related stress and its correlates among gay and bisexual male adolescents of predominantly Black and Hispanic background. *Journal of Community Psychology* 24:136–159.

Rosenberg, S., and Gara, M. (1985) The multiplicity of personal identity. In: Shaver, P.R. (ed) *Self, situations, and social behavior: review of personality and social psychology*. Sage Publications, Beverly Hills, CA, pp. 87–113.

Ross, M.W. (1985) Actual and anticipated societal reaction to homosexuality and adjustment in two societies. *Journal of Sex Research* 21:40–55.

Ross, M.W., and Rosser, S.B.R. (1996) Measurement and correlates of internalized homophobia: a factor analytic study. *Journal of Clinical Psychology* 52:15–21.

Rosser, B., Metz, M., Bockting, W., and Buroker, T. (1997) Sexual difficulties, concerns and satisfaction in homosexual men: an empirical study with i mplications for HIV prevention. *The Journal of Sex and Marital Therapy* 23:61–73.

Rotheram-Borus, M.J., and Fernandez, M.I. (1995) Sexual orientation and developmental challenges experienced by gay and lesbian youths. *Suicide and Life-Threatening Behavior* 25:26–34.

Safe Schools Coalition of Washington. (1999) *Eighty-three thousand youth: selected findings of eight population-based studies as they pertain to anti-gay harassment and the safety and well-being of sexual minority students*. Safe Schools Coalition of Washington, Seattle.

Shade, B.J. (1990) Coping with color: the anatomy of positive mental health. In: Ruiz, D.S. (ed) *Handbook of mental health and mental disorder among Black Americans*. Greenwood Press, New York.

Shidlo, A. (1994) Internalized homophobia: conceptual and empirical issues in measurement. In: Greene, B., and Herek, G.M. (eds) *Lesbian and gay psychology: theory, research and clinical applications*, Vol. 1. Sage, Thousand Oaks, CA, pp. 176–205.

Siegel, K., and Epstein, J.A. (1996) Ethnic-racial differences in psychological stress related to gay lifestyle among HIV-positive men. *Psychological Reports* 79:303–312.

Smart, L., and Wegner, D.M. (2000) The hidden costs of stigma. In: Heatherton, T.F., Kleck, R.E., Hebl, M.R., and Hull, J.G. (eds) *The social psychology of stigma*. Guilford Press, New York, pp. 220–242.

Smith, A.J., and Siegel, R.F. (1985) Feminist therapy: redefining power for the powerless. In: Rosewater, L.R., and Walker, L.E.A. (eds) *Handbook of feminist therapy: women's issues in psychotherapy*. Springer, New York.

Smyth, J.M., Stone, A.A., Hurewitz, A., and Kaell, A. (1999) Effects of writing about stressful experiences on symptom reduction in patients with asthma or rheumatoid arthritis. *Journal of the American Medical Association* 281:1304–1309.

Steele, C.M. (1997) A threat in the air: how stereotypes shape intellectual identity and performance. *The American Psychologist* 52:613–629.

Steele, C.M., and Aronson, J. (1995) Stereotype threat and the intellectual test performance of African Americans. *Journal of Personality and Social Psychology* 69:797–811.

Stiles, W.B. (1995) Disclosure as a speech act: is it psychotherapeutic to disclose? In: Pennebaker, J.W. (ed) *Emotion, disclosure, & health*. American Psychological Association, Washington, DC, pp. 71–91.

Stokes, J.P., and Peterson, J.L. (1998) Homophobia, self-esteem, and risk for HIV among African American men who have sex with men. *Aids Education and Prevention* 10:278–292.

Swim, J.K., Hyers, L.L., Cohen, L.L., and Ferguson, M.J. (2001) Everyday sexism: evidence for its incidence, nature, and psychological impact from three daily diary studies. *Journal of Social Issues* 57:31–53.

Szymanski, D.M., and Chung, Y.B. (2001) The lesbian internalized homophobia scale: a rational/theoretical approach. *Journal of Homosexuality* 41:37–52.

Thoits, P. (1985) Self-labeling processes in mental illness: the role of emotional deviance. *American Journal of Sociology* 91:221–249.

Thoits, P. (1991) On merging identity theory and stress research. *Social Psychology Quarterly* 54:101–112.

Thoits, P. (1999) Self, identity, stress, and mental health. In: Aneshensel, C.S., and Phelan, J.C. (eds) *Handbook of the sociology of mental health*. Kluwer Academic/Plenum Publishers, New York, pp. 345–368.

Troiden, R.R. (1989) The formation of homosexual identities. *Journal of Homosexuality* 17:45–73.

Twenge, J.M., and Crocker, J. (2002) Race and self-esteem: meta-analyses comparing Whites, Blacks, Hispanics, Asians, and American Indians and comment on Gray-Little and Hafdahl (2000). *Psychological Bulletin* 128:371–408.

U.S. Department of Health and Human Services. (2000) *Healthy people 2010: understanding and improving health*. U.S. Department of Health and Human Services, Government Printing Office, Washington, DC.

Waldo, C.R. (1999) Working in a majority context: a structural model of heterosexism as minority stress in the workplace. *Journal of Counseling Psychology* 46:218–232.

Weinberg, M.S., and Williams, C.J. (1974) *Male homosexuals: their problems and adaptations*. Oxford University Press, New York.

Williamson, I.R. (2000) Internalized homophobia and health issues affecting lesbians and gay men. *Health Education Research* 15:97–107.

Woolfolk, R.L., Novalany, J., Gara, M.A., Allen, L.A., and Polino, M. (1995) Self-complexity, self-evaluation, and depression: an examination of form and content within the self-schema. *Journal of Personality and Social Psychology* 68:1108–1120.

11

Determinants of Health Among Two-Spirit American Indians and Alaska Natives

Karen C. Fieland, Karina L. Walters, and Jane M. Simoni

1 Introduction

In comparison to other racial/ethnic groups, American Indians and Alaska Natives (AIANs or "Natives") suffer from glaring disparities in health-related resources and outcomes. Specifically, morbidity due to violence and substance use is higher and overall mortality is greater (Indian Health Service [IHS], 2001). AIANs who identify as gay, lesbian, bisexual, or transgender (GLBT) or with the modern roughly equivalent Native term "two-spirit" (hereafter collectively referred to as "two-spirits") face additional stressors associated with negotiating their dual oppressed statuses. They often confront heterosexism from Natives and racism from GLBTs. Not surprisingly, two-spirits are thought to be at even greater risk for adverse health outcomes than other Natives (Walters, 1997; Walters et al., 2001). Preliminary empirical evidence supports the notion that two-spirits experience disproportionately greater anti-gay as well as anti-Native violence, including sexual and physical assault during childhood and adulthood (Walters et al., 2001; Simoni et al., 2004a) and historical trauma (Balsam et al., 2004)—experiences that are typically linked to adverse health and psychosocial functioning. Despite the considerable heterogeneity both within and across the more than 562 federally recognized tribes in the United States, the universal experience of colonization has created a shared history for two-spirit people, shaping distinctive conditions of health risk and resilience.

The health problems of AIANs in general and two-spirits in particular are not simply an artifact of Native genetics, culture, or way of life.

Rather, historical and contemporary trauma in concert with sociodemographic vulnerabilities have interacted to undermine the physical and mental health of indigenous populations (Walters & Simoni, 2002). Precisely how these factors affect the health of two-spirits has yet to be empirically evaluated. Indeed, public health research and practice has given scant attention to AIAN populations and has virtually ignored two-spirits: There are no comprehensive reviews of two-spirit health or health-related issues and few empirical studies of even modest scope.

The major aim of this chapter is to stimulate work in the area of two-spirit health by providing a foundation for the conceptualization of two-spirit health risks and resilience. We review the available literature, highlight major gaps in the knowledge base, and provide directions for future research. We first provide an overview of the historical experience of two-spirit people and of the literature on Native health, including morbidity and mortality statistics. We then present the "indigenist" stress-coping model of Walters et al. (2002) as a framework by which to conceptualize how historical, structural, interpersonal, and cultural factors affect two-spirit health outcomes. Research related to some of these health-determining factors is then reviewed. Given the dearth of studies focusing on two-spirits, we refer mainly to studies of AIANs and other people of color as well as GLBT populations, which are almost exclusively non-Native. We conclude with a list of "decolonizing" strategies for future research on two-spirit health.

2 Two-Spirits: Historical Overview

Native worldviews generally do not involve strict binary categories reflected in the Western *weltanshauung*, according to which male is contrasted with female, gay with straight. Instead, they include a fluid conception of self, community, time, and space that permeates cultural norms and linguistic understanding of the self in relation to ancestors, contemporary community, and future generations (Walters et al., 2001). Appreciation of this nonlinear perspective is critical to understanding Native concepts of gender and sexuality, which lack meaningful equivalents in the West (Tafoya, 1992).

Historically, Native societies incorporated gender roles beyond male and female. Individuals embracing "third" or "fourth" genders may have dressed; assumed social, spiritual, and cultural roles; or engaged in sexual and other behaviors not typically associated with members of their biologic sex. From the community's perspective, the fulfillment of social or ceremonial roles and responsibilities was a more important defining feature of gender than sexual behavior or identity. Although often referred to as "two-spirits" today, there were tribe-specific terms for these individuals, including *heemaneh* (among the Cheyenne), *Miati* (Hidatsa), *Winkte* (Oglala Lakota), and *Agokwe* (Ojibway) for men and *Tw!inna'ek* (Klamath), *suku* (Maidu), *Brumaiwi* (Couer d'Alene), and *Kwido'* or *kweedo'* (Tewa) for women.

Two-spirit men generally had sexual liaisons and partnerships with men and women. These ranged from brief sexual encounters to culturally sanctioned marriages to other males, which could be polygamous, monogamous, or part of a series of marriages (Lang, 1998). For example, among the Aleuts, marriages between a man and a *shupan* were commonplace, although typically the *shupan* would be a "wife" who was second to a biologic woman (Lang, 1998). Among the Nevada Shoshoni, a marriage between a *tangowaiipü* (two-spirit woman) and a Shoshoni woman also would be sanctioned, although the *moroni noho* (two-spirit women) of the Paiute people typically remained single. Two-spirit marriages or partnerships were viewed as unions with a third-gendered person; therefore, they were not viewed as "homosexual" but, rather, as "hetero-gendered" (Lang, 1998).

Although there were exceptions, many of the individuals who embodied "alternative" gender roles or sexual identities were integrated within their community, often occupying highly respected social and ceremonial roles (Medicine, 1988; Brown, 1997; Little Crow et al., 1997). In her review of more than 125 tribal cultures, Lang (1998) noted that two-spirit men were generally held in high esteem and thought to be endowed with spiritual or medicinal powers.

The Western lens through which early anthropologists judged Native gender roles and sexuality was fraught with ethnocentric biases, leading to their confounding gender roles with sexual orientation. Early anthropologic reports employed the term *berdache* to describe Native people whose gender role varied from Western conventions. The term is offensive to AIANs because of its colonial origins and purely sexual connotations: it is a non-Native word of Arabic origin (i.e., *berdaj*), which refers to male slaves who served as anally receptive prostitutes (Jacobs et al., 1997; Thomas & Jacobs, 1999). More contemporary anthropologists created the terms "women-men" to describe men who assumed gender roles and behaved in ways more commonly associated with women and "men-women" to describe women who assumed gender roles and behaved in ways more commonly associated with men (Lang, 1998).

Western colonization and Christianization of Native cultures included attacks on traditional Native conceptions of gender and sexual identity. Missionaries in boarding schools and government agents on reservations enforced conformity to the European and Christian binary, anatomically based gender system that dictated "proper" dress, appearance, and social and work roles. This colonizing process succeeded in undermining traditional ceremonial and social roles for two-spirits in many tribal communities. The cultural genocide (i.e., ethnocide) resulting from Christianization (Tinker, 1993) replaced traditionally accepting and inclusive tribal traditions toward two-spirits with systems of oppression and shaming condemnation, giving rise to internalized heterosexism and homophobia in Native communities. A movement toward retraditionalization has begun to reverse this destructive process. Begun during the Red Power movement of the 1970s, retraditionalization involves reembracing traditional practices and is the impetus for such programs as language revitalization.

The conflation of gender and sexual orientation resulting from Western misinterpretations of Native traditions was partially corrected by introduction of the pan-Indian term "two-spirit." Adopted in 1990 at the third annual spiritual gathering of GLBT Natives, the term derives from the northern Algonquin word *niizh manitoag*, meaning "two spirits," and refers to the inclusion of both feminine and masculine components in one individual (Anguksuar, 1997). The creation of a two-spirit identity, according to Native activists, is an attempt to reinform, recreate, and retraditionalize the contemporary Native GLBT experience according to affirming historical practices (Walters et al., 2001). It is inclusive of different tribal histories, ceremonial and social statuses, and contemporary gender and sexual identities, allowing AIANs to align with ancestral traditions while simultaneously enacting political resistance to Eurocentric hegemony in non-Native GLBT communities (Walters et al., 2001).

The term "two-spirit" is not easily translated into indigenous languages (e.g., in Navajo it means literally "being possessed"). Neither is the term uniformly employed or widely accepted among Natives. To some AIANs, the term refers to a person with a GLBT orientation. To others, it denotes an individual with tribally specific spiritual, social, and cultural roles that are not defined at all by sexual orientation or gender role. Still other Natives employ the term in a highly contextualized way. For example, one Navajo activist refers to himself as *n'dleeh* when interacting with other Navajos, as "two-spirit" when interacting with non-Navajo Natives, and as "gay" when interacting with non-Native GLBT individuals.

The activism, resilience, and strength that two-spirit community members display are even more remarkable in light of their uniquely stressful status. Their loss of acceptance and position among their indigenous communities is exacerbated by the lack of understanding from the GLBT community. Buffeted by heterosexism in their Native communities and racism in the GLBT community, they often lack support for embracing and consolidating their racial/ethnic and gender/sexual identities.

3 Overview of Native Health

Most large epidemiologic health studies conducted in the United States ignore AIANs. Few studies specifically address Native health, and data on two-spirits are even scarcer. The little information that is available paints a troubling picture of Native health. Following is an overview of this literature, with reference to two-spirits or GLBT populations where available. Specifically, we consider morbidity and mortality, mental health, and substance use as well as human immunodeficiency virus (HIV) infection and other sexually transmitted infections (STIs).

3.1 Morbidity and Mortality

Native men have rates of chronic disease factors higher than those for men in any other ethnic/racial minority group (Centers for Disease

Control and Prevention [CDC], 2003b). In particular, Native men have the highest rates of obesity, smoking, cardiovascular disease, hypertension, high cholesterol, and diabetes; and Native women have the highest rates of obesity, smoking, cardiovascular disease, and diabetes and the second highest rates (after African American women) of hypertension and high cholesterol (CDC, 2003b). Moreover, a higher proportion of Native women and men report having three or more chronic disease risk factors than do African Americans, Hispanics, or Asians (CDC, 2003b).

Although there are no specific data for two-spirit women, data on women in general suggest that two-spirit women may have more chronic disease risk, in particular for cardiovascular disease, than heterosexual Native women. Compared to heterosexual women, lesbian and bisexual women have higher prevalence rates of tobacco and heavy alcohol use and are more likely to be overweight (Aaron et al., 2001; Gruskin et al., 2001; Mays et al., 2002).

In terms of mortality rates, nearly one-fourth (23.3%) of Native men die by age 34 and nearly one-half (46.6%) by age 54 (IHS, 2001). Compared to women in the general population, Native women have higher death rates (per 100,000) due to diabetes (22.4 vs. 45.4), accidents (22.0 vs. 38.1), chronic liver disease and cirrhosis (6.1 vs. 20.5), alcohol abuse (3.5 vs. 20.3), and suicide (4.4 vs. 5.2) (CDC, 2001a). Moreover, Native women are second only to African American women in terms of death rates (per 100,000) due to homicide (4.8 vs. 9.0) and drug abuse (4.7 vs. 4.8) (CDC, 2001a).

3.1.1 Cancer

Cancer is the second leading cause of death for Native females and the third leading cause of death for Native males (IHS, 1999a). The top cancers afflicting AIAN men (prostate) and AIAN women (breast) parallel those for Whites (Paltoo & Chu, 2004). Although AIANs experience these cancers at lower rates, they are more likely to die from them once they are diagnosed. Native women have the youngest mean age (54 years) for breast cancer diagnosis of all racial groups (56–62 years) and the poorest survival rates (Li et al., 2003). Poor survival rates are due in part to low rates of preventive screening. Of all races, AIAN women had the lowest rates of mammogram screening during the last 1- and 2-year periods (Ward et al., 2004).

Two-spirit women may be at even greater risk. In a study comparing primarily White lesbians with their heterosexual sisters, lesbians had significantly higher rates of breast cancer (Dibble et al., 2004).

Compared to Whites, AIAN females and males have higher incidence rates of gallbladder, liver, stomach, and kidney cancers (Paltoo & Chu, 2004). For all cancers combined, AIANs have lower mortality rates than the general U.S. population. However Natives with cancer have disproportionately lower 5-year survival rates than Whites (Ward et al., 2004); for all cancers combined, AIAN women [relative risk (RR) 1.54] and men (RR 1.69) had the highest 5-year relative risk of death among all ethnic/racial groups (Jemal et al., 2004). Compared to all races, the highest 5-year relative risk of death for AI men is for cancer of the larynx, prostate, and stomach, and for women it is cancer of the colon/rectum, stomach, and urinary bladder (Jemal et al., 2004). Cancer rates vary greatly across regions, illustrating the heterogeneity in Native populations. For example, lung cancer mortality rates per 100,000 in Alaska (78.1) and the Northern Plains (96.9) were higher than the combined U.S. rate (57.8), whereas those in the Southwest (14.1), Pacific Coast (39.5), and East (37.0) were lower (CDC, 2003a). These trends also exist for colorectal cancer and all cancers combined (CDC, 2003a).

3.1.2 Diabetes

Diabetes is a scourge among Natives. It is the fourth leading cause of death for female AIANs and the sixth leading cause of death for male AIANs (IHS, 1999a). Natives are more than twice as likely to be diagnosed with diabetes as their White counterparts (American Diabetes Association [ADA], 2004). Diabetes-related disorders occur more often among AIANs than other populations; for example, amputation rates among Natives are three to four times higher than among the general population (ADA, 2004).

3.1.3 Accidents and Injuries

Accidents are the second leading cause of death among Native males and the third leading cause of death among Native females (IHS, 1999a). When compared to White females and all U.S. females, Native female death rates for accidents are higher for all age groups (IHS, 1999b). Compared to Native females, Native males over the age of 20 are twice as likely to die from a car accident or from fire or burn injuries, three times as likely to be murdered, and nearly five times as likely to drown (CDC, 2003c). In fact, Native males aged 15 to 19 years have higher rates for motor vehicle accidents, firearm-related deaths, homicides, suicides, and drownings than the general population (IHS, 1997).

3.2 Mental Health

3.2.1 Suicidality

Native rates of death by suicide are 1.5 times greater than those for the United States population overall (Wallace et al., 1996). Suicide is the fifth leading cause of death among Native males and the tenth leading cause of death among Native females (IHS, 1999a). Among women aged 25 to 44 years, AIANs had the highest suicide rate in 2000 (National Women's Health Information Center, 2003). Native males under age 19 years have suicide rates that are two to eight times higher than their non-Native peers (IHS, 1997). From 1979 to 1992, AIAN males aged 15 to 24 years accounted for 64% of all AIAN suicides (National Center for Injury Prevention and Control [NCIPC], 2002). Compared to Native females, Native males over 20 years of age are four times more likely to commit suicide (CDC, 2003c). Data on suicide attempts also indicate greater risk for Natives than non-Natives. Specifically, 32.2% of AIAN females reported suicide attempts in the previous 12 months (White 10.5%; African American 9.7%), as did 22.2% of AIAN males (White 4%; African American 5.2%) (Frank & Lester, 2002).

Two-spirit Natives are at particularly high risk for suicidality. Monette et al., (2001) found 32% of two-spirit males had attempted suicide. In a study of primarily nonheterosexually identified urban males, AIANs reported a much higher prevalence rate for suicide attempts than the sample overall (30% vs. 12%) (Paul et al., 2002), with AIAN males under the age of 25 years at particular risk (25% had attempted suicide compared to 8% of their non-Native counterparts). Two-spirit women also report significantly greater suicidality than their White GLBT counterparts (Morris et al., 2001). Because both Native (vs. non-Native) youth and GLBT (vs. non-GLBT) youth are at increased risk for suicidality (Safren & Heimberg, 1999; Halpert, 2002) two-spirit youth are particularly vulnerable.

3.2.2 Anxiety and Mood Disorders

Robin et al. (1996) described four epidemiologic studies conducted during the 1990s that revealed higher rates of mental health disorders among Natives compared to the general U.S. population; depression was the most commonly reported lifetime disorder. Compared to their heterosexual counterparts, GLBT individuals have higher prevalence rates of anxiety and mood disorders (Gilman et al., 2001; Meyer, 2003). Co-morbidity of these disorders is higher among both gay/bisexual men (19.6%) and lesbian/bisexual women (23.5%) than among their heterosexual peers (5.0% and 7.7%, respectively) (Cochran et al., 2003). In an urban community-based sample, two-spirits reported significantly more anxiety and symptoms of posttraumatic stress than their heterosexual Native peers, although rates of depressive symptomatology were comparable (Balsam et al., 2004). Although AIANs are as likely to develop posttraumatic stress disorder (PTSD) after trauma exposure as their non-Native peers, AIANs experience higher levels of trauma exposure, which increases their risk of developing PTSD, with prevalence as high as 25.4% documented among AIAN women (Robin et al., 1997a).

3.3 Substance Use

3.3.1 Alcohol Use

Prevalence rates of alcohol abuse vary widely among tribal nations and urban Native communities (Gray & Nye, 2001). A bimodal drinking pattern has been documented, however, with high percentages of both abstainers and heavy drinkers (May & Smith, 1988; May, 1995). In a study of adults in 2000, more AIANs reported being abstainers than did Whites (50.7% vs. 35.1%), yet AIANs had the highest binge (26.2%) and heavy drinking (7.2%) rates (National Center for Health Statistics [NCHS], 2002). Native males have higher rates of abusive and chronic drinking than Native females, and alcohol is involved in 27% of all Native male deaths. Overall, AIANs are nearly five times more likely than non-Natives to die from alcohol-related causes (NCHS, 1999).

In one of the few studies comparing two-spirits and other Natives, Balsam et al. (2004) reported that two-spirits reported having their first drink at an earlier age (12.6 vs. 14.7 years) and were more likely to report drinking to manage moods and to relax, to make friends, and to decrease feelings of inferiority. However, the two groups did not differ in terms of current drinking status, with about 19% in each group reporting moderate to heavy drinking.

3.3.2 Illicit Drug Use

There is a dearth of reliable data on illicit substance use among AIANs, with more data on youths than adults (Walters et al., 2002). The available data, however, clearly indicate greater substance use among Natives than non-Natives. In 1999, more AIANs age 12 years and older reported ever using illicit drugs (51%) than any other racial/ethnic group (20.8–42.2%) (Substance Abuse and Mental Health Services Administration [SAMHSA], 2000). Moreover, more Natives 12 to 17 years old reported using illicit drugs during the past year than did non-Natives in this age group (30.5% vs. 13–26%). Compared to non-AIANs, AIAN 12th graders were much more likely to have used marijuana, cocaine, stimulants, and psychedelics during the past month. Mortality data demonstrate the deleterious effect of drug use on AIANs. The age-adjusted mortality from drugs for AIANs is 18% higher than for the U.S. population, rising from 3.4 deaths per 100,000 in 1979–1981 to 5.3 deaths per 100,000 in 1992–1994 (IHS, 1999a). Drug use among two-spirits has been inadequately documented. However, Balsam et al. (2004) reported that two-spirits were more likely than other Natives to have used illicit drugs other than marijuana (78.3% vs. 56.0%).

3.4 Sexual Behavior and HIV/STI Risk

3.4.1 Sexuality and Sexual Behavior

The empirical research on sexuality and sexual orientation among AIANs comprises only a few studies (Saewyc et al., 1996, 1998a,b). Overall, they indicate that Native youth are more likely than non-Native youth to report GLBT and "unsure" sexual identities and that Native GLBT youth report high rates of unprotected sex, early sexual activity onset, and history of abuse that place them at risk for exposure to HIV and other STIs. Specifically, GLBT-identified Native youth were more likely than their heterosexual peers to engage in heterosexual intercourse before age 14, with GLBT girls just as likely as their heterosexual peers to become pregnant. This "functional bisexuality" (i.e., heterosexual sexual behavior among self-identified GLBTs) has been observed among Natives elsewhere (Tafoya & Rowell, 1988). Tafoya (1996) hypothesized that this apparent fluidity in sexual relationships may reflect the less restrictive gender roles historically associated with two-spirits.

3.4.2 Sexually Transmitted Infections

The AIANs are second only to African Americans in terms of incidence rates for gonorrhea and *Chlamydia* infection. They are 4 times more likely to be diagnosed with gonorrhea, 5.5 times more likely to be diagnosed with *Chlamydia*, and 6 times more likely to be diagnosed with syphilis than Whites (CDC, 2004a). Additionally, AIANs who are infected with HIV are more likely than non-AIANs also to be infected with other STIs (Diamond et al., 2001).

Increased rates of gonorrhea and syphilis among men who have sex with men (MSM) have coincided with a recent rise in high-risk sexual behavior (CDC, 2000; Fox et al., 2001; Chen et al., 2002). Although women who have sex exclusively with women are given little attention in STI and HIV research, one study noted an STI prevalence of 13% among this group, which the authors attributed to a low level of regular STI testing (10%) (Bauer & Welles, 2001). There are no data on STI rates among AIAN women (J. Marrazzo, personal communication, October 10, 2004).

3.4.3 HIV/AIDS Surveillance Data

According to data from the CDC (2004b), the absolute number of acquired immunodeficiency syndrome (AIDS) cases among AIAN is rather low; however, in the relatively small population of AIANs in the United States, these translate into AIDS incidence rates (per 100,000) of 16.9 for men and 5.8 for women, which, though lower than those for African Americans and Latinos, are 1.5 times higher than the rates for Whites. Moreover, these rates are increasing. From 1996 to 2001, AIDS incidence and AIDS-related mortality decreased among all racial/ethnic groups except AIANs (CDC, 2001b). Five-year increases in AIDS incidence for MSM were higher for AIANs (53%) than African Americans (45%) or Latinos (23%) (Sullivan et al., 1997). HIV transmission among young AIAN females is on the rise as well (CDC, 1998).

Even more disturbingly, the CDC data are likely underestimates, as health organizations often fail to identify AIANs correctly (Bertolli et al., 2004). Metler et al., (1991) suggested that misclassification might be particularly prevalent in off-reservation areas. Indeed, a review of 6500 records at Los Angeles County community-based organizations located 60 AIAN clients with AIDS, only 6 of whom had been reported as Native to the public health authorities (Lieb et al., 1992). In a community-based survey of 71 AIAN males in New York City, 10% of two-spirit men and 6% for heterosexual men reported having HIV/AIDS (Simoni et al., 2004a), figures much larger than expected based on CDC data.

According to the latest available data, adult and adolescent males accounted for 83% of all AIDS cases among AIANs reported through 2002 (CDC, 2004b). The top transmission categories are MSM (55%), MSM/injection drug use (IDU) (17%), and IDU (16%). The MSM/IDU exposure category for AIAN male AIDS cases (17%) and HIV (12%) is larger than it is for all other racial/ethnic groups (4–8% for AIDS and 2–7% for HIV). Based on data from the 30 areas where confidential name-based HIV infection reporting occurs, 17% of Native male MSM/IDUs were living with AIDS by the end of 2002 compared to 5% to 9% of MSM/IDUs in other racial/ethnic groups. Similarly, the percentage of AIDS cases attributable to IDU among AIAN women (in 2002 it was 31%; cumulatively, it was 43%) is greater than among White (30%/41%), Black/African American (19%/38%), or Hispanic (21%/38%) women (CDC, 2004b).

3.4.4 Condom Use

The scant data available for Natives in both Canada and the United States demonstrate inconsistent condom use and considerable risk for HIV and other STIs (Metler et al., 1991; Conway et al., 1992; Fenaughty et al., 1994; Myers et al., 1997; Walters et al., 2000). In a study of 13,454 AIAN youth, only 49% of males reported using condoms during sex (Blum et al., 1992). Among 100 urban Natives, 73% of those reporting sexual activity during the past 6 months engaged in vaginal or anal sex without a condom (Walters et al., 2000).

3.4.5 HIV Sexual Risk and Substance Use

Only recently has research begun to address the co-occurrence of substance use and risky sex (Duran & Walters, 2004). IDU, in particular, has been established as an important risk factor for HIV infection among AIANs (Tafoya, 1989; Loecker et al., 1992). In a multiethnic study of males and females in Washington State, 3% of 3039 injection drug users entering treatment tested positive for HIV. Gay or bisexual men had the highest prevalence (37%); heterosexual men had a substantially lower rate (2%). After adjusting for sexual orientation, HIV prevalence was 3.6 times greater for AIANs than for Whites (Harris et al., 1993). Preliminary research indicates that urban Native drug users are at greater risk for HIV infection than their reservation counterparts owing to trading sex for money, drugs, or housing as well as practicing unprotected sex (Fisher et al., 2000; Stevens et al., 2000). In one study of Native drug users, 50% reported drinking until drunk and engaging in unprotected sexual intercourse while in a blackout state (Baldwin et al., 2000). In another study, the combination of alcohol and crack use was more strongly related to unprotected sex, sex with strangers, and other high-risk sexual behaviors than crack use alone (Baldwin et al., 1999). In addition, among 100 urban Native New Yorkers, preliminary evidence indicated that respondents who engaged in sex while drunk or high were 14.34 times more likely to engage in risky sexual behaviors than those who had not engaged in sex while drunk or high (Walters et al., 2000). Finally, in a medical review study, HIV-positive Native men were more likely than HIV-positive non-Native men to report both IDU and unprotected sex with other men (32% vs. 14%) (Diamond et al., 2001). Among Native women, research indicates that substance use, in particular IDU, may mediate the relationship between trauma and sexual risk behaviors (Walters & Simoni, 1999; Simoni et al., 2004b).

4 "Indigenist" Stress-Coping Model

As noted by Walters and colleagues (2002), most of the theoretical and empirical work on stress and coping processes reflects firmly entrenched Eurocentric values and paradigms. When researchers uncritically accept these models, they risk unintentionally reenacting colonial processes and ultimately compromising the validity of their work. To increase its cultural relevance and practice utility, research on AIAN populations must consider the sociohistorical context and assess its impact on biologic, psychological, social, cultural, and spiritual functioning at the level of the AIAN individual, the family, and the tribal community. Such an approach has the potential to produce novel findings, unleashing a liberating research dynamic into the field.

Failure to account for the historical and contemporary social context can lead to distorted perceptions of Native communities and unintentional pathologizing of individuals (Browne & Fiske, 2001). Any valid explanation for the marked health disparities between Natives and non-Natives must incorporate data on Natives' exorbitant rates of poverty, unemployment, and educational deficits as well as their experience of the traumatic effects of racism and discrimination, both historically and contemporarily. The influence of cumulative adversity on physical and mental health outcomes cannot be underestimated (Turner & Lloyd, 1995). Many health problems are directly related to AIANs' colonized status and associated environmental, institutional, and interpersonal discrimination and associated stress (Walters et al., 2002).

Our theorizing in this area has culminated in the "indigenist" stress-coping model (Walters & Simoni, 2002; Walters et al., 2002), which is situated conceptually in a Fourth World framework that builds on the work of Dinges and Joos (1988) and Krieger (1999). Indigenist and Fourth World perspectives acknowledge the colonized position of indigenous communities in the United States and therefore emphasize the importance of including in any health analysis the socio-political-historical-environmental context in which health behaviors occur.

Specifically, the model (summarized in Figure 11.1 and described in the following sections) posits a relation between ecosocial stressors

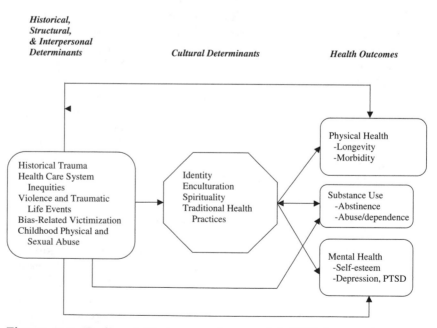

Figure 11.1 "Indigenist" stress-coping model: HIV, human immuno-deficiency virus; PTSD, posttraumatic stress disorder.

and health outcomes that is moderated by cultural buffers (i.e., identity, enculturation, spirituality, traditional health practices). From an indigenous world-view, these cultural moderators are aspects of a holistic existence that maintains good health. As a stress-coping framework, the model identifies the experience of colonization as an organizing principle from which to understand health outcomes and culturally specific risk and health-promoting behaviors.

Although the model was developed for all AIANs, it can serve as a framework for understanding health outcomes among two-spirit AIANs specifically by considering factors unique to their experience. For example, bias-related victimization should take into account sexual orientation bias crimes; and with respect to identity, an affirming two-spirit identity should be assessed.

5 Historical, Structural, and Interpersonal Determinants of Two-Spirit Health

Two-spirit health is affected by contemporary structural and interpersonal factors as well as historic events. The following determinants are reviewed below: historical trauma, health care system inequities, and interpersonal factors such as violence and traumatic life events, bias-related victimization, and childhood physical and sexual abuse. These determinants are not discrete circumstances but interrelated legacies of colonization. The categories are not meant to be mutually exclusive or exhaustive. Rather, they reflect the current state of research, which is often reported in terms of these constructs. We conclude this section with data on the specific links between interpersonal determinants and adverse health outcomes.

5.1 Historical Trauma

During the five centuries since European contact, AIANs have endured a succession of traumatic assaults on their tribal nations, their families, and their individual physical, spiritual, and psychological integrity. These assaults include massacres such as at Wounded Knee in 1890, during which mutilation of corpses was commonplace; abrupt displacement or relocation to inhospitable reservations; systematic ethnocide, including the prohibition of indigenous religions and ceremonies via the U.S. Court of Indian Offenses (1890); removal of Native children from their families and forced placement in punitive boarding schools; and experimental medical procedures, including eye surgery and involuntary sterilization (Walters & Evans-Campbell, 2004).

Native scholars and community healers conceptualize these assaults as a soul or spirit wound in indigenous communities (Duran et al., 1998). Enforced suppression of Native grieving and healing practices has stifled healing of this soul wound (Yellow Horse Brave Heart & DeBruyn, 1998), which manifests in the current social conditions and ill health of Native peoples (Duran & Duran, 1995).

Researchers are just now empirically examining the effects of historical trauma on wellness outcomes. Preliminary results from a study of

143 American Indian adults in the upper Midwest indicated frequent thoughts pertaining to historical losses and associated anxiety/depression and anger/avoidance symptoms (Whitbeck et al., 2004).

5.2 Healthcare System Inequities

The inequities in the current healthcare systems were summarized by the U.S. Commission on Civil Rights (2004) as follows: "Persistent discrimination and neglect continue to deprive Native Americans of a health system sufficient to provide health care equivalent to that provided to the vast majority of Americans" (p. 6). AIANs are disadvantaged by the current health care delivery system with respect to at least three factors: stigma and provider discrimination, geographic isolation, and inadequate insurance coverage.

Service providers and two-spirit people have identified sexual orientation stigma and fears of being "outed" as significant barriers to two-spirit service utilization from AIAN community services (Walters et al., 2001). Fears of discrimination due to sexual orientation have deterred two-spirit men from accessing health services (37%) and social services (29%); and parallel fears of discrimination due to "being Native" have deterred access to health (28%) and social services (25%) (Monette et al., 2001).

Geographic isolation from reservation-based services precludes most AIANs from adequately utilizing the health services to which they are entitled. IHS policy states that most of the care offered should be dedicated to AIANs living on or near reservations. As a result of these geographic barriers, only 20% of AIAN people surveyed in one study reported using IHS services in 1997 (Brown et al., 2000). For urban-dwelling Natives, the comparable figure is only 10% (Burhansstipanov, 2000). Although more than half of all AIAN people live in urban areas, just 1% of the $2.6 billion IHS budget is allocated to urban Indian health programs. Services from the few urban-based IHS facilities are limited primarily to the provision of health information and referrals (Forquera, 2001). Many urban Indians jeopardize their health by waiting until they are severely ill before returning to their reservations or tribal jurisdiction areas to access IHS services.

Nationally, the percentage of AIANs who lack medical insurance (24.5%) is higher than for any other racial/ethnic group and more than two times higher than for Whites (10.8%) (Bolen et al., 2000). One in three AIANs who is uninsured does not have a regular source of care (Brown et al., 2000). A recent study of Ryan White Comprehensive AIDS Resources Emergency Act-funded providers in five geographic areas indicated few differences in service-utilization patterns and health outcomes among HIV-positive AIANs and their counterparts from other racial/ethnic groups, suggesting that once AIANs surmount barriers to care, they are just as likely to benefit as others (Ashman et al., 2004).

5.3 Violence and Traumatic Life Events

According to U.S. Bureau of Labor Statistics, AIANs experience disproportionate levels of violence (Greenfeld & Smith, 1999). Their rate of violent victimization (124/1000) is higher than the rates for African Americans (61/1000), Whites (49/1000), and Asians/Pacific Islanders (29/1000). Moreover, class and income have little to no buffering effect on these rates: At every income level, AIANs have a 2.0 to 2.5 times higher rate of victimization than other ethnic/racial groups. The rate of violent assaults for Native men is twice that for all males, and Native women experience violent assaults at a rate nearly 50% higher than that reported by African American males. These figures are supported by results from a series of community-based studies among AIAN men and women in New York City, where almost half of the participants reported some form of lifetime trauma, such as physical or sexual assault by a family member or stranger (Walters & Simoni, 1999; Walters et al., 2000; Simoni et al., 2004b).

Two studies have directly compared rates of victimization among two-spirit and other urban AIANs. In a sample of 71 Native men, sexual and physical abuse or assault trauma was higher among the two-spirits than other men (Simoni et al., 2004a). In a sample of 179 men and women, there were no differences in lifetime physical or sexual assault between the two-spirits and the rest of the sample (Balsam et al., 2004).

AIANs experience more traumatic events than the general U.S. population (Robin et al., 1997b). Results of three studies including 447 AIANs aged 8 to 20 years indicated that 51% to 62% experienced at least one major traumatic event (e.g., shooting, overdose, car accident, rape) (Manson et al., 1996). Among the Natives who experienced a traumatic event, 50.0% to 87.4% reported active PTSD symptomatology and 52% met criteria for an additional mental disorder.

5.4 Bias-Related Victimization

Although accurate bias-related crime rates are difficult to estimate because GLBT individuals are less likely to report hate crimes because of sexual orientation than nonbias criminal victimization (Herek et al., 1999), research suggests sexual minority youth are at increased risk for victimization and exposure to extreme violence compared to their heterosexual peers (Russell et al., 2001). Among high-school youth, sexual minority status was associated with property victimization and being threatened with a weapon (Garofalo et al., 1998).

Two-spirits, who face racism in the GLBT community and heterosexism in their tribal communities, are at compounded risk for discrimination and violent victimization (Jacobs & Brown, 1997; Brotman et al., 2002). In a tragic example, in 2001 Fred Martinez, Jr., a 16-year old two-spirit Navajo, was beaten to death in a bias-motivated crime in Cortez, Colorado (Norrell, 2001). In a small study of urban two-spirits, violence due to sexual orientation bias in terms of verbal insults (100%), threats of attack (79%), physical assaults (36%), assaults with a weapon (36%), and sexual assault (29%) (Walters et al., 2001) exceeded rates reported by predominantly White GLBTs for sexual (3–7%) or physical (5–13%) assault (Herek et al., 1999). In a Canadian study, two-spirit men reported high rates of racism (44%), homophobia (38%), HIV discrimination (32%) and gay bashing (33%) (Monette et al., 2001).

5.5 Childhood Physical and Sexual Abuse

Results from the few empirical studies that document the rates of childhood victimization among AIAN indicate that Native children are more likely to be abused and neglected than White children (National Indian Justice Center [NIJC], 1990; Libby et al., 2004). Specifically, in a reservation-based sample in the Southwest, 2.4% of males and 12.7% of females experienced sexual abuse prior to the age of 15 (Kunitz et al., 1998; Kunitz & Levy, 2000). In another study, 14% of the Native males reported childhood sexual abuse prior to the age of 16 (Robin et al., 1997a), a rate higher than that reported for non-Native males (Haugaard & Reppucci, 1988). In a more recent study of AIAN adults from two tribes, the prevalence of childhood physical abuse was approximately 7% for both sexes; childhood sexual abuse was higher for females than males (7.15–7.65% vs. 84.0–2.3%) (Libby et al., 2004).

Large-scale studies of multiethnic MSM populations have found relatively high rates of self-reported childhood sexual abuse, ranging from 21.6% to 34.0% (Doll et al., 1992; Tjaden et al., 1999; Kalichman et al., 2001; Paul et al., 2001). These rates appear higher than the 10% to 15% found among men in the general population (Kessler et al., 1997; MacMillan et al., 2001). Indeed, studies that have directly compared sexual minority men to heterosexual men have found significantly higher rates among the former (e.g., Tjaden et al., 1999; Tomeo et al., 2001; Balsam et al., 2004b). Gay male youth who were open about their sexual orientation and who had a history of gender-atypical behavior were more likely to be physically victimized than lesbian or bisexual youth (D'Augelli et al., 2002).

We could locate only one empirical study of AIAN adults examining abuse by sexual orientation. Balsam et al. (2004), in a study of 179 AIAN men and women in New York City, reported that two-spirit participants reported significantly higher rates of childhood physical abuse than their heterosexual counterparts (48% vs. 25%). Among reservation-based AIAN adolescent males, gay/bisexual-identified adolescents had significantly higher rates of childhood physical and sexual abuse than their heterosexual peers (Saewyc et al., 1998b).

5.6 Interpersonal Determinants and Health Outcomes

As specified in the Model (Fig. 11.1), violence, victimization, and abuse have direct and indirect effects on AIAN health outcomes. There is a considerable body of empirical research documenting these adverse health outcomes; however, much of the research involves general population surveys, or it targets at-risk subgroups that include few AIANs. The data on sexual minorities and two-spirits specifically are rare.

Research conducted with primarily non-Native samples indicates that people exposed to violence and victimization are at risk for physical and mental health problems, including PTSD, depression, anxiety, and substance use (Breslau et al., 1991; Fullilove et al., 1993; Veenema,

2001; Coker et al., 2002; Johnson et al., 2002; Ceballo et al., 2003; Hourani et al., 2003; Kilpatrick & Acierno, 2003). Among AIAN youth in particular, victimization has been shown to lead to substance abuse (Jones et al., 1997).

Few studies have focused on the effects of bias-related victimization specifically, although Herek and colleagues (1999) reported that sexual orientation bias crimes resulted in significantly elevated symptoms of traumatic stress, depression, and anxiety, which persisted well beyond the time of the event. There is more research on the psychological and physical costs of being a target of discrimination among racial minorities, which points clearly to its deleterious effects on psychological well-being (Williams & Williams-Morris, 2000) and physical health (Harrell et al., 2003), leading to an increased risk of negative self-reported health status, high blood pressure, and depression (Krieger & Sidney, 1996; Schultz et al., 2001; Gee, 2002; Karlsen & Nazroo, 2002). Research on Latino gay and bisexual men indicates that social discrimination in the form of homophobia and racism is linked to increased anxiety, depression, and suicidality (Diaz et al., 2001). Among reservation- based AIAN adults, discrimination has been shown to be significantly associated with depression (Whitbeck et al., 2002).

Research on the effects of childhood physical and sexual abuse has identified three major adverse outcomes: psychopathology, substance use, and sexual risk behaviors. Sexual abuse is related to higher levels of depression among clinical and nonclinical samples (Finkelhor, 1984) and to greater psychopathology among AIANs specifically (Robin et al., 1997a). Links to substance abuse have been documented for the general population (Thompson et al., 2004), and preliminary research indicates that these links also exist among AIAN men (Flanigan, 1990; Stewart, 1996; Libby et al., 2004) and gay/bisexual men (Doll et al., 1992; Ratner et al., 2003). Among women in the general population, two reviews support the association between childhood sexual and physical abuse and alcohol and drug problems during adulthood (Langeland & Hartgers, 1998; Simpson & Miller, 2002). Among urban AIAN women specifically, abuse and assault have been linked with IDU (Walters & Simoni, 1999; Simoni et al., 2004b). Evidence for the association between childhood abuse and later sexual risk behaviors exists for men in the general population (Bensley et al., 2000), women (Koenig et al., 2004), and MSM (Doll et al., 1992; Paul et al., 2001; Relf et al., 2004), as well as Native men (Robin, et al., 1997a; Libby et al., 2004), Native women (Walters & Simoni, 1999; Simoni et al., 2004b), and Native youth (Kaufman et al., 2004).

6 Cultural Determinants of Two-Spirit Health

Not all AIANs exposed to trauma-related stressors experience adverse health outcomes. What cultural factors might serve to buffer the effects of traumatic stressors? Empirical studies among non-Natives have identified identity (Scheier et al., 1997; Townsend & Belgrave, 2000), Afrocentricity (Belgrave et al., 1997), traditionalism (Cuadrado &

Lieberman, 1998), and religiosity and spirituality (Corwin & Benda, 2000) as critical moderating factors in the trauma–health consequences relation. Emerging research among AIANs indicates that the very aspects of Native culture targeted by colonial persecution (i.e., identity, spirituality, traditional health practices) may serve as sources of resistance and resilience (Walters et al., 2002; Whitbeck et al., 2004). Although research is just beginning to examine these links empirically, community wellness efforts have already identified these cultural factors as key to good health outcomes.

6.1 Identity

Although race or ethnicity can be the basis for discrimination, a positive racial/ethnic identity can mitigate discrimination's impact (Noh et al., 1999). Various frameworks have been proposed to describe identity development processes among non-Natives (Walters et al., 2002). Native researchers have focused on bicultural identities (Moran et al., 1999), orthogonal identities (Oetting and Beauvais, 1990–1991), and identity attitude development (Walters, 1999). Although the empirical findings are mixed, AIAN identity, regardless of how it is conceptualized, tends to function as a moderator for both risk and resilience. For example, among urban Indians who were previously heavy drinkers, ethnic identity was identified as key to establishing an abstinent lifestyle (Spicer, 2001). Additionally, internalized or externalized oppressive identity attitudes among a community sample of 332 AIAN in the Los Angeles area accounted for 10% to 21% of the variance in self-esteem, depression, anxiety, and interpersonal sensitivity (Walters, 1999).

Two-spirits, like other GLBTs of color, must reconcile competing demands from the dominant society, the GLBT community, and their own racial/ethnic groups to develop healthy self and group identities. [See related-research on AIAN (Walters, 1998), African Americans (Icard, 1986; Loicano, 1989), Mexican Americans (Espin, 1987; Morales, 1989), and Asian Americans (Chan, 1989).] Researchers studying GLBTs of color tend to combine racial identity attitude models that capture the development of positive attitudes toward one's own group (e.g., Cross, 1978; Atkinson et al., 1983) with GLBTs or "coming out" models that focus on the coming to terms with the realization of being a sexual minority (e.g., Cass, 1984). Walters (1998), elaborating on the work of Morales (1989), proposed an 2 × 2 identity matrix, according to which attitudes toward one's own ethnic group and attitudes toward GLBTs as a group are each separately rated as either positive or negative.

6.2 Enculturation

Enculturation, in contrast to acculturation, refers to the process by which individuals learn or reimmerse themselves in their cultural heritage, norms, and behaviors within a contemporary context. Many researchers have suggested that identity alone cannot capture the multidimensional nature of cultural experience and have proposed that enculturation may yield crucial information with respect to cultural protective processes (Walters, 1999; Walters et al., 2002). Preliminary evidence suggests that enculturation can mitigate the effects of a risk factor (e.g., trauma) or enhance the effects of another buffer (e.g., identity) to decrease risk for poor health outcomes (Zimmerman et al., 1998). For example, participation in traditional activities buffered the impact of perceived discrimination on depressive symptoms among AIANs (Whitbeck et al., 2002), and a self-governing community was found to be the most significant protective factor against suicide among AIAN youth in Canada (Chandler & Lalonde, 1998).

For two-spirits, enculturation in the form of retraditionalizaton may be a particularly powerful process because of the denigration of their formally elevated status in many tribal communities. In urban settings, participation in the Native community has helped strengthen tribal identity, affiliation, and enculturation among urban AIANs (Straus & Valentino, 2001). For some urban two-spirits, development of a positive two-spirit community may facilitate the process of retraditionalization, although this has yet to be empirically documented.

6.3 Spirituality

A growing body of literature indicates that religiosity and spirituality are predictive of good health-related outcomes (Hill & Pargament, 2003)—including decreased levels of anxiety, depression, perceived stress, and alcohol intake—and improved quality of life (Underwood & Teresi, 2002). Spiritual coping was significantly associated with enhanced mental health among HIV-positive racial/ethnic minority women (Simoni et al., 2002) and gay men (Woods et al., 1999). Research also indicates that spirituality buffers racial stress among African Americans (Bowen-Reid & Harrell, 2002).

During the development of their religious and spiritual identities, GLBT individuals often face discrimination and oppression due to Christian influences. Two-spirits, like other AIANs, may respond by adopting an inclusive approach to their spirituality that comprises traditional tribal, pan-Indian, and Christian influences. In one study of an urban community-based sample, two-spirits reported participation in spiritual and cultural AIAN activities to the same extent as their heterosexual peers (Balsam et al., 2004). Most of the individuals in both groups reported that their traditional spiritual tribal beliefs or cultural practices were very important, and an even greater number of two-spirits than heterosexual AIANs reported that spirituality was extremely important in their lives.

6.4 Traditional Health Practices

Traditional Native health practices are ways of coping with disease that are consistent with a resilient stance supporting transformation and growth in the context of adversity (Waldram, 2000; Walsh, 2002). Based on an indigenous worldview emphasizing harmony and balance, many traditional health practices involve community participation in the healing process (e.g. sweat lodge, Native American Church, pipe ceremony, Sun Dance). Indeed, health prevention interventions have been most successful when they have incorporated cultural processes and community participation (Joe, 2001). Both urban and reservation-based AIANs report using traditional health practices in conjunction with Western biomedical approaches to health (Waldram, 1990; Kim and Kwok, 1998; Marbella et al., 1998; Buchwald et al., 2000; Storck et al., 2000; Gurley et al., 2001), often viewing traditional medicine as treating the underlying cause (e.g., violation of a cultural taboo) and Western medicine as treating the symptoms (Buchwald et al., 2000).

Urban AIANs have access to Native-specific health practices that incorporate sobriety, healthy life-styles, and community responsibility. As urban two-spirits appear to have higher rates of lifetime alcohol abuse and higher rates of posttraumatic stress than their heterosexual counterparts (Balsam et al., 2004), they are likely candidates for seeking healing through traditional AIAN practices. However, because of discriminatory experiences in the U.S. health care systems and heterosexist attitudes among some traditional healers, two-spirits may not be open about their identity or speak honestly about all their health practices during the course of their treatment (Marbella et al., 1998; Buchwald et al., 2000).

7 "Decolonizing" Strategies Recommended for Researchers

Public health researchers aiming to reduce health disparities with respect to AIANs and to address the concerns of two-spirit individuals in particular must adopt a "decolonizing" perspective. A "decolonizing" outlook displays an appreciation for the experience of colonialization that two-spirits have endured and an active attempt to interact in ways that counters oppressive experience (Walters et al. 2002). Three specific decolonizing strategies for researchers are described below (mental health practitioners should refer as well to Evans-Campbell and Walters, 2004). These guidelines aim to instigate further work; they are certainly not exhaustive.

7.1 Increase the Visibility of Two-Spirits and Other Natives in Health Research

Inadequate information on or, more commonly, underestimation of AIAN morbidity and mortality is common due to the lack of AIAN research participants, the failure to include a discrete category for AIANs when they do participate, and racial misclassification in health research studies (Burhansstipanov & Satter, 2000; Stehr-Green et al., 2002), the last of which affects AIANs more often than any other racial/ethnic group (Kelly et al., 1996; Boehmer et al., 2002). Health information on AIANs who live in urban settings, as do most Natives, is particularly lacking. Reflective of this knowledge gap, there are no baseline data on AIANs for 61% of the Healthy People objectives (Burhansstipanov & Satter, 2000).

GLBT individuals also suffer from invisibility in health research, as they are often ignored or relegated exclusively to HIV-related studies (Boehmer, 2002). The paucity of health data was an institutional barrier with respect to the inclusion of GLBT health priorities in the Healthy People 2010 objectives (Meyer, 2001). When GLBT individuals are studied, race is rarely included as a discrete demographic factor—less than 15% of the time according to Boehmer (2002)—obscuring potentially important discrepancies across race/ethnicity.

Much of our knowledge of two-spirit people derives from preliminary studies or data that has been synthesizes from studies of the broader groups of AIANs and GLBTs. Most studies involving either AIANs of diverse sexual orientations or multiethnic samples of GLBT do not include two-spirit people as a discrete subgroup (Boehmer, 2002).

The invisibility of indigenous health statistics has been conceptualized as the "final colonization" (Houghton, 2002). Indeed, the lack of any national epidemiological studies addressing health issues relative to AIAN and two-spirit populations undermines health promotion and disease prevention efforts at federal, tribal, state, and local levels. In a vicious cycle of neglect, the dearth of empiric data makes it difficult to write competitive applications seeking to secure funding for future research. To counter some of this invisibility, researchers need to oversample AIAN and two-spirit participants to ensure equitable representation of their voices in health research efforts.

7.2 Conduct Community-Based Empiric Studies in Native Communities that Employ a Fourth-World Perspective

It is imperative that researchers work directly with community leaders, elders, and tribal members throughout all phases of their research on AIAN issues. Not only is this sound empowerment and community-based research practice, but it ensures the cultural integrity of the findings as well as relevance to the Native community. We are currently working to validate the "indigenist" stress-coping model, but more work is needed. With respect to two-spirits, research is lacking on parenting issues and other family-based concerns. We need studies of "lateral" oppression, which is the discrimination two-spirits experience within Native communities, such as when they are "outed" or excluded from community events because of their sexual orientation. Research on whether historical trauma or more proximate discriminatory experiences contribute to health conditions among AIANs is needed to guide intervention efforts. Finally, we need more translation research that can stimulate the development of culturally acceptable and efficacious programs in Native communities.

7.3 Develop Understanding of Justifiable Native Mistrust

Studies show that AIANs often harbor high levels of mistrust toward government institutions, health care systems, and research efforts (Evans-Campbell, 2000). For example, many Native parents believe that a child taken into the foster care system will never be released, and one-third of the Native men in an urban sample reported believing that AIDS was a form of germ warfare against Native people (Simoni et al., 2004a). High levels of institutional mistrust are not surprising given the experiences of Natives with IHS and academic institutions (Duran & Walters, 2004). Researchers therefore should be prepared to encounter distrustful attitudes. However, instead of viewing this mistrust as a hostile reaction, they should anticipate it, understand it, and even reframe it as a healthy reaction to what in other historical circumstances would have been a viable threat.

8 Summary

Two-spirit individuals constitute a diverse segment of contemporary Native communities, some embracing a modern GLBT identity and others self-identifying as heterosexual while incorporating aspects of both male and female gender roles in their daily lives. Historically embraced in many tribal communities, they have seen their sacred ceremonial roles and community responsibilities suppressed or eradicated by colonization and Christianization; traditionally affirming tribal attitudes have nearly vanished.

Two-spirits have been all but ignored in public health research. The few data available suggest that they are at considerable risk for adverse health outcomes. There are reports that chronic, repeated, or prolonged trauma is associated with psychological numbing and denial and may be more damaging than a single traumatic event (Terr, 1991; Williams et al., 1997). They suggest that two-spirits, who experience intergenerational trauma in their communities as well as heterosexism from Native communities and racism in GLBT communities, are particularly vulnerable.

An "indigenist" stress-coping model was presented as an organizing framework from which to conceptualize influences on two-spirit health. Historical traumatic events and data on current societal stressors, including health care system inequities, violence and traumatic life events, bias-related victimization, and childhood physical and sexual abuse, were reviewed to contextualize the condition of two-spirits as a colonized people still living under siege. We presented an overview of the research documenting an association between these health determinants and adverse physical and mental health outcomes. Incorporating a strengths-based perspective, the model points to four cultural factors that act to buffer the relation between these life stressors and adverse health outcomes: identity, enculturation, spirituality, traditional health practices. Finally, recommendations for further culturally sensitive work in this area were provided. Although, as we emphasized throughout this chapter, the empiric research on the determinants of two-spirit health outcomes is limited, we hope we have provided researchers and practitioners with a solid foundation concerning Native health issues in general and two-spirit health issues in particular—one that informs current efforts as well as inspires further work.

Finally, our emphasis on the vulnerabilities of two-spirit individuals should not detract from a strengths-based approach toward this community. Despite their exposure to traumatic conditions, many two-spirit people do not engage in drug use or other high-risk behaviors; and they experience good physical and mental health. The continued survival, health, and wellness of two-spirit persons are signs of their resilience, offering hope for their healing and the increased welfare of all Native communities until the seventh generation and beyond.

Acknowledgments: This work was supported in part by National Institute of Mental Health grant RO1 MH65871 to Karina L. Walters and National Institute of Mental Health Prevention training grant T32MH20010.

References

Aaron, D.J., Markovic, N., Danielson, M.E., Honnold, J.A., Janosky, J.E., and Schmidt, N.J. (2001) Behavioral risk factors for disease and preventive health practices among lesbians. *American Journal of Public Health* 91:972–975.

American Diabetes Association (ADA). (2004) *Diabetes statistics for Native Americans.* Retrieved August 2004 from www.diabetes.org.

Anguksuar [LaFortune, R.] (1997) A postcolonial perspective on Western [mis]conceptions of the cosmos and the restoration of indigenous taxonomies. In: Jacobs, S.E., Thomas, W., and Lang S. (eds) *Two-spirit people: Native American gender identity, sexuality, and spirituality.* University of Illinois Press, Chicago, pp. 217–222.

Ashman, J.J., Pérez-Jiménez, D., and Marconi, K. (2004) Health and support service utilization patterns of American Indians and Alaska Natives diagnosed with HIV/AIDS. *AIDS Education and Prevention* 16:238–249.

Atkinson, D., Morten, G., and Sue, D. (1983) *Counseling American minorities.* W.C. Brown, Dubuque, IA.

Baldwin, J.A., Trotter, R.T., Martinez, D., Stevens, S.J., John, D., and Brems, C. (1999) HIV/AIDS risks among Native American drug users: key findings from focus group interviews and implications for intervention strategies. *AIDS Education and Prevention* 11:279–292.

Baldwin, J.A., Maxwell, C.J., Fenaughty, A.M., Trotter, R.T., and Stevens, S.J. (2000) Alcohol as a risk factor for HIV transmission among American Indian and Alaska Native drug users. *American Indian and Alaska Native Mental Health Research* 9(1):1–16.

Balsam, K.F., Huang, B., Fieland, K.C., Simoni, J.M., and Walters, K.L. (2004). Culture, trauma, and wellness: a comparison of heterosexual and lesbian, gay, bisexual and two-spirit Native Americans. *Cultural Diversity and Ethnic Minority Psychology* 10:287–301.

Bauer, G.R., and Welles, S.L. (2001) Beyond the assumptions of negligable risk: sexually transmitted diseases and women who have sex with women. *American Journal of Public Health* 91:1282–1286.

Belgrave, F., Townsend, T.B., Cherry, V.R., and Cunningham, D.M. (1997) The influence of an Afrocentric world-view and demographic variables on drug knowledge, attitudes, and use among African American youth. *Journal of Community Psychology* 25:421–433.

Bensley, L.S., Van Eenwyk, J., and Simmons, K.W. (2000) Self-reported childhood sexual and physical abuse and adult HIV-risk behaviors and heavy drinking. *American Journal of Preventive Medicine* 18:151–158.

Bertolli, J., McNaghten, A.D., Campsmith, M., Lee, L.M., Leman, R., Bryan, R.T., and Buehler, J.W. (2004) Surveillance systems monitoring HIV/AIDS and HIV risk behaviors among American Indians and Alaska Natives. AIDS Education and Prevention 16:218–237.

Blum, R.W., Harmon, B., Harris, L., Bergeisen, L., and Resnick, M.D. (1992) American Indian-Alaska Native youth health. *Journal of the American Medical Association* 267:1627–1644.

Boehmer, U. (2002) Twenty years of public health research: Inclusion of lesbian, gay, bisexual and transgender populations. *American Journal of Public Health* 92:1125–1130.

Boehmer, U., Kressin, N.R., Berlowitz, D.R., Christiansen, C.L., Kazis, L.E., and Jones, J.A. (2002) Self-reported vs administrative race/ethnicity data and study results. *American Journal of Public Health* 92:1471–1473.

Bolen, J.C., Rhodes, L., Powell-Griner, E.E., Bland, S.D., and Holtzman, D. (2000) State-specific prevalence of selected health behaviors by race and ethnicity—behavioral risk factor surveillance system, 1997. *MMWR Surveillance Summaries* 49(SS02).

Bowen-Reid, T.L., and Harrell, J.P. (2002) Racist experiences and health outcomes: an examination of spirituality as a buffer. *Journal of Black Psychology* 28(1):18–36.

Breslau, N., Davis, G.C., Andreski, P., and Peterson, E. (1991) Traumatic events and posttraumatic stress disorder in an urban population of young adults. *Archives of General Psychiatry* 48:216–222.

Brotman, S., Ryan, B., Jalbert, Y., and Rowe, B. (2002) Reclaiming space-regaining health: the health care experiences of two-spirit people in Canada. *Journal of Gay and Lesbian Social Services: Issues in Practice, Policy and Research* 14:67–87.

Brown, E.R., Ojeda, V.D., Wyn, R., and Levan, R. (2000) *Racial and ethnic disparities in access to health insurance and health care.* UCLA Center for Health Policy Research and Kaiser Family Foundation, Los Angeles.

Brown, L.B. (1997) Women and men, not-men and not-women, lesbians and gays: American Indian gender style alternatives. *Journal of Gay and Lesbian Social Services* 6(2):5–20.

Browne, A.J., and Fiske, J. (2001) First Nations women's encounters with mainstream health care services. *Western Journal of Nursing Research* 23: 126–147.

Buchwald, D., Beals, J., and Manson, S.M. (2000). Use of traditional health practices among Native Americans in a primary care setting. *Medical Care* 38:1191–1199.

Burhansstipanov, L. (2000) Urban Native American health issues. *Cancer Supplement* 88:1207–1213.

Burhansstipanov, L., and Satter, D.E. (2000) Office of management and budget racial categories and implications for American Indians and Alaska Natives. *American Journal of Public Health* 90:1720–1723.

Cass, V.C. (1984) Homosexual identity formation: testing a theoretical model. *Journal of Sex Research* 20:143–167.

Ceballo, R., Ramirez, C., Hearn, K.D., and Maltese, K.L. (2003) Community violence and children's psychological well-being: does parental monitoring matter? *Journal of Clinical Child and Adolescent Psychology* 32:586–592.

Centers for Disease Control and Prevention (CDC). (1998) HIV/AIDS among American Indians and Alaskan Natives—United States, 1981–1997. *MMWR, Morbidity and Mortality Weekly Report* 47(8):154–160.

Centers for Disease Control and Prevention (CDC). (2000) *Tracking the hidden epidemics: trends in STDS in the United States.* CDC, Atlanta.

Centers for Disease Control and Prevention (CDC). (2001a) Death rates and number of deaths by state, race, sex, age, and cause, 1994–1998. CDC, Atlanta.

Centers for Disease Control and Prevention (CDC). (2001b) *HIV/AIDS surveillance report*. 13(2). CDC, Atlanta.

Centers for Disease Control and Prevention (CDC). (2003a) Cancer mortality among American Indians and Alaska Natives—United States, 1994–1998. *MMWR, Morbidity and Mortality Weekly Report* 52(30):704–707.

Centers for Disease Control and Prevention (CDC). (2003b) Health status of American Indians compared with other racial/ethnic minority populations—selected states, 2001–2002. *MMWR, Morbidity and Mortality Weekly Report* 52(47):1148–1152.

Centers for Disease Control and Prevention (CDC). (2003c) Web-based injury statistics query and reporting system (WISQARS). Available from: www.cdc.gov/ncipc/wisqars.

Centers for Disease Control and Prevention (CDC). (2004a) *Fact sheet: racial/ethnic health disparities*. Retrieved August 2004.

Centers for Disease Control and Prevention (CDC). (2004b) *HIV/AIDS surveillance supplemental report: cases of HIV infection and AIDS in the United States, by race/ethnicity, 1998–2002*, 10(1). CDC, Atlanta.

Chan, C. (1989) Issues of identity development among Asian-American lesbians and gay men. *Journal of Counseling and Development* 68(1):16–20.

Chandler, M.J., and Lalonde, C. (1998) Cultural continuity as a hedge against suicide in Canada's First Nations. *Transcultural Psychiatry* 35:191–219.

Chen, S.Y., Gibson, S., Katz, M.H., Klausner, J.D., Dilley, J.W., Schwarcz, S.K., Kellogg, T.A., and McFarland, W. (2002) Continuing increases in sexual risk behavior and sexually transmitted disesases among men who have sex with men: San Francisco, Calif, 1999–2001. *American Journal of Public Health* 92:1387–1388.

Cochran, S.D., Sullivan, J.G., and Mays, V.M. (2003) Prevalence of mental disorders, psychological distress, and mental health services use among lesbian, gay, and bisexual adults in the United States. *Journal of Consulting and Clinical Psychology* 71:53–61.

Coker, A.L., Davis, K.E., Arias, I., Desai, S., Sanderson, M., Brandt, H.M., and Smith, P.H. (2002) Physical and mental health effects of intimate partner violence for men and women. *American Journal of Preventive Medicine* 23:260–268.

Conway, G.A., Ambrose, T.J., Chase, E., Hooper, E.Y., Helgerson, S.D., Johannes, P., Epstein, M.R., McRae, B.A., Munn, V.P., Keevama, L., et al. (1992) HIV infection in American Indians and Alaska Natives: surveys in the Indian Health Service. *Journal of Acquired Immune Deficiency Syndromes* 5:803–809.

Corwin, R.F., and Benda, B.B. (2000) Religiosity and church attendance: the effects on use of "hard drugs" controlling for sociodemographic and theoretical factors. *International Journal of Psychology of Religion* 10:241–258.

Cross, W. (1978) The Thomas and Cross models of psychological nigrescence: a literature review. *Journal of Black Psychology* 4:13–31.

Cuadrado, M., and Lieberman, L. (1998) Traditionalism in the prevention of substance misuse among Puerto Ricans. *Substance Use Misuse* 33:2737–2755.

D'Augelli, A.R., Pilkington, N.W., and Hershberger, S.L. (2002) Incidence and mental health impact of sexual orientation victimization of lesbian, gay, and bisexual youths in high school. *School Psychology Quarterly* 17:148–167.

Diamond, C., Davidson, A., Sorvillo, F., and Buskin, S. (2001) HIV-infected American Indians/Alaska Natives in the western United States. *Ethnicity & Disease* 11:633–644.

Diaz, R.M., Ayala, G., Bein, E., Henne, J., and Marin, B.V. (2001) The impact of homophobia, poverty, and racism on the mental health of gay and bisexual Latino men: findings from 3 US cities. *American Journal of Public Health* 91:927–932.

Dibble, S.L., Roberts, S.A., and Nussey, B. (2004) Comparing breast cancer risk between lesbians and their heterosexual sisters. *Women's Health Issues* 14:60–68.

Dinges, N.G., and Joos, S.K. (1988) Stress, coping, and health: models of interaction for Indian and Native populations. *Behavioral Health Issues among American Indians and Alaska Natives: Explorations of the Frontiers of the Biobehavioral Sciences* 1:8–64.

Doll, L.S., Joy, D., Bartholow, B.N., Harrison, J.S., Bolan, G., Douglas, J.M., Saltzman, L.E., Moss, P.M., and Delgado, W. (1992) Self-reported childhood and adolescent sexual abuse among adult homosexual bisexual men. *Child Abuse and Neglect* 16:855–864.

Duran, B., and Walters, K.L. (2004) HIV/AIDS prevention in "Indian Country": current practice, indigenist etiology models, and postcolonial approaches to change. *AIDS Education and Prevention* 16:187–201.

Duran, E., and Duran, B. (1995) *Native American postcolonial psychology*. State University of New York Press, Albany.

Duran, E., Duran, B., Yellow Horse Brave Heart, M., and Yellow Horse-Davis, S. (1998) Healing the American Indian soul wound. In: Danieli, Y. (ed) *International handbook of multigenerational legacies of trauma*. Plenum, New York, pp. 341–354.

Espin, O. (1987) Issues of identity in the psychology of Latina lesbians. In: Boston Lesbian Psychologies Collective (ed) *Lesbian psychologies: explorations and challenges*. University of Illinois Press, Urbana, pp. 35–51.

Evans-Campbell, T. (2000) *Perceptions of and attitudes toward child neglect among urban American Indians Los Angeles*. Doctoral dissertation, University of California, Los Angeles.

Evans-Campbell, T., and Walters, K.L. (2004) Catching our breath: a decolonization framework for healing indigenous families. In: Fong, R., McRoy, R., and Hendricks, C.O. (eds) *Intersecting child welfare, substance abuse, and family violence: culturally competent approaches*. CSWE Publications, Alexandria, VA.

Fenaughty, A.M., Fisher, D.G., MacKinnon, D.P., Wilson, P.I., and Cagle, H.H. (1994) Predictors of condom use among Alaska Natives, White and Black drug users in Alaska. *Arctic Medicine Research 53*.

Finkelhor, D. (1984) *Child sexual abuse, new theory and research*. Free Press, New York.

Fisher, D.G., Fenaughty, A.M., Paschane, D.M., and Cagle, H.H. (2000) Alaska Native drug users and sexually transmitted disease: results of a five-year study. *American Indian and Alaska Native Mental Health Research* 9:47–57.

Flanigan, B.J. (1990) The social context of alcohol consumption prior to female sexual intercourse. *Journal of Alcohol and Drug Education* 36:97–113.

Forquera, R. (2001) *Urban Indian health*. The Henry J Kaiser Family Foundation, Menlo Park, CA.

Fox, K.K., del Rio, C., Holmes, K.K., Hook, E.W. III, Judson, F.N., Knapp, J.S., Procop, G.W., Wang, S.A., Whitlengton, W.L., and Levine, W.C. (2001) Gonorrhea in the HIV era: a reversal in trends among men who have sex with men. *American Journal of Public Health* 91:959–964.

Frank, M.L., and Lester, D. (2002) Self-destructive behaviors in American Indian and Alaska Native high school youth. *American Indian and Alaska Native Mental Health Research* 10(3):24–32.

Fullilove, M.T., Fullilove, R.E., Smith, M., Winkler, K., Michael, C., Panzer, P.G., and Wallace, R. (1993) Violence, trauma, and post-traumatic stress disorder among women drug users. *Journal of Traumatic Stress* 6:533–543.

Garofalo, R., Wolf, R.C., Kessel, S., Palfrey, J., and DuRant, R.H. (1998) The association between health risk behaviors and sexual orientation among a school-based sample of adolescents. *Pediatrics* 101:895–902.

Gee, G.C. (2002) A multilevel analysis of the relationship between institutional and individual racial discrimination and health status. *American Journal of Public Health* 92(4):615–623.

Gilman, S.E., Cochran, S.D., Mays, V.M., Hughes, M., Ostrow, D., and Kessler, R.C. (2001) Risk of psychiatic disorders among individuals reporting same-sex sexual partners in the National Comorbidity Survey. *American Journal of Public Health* 91:933–939.

Gray, N., and Nye, P.S. (2001) American Indian and Alaska Native substance abuse: comorbidity and cultural issues. *American Indian and Alaska Native Mental Health Research* 10(2):67–84.

Greenfeld, L.A., and Smith, S.K. (1999). *American Indians and crime* (no. NCJ 173386 BJS Publication). U.S. Department of Justice, Washington, DC.

Gruskin, E.P., Hart, S., Gordon, N., and Ackerson, L. (2001) Patterns of cigarette smoking and alcohol use among lesbians and bisexual women enrolled in a large health maintenance organization. *American Journal of Public Health* 91:976–979.

Gurley, D., Novins, D.K., Jones, M.C., Beals, J., Shore, J.H., and Manson, S.M. (2001) Comparative use of biomedical services and traditional healing options by American Indian veterans. *Psychiatric Services* 52(1):68–74.

Halpert, S.C. (2002) Suicidal behavior among gay male youth. *Journal of Gay and Lesbian Psychotherapy* 6(3):53–79.

Harrell, J.P., Hall, S., and Taliaferro, J. (2003) Physiological responses to racism and discrimination: an assessment of the evidence. *American Journal of Public Health* 93:243–248.

Harris, N.V., Thiede, H., McGough, J.P., and Gordon, D. (1993) Risk factors for HIV infection among injection drug users: results of blinded surveys in drug treatment centers, King County, Washington 1988–1991. *Journal of Acquired Immune Deficiency Syndromes* 6:1275–1282.

Haugaard, J.J., and Reppucci, N.D. (1988) *The sexual abuse of children: a comprehensive guide to current knowledge and intervention strategies.* Jossey-Bass, San Francisco.

Herek, G.M., Gillis, J.R., and Cogan, J.C. (1999) Psychological sequelae of hate-crime victimization among lesbian, gay, and bisexual adults. *Journal of Consulting and Clinical Psychology* 67:945–951.

Hill, P.H., and Pargament, K.I. (2003) Advances in the conceptualization and measurement of religion and spirituality: implications for physical and mental health research. *American Psychologist* 58(1):64–74.

Houghton, F. (2002) Misclassification of racial/ethnic minority deaths: the final colonization. *American Journal of Public Health* 92:1386.

Hourani, L.L., Yuan, H., and Bray, R.M. (2003) Psychological and health correlates of types of traumatic event exposures among U.S. military personnel. *Military Medicine* 168:736–743.

Icard, L. (1986) Black gay men and conflicting social identities: sexual orientation versus racial identity. *Journal of Social Work and Human Sexuality: Social Work Practice in Sexual Problems [special issue]* 4(1/2):83–93.

Indian Health Service (IHS). (1997) *Trends in Indian health, 1996.* U.S. Department of Health and Human Services, Public Health Service, Indian Health Service, Office of Planning, Evaluation, and Legislation, Division of Program Statistics, Rockville, MD.

Indian Health Service (IHS). (1999a) *Trends in Indian health, 1998–99.* U.S. Department of Health and Human Services, Indian Health Service, Office of Public Health, Program Statistics Team, Rockville, MD.

Indian Health Service (IHS). (1999b) *Indian health focus: Women.* U.S. Department of Health and Human Services, Indian Health Service, Office of Public Health, Program Statistics Team, Rockville, MD.

Indian Health Service (IHS). (2001) *Regional differences in Indian health, 2000–2001.* U.S. Department of Health and Human Services, Indian Health Service, Office of Public Health, Program Statistics Team, Rockville, MD.

Jacobs, M.A., and Brown, L.B. (1997) American Indian lesbians and gays: an exploratory study. *Journal of Gay and Lesbian Social Services* 6:29–41.

Jacobs, S.E., Thomas, W., and Lang, S. (1997) Introduction. In: Jacobs, S.E., Thomas, W., and Lang, S. (eds) *Two-spirit people: Native American gender identity, sexuality, and spirituality.* University of Illinois Press, Urbana, pp. 1–18.

Jemal, A., Clegg, L.X., Ward, E., Ries, L.A.G., Wu, X., Jamison, P.M., Wingo, P.A., Howe, H.L., Anderson, R.N., and Edwards, B.K. (2004) Annual report to the nation on the status of cancer, 1975–2001, with a special feature regarding survival. *Cancer* 101:3–27.

Joe, J.R. (2001) Out of harmony: health problems and young Native American men. *Journal of American College Health* 49:237–250.

Johnson, R.M., Kotch, J.B., and Catellier, D.J. (2002) Adverse behavioral and emotional outcomes from child abuse and witnessed violence. *Child Maltreatment* 7:179–186.

Jones, M.C., Daughinais, P., Sack, W.H., and Somervell, P.D. (1997) Trauma-related symptomatology among American Indian adolescents. *Journal of Traumatic Stress* 10:163–173.

Kalichman, S.C., Benotsch, E., Rompa, D., Gore-Felton, C., Austin, J., Luke, W., DiFonzo, K., Buckles, J., Kyomugisha, F., and Simpson, D. (2001) Unwanted sexual experiences and sexual risks in gay and bisexual men: associations among revictimization, substance use and psychiatric symptoms. *Journal of Sex Research* 38(1):1–9.

Karlsen, S., and Nazroo, J.Y. (2002) Relation between racial discrimination, social class, and health among ethnic minority groups. *American Journal of Public Health* 92:624–631.

Kaufman, C., Beals, J., Mitchell, C., Lemaster, P., and Fickenscher, A. (2004) Stress, trauma, and risky sexual behavior among American Indians in young adulthood. *Culture, Health, and Sexuality* 6:301–318.

Kelly, J.J., Chu, S.Y., Diaz, T., Leary, L.S., Buehler, J.W., The AIDS Mortality Project Group (1996) Race/ethnicity misclassification of persons reported with AIDS. *Ethnicity and Health* 1(1):87–94.

Kessler, R.C., Crum, R.M., Warner, L.A., Nelson, C.B., Schulenberg, J., and Anthony, J.C. (1997) Lifetime co-occurrence of DSM-III-R alcohol abuse and dependence with other psychiatric disorders in the National Comorbidity Survey. *Archives of General Psychiatry* 54:313–321.

Kilpatrick, D.G., and Acierno, R. (2003) Mental health needs of crime victims: epidemiology and outcomes. *Journal of Traumatic Stress* 16:119–132.

Kim, C., and Kwok, Y.S. (1998) Navajo use of Native healers. *Archives of Internal Medicine* 158:2245–2249.

Koenig, L.J., Doll, L.S., and O'Leary, A. (2004) *From child sexual abuse to adult sexual risk: trauma, revictimization, and intervention.* American Psychological Association, Washington, DC.

Krieger, N. (1999) Embodying inequality: a review of concepts, measures, and methods for studying health consequences of discrimination. *International Journal of Health Services* 29:295–352.

Krieger, N., and Sidney, S. (1996) Racial discrimination and blood pressure: the CARDIA study of young black and white adults. *American Journal of Public Health* 86:1370–1378.

Kunitz, S.J., and Levy, J.E. (eds). (2000) *Drinking, conduct disorder, and social change: Navajo experiences.* Oxford University Press, London.

Kunitz, S.J., Levy, J.E., McCloskey, J., and Gabriel, K. R. (1998) Alcohol dependence and domestic violence as sequelae of abuse and conduct disorder in childhood. *Child Abuse & Neglect* 22:1079–1091.

Lang, S. (1998) *Men as women, women as men: changing gender in Native American cultures* (J.L. Vantine, trans.). University of Texas Press, Austin.

Langeland, W., and Hartgers, C. (1998) Child sexual and physical abuse and alcoholism: a review. *Journal of Studies on Alcohol* 59:336–348.

Li, C.I., Malone, K.E., and Daling, J.R. (2003) Differences in breast cancer stage, treatment, and survival by race and ethnicity. *Archives of Internal Medicine* 163:49–56.

Libby, A.M., Orton, H.D., Novins, D.K., Spicer, P., Buchwald, D., Beals, J., Manson, S.M., AI-SUPERPFP Team. (2004) Childhood physical and sexual abuse and subsequent alcohol and drug use disorders in two American-Indian tribes. *Journal of Studies on Alcohol* 65:74–83.

Lieb, L.E., Conway, G.A., Hedderman, M., Yao, J., and Kerndt, P.R. (1992) Racial misclassification of American Indians with AIDS in Los Angeles County. *Journal of Acquired Immune Deficiency Syndromes* 5:1137–1141.

Little Crow, Wright, J.A., and Brown, L.A. (1997) Gender selection in two American Indian tribes. *Journal of Gay and Lesbian Social Services* 6(2):21–28.

Loecker, G., Smith, D.A., Smith, L., and Bunger, P. (1992) HIV associated risk factors: a survey of a troubled adolescent population. *South Dakota Journal of Medicine* 45(4):91–94.

Loicano, D.K. (1989) Gay identity issues among Black Americans: racism, homophobia, and the need for validation. *Journal of Counseling and Development* 68:21–25.

MacMillan, H.L., Fleming, J.E., Streiner, L.D., Lin, E., Boyle, M.H., Jamieson, E., Duku, E.K., Walsh, C.A., Wong, M.Y., and Beardslee, W.R. (2001) Childhood abuse and lifetime psychopathology in a community sample. *American Journal of Psychiatry* 158:1878–1883.

Manson, S.M., Beals, J., O'Nell, T., Piasecki, J., Bechtold, D., Keane, E., and Jones, M. (1996) Wounded spirits, ailing hearts: PTSD and related disorders among American Indians. In: Marsella, A.J., Friedman, M.J., Gerrity, E.T., and Scurfield, R.M. (eds) *Ethnocultural aspects of posttraumatic stress disorder: issues, research, and clinical applications.* American Psychological Association, Washington, DC, pp. 255–283.

Marbella, A.M., Harris, M.C., Diehr, S., Ignace, G., and Ignace, G. (1998) Use of Native American healers among Native American patients in an urban Native American health center. *Archives of Family Medicine* 7:182–185.

May, P.A. (1995) The prevention of alcohol and other drug abuse among American Indians: a review and analysis of the literature. In: Langton, P.A. (ed) *The challenge of participatory research: preventing alcohol-related problems in ethnic communities.* NIAAA/CSAP Monograph No. 3. Cultural Competence Series. U.S. Department of Health and Human Services, CSAP, Bethesda, pp. 185–241.

May, P.A., and Smith, M.B. (1988) Some Navajo Indian opinions about alcohol abuse and prohibition: a survey and recommendations for policy. *Journal of Studies in Alcohol* 49:324–334.

Mays, V.M., Yancey, A.K., Cochran, S.D., Weber, M., and Fielding, J.E. (2002) Heterogeneity of health disparities among African American, Hispanic, and

Asian American women: unrecognized influences of sexual orientation. *American Journal of Public Health* 92:632–639.

Medicine, B. (1988) "Warrior women"—sex role alternatives for Plains Indian women. In: Albers, P., and Medicine, B. (eds) *The hidden half: studies of Plains Indian women.* University Press of America, New York, pp. 267–280.

Metler, R., Conway, G.A., and Stehr-Green, J. (1991) AIDS surveillance among American Indians and Alaska Natives. *American Journal of Public Health* 81:1469–1471.

Meyer, I.H. (2001) Why lesbian, gay, bisexual, and transgender public health. *American Journal of Public Health* 91:856–859.

Meyer, I.H. (2003) Prejudice, social stress, and mental health in lesbian, gay, and bisexual populations: conceptual issues and research evidence. *Psychological Bulletin* 129:674–697.

Monette, L., Albert, D., and Waalen, J. (2001) *Voices of two-spirited men: a survey of aboriginal two-spirited men across Canada.* 2-Spirited People of the 1st Nations, Toronto.

Morales, E.S. (1989) Ethnic minority families and minority gays and lesbians. *Marriage and Family Review* 14:217–239.

Moran, J.R., Fleming, C.M., Somervell, P., and Manson, S.M. (1999) Measuring bicultual ethnic identity among American Indian adolescents: a factor analytic study. *Journal of Adolescent Research* 14:405–426.

Morris, J.F., Waldo, C.R., and Rothblum, E.D. (2001) A model of predictors and outcomes of outness among lesbian and bisexual women. *American Journal of Orthopsychiatry* 71:61–71.

Myers, T., Bullock, S.L., Calzavara, L.M., Cockerill, R., and Marshall, V.W. (1997) Differences in sexual risk-taking behavior with state of inebriation in an aboriginal population in Ontario, Canada. *Journal of Studies on Alcohol* 58:312–322.

National Center for Health Statistics (NCHS). (1999) Alcohol consumption by state, race/ethnicity, sex, and age, 1997–1999. National Vital Statistics Reports, National Vital Statistics System, United States, Washington, DC.

National Center for Health Statistics (NCHS). (2002) *Health, United States, 2002 with chartbook on trends in the health of Americans* (No. 1232). U.S. Government Printing Office [DHHS], Washington, DC.

National Center for Injury Prevention and Control (NCIPC). (2002) *Suicide in the United States.* Accessed at: www.cdc.gov/ncipc/default.htm.

National Indian Justice Center (NIJC). (1990) Child abuse and neglect in American Indian and Alaska Native communities and the role of the Indian Health Service. Unpublished final report, U.S. Department of Health and Human Services.

National Women's Health Information Center (NWHIC). (2003) *Frequently asked questions abouth health problems in American Indian/Alaska Native women.* Retrieved August 2004 from 4woman.gov.

Noh, S., Beiser, M., Kaspar, V., Hou, F., and Rummens, J. (1999) Perceived racial discrimination, depression, and coping: a study of Southeast Asian refugees in Canada. *Journal of Health and Social Behavior* 40:193–207.

Norrell, B. (2001, August 1). *Mother of murdered Navajo teen says it was a hate crime.* Indian Country Today, from http://www.indiancountry.com.

Oetting, E.R., and Beauvais, F. (1990–1991) Orthogonal cultural identification theory: the cultural identification of minority adolescents. *International Journal of Addiction* 25(5A–6A):655–685.

Paltoo, D.N., and Chu, K.C. (2004) Patterns in cancer incidence among American Indians/Alaska Natives, United States, 1992–1999. *Public Health Reports* 119:443–451.

Paul, J.P., Catania, J., Pollack, L., and Stall, R. (2001) Understanding childhood sexual abuse as a predictor of sexual risk-taking among men who have sex with men: the Urban Men's Health Study. *Child Abuse and Neglect* 25:557–584.

Paul, J.P., Catania, J., Pollack, L., Moskowitz, J., Canchola, J., Mills, T., et al. (2002) Suicide attempts among gay and bisexual men: lifetime prevalence and antecedents. *American Journal of Public Health* 92:1338–1345.

Ratner, P.A., Johnson, J.L., Shoveller, J.A., Chan, K., Martindale, S.L., Schilder, A.J., et al. (2003) Non-consensual sex experienced by men who have sex with men: prevalence and association with mental health. *Patient Education and Counseling* 49:67–74.

Relf, M.V., Huang, B., Campbell, J., and Catania, J. (2004) Gay identity, interpersonal violence, and HIV risk behaviors: an empirical test of theoretical relationships among a probability-based sample of urban men who have sex with men. *Journal of the Association of Nurses in AIDS Care* 15(2):14–26.

Robin, R.W., Chester, B., and Goldman, D. (1996) Cumulative trauma and PTSD in American Indian communities. In: Marsella, A.J., Friedman, M.J., Gerrity, E.T., and Scurfield, R.M. (eds) *Ethnocultural aspects of posttraumatic stress disorder: issues, research, and clinical applications.* American Psychological Association, Washington, DC, pp. 239–254.

Robin, R.W., Chester, B., Rasmussen, J.K., Jaranson, J.M., and Goldman, D. (1997a) Factors influencing utilization of mental health and substance abuse services by American Indian men and women. *Psychiatric Services* 48:826–834.

Robin, R.W., Chester, B., Rasmussen, J.K., Jaranson, J.M., and Goldman, D. (1997b) Prevalence and characteristics of trauma and posttraumatic stress disorder in a southwestern American Indian community. *American Journal of Psychiatry* 154:1582–1588.

Russell, S.T., Franz, B.T., and Driscoll, A.K. (2001) Same-sex romantic attraction and experiences of violence in adolescence. *American Journal of Public Health* 91:903–906.

Saewyc (Carlson), E.M., Bearinger, L.H., Skay, C.L., Resnick, M.D., and Blum, R.W. (1996) Demographic of sexual orientation among Native American adolescents. *Journal of Adolescent Health* 18:137.

Saewyc, E.M., Skay, C.L., Bearinger, L.H., Blum, R.W., and Resnick, M.D. (1998a) Demographics of sexual orientation among American Indian adolescents. *American Journal of Orthopsychiatry* 68:590–600.

Saewyc, E.M., Skay, C.L., Bearinger, L.H., Blum, R.W., and Resnick, M.D. (1998b) Sexual orientation, sexual behaviors, and pregnancy among American Indian adolescents. *Journal of Adolescent Health* 23:238–247.

Safren, S.A., and Heimberg, R.G. (1999) Depression, hopelessness, suicidality, and related factors in sexual minority and heterosexual adolescents. *Journal of Consulting and Clinical Psychology* 67:859–866.

Scheier, L.M., Botvin, G.J., Diaz, T., and Ifill-Williams, M. (1997) Ethnic identity as a moderator of psychosocial risk and adolescent alcohol and marijuana use: concurrent and longitudinal analysis. *Journal of Child Adolescent Substance Abuse* 6(1):21–47.

Schultz, A., Parker, E., Israel, B., and Fisher, T. (2001) Social context, stressors, and disparities in women's health. *Journal of the American Medical Women's Association* 56:143–150.

Simoni, J., Walters, K., Balsam, K., and Meyers, S.B. (2004a) Victimization, substance use, and HIV risk behaviors among American Indian men in New York City. Unpublished observations.

Simoni, J.M., Martone, M.G., and Kerwin, J.F. (2002) Spirituality and psychological adaptation among women with HIV/AIDS: implications for counseling. *Journal of Counseling Psychology* 49:139–147.

Simoni, J.M., Sehgal, S., and Walters, K.L. (2004b) Triangle of risk: urban American Indian women's sexual trauma, injection drug use, and HIV sexual risk behaviors. *AIDS and Behavior* 8(1):33–45.

Simpson, T.L., and Miller, W.R. (2002) Concomitance between childhood sexual and physical abuse and substance use problems: a review. *Clinical Psychology Review* 22(1):27–77.

Spicer, P. (2001) Culture and the restoration of self among former American Indian drinkers. *Social Science and Medicine* 53:227–240.

Stehr-Green, P., Bettles, J., and Robertson, L.D. (2002) Effect of racial/ethnic misclassification of American Indians and Alaskan Natives on Washington state death certificates, 1989–1997. *American Journal of Public Health* 92:443–444.

Stevens, S.J., Estrada, A.L., and Estrada, B.D. (2000) HIV drug and sex risk behaviors among American Indian and Alaska Native drug users: gender and site differences. *American Indian and Alaska Native Mental Health Research* 9(1):33–46.

Stewart, S.H. (1996) Alcohol abuse individuals exposed to trauma: a critical review. *Psychological Bulletin* 120:83–112.

Storck, M., Csordas, T.J., and Strauss, M. (2000) Depressive illness and Navajo healing. *Medical Anthropological Quarterly* 14:571–597.

Straus, T., and Valentino, D. (2001) Retribalization in urban Indian communities. In: Lobo, S., and Peters, K. (eds) *American Indians and the urban experience*. Altamira Press, Walnut Creek, CA, pp. 85–94.

Substance Abuse and Mental Health Services Administration (SAMHSA). (2000) *Summary findings from the National Household Survey on Drug Abuse, 1999 and 2000*. Department of Health and Human Services (US), Office of Applied Studies, Substance Abuse and Mental Health Services Administration, Rockville, MD.

Sullivan, P.S., Chu, S.Y., Fleming, P.L., and Ward, J.W. (1997) Changes in AIDS incidence for men who have sex with men, United States 1990–1995. *AIDS* 11:1641–1646.

Tafoya, T. (1989) Pulling coyote's tale: Native American sexuality and AIDS. In: Mays, V.M., and Albee, G.W. (eds) *Primary prevention of AIDS: psychological approaches; primary prevention of psychopathology*, Vol. 13. Sage, Thousand Oaks, CA, pp. 280–289.

Tafoya, T. (1992) Native gay and lesbian issues: the two-spirited. In: Berzon, B. (ed) *Positively gay: new approaches to gay and lesbian life*. Celestial Arts Publishing, Berkeley, CA.

Tafoya, T., and Rowell, R. (1988) Counseling gay and lesbian Native Americans. In: Shernoff, M., and Scott, W. (eds) *The sourcebook on lesbian/gay health care*. National Lesbian and Gay Health Foundation, Washington, DC.

Tafoya, T.N. (1996) Native two-spirit people. In: Cabaj, R.P., and Stein, T.S. (eds) *Textbook of homosexuality and mental health*. American Psychiatric Association, Washington, DC: pp. 603–617.

Terr, L.C. (1991) Childhood traumas: an outline and overview. *American Journal of Psychiatry* 148:10–20.

Thomas, W., and Jacobs, S.E. (1999) "... And we are still here": from *berdache* to two-spirit people. *American Indian Culture and Research Journal* 23:91–107.

Thompson, M.P., Kingree, J.B., and Desai, S. (2004) Gender differences in long-term health consequences of physical abuse of children: data from a nationally representative survey. *American Journal of Public Health* 94:599–604.

Tinker, G.E. (1993) *Missionary conquest: the gospel and Native American cultural genocide*. Fortress Press, Minneapolis.

Tjaden, P., Thoeness, N., and Allison, C.J. (1999) Comparing violence over the life span in samples of same-sex and opposite-sex cohabitants. *Violence and Victims* 14:413–425.

Tomeo, M.E., Templer, D.I., Anderson, S., and Kotler, D. (2001) Comparative data of childhood and adolescence molestation in heterosexual and homosexual persons. *Archives of Sexual Behavior* 30:535–541.

Townsend, T.G., and Belgrave, F.Z. (2000) The impact of personal identity and racial identity on drug attitudes and use among African American children. *Journal of Black Psychology* 26:421–433.

Turner, R.J., and Lloyd, D.A. (1995) Lifetime traumas and mental health: the significance of cumulative adversity. *Journal of Health & Social Behavior* 36:360–376.

Underwood, L.G., and Teresi, J.A. (2002) The daily spiritual experience scale: development, theoretical description, reliability, exploratory factor analysis, and preliminary construct validity using health-related data. *Annals of Behavioral Medicine* 24:22–33.

U.S. Commission on Civil Rights. (2004, July 2). Broken promises: evaluating the Native American health care system. Retrieved August 2004 from http://www.usccr.gov/pubs/nahealth/nabroken.pdf.

Veenema, T.G. (2001) Children's exposure to community violence. *Journal of Nursing Scholarship* 33:167–173.

Waldram, J.B. (1990) The persistence of traditional medicine in urban areas: the case of Canada's Indians. *American Indian and Alaska Native Mental Health Research* 4:9–29.

Waldram, J.B. (2000) The efficacy of traditional medicine: current theoretical and methodological issues. *Medical Anthropological Quarterly* 14:603–625.

Wallace, L.J.D., Calhoun, A.D., Powell, K.E., O'Neil, J., and James, S.P. (1996) Homicide and suicide among Native Americans, 1979–1992. *Violence Surveillance Summary Series* No. 2.

Walsh, F. (2002) A family resilience framework: innovative practice applications. *Family Relations* 51:130–137.

Walters, K.L. (1997) Urban lesbian and gay American Indian identity: implications for mental health service delivery. *Journal of Gay and Lesbian Social Services* 6(2):43–65.

Walters, K.L. (1998) Negotiating conflicts in allegiances among lesbians and gays of color: reconciling divided selves and communities. In: Mallon, G.P. (ed) *Foundations of social work practice with lesbian and gay persons.* Harrington Park Press/Haworth Press, Binghamton, NY, pp. 47–75.

Walters, K.L. (1999) Urban American Indian identity attitudes and acculturative styles. *Journal of Human Behavior and Social Environment* 2:163–178.

Walters, K.L., and Evans-Campbell, T. (2004, February). Measuring historical trauma among urban American Indians. Presented at the University of New Mexico, School of Medicine, Albuquerque, NM.

Walters, K.L., and Simoni, J.M. (1999) Trauma, substance use, and HIV risk among urban American Indian women. *Cultural Diversity and Ethnic Minority Psychology* 5:236–248.

Walters, K.L., and Simoni, J.M. (2002) Reconceptualizing native women's health: an "indigenist" stress-coping model. *American Journal of Public Health* 92:520–524.

Walters, K.L., Simoni, J.M., and Harris, C. (2000) Patterns and predictors of HIV risk among urban American Indians. *American Indian and Alaska Native Mental Health Research* 9(2):1–21.

Walters, K.L., Simoni, J.M., and Horwath, P.F. (2001) Sexual orientation bias experiences and service needs of gay, lesbian, bisexual, transgendered, and two-spirited American Indians. *Journal of Gay and Lesbian Social Services* 13:133–149.

Walters, K.L., Simoni, J.M., and Evans-Campbell, T. (2002) Substance use among American Indians and Alaska Natives: incorporating culture in an "indigenist" stress-coping paradigm. *Public Health Reports* 117(Suppl 1): S104–S117.

Ward, E., Jemal, A., Cokkinides, V., Singh, G.K., Cardinez, C., Ghafoor, A., and Thun, M. (2004) Cancer disparities by race/ethnicity and socioeconomic status. *Cancer Disparities* 54(2):78–93.

Whitbeck, L.B., Adams, G.W., Hoyt, D.R., and Chen, X. (2004) Conceptualizing and measuring historical trauma among American Indian people. *American Journal of Community Psychology* 33:119–130.

Whitbeck, L.B., McMorris, B.J., Hoyt, D.R., Stubben, J.D., and LaFromboise, T. (2002) Perceived discrimination, traditional practices, and depressive symptoms among American Indians in the Upper Midwest. *Journal of Health and Social Behavior* 43:400–418.

Williams, D.R., and Williams-Morris, R. (2000) Racism and mental health: the African American experience. *Ethnicity and Health* 5:243–268.

Williams, D.R., Yu, Y., Jackson, J.S., and Anderson, N.B. (1997) Racial differences in physical and mental health: socioeconomic status, stress, and discrimination. *Journal of Health Psychology* 2:335–351.

Woods, T.E., Antoni, M.H., Ironson, G.H., and Kling, D.W. (1999) Religiosity is associated with affective and immune status in symptomatic HIV-infected gay men. *Journal of Psychosomatic Research* 46:165–176.

Yellow Horse Brave Heart, M., and DeBruyn, L.M. (1998) The American Indian holocaust: healing historical unresolved grief. *American Indian and Alaska Native Mental Health Research* 8(2):56–78.

Zimmerman, M.A., Ramirez, J., Washienko, K.M., Walter, B., and Dyer, S. (1998) Enculturation hypothesis: exploring direct and protective effects among Native American youth. In: McCubbin, H.I., Thompson, E.A., Thompson, A.I., and Fromer, J.E. (eds) *Resiliency in Native American and immigrant families.* Sage, Thousand Oaks, CA, pp. 199–220.

"I Don't Fit Anywhere": How Race and Sexuality Shape Latino Gay and Bisexual Men's Health

Jesus Ramirez-Valles

1 Introduction

Society's negative views toward homosexuality continue to decline, although gay, lesbian, and transgender people in the United States experience stigma (Weitz, 1991; Herek, 1999; Kaiser Foundation, 2001; Loftus, 2001). The stigma of homosexuality has serious consequences for many gay men, such as stress, low self-esteem, suicide, unemployment, and dislocation (Cochran & Mays, 2000; Link & Phelan, 2001; Mays & Cochran, 2001; Paul et al., 2002). The AIDS epidemic has intensified this stigma (Herek, 1999). Moreover, stigma of homosexuality may be particularly critical for ethnic minorities, such as Latino gay men, because of the added racial discrimination (Diaz, 1998; Finch et al., 2000; Ramirez-Valles et al., 2005).

The purpose of this chapter is to analyze the means by which racial and homosexual stigmas shape the health and lives of Latino gay and bisexual men and transgender persons (GBT). The first section discusses the homosexual stigma, and the second focuses on racial stigma. Stigma refers to a labeling of individuals or groups in a way that discredits them (Goffman 1963). It is a process by which differences between groups of people are enacted and labeled; undesirable characteristics are attached to the labeled group; a social separation is created between the labeled and the labeling group; and the labeled group is subjected to discriminatory practices (Link et al., 1997; Link & Phelan, 2001; Meyer, 2003). The stigma process is usually initiated by a dominant group against a minority or oppressed group.

Among Latino gay and bisexual men, including those living with human immunodeficiency virus/acquired immunodeficiency syndrome (HIV/AIDS), it is difficult to disentangle how, and with what effects, the homosexual and race stigma function (Ramirez-Valles et al., 2005). This group is stigmatized not only because of their sexual orientation and assigned racial group but also because of HIV/AIDS. The

HIV/AIDS epidemic, unfortunately, has expanded the stigma of homo-sexuality and race by adding new attributes: illness, death, drug use, promiscuity (Alonzo & Reynolds, 1995; Herek, 1999; CDC, 2001). Two decades after the onset of the AIDS epidemic, its stigma has not decreased (Herek, 2002). Although some of the stigmatizing attitudes have declined, many individuals still believe that people with AIDS are responsible for their own illness (Herek, 1999, 2002) and associate HIV/AIDS with homosexuality, immigration, and skin color (e.g., brown or black).

Those three stigmas are conceptually independent but are related theoretically and empirically. For instance, gay men's perception and experiences of family rejection, although based on the homosexual stigma, might have been intensified by the HIV/AIDS epidemic. Like-wise, Latino gay men's experiences of race stigma may have increased owing to the public's association of HIV/AIDS with ethnic minorities and immigrant groups in the United States.

Among Latino gay and bisexual men, the HIV/AIDS stigma is also widespread (Diaz & Ayala, 2001). In a national study of Latino gay men (Diaz, 2003), almost half of the HIV-negative participants reported that HIV-positive individuals are to blame for the spread of the disease. Nearly half of the HIV-positive participants had experienced unfair treatment, and 45% indicated that they had to hide their serostatus to be accepted by family and friends. HIV-positive respondents also report that the disease affects their social and sexual lives more than other life domains. In addition, the experience of the HIV stigma is associated with social isolation and low self-esteem (Diaz, 2003). Those stigmas, furthermore, work as social markers that create boundaries among groups and identities based on race and sexuality discourses (Watney, 1989; Crawford, 1994). Race and the identities derived from it are not biologic or genetic categories but social concepts, which usually draw on the biologic sciences (and medicine and public health) for val-idation (Cooper & David, 1986). Race, in the particular case of the United States, is the product of the political economy (rather than skin color) of that country during the nineteenth and twentieth centuries (Roediger, 1991). Racism is perhaps a more useful concept than race if we wish to examine how individuals' social location affects their health. Racism is an exclusion process based on discourses and prac-tices of inferiorization (Anthias, 1990). It is based on socially con-structed physical and biologic differences, which are used to define groups and place them in a social structure of inequality (Wolpe, 1986).

Likewise, and borrowing from Foucault's work (1990), I view homo-sexuality and gayness as socially constructed concepts. Being gay (or man and woman, for that matter) is not based on biologic, genetic, or psychological traits. The category of gay, and gay man in particular, is relatively new, emerging from the discourse of sexuality. This dis-course, fashioned in large by medicine, psychiatry, and psychology, defines identities based on presumed sexual differences and desires (Scott, 1986; Foucault, 1990; Sawicki, 1991). To call oneself a gay man is thus the result of a subjective reflection in the context of historically bounded notions (and norms) of sexuality, femininity, and masculinity (Taylor, 1989; Chauncey, 1994; Cerulo, 1997; Hawkesworth, 1997).

2 Homosexual Stigma

The homosexual and racial stigmas may cause a variety of negative health outcomes (Krieger, 1990; Meyer, 1995; Kessler et al., 1999; Williams et al., 2003). Stigma based on homosexuality, or homophobia, has been found to be associated with depression, low self-esteem, and sexual risk behavior among white and Latino gay men (Meyer, 1995; Frable et al., 1997; Williamson, 2000; Diaz et al., 2001; Huebner et al., 2002; Ramirez-Valles et al., 2005).

In a national random sample of self-identified lesbians, gays, and bisexuals, 74% reported experiences of prejudice and discrimination based on sexual orientation, and 32% reported having been targets of physical violence (Kaiser Family Foundation, 2001). In addition, 80% of respondents believe that there is "a lot" of prejudice and discrimination attributed to sexual orientation (Kaiser Family Foundation, 2001). Likewise, a recent report of stigma on college campuses in the United States found that 30% of respondents recounted experiences of harassment due to sexual orientation or gender identity during the past 12 months (Rankin, 2003).

Stigmatizing attitudes toward sexual orientation may be more prevalent in Latino communities than in other communities. Latinos tend to be less supportive of civil liberties for homosexuals than Whites and African-Americans (Bonilla & Porter, 1990). In a recent national survey, 72% of Latinos thought that sex between two adults of the same sex is unacceptable compared to 59% of Whites (Pew Hispanic Center/Kaiser Family Foundation, 2003). Acculturation to the United States intensifies these attitudes, and the difference becomes more pronounced for Spanish-speaking Latinos than for English-speaking Latinos (81% vs. 60%) (Pew Hispanic Center/Kaiser Family Foundation, 2003). Moreover, factors associated with greater stigmatization, such as high religiosity and strong support of traditional gender roles, remain common in Latino communities (Herek, 1999).

In a major study of Latino gay men living in New York City, Miami, and Los Angeles (Diaz & Ayala, 2001), most men reported experiences of stigmatization due to their sexual orientation. Altogether, 64% of the participants in this probabilistic sample indicated that they were verbally abused during childhood, and 71% noted hearing that gay people grow old alone. In addition, 70% expressed having thought that their homosexuality hurts their families, and 64% reported that they have pretended to be straight to gain acceptance. Diaz and colleagues (2001) also found those experiences of homophobia to be negatively associated with mental health. Moreover, the stigmas of homosexuality and

Table 1. Distribution of Perceived, Internalized, and Experienced Sexual Orientation Stigma Among Latino Gay and Bisexual Men and Transgender Persons in Chicago and San Francisco, 2004 ($n = 643$)

Parameter	Strongly agree/ agree (%)
Perceived*	
Many people believe that gay individuals have psychological problems.	56
Many people look down on gay individuals.	62
Many employers would look down on an effeminate man regardless of qualifications.	61
Many Latinos do not see gay individuals as real men.	77
Most families would be disappointed to have a gay son.	76
Many people believe that gay individuals are promiscuous.	77
Many people believe that gay individuals should not raise children.	76
Internalized*	
I am glad to be gay.	34
I have tried to stop being attracted to men.	31
Men who look or act too effeminate make me feel uncomfortable.	37
It is important for me to look and behave in a masculine way.	49
I am comfortable with people knowing about my sexual orientation.	37
Gay people are promiscuous.	37
I try to look masculine in order to avoid people's rejection.	35

Parameter	Once to many times (%)
Experienced[†]	
Had heard people making negative remarks about gay people.	90
Had been treated differently in social situations.	58
While growing up, was made fun of or called names by family.	67
While growing up, other kids made fun of him or called him names.	82
While growing up, was pushed around or beaten up.	58
As an adult, had to pretend that he is straight to be accepted.	69
Had moved away from friends and family.	49
Family had ignored or refused to acknowledge sexual orientation.	61

*The original scale ranged from strongly disagree to strongly agree.
[†]The original scale ranged from never to many times.

race were significantly associated with a higher rate of unprotected anal intercourse with a nonmonogamous recent partner and higher substance use during the last 6 months (Diaz et al., 2001).

Similar patterns are reported by HIV-positive Latino gay men. Zea and colleagues (R01MH60545, personal communication, July 21, 2003) found that among their HIV-positive male sample 68% reported being called names at least once during childhood because of their feminine appearance, and 67% reported such experiences during their adult years. In addition, 34% of these Latino men reported being beaten or hit at least once in their lifetime because of their sexual orientation, 34% recounted being harassed by the police at least once, and 35% believed they had lost a job or career opportunity at least once because of their sexual orientation. Furthermore, this sexual orientation stigma experienced by HIV-positive Latino men is positively associated with depression and loneliness and negatively associated with self-esteem (Ramirez-Valles et al., 2005).

Evidence of the predominance of stigma of homosexuality was further supported and extended in a study by Ramirez-Valles (2005a) conducted in Chicago and San Francisco. The study included a sample of 643 (320 in Chicago and 323 in San Francisco) Latino GBTs recruited using respondent-driven sampling (Ramirez-Valles et al., 2005). Unlike previous studies, measures of the sexual orientation stigma comprised three areas: experienced, perceived, and internalized. Table 1 shows the distribution for selected items in each of those three areas. The three subscales have good reliability (Cronbach $\alpha > 0.80$) and are correlated but are independent of each other. Perceptions are relatively higher than experiences and internalization. The latter has the lowest levels of the three areas. Thus, these data suggest that Latino GBTs are very aware of society's' negative attitudes toward homosexuality, but their levels of internalization are moderate. Furthermore, the most common forms of stigmatization they have experienced include verbal remarks and mockery, especially during childhood.

3 Community Involvement and Stigma

Many gay men, including those living with HIV/AIDS, confront the stigma and avoid some of its negative consequences (Ramirez-Valles, 2002). Some research indicates that activism and volunteerism, such as participation in the AIDS movement, may help gay men develop a positive sense of themselves and thus buffer the stigma (Kobasa, 1991; Weitz, 1991).

Community involvement refers to unpaid work on behalf of others, or for a collective good, outside the home and the family (Ramirez-Valles, 2002). This includes concepts such as volunteering, activism, and informal help. For gay men, community involvement has been vital because it has provided social integration and a means for social action in light of the AIDS epidemic and rejection from families and coworkers (Kobasa, 1991; Turner et al., 1993; Cantu, 2000).

Community involvement, particularly in AIDS and gay causes, may have positive effects on Latino gay men's health (Ramirez-Valles, 2002). Community involvement has been linked to psychological well-being among gay men, including self-esteem, social support, and self-efficacy (Chambre, 1991; Bebbington & Gatter, 1994; Smith, 1994, 1997; Wolfe, 1994; Ouellette et al., 1995; Frable et al., 1997; Stewart & Weinstein, 1997; Altman et al., 1998; Rietschlin, 1998; Waldo et al., 1998; Moen & Fields, 1999; Allahyari, 2000; Thoits & Hewitt, 2001; Omoto & Snyder, 2002).

Although Latino gay men may have been less involved in the gay and AIDS movements than their White peers two decades ago, it is difficult to compare their current levels of community involvement (Valentgas et al., 1990; Omoto & Snyder, 1995). For instance, in a convenient sample from three cities in the Southwest (i.e., Austin, Phoenix, Albuquerque), Ferrer and colleagues (2002) found rates of volunteering in HIV/AIDS and gay issues to be higher among White gay men (26%) than among their Latino peers (20%). In another study based on a probabilistic sample of Latino gay men in Los Angeles, Miami, and

New York City, the percentages were higher, ranging from 37% in the first city to 63% in the third city (Ramirez-Valles & Diaz, 2005). These differences could be attributed to the measurement in addition to the evident geographic variation. The study in the Southwest assessed only volunteer work (e.g., yes/no) on HIV/AIDS and gay issues during the last 12 months. The study in the metropolitan areas included the current level of involvement (e.g., definitely yes to definitely no) in gay and Latino organizations.

There is some evidence, albeit limited, of the positive effects of community involvement on Latino gay men's well-being (Ramirez-Valles & Brown, 2003). In the aforementioned study in the Southwest, volunteering for HIV/AIDS activities was only minimally associated with gay identity openness but not to self-esteem or social support after controlling for demographic variables and HIV status (Ferrer et al., 2002). In the study of Latino gay men in Los Angeles, Miami, and New York City, community involvement in HIV/AIDS- and gay-related issues slightly offset the negative effects of experienced sexual orientation stigma on social support and self-esteem (Ramirez-Valles & Diaz, 2005). Neither of those studies found support for moderating effects (e.g., interaction between sexual orientation stigma and community involvement) or mediating effects (e.g., between experienced sexual orientation stigma and self-esteem) of community involvement.

There are also some data on the positive effects of community involvement among Latino HIV-positive men. In a study of HIV-positive Latino gay and bisexual men living in New York City and Washington, DC, we tested whether community involvement buffered the effects of stigma on mental health (Ramirez-Valles et al., 2005). We measured community involvement using a frequency index of involvement in AIDS and gay organizations during the last 12 months. Homosexual stigma was measured only as experienced stigma using items from Diaz's scale (Diaz et al., 2001).

Experienced stigma attributed to homosexuality was negatively associated with self-esteem but positively associated with depression and loneliness. Community involvement, however, compensated for those positive associations with depression and loneliness. Community involvement also buffered the association between stigma and self-esteem. For individuals with low involvement, experienced stigma was negatively associated with self-esteem. For the men reporting high involvement in AIDS and gay organizations, increases in experienced stigma were related to increases in self-esteem. Thus, HIV-positive Latino gay men who are highly involved in AIDS and gay organizations may report high self-esteem because they see themselves as victims of discriminatory practices rooted in the prejudice of others. They are aware of the stigma but attribute it to society's prejudice because they have adopted the agenda of the AIDS and gay organizations (e.g., fighting society's stigma assigned to homosexuality and AIDS). In addition, HIV-positive Latino gay men who are highly involved may report higher levels of self-esteem than those who are less involved because community involvement fosters intragroup comparisons, as it brings peers (e.g., Latino gay or HIV-positive men) together.

4 Racial Stigma

Latino (or Hispanic, Chicano) is a socially constructed concept, or category, when referring to a group. Its existence and meanings are contingent on a particular social and historical context, which in this instance is the racial system in the United States. To think of Latino as a social construct is not to deny the actual consequences its use has on the individuals categorized as such. One of the most significant consequences is the stigma and the discriminatory practices exercised upon people referred to as Latinos.

In the United States, Latino is used as a label to categorize people, usually thought of as a race, ethnic group, or minority. As Foucault (1973) proposed, labels such as this one are created to manage populations. One of the features of power is to create and name the other (e.g., people not defined as White and thought of as different) through such labels. In doing so, it reduces human complexity to a set of characteristics or a stereotype, which then becomes an identity. The creation of this Latino identity, however, cannot be attributed solely to what is usually thought of as the sites of power, namely, state institutions and the mostly White male ruling group. Individuals and groups categorized as Latinos have also been active participants in the creation and maintenance of such identity (Skerry, 1993).

The use of Latino is not unambiguous, from the perspective of either lay people or state institutions (e.g., census). Both frequently equate Latino with race, ethnicity, or minority status (Skerry, 1993). Latino as a racial group quickly becomes empty—not when we see the enormous variation of so-called races included in the Latino category but when we think of race as a social construct. Race does not exist as a homogeneous group of people sharing a particular set of genes or physiological features (Williams et al., 1994). Races, like "black" and "white," are only the product of social factors in a context of power relations and in a given historical time (Roediger, 1991). In the United States, race has been created through state regulations, such as segregated schooling and housing programs, and through daily life practices such as attitudes, harassment, and verbal abuse (Krieger et al., 1993).

Although the dominant discourse promotes and uses labels or identities based on assumed racial or ethnic differences, it does not mean that individuals take on those labels (Fraser, 1989). Individuals do have some freedom to negotiate how (if at all) and when they use an identity such as Latino. The ambiguity and contradictions characteristic of the label Latino (or Hispanic) allow variation in the way people use it and even the possibility of rejecting its use. Escaping a racial identity, however, is nearly impossible in a society based on assumed racial differences.

The way individuals interact with the dominant racial discourse to define themselves is exemplified by life history data collected from Latino GBTs activists from San Francisco and Chicago (Ramirez-Valles, 2005b). For example, Ignacio, a 19 year-old activist, was born and raised in the Midwest. Because his Spanish is limited, his high school peers would tell him that he was not Latino. "I don't fit anywhere," is the conclusion Ignacio reached.

When I was in high school, I would always get, "Oh you're not Mexican." "You're not Mexican enough." And I was like, What is it to be Mexican? "How come you never speak Spanish?" My own philosophy is [that] I'm Mexican and that has nothing to do with it. Like, what is it to dress Mexican? So in high school and in college, I distanced myself from the Latino community simply because I'd get shunned a lot, or I'd get a lot of "you're gay." I'd get shunned and then I just don't want that. I'm trying to work on it, but I feel very uncomfortable talking to Latino heterosexuals. I have this stereotype of Latino men, that I feel they're going to be very macho and I just feel uncomfortable, but I'm working on that. Now, I'm in the moment of getting back into my Latino community. I know I could fit in. I want to see how I can better myself, and how I can help that community and work with the gay community too. I am Latino and gay, there's nothing wrong with that. Now I'm into my poetry stage. I did some readings with a room full of Latinos and Latinas. They loved it. One poem was very queer, another one was titled "What is it to be Mexican?" I was proud of them. They loved the poems and that just felt good. So at that moment I felt like this is me and it can work. I felt accepted. I was, wow! It's like being happy.

Language, like Spanish, is used by both outsiders and insiders as a marker of ethnicity or race. Language is, after skin color, the most salient indicator of group membership. If someone is perceived as Latino, he is expected to speak Spanish. If he does not, he is not a "real" Latino. This may cause an identity conflict for many individuals such as Ignacio. He did not socialize with Latinos during his childhood and adolescent years. He felt rejected, first, because he did not speak the language and, later, because of his homosexuality. Now, as a young adult, Ignacio is working to become a "Latino" and incorporate such identity into his gay identity. He, like many other first generation immigrants from Latin America do, has sought out others to create and validate his own identity as a Latino. Yet, as Ignacio explains, this does not completely resolve the identity question, as one continually has to explain to oneself and to others what Latino means.

I think the term Hispanic is very Euro-centric. We're not Indian and we're not African-American. We're not indigenous or African-American, but some people are and others aren't. Not everyone's from Spain. So that's what I grew up with. In high school and in grade school my question was, "Which one do I check? Hispanic?" I think many people use that term not knowing what it means. Just because that's brainwashed. Not brainwashed, but just because it's so common. So, I use Latino just to encompass everyone, "*la raza de Latin America*." I say Latino-Latina, and for me I'd say Chicano. That's my identity. I'm Chicano because I am American and I don't deny that. But I am Mexican too. I have to realize that, and I'm learning, but I don't fit in anywhere. . . . If someone asks "What ethnicity are you?" I'd reply, "I'm Chicano." Or I usually say Latino, depending on what community I'm in. If someone is white, I'd be Latino, and . . . well, Chicano. But then they'd ask, "What is that?" "It's Mexican-American," I'd have to explain. For me, I'm Mexican, but I'm not Mexican. I will never be seen as a Mexican. Then I'm American, but I'm not white American. I don't know . . . But I love America and I love Mexico . . . I remember when I was a kid, I wouldn't use the color brown, because it was an ugly color. I'm brown. And I accept that and I'm Chicano and I'm learning about my culture. But I'm living in America.

Ignacio's struggle to make sense of himself in the context of United States' society and culture illustrates the interactive process by which individuals take on identities promoted by the dominant discourse. It reflects the dilemmas, conflicts, and consequences of adopting a label to define the self. Moreover, Ignacio's example shows the ambiguity and contradictions inherent in the label Latino.

4.1 The Experience of Race

One of the most enduring and painful marks of racism is the verbal and nonverbal actions individuals experience because they are considered different and inferior. Actions such as insults, segregation, and mistreatment leave permanent scars in the self. The size and pain of the scars may change as time passes, sometimes becoming invisible and numb, but they never disappear. They remain as constant reminders of who one is and of one's relation with the outside world—the offender. The scars permeate the way one sees oneself and the outside world.

The acts of racism, verbal and nonverbal, also constitute the ways in which race is expressed and sustained. That is, when we insult a person because of her or his brown skin color, we are enacting race as the idea of difference. At the same time, we are reproducing the racial system in which we live and that gave origin to that insult.

Table 2 presents data on racial stigma from Latino GBTs in San Francisco and Chicago (Ramirez-Valles, 2005a). Data were collected on three areas of stigma: experienced, perceived, internalized. The three subscales demonstrated good psychometric properties and independence from each other. Similar to sexual orientation stigma, perceptions are relatively higher than experiences and internalization; and internalization of racial stigma is somewhat low.

In the Latino gay activists study (Ramirez-Valles, 2005b), almost all ($n = 80$) participants reported experiencing racism at some point in their lives—independent of whether they are immigrants or U.S. natives. Their experiences included verbal insults, distancing or isolation, harassment, and mistreatment. Although these experiences are very common among these activists, they are not as pervasive or salient as the experiences attributed to homosexuality discussed above. The latter are more numerous and more painful to recount than the former. This may be the result of the relationship between the victim and the offender. In the case of the homosexual stigma much of the

Table 2. Distribution of Perceived, Internalized, and Experienced Racial Stigma Among Latino Gay and Bisexual Men and Transgender Persons in Chicago and San Francisco, 2004 ($n = 643$)

Parameter	Strongly agree/ agree (%)
Perceived*	
Many employers would prefer to hire a white person rather than a Latino.	47
Many people treat whites with more respect than Latinos.	69
Latinos who are light-skinned are treated better than those who are dark-skinned.	57
Many people do not like it when Latinos speak Spanish.	68
Many people believe that Latinos are an inferior ethnic group.	61
Many people believe that Latinos are more violent or more likely to commit a crime than white people.	63
Many people are surprised by successful Latinos.	79
Internalized*	
Latinos are partially to blame for people's negative attitudes toward them.	41
Most Latinos are involved in gangs and crime.	19
I sometimes feel ashamed of being Latino.	9
I sometimes feel embarrassed by the way Latinos look and act.	38
As a Latino, I sometimes feel undesirable or unattractive.	13
I prefer to date white people rather than Latinos.	16

Parameter	Once to many times (%)
Experienced†	
Have been treated differently in the workplace because of being Latino.	67
White growing up, was treated differently because of accent or because did not speak English well.	28
As an adult, have been treated differently because of accent or because do not speak English well.	61
Have felt uncomfortable in a gay bar or club because of being Latino.	41
Potential romantic or sexual partners have taken more interest in his race than in who he is as a person.	62
Have been treated with less respect than others because of being Latino.	66

*The original scale ranged from strongly disagree to strongly agree.
†The original scale ranged from never to many times.

stigmatization comes from family and friends, whereas stigmatization caused by skin color or language usually comes from a more distant individual, such as teachers and classmates, but rarely from family and friends. The experiences of racism are particularly salient as individuals enter the outside, larger social world: that is, when children move from the usually monoethnic and monolingual environment of family and neighborhood to a multiethnic (if not white only) milieu, such as school. The life history from one activist, Abraham, provides an example of how bilingual education works to create and reproduce racial stigma (Ramirez-Valles, 2005b).

Abraham was born in New York City but spent some time in Puerto Rico because his parents were originally from there. As a child, he was sent to bilingual education because his English was not "very good." Like others who have gone through such a system, he describes this experience as "horrible."

I didn't speak very good English. I had an accent. The English I already had was a New York accent. On top of that being in Puerto Rico for a year or so I was already speaking Spanish. I remember having to be held back in a bilingual class. Bilingual then was horrible. It was in the basement and you were separated. You were just with a few other kids and it was like in the dingy room and it didn't make you feel really good. I remember I was pretty big already, because I was held back just because I didn't speak English, whether properly or not. I should have been in first grade and I wasn't.

The official discourse would say that the purpose of bilingual education, or any type of "special" education, is to promote advancement and integration. What Abraham experienced, however, is separation, which is a form of stigmatization similar to segregation. Separation can also be thought of as a social distancing between the "normal" students and the "special," or "not-normal," students. One consequence of this special treatment is the sense of being different and "less" than others. As Abraham poignantly said, he was in a "basement." It makes children question their abilities and, furthermore, their sense of who they are. Because people such as Abraham come to believe that others (the outside world) think they are not good enough, they strive to demonstrate otherwise.

One of the things I got to realize looking back was the language thing and I always used to think I had a problem speaking English because I was Puerto Rican. I remember in school the teacher would always correct me. It turns out, it was not that I didn't speak English properly. She was correcting my New York English to Chicago English. So I always thought I had a speaking problem. I think those sort of things created a lot of confusion. I used to think, "am I smart?" I think it did affect me, and I always had to prove that I was smart.

When I was leaving Puerto Rico to come back to the States, I would say "I wanted to buy English." "I'm going to English," because I was going to speak English. My grandparents always spoke to me in Spanish and funny that now my Spanish is horrible. It's almost like whatever I knew I forgot. After a while and being here for so long, I didn't need to use it. My mother would speak English, for the most part, although constantly peppered with Puerto Rican Spanish. That got me into trouble too, because I thought some words were Spanish, but I'd be corrected, "no, that's only for Puerto Ricans." Then that becomes a problem later, when I try to go back into Spanish. This is the language that proved to be a major issue in my life, actually. It has a lot to do with identity. In fact, identity has become a major issue for me especially when I was growing up.

Bilingual education not only separated Abraham from his peers and discredited his skills, it also questioned his sense of being Puerto Rican. The message Abraham got was that being Puerto Rican was not good. His problem was being Puerto Rican. Yet, in learning English, he lost his native language. Language is not simply a skill or a tool to communicate. It is the means by which culture is transmitted and the means to construct one's world or reality. As Freire (1986) would put it, through language one comes to name and own one's world.

This is why language, as "Puerto Rican Spanish," is the basis for Abraham's identity and the target of bilingual education in a racial system.

Rejection, another form of stigmatization commonly experienced by these GBT activists, is frequently based on skin color and language. Moreover, rejection is usually linked with insults, another form of stigmatization. The insult, or name-calling, is used to degrade, mark a difference, and, as a consequence, to reject. When a person is called a "beaner," as Gonzalo illustrates next, he or she is been referred to as someone who eats beans and hence is poor. That, in and of itself, works as an insult, which also denotes rejection.

I wasn't spoken to here because I was a Mexican. I was a beaner. That's what they would call me. So pretty soon, after about a year, I learned not to associate with white people. When school was out, we moved to a city, which was bigger and more diverse. The neighborhood that we were living was very diverse. I didn't want to associate with white people, because to them I was a Beaner, and I was this and I was that. Asian people wouldn't associate with me because I didn't speak their language and I was prohibited from talking to the black kids.

Gonzalo grew up in a small town in California. His parents came to the United States to improve their financial situation. When they arrived, they were the only family in town. The other migrant workers were all adults and single. Gonzalo thus felt isolated at an early age. When he started school, he barely spoke any English, and none of the teachers was bilingual. "I felt pretty weird," Gonzalo recollects. "It felt isolating. I've never seen so many White people in my life." The rejection that was implicit in the insult increased Gonzalo's isolation and sense of being different, which he eventually internalized. Gonzalo learned he was not welcome by White people.

The separation created by bilingual education, the insults, and the mockery are part of the adversity endured by these activists. These experiences are attributed largely to their skin color and language and to a lesser extent their ethnicity. They are some of the means by which the idea of race and difference is enacted. Being Latino, as another activist puts it, "is in many ways like being gay. It is to be outside the larger society. Sometimes it is harder than being gay. One can hide the gay part, but the color of your skin is very visible." The experiences of stigmatization that are based on the idea of race, like those attributed to homosexuality, are particularly salient during childhood and adolescence. Stigmatization based on race is magnified when individuals leave the confines of a small, homogeneous (e.g., same language and ethnicity) group, such as the family and the neighborhood and enter a larger, mostly white setting. In the words of the same activist, "I didn't care about skin color when I was younger, maybe because I was in an enclosed and mostly Hispanic community. But as I step in the outside world, I notice it more. And I know that many people look first at the color of my skin."

4.2 The White Gay Ghetto

Humberto, one of the activists in the aforementioned study by Ramirez-Valles (2005b), reported that he never felt discriminated against because of his physical appearance until he moved to San Francisco and began visiting gay bars. "There's really, really a lot of racism." He noted, "But it's not directed at you that much. But you feel it. Here, it's thrown at you." Forty-seven year-old Humberto was born in the United States and raised in California. He speaks sharply of the rejection and alienation he has experienced in mainstream gay circles because he is not perceived as Caucasian. His experience is not unique. Many of these activists speak of the racial discrimination and segregation that exists in bars, clubs, and organizations in the Bay Area, Chicago, New York, Miami, Washington, DC, and other large cities in the country.

The racism experienced by the Latino GBT activists is not always explicit or overt, such as with insults and segregation. It frequently takes place in an implicit manner. "You feel it," Humberto noted. It is perceived in the atmosphere created by the dominant presence of White men, the little interaction between White men and the few non-White men, and, in the words of Isidro, an activist, by the "body and gym culture."

Humberto also recounted the most palpable forms of stigmatization that he experienced in gay bars, such as being ignored and hearing racial derogatory comments.

When I first started going to the bars, it took me a lot to walk into one. 'Cause basically they were all White. When I finally got comfortable and went in, they wouldn't serve me. I would just stand there, and stand there, and stand there. They would totally ignore me. They would help everybody around the side. Until they would come up and say, "What's going on?" I'd tell them and they'd go get the drink.

I never felt that before. Not like that. People talking about Jews and Mexicans and this and that. It got to the point where I'd be in the bar and they'd be talking "Oh did you see those Mexicans?" I'm standing there and I'm going like, "Okay." I didn't know whether to say something or not. I just felt smaller, and smaller, and smaller. Where I didn't move. I felt that if I left, they've won. I just stood there. I just stood there and ignored. It hasn't happened as much anymore. I think because I've been conditioned now. I don't pay attention.

Another activist, Felipe, further suggested that the segregation in gay communities is not only based on skin color but also on social class.

I'm not into going to the gay *barrio*, either here or in other cities I have visited. Everywhere, the neighborhoods are what I'd call White ghetto. A gay White ghetto, that's what it represents for me. I'd even call it an upper-middle-class gay White ghetto. It is about race but also is about social class. Of course, every once in a while I'd go to a coffee shop or restaurant there, but I don't think it is my neighborhood. As a Latino and as a gay man, it doesn't do it for me.

Other activists in this group of GBTs would agree with this assessment, but Felipe is the only one who articulated this explicitly. Recall that many of these activists are immigrants; and although some of them belong to a middle class stratum, few can afford homes in the (mostly) gay neighborhoods of Chicago and San Francisco. The cost of housing in those gay neighborhoods is among the most expensive in both cities.

Social class thus intensifies the racial segregation in gay communities. Race and social class converge to form, in the eyes and realities of these GBTs, a gay culture that is White and middle class. The stigmatization emerging from such gay culture toward those of colored skin and broken English has isolated and alienated many of these activists. Yet, they participate in the dominant gay culture, and in some instances they employ the widespread racialized views of Latinos to their own advantage. One example found among these GBTs is the use of their "Latino" outlook to attract gay White men. That is, they "play" the exoticism of Latinos, as Luigi described it.

When I lived in San Diego, I started meeting White men who liked my eyes, my hair, and my cock. They liked the way I looked; my hairy body. I played that for a while. I don't play it any more. I want to be seen as an entire person now. I want to be seen for my mind as well. It was fun for a while. I'm not going to say I didn't play the card. I outgrew it very quickly.

Luigi's approach—to play the "race card"—is somewhat contradictory. On the one hand, it intensifies instead of questions the stigmatizing attitudes and actions toward Latino GBTs. It also makes the act, rather than Luigi, a part of the gay culture and its stigmatization of Latinos. On the other hand, Luigi is conscious of the fact that he is playing the "race card." He knows that he can use it when he wishes—to a certain extent. He also is aware that such an approach objectifies him and is founded on racist stereotypes. Thus he has some control over being objectified. As a result, the stigmatization may not be as damaging (if at all) at the personal level, as an insult.

5 Summary

The stigma of homosexuality and race are part of Latino GBTs lives, beginning early in childhood. Many Latino GBTs grow up knowing they are different and are valued less than others. Many grow up feeling rejected and alienated. The stigma they have experienced, and continue to experience, contributes to a variety of negative outcomes, such as poverty, truncated education, unemployment, depression, suicide, substance use, and risky sexual behavior. During the course of their lives, however, some Latino GBTs are able to cope with, or confront, racial and homosexual stigmas. They are able to prevent or redress the negative effects of the stigma. Community involvement, in the form of activism and volunteerism, in particular plays a significant role in buffering and preventing the negative effects of the stigma.

Unfortunately, research is scarce, and the available studies have limitations. Most of the studies available are (understandable) narrowly focused on HIV/AIDS, rely on cross-sectional data, and use different measures to make valid comparisons. Those shortcomings prevent us from fully comprehending the Latino GBT's health needs and strengths.

It is quite evident from the available literature that we need to increase our efforts to understand the health status of Latino GBTs. Most current studies have justifiably focused on HIV, AIDS, and substance use. Without ignoring those issues, we need to broaden the health issues to a comprehensive concept of health. For instance, one clear implication from the studies reviewed here is that interventions are needed to halt the stigmatization of nonconforming gender behavior and ethnic minorities. These interventions must be oriented to the sources of the stigma, rather than the victims. They also need to go beyond the popular but ineffective discourse of cultural sensitivity and tolerance. Such interventions may have to address structural and institutional practices (e.g., education, media) that label GBTs and minorities as inferior citizens.

Future research efforts, however, need to address basic questions about the meanings of homosexuality, gayness, and race. Health research, for the most part, has overlooked those concepts and restricted the work to ambiguous definitions (e.g., gay men, men who have set with men, Latinos). Researchers rarely pause to think and question, for instance, what "gay men" means or who comes under the category of "Latino." To undertake this endeavor, health researchers may need to work closely with those from the humanities and social sciences. In addition, they should embrace theoretical frameworks, rather than focus exclusively on data, to guide the formulation of research questions and the problem of racial and sexuality-based categories.

Acknowledgments: This study was funded by a National Institute of Mental Health grant to Jesus Ramirez-Valles (MH62937-01).

References

Allahyari, R.A. (2000) *Visions of charity: volunteer workers and moral community.* D. University of California Press, Berkeley.

Alonzo, A.A., and Reynolds, N.R. (1995) Stigma, HIV, and AIDS: an exploration and elaboration of the illness trajectory surrounding HIV infection and AIDS. *Social Science and Medicine* 41:303–315.

Altman, D.G., Feighery, E., Robinson, T.N., Haydel, K.F., Strausberg, L., Lorig, K., and Killen, J.D. (1998) Psychological factors associated with youth involvement in community activities promoting heart health. *Health Education and Behavior* 25:489–500.

Anthias, F. (1990) Race and class revisited—conceptualizing race and racism. *Sociological Review* 38:19–42.

Bebbington, A.C., and Gatter, P.N. (1994) Volunteers in an HIV social care organization. *AIDS Care* 6:571–585.

Bonilla, L., and Porter, J. (1990) A comparison of Latino, Black, and non-Hispanic White attitudes toward homosexuality. *Hispanic Journal of Behavioral Sciences* 12:437–452.

Cantu, L. (2000) *Entre hombres/between men: Latino masculinities and homosexualities.* Sage, Thousand Oaks, CA.

Centers for Disease Control and Prevention (CDC). (2001) *HIV prevention strategic plan through 2005.* CDC, Atlanta.

Cerulo, A.K. (1997) Identity construction: new issues, new directions. *Annual Review of Sociology* 23:385–409.

Chambre, S.M. (1991) Volunteers as witness: the mobilization of AIDS volunteers in New York City, 1981–1988. *Social Services Review* 65:531–547.

Chauncey, G. (1994) *Gay New York: gender, urban culture, and the making of the gay male world, 1890–1940.* Basic Books, New York.

Cochran, S.D., and Mays, V.M. (2000) Lifetime prevalence of suicide symptoms and affective disorders among men reporting same-sex sexual partners: results from NHANES III. *American Journal of Public Health* 90:573–578.

Cooper, R., and David, R. (1986) The biological concept of race and its application to epidemiology. *Journal of Health Politics Policy and Law* 11:97–116.

Crawford, R. (1994) The boundaries of the self and the unhealthy other: reflections on health, culture and AIDS. *Social Science & Medicine* 38:1347–1365.

Diaz, R.M. (1998) *Latino gay men and HIV: culture, sexuality, and risk behavior.* Routledge, New York.

Diaz, R.M. (2003) In our own backyard: HIV/AIDS stigmatization in the Latino gay community. In: Teunis, N. (ed) *Sexual inequalities: essays from the field.*

Diaz, R.M., and Ayala, G. (2001) *Social discrimination and health: the case of Latino gay men and HIV risk.*

Diaz, R.M., Ayala, G., Bein, E., Henne, J., and Marin, B.V. (2001) The impact of homophobia, poverty, and racism on the mental health of gay and bisexual Latino men: findings from 3 US cities. *American Journal of Public Health* 91:927–932.

Ferrer, L.M., Ramirez-Valles, J., Kegeles, S., and Rebehook, G. (2002) Community involvement and HIV/AIDS among young gay/bisexual men. Presented at the XIV International AIDS Conference, Barcelona.

Finch, B.K., Kolody, B., and Vega, W.A. (2000) Perceived discrimination and depression among Mexican-origin adults in California. *Journal of Health and Social Behavior* 41:295–313.

Foucault, M. (1973) *The order of things: an archeology of the human sciences.* Vintage Books, New York.

Foucault, M. (1990/1976) *The history of sexuality: an introduction*, Vol. 1. Vintage Books, New York.

Frable, D.E., Wortman, C., and Joseph, J. (1997) Predicting self-esteem, well-being, and distress in a cohort of gay men: the importance of cultural stigma, personal visibility, community networks, and positive identity. *Journal of Personality* 65:599–624.

Fraser, N. (1989) *Unruly practices: power, discourse and gender in contemporary social theory.* University of Minnesota Press, Minneapolis.

Freire, P. (1986) *The pedagogy of the oppressed.* Continuum.

Goffman, E. (1963) *Stigma.* Prentice-Hall, Englewood Cliffs, NJ.

Hawkesworth, M. (1997) Confounding gender. *Signs* 22:648–685.

Herek, G.M. (1999) AIDS and stigma. *American Behavioral Scientist* 42:1102–1112.

Herek, G.M. (2002) HIV-related stigma and knowledge in the United States: prevalence and trends, 1991–1999. *American Journal of Public Health* 92:371–377.

Huebner, D.M., Davis, M.C., Nemeroff, C.J., and Aiken, L.S. (2002) The impact of internalized homophobia on HIV preventive interventions. *American Journal of Community Psychology* 30:327–348.

Kaiser Family Foundation. (2001) *Inside-OUT: a report on the experiences of lesbians, gays and bisexuals in America and the public's views on issues and policies related to sexual orientation*. Kaiser, Meno Park, CA.

Kessler, R.C., Mickelson, K.D., and Williams, D.R. (1999) The prevalence, distribution, and mental health correlates of perceived discrimination in the United States. *Journal of Health & Social Behavior* 40:208–230.

Kobasa, S.C.O. (1991) AIDS volunteering: links to the past and future prospects. In: Nelkin, D., Willis, D., and Parris, S. (eds) *A disease of society: cultural and institutional responses to AIDS*. Cambridge University Press, Cambridge, pp. 172–188.

Krieger, N. (1990) Racial and gender discrimination: risk factors for high blood pressure? *Social Science and Medicine* 30:1273–1281.

Krieger, N., Rowley, D., Herman, A., Avery, B., and Phillips, M. (1993) Racism, sexism, and social class: implications for studies of health, disease, and well-being. *American Journal of Preventive Medicine* 9(Suppl 9):82–122.

Link, B.G., and Phelan, J.C. (2001) Conceptualizing stigma. *Annual Review of Sociology* 363–385.

Link, B.G., Struening, E.L., Rahav, M., Phelan, J.C., and Nuttbrock, L. (1997) On stigma and its consequences: evidence from a longitudinal study of men with dual diagnoses of mental illness and substance abuse. *Journal of Health and Science Social Behavior* 38:177–190.

Loftus, J. (2001) America's liberalization in attitudes toward homosexuality, 1973 to 1998. *American Sociological Review* 66:762–782.

Mays, V.M., and Cochran, S.D. (2001) Mental health correlates of perceived discrimination among lesbian, gay and bisexual adults in the United States. *American Journal of Public Health* 91:1869–1876.

Meyer, I.H. (1995) Minority stress and mental health in gay men. *Journal of Health and Social Behavior* 36:38–56.

Meyer, I.H. (2003) Prejudice, social stress, and mental health in lesbian, gay, and bisexual populations: conceptual issues and research evidence. *Psychological Bulletin* 129(5):674–697.

Moen, P., and Fields, S. (1999, August) Retirement and well-being: does community participation replace paid work? Presented at the American Sociological Association, Chicago.

Omoto, A.M., and Snyder, M. (1995) Sustained helping without obligation: motivation, longevity of service, and perceived attitude change among AIDS volunteers. *Journal of Personality & Social Psychology* 68:333–356.

Omoto, A.M., and Snyder, M. (2002) Considerations of community: the context and process of volunteerism. *American Behavioral Scientist* 45:846–867.

Ouellette, S.C., Cassel, B.J., Maslanka, H., and Wong, L.M. (1995) GMHC volunteers and the challenges and hopes for the second decade of AIDS. *AIDS Education and Prevention* 7(Suppl.):64–79.

Paul, J.P., Catania, J., Pollack, L., Moskowitz, J., Canchola, J., Mills, T., Binson, D., and Stall, R. (2002) Suicide attempts among gay and bisexual men: lifetime prevalence and antecedents. *American Journal of Public Health* 2002;92: 1338–1345.

Pew Hispanic Center/Kaiser Family Foundation. (2003) *2002 National Survey of Latinos*.

Ramirez-Valles, J. (2002) The protective effects of community involvement for HIV risk behavior: a conceptual framework. *Health Education Research* 17:389–403.

Ramirez-Valles, J. (2005a) 2 Communidades Study. Unpublished data.

Ramirez-Valles, J. (2005b) What activists are made of: the lives of Latino gay men and transgender persons in the times of AIDS. Unpublished manuscript.

Ramirez-Valles, J., and Brown, A.U. (2003) Latino's community involvement in HIV/AIDS: organizational and individual perspectives on volunteering. *AIDS Education and Prevention* 15(Suppl A):90–104.

Ramirez-Valles, J., and Diaz, R.M. (2005) Public health, race, and the AIDS movement: the profile and consequences of Latino gay men's community involvement. In: Omoto, A.M. (ed) *Processes of community change and social action.* Lawrence Erlbaum, Mahwah, NJ.

Ramirez-Valles, J., Fergus, S., Reisen, C.A., Poppen, P.J., and Zea, M.C. (2005) Confronting stigma: community involvement and psychological well-being among HIV-positive Latino gay men. *Hispanic Journal of Behavioral Sciences* 27:101–119.

Rankin, S.R. (2003) *Campus climate for gay, lesbian, bisexual, and transgender people: a national perspective.* The National Gay and Lesbian Task Force Policy Institute, New York.

Rietschlin, J. (1998) Voluntary association membership and psychological distress. *Journal of Health and Social Behavior* 39:348–355.

Roediger, D.R. (1991) *The wages of witheness: race and the making of the working class.* Verso, London.

Sawicki, J. (1991) *Disciplining Foucault, feminism, power, and the body.* Routledge, New York.

Scott, J. (1986) Gender: a useful category of historical analysis. *American Historical Review* 91:1053–1075.

Skerry, P. (1993) *Mexican Americans: the ambivalent minority.* Harvard University Press, Cambridge, MA.

Smith, H.D. (1994) Determinants of voluntary association, participation and volunteering: a literature review. *Nonprofit and Voluntary Sector Quarterly* 23:243–263.

Smith, H.D. (1997) Grassroots associations are important: some theory and a review of the impact literature. *Nonprofit and Voluntary Sector Quarterly* 26:269–306.

Stewart, E., and Weinstein, R.S. (1997) Volunteer participation in context: motivations and political efficacy within three AIDS organizations. *American Journal of Community Psychology* 25:809–837.

Taylor, C. (1989) *Sources of the self: the making of the modern identity.* Harvard University Press, Cambridge, MA.

Thoits, P.A., and Hewitt, L.N. (2001) Volunteer work and well-being. *Journal of Health and Social Behavior* 42(June):115–131.

Turner, H.A., Hays, R.B., and Coates, T.J. (1993) Determinants of social support among gay men: the context of AIDS. *Journal of Health and Social Behavior* 34:37–53.

Valentgas, P., Bynum, C., and Sierler, S. (1990) The buddy volunteer commitment in AIDS care. *American Journal of Public Health* 80:1378–1380.

Waldo, C.R., Kegeles, S.M., and Hays, R.B. (1998) Self-acceptance of gay identity decreases sexual risk behavior and increases psychological health in U.S. young gay men. Presented at the 12th World AIDS Conference, Geneva.

Watney, S. (1989) Missionary positions: AIDS, Africa, and race. *Differences* 1:83–100.

Weitz, R. (1991) *Life with AIDS.* Rutgers University Press, New Brunswick, NJ.

Williams, D., Lavizzo-Mourey, R., and Warren, R. (1994) The concept of race and the health status in America. Public Health Reports.

Williams, D.R., Neighbors, H.W., and Jackson, J.S. (2003) Racial/ethnic discrimination and health: findings from community studies. *American Journal of Public Health* 93:200–208.

Williamson, I.R. (2000) Internalized homophobia and health issues affecting lesbians and gay men. *Health Education Research* 15:97–107.

Wolfe, M. (1994) The AIDS coalition to unleash power (ACT UP): a direct model of community research for AIDS prevention. In: Van Vugt, J.P. (ed) *AIDS prevention and services: community based research*. Begin & Garvey, Westport, CT.

Wolpe, H. (1986) Class concepts, class struggle, and racism. In: Rex, J., and Mason, D. (eds) *Theories of race and ethnic relations*. Cambridge University Press, Cambridge, UK pp. 110–130.

13

Black LGB Health and Well-Being

Juan Battle and Martha Crum

1 Introduction

Two landmark publications during the mid-1970s, Thomas McKeown's *The Modern Rise of Population* (1976) and John Cassel's "The contribution of the social environment to host resistance" (1976), helped rekindle interest in how social factors influence health. Realization that communities and social structures affect the health of populations and affect them differentially was not new. Associations between poverty and ill health are centuries old and were key to the activist-oriented U.S. public health movement at the turn of the twentieth century. However, the ascendancy of the germ theory during the last decades of the nineteenth century dampened interest in poverty and other socially constructed conditions as significant pathways to ill health. However "wrong" the theory of miasma—that disease was caused by the fetid air produced by the overcrowded and unsanitary conditions of the urban poor—the theory at least focused public health initiatives on improving the lives of economically marginalized people. With its decline, health initiatives moved from living conditions to the laboratory.

As chronic disease began to surpass infectious disease as a source of morbidity and mortality in industrialized countries, epidemiologists and academic medicine more broadly elevated the role of the "host" in the "host–agent–environment" paradigm of disease, with an emphasis on individual-level behavioral risk factors. Yet as critics have pointed out, this emphasis was completely decontextualized from how both host and environment are shaped by social and material factors (Pearce, 1996; Susser & Susser, 1996; Kreiger, 2000b). Although a recent resurgent interest in social causation of disease is attempting to break the intellectual lock that the "risk factor" paradigm has had on the epidemiologic scholarship (and, importantly, on interventions), the field is still dominated by more individualistic approaches to understanding health and disease.

Interest in social causes of disease has been especially important to the Black[1] population and more recently to the lesbian, gay, and bisexual populations. Compared to Whites, Black people suffer from excess morbidity and mortality across a broad spectrum of diseases, including diabetes, hypertension and other cardiovascular disease, human immunodeficiency virus infection/acquired immunodeficiency disease (HIV/AIDS), renal disease, and many common cancers (Kreiger et al., 1993; Kaufman et al., 1997; Schultz et al., 2000). Research on health disparities affecting lesbian, gay, and bisexual (LGB) people has focused primarily on mental health issues and HIV/AIDS, with more recent scholarship attempting to understand health disparities more broadly. Research on health disparities affecting the intersection of these two stigmatized populations—Black LGBs—is almost nonexistent.

Social epidemiologists have developed comprehensive models to explain how social marginalization compromises the physical or mental health of marginalized people (Kreiger, 2001; Link & Phelan, 2001). These models are similar in scope and dimension to how other scholars have conceptualized the effects of racism on the health of Black Americans (Clark et al., 1999; Jones, 2000). Empirical work informed by these models is in its infancy. Studies on health effects of perceived discrimination, for example, have tended to focus on mental health rather than physical health (Kreiger, 2000a). There is little work on the health effects of structural inequality. Studies on social causation compete for institutional support with the better-funded individual-behavior paradigm, where diseases such as HIV/AIDS, diabetes, and cardiovascular health are perceived, in varying degree, to be a function of individual life-style choices, leading to interventions focused on individual behavioral change. As a relatively small community, one might be tempted to dismiss Black LGBs as a serious object of academic inquiry. From a standpoint theory point of view (Collins, 2003) however, this population is of particular interest because it stands at the intersection of multiple stigmatized populations. To understand the health consequences of marginalization is to understand just how high are the individual and social costs of discrimination in its multifarious forms. To understand the pathways through which marginalization expresses itself physiologically and psychologically is to understand potential points of intervention. To understand if and how Black LGB identity can mediate the negative health effects of marginalization and empower Black LGBs in the struggle against oppression is to understand how to unleash a powerful resource not only for Black LGBs but potentially for LGBs, for Blacks, and for other marginalized groups. It

---

[1]Throughout this text, we will use the term *Black* to refer to people of African Diaspora, and to such populations that reside within the United States. To some, African Americans are a subgroup within the larger Black community. Because our discussion purposely includes those who may be first-generation immigrants or who, for whatever reason, do not identify as African American, we employ the term "Black." Furthermore, we capitalize it to distinguish the racial category and related identity from the color. Similarly, we capitalize the word *White* when referring to race.

is this latter point that underscores the standpoint theorists' position that the most marginalized may well have the most to teach us.

This chapter reviews some of the major works on health and marginalization and on identity and health, both theoretical and empirical. After assessing the significance of the literatures for the health and well-being of Black LGBs, we return to the issue of how the experiences of Black LGBs can inform larger struggles for freedom.

2 Pathways to Ill Health and Reduced Life Chances

There is a long tradition of scholarship on stigma and its adverse consequences for the stigmatized (Allport, 1954/1979; Goffman, 1963; Crocker & Major, 1989; Crocker et al., 1998). More recently, scholars have begun to hypothesize and test a variety of pathways through which stigma, and its consequent marginalization, leads to poorer health and well-being. The most comprehensive models (Clark et al., 1999; Jones, 2000; Kreiger, 2001; Link & Phelan, 2001) tend to include three major pathways: disadvantageous social structures, perceived discrimination, and internalization of stigma.

Structural pathways include what is known in the literature on race inequality as institutionalized racism. This is conceptualized as compromised access to material well-being and power as a function of race (Jones, 2000). Thinking more broadly about stigmatized groups, we might think of these structural factors as the unique contribution to reduced chances for health, well-being and longevity that accrues from being subject to a particular "ism," in the hypothetical case where the person had no idea he or she was a member of the group subject to the "ism." In other words, the effects of this type of "ism" do not have to be seen or perceived to be felt. For example, both Black men and gay men, as populations, are disadvantaged in the labor market, and this disadvantage goes beyond differential educational achievement (itself a marker of institutionalized racism) (Badgett, 1995; Darity et al., 1996; Darity, 1998). Segregation has also been associated with higher mortality (Collins & Williams, 1999). Structural determinants affect people's material environments, regardless of how any specific event or trend is "interpreted." The environment then becomes the pathway—through differential exposure to pollution, crime, neighborhood services, food availability, good schools, information, and the like—to the health disparity.

The link between health and perceived discrimination, on the other hand, is largely conceptualized in terms of social psychological processes in which the perceived discrimination is experienced as a stigma-related stressor. An important part of this conceptualization is the coping resources or styles a given individual uses to mediate stigma-related stressors. Too exclusive a reliance on this model, however, has been criticized as overly individualistic (Kreiger, 2001; Link & Phelan, 2001). Kreiger, for example, has argued that "the study of why some people swim well and others drown when tossed into a river displaces the study of who is tossing whom into the current—and what else might be in the water" (Kreiger, 2001, p. 670).

The psychosocial paradigm of perceived discrimination initially focused on mental health outcomes and disparities. More recently, the stress paradigm from the medical literature has been incorporated into the discrimination effects framework for a richer, more multidimensional understanding of the effects of perceived discrimination. In the medical literature, chronic stress is hypothesized to have a direct pathogenic pathway to physical disease (Sapolsky, 1994; McEwen, 1998; Solarz, 1999) and thus to physical health disparities. Whether the pathways from perceived discrimination to ill health are physiologic, psychological, or both, a key component is that the discrimination is personally mediated. In other words, this type of "ism" follows from someone interpreting or experiencing a particular act, behavior, or event as discriminatory.

Finally, internalized "isms" have been posited as having ill effects on the health and well-being of marginalized people through lowered self-esteem and consequent mental health morbidity. This literature traces its roots to the social interaction theory, particularly the "looking glass theory," where the self concept is at least in part constructed from a reflection of how others see you (Mead, 1934; Cooley, 1956). As we shall see in looking specifically at Black and LGB populations, this theory has worked in unexpected and differential ways for these two populations, perhaps as a function of conceptual subtleties in different types of stigma first identified by Goffman (1963).

The distinctions between structural and psychosocial pathways are not always clear-cut, particularly as they interact across time and the life course. Although we highlight research involving structural determinants, perceived discrimination, and internalization of stigma, it is important to understand that marginalization does not "travel" in single pathways, nor does it result in single "outcomes." Link and Phelan (2001) noted that most research on stigma proceeds by looking at one stigma and one outcome at a time. They argued, however, that stigma affects many life chances and that any particular outcome is affected by multiple stigmatizing circumstances. Therefore, they caution that stigma processes have a "dramatic and probably a highly underestimated impact" on life chances (p. 381), a caution that is likely to apply to Black LGBs.

2.1 Structural Determinants of Health

Social and economic determinants provide structural pathways for the systematic shaping of life chances. Skyrocketing asthma rates in Harlem, New York, for example, are not the direct result of individuals making decisions based on racial or ethnic stereotypes. Rather, they are the result of, among other things, poverty and segregation. The maze of pathways that leads to elevated asthma rates among Harlem youth likely includes substandard housing (which tends to have high rodent and roach infestation and therefore a high density of rodent and roach feces—triggers for asthma attacks); city planning practices that have resulted in a disproportionate number of the city's bus terminals being housed in the immediate vicinity, creating excess smog and air pollution (also a trigger for asthmatics); high crime rates, which keep the children of concerned parents and guardians off the streets and "safely" cloistered in their toxic home environments; and lack of employment opportunity, which keep large portions of the population medically uninsured and therefore less likely to have access to the preventive and educational resources so crucial to managing chronic health conditions (Epstein, 2003).

Understanding disparities in socioeconomic status and how those disparities manifest in the material and social environment is a crucial context for understanding disparities in health. Social and economic determinants provide a key pathway between racism and Black Americans' disadvantaged health outcomes. To the degree these Black/White disparities exist in the larger population, it stands to reason they also exist in the LGB community.

The Council on Economic Advisors for the President's Initiative on Race (1998) has documented just how disadvantaged Black men are vis-à-vis the labor market. Black men have experienced unemployment rates that are roughly twice as high as those for White men over the past 50 years. Among the college-educated, Black men are four times more likely to experience unemployment compared to Whites, and the Black male labor force participation rate has declined at a faster rate than that of White men. Furthermore, the Black/White household income gap has remained remarkably stable since the 1950s, and Black men working full time still earn only 74% of the median full-time wages of White men (Sigelman & Welch, 1991; Hacker, 1993; Business Week, 2003). Additionally, analysis of the Black/White differential in socioeconomic status has shown strong and persistent effects for both social capital (lower attainment levels of income-related characteristics such as education, occupational status, metropolitan location, and English fluency, among others) and for labor market discrimination (lower returns for the same level of attainment of income-related characteristics) (Darity, 1998).

The impact of the socioeconomic status disadvantage on the health of Black Americans is likely to be underestimated in the health disparities literature. Some social scientists have argued that much of the "cause" of health disparities in the literature that has traditionally been attributed to race is in fact attributable to differential socioeconomic status (Kaufman et al., 1997; Kreiger, 2000a). This is because conventional "controls" for socioeconomic status include crude categorizations, such as above or below the poverty line, and do not take into consideration that Blacks are considerably poorer than Whites *within* the ordinal categories typically associated with socioeconomic status analyses. Thus many analyses are flawed by residual confounding, erroneously pointing to "racial differences" and leading to a search for genetic causal factors to explain disparities. Other scholars have shown that there are substantial differences in wealth between Blacks and Whites that are not captured by using income alone to define socioeconomic status (Oliver & Shapiro, 1997). Conley (1999) showed that controlling for wealth attenuates (sometimes to zero) or actually reverses the direction of race disparities in multiple domains of social life, such as educational achievement, out-of-wedlock childbirths, labor market participation, and employment. However, his work does not explore race-related disparities in health.

It is less clear what role social and economic determinants play in the health of the LGB population. Until recently, reliable population level data on LGBs were nearly impossible to get, making socioeconomic comparisons difficult. In response to the HIV/AIDS epidemic, questions on sexual behavior and orientation were added to some large-scale national studies, but they were more often added for men and often resulted in small samples of homosexually active respondents, thus providing little statistical power to detect effects (Cochran & Mays, 2000). Issues related to definition hinder comparisons further. Some studies use a behavioral history of same-sex partners to identify gay/bisexual populations, whereas others use self-reported identity measures (e.g., gay, lesbian, bisexual, queer). Although most men who self-identify as gay or bisexual are "captured" by screening techniques based on sexual behavior history, the reverse is not true. That is, slightly less than half of the men who report at least some adult same-sex behavior self-identify as gay, homosexual, or bisexual (Cochran & Mays, 2000). Nonetheless, several studies, both population-based and those with convenience samples, show a consistent, if directional tendency for higher education and lower income among gay-identified men compared to the national population (Herek & Glunt, 1995; Cochran & Mays, 2000; Gilman et al., 2001; Cochran et al., 2003).

The visibility of openly gay men in Hollywood and more broadly in the arts may have contributed to a popular perception of the gay community as affluent. Badgett (2000), in her analysis of marketing and promotional efforts that characterized the gay community as an untapped affluent market, has shown that the data profiles packaged by Simmons Market Research Bureau and other marketing research companies were based on convenience samples from such outlets as gay-targeted media, gay political organizations, mail order companies, and credit card companies. By contrast, Badgett's (1995) analysis of a random sample of behaviorally LGB men and women from the 1989–1991 General Social Survey conducted by the University of Chicago's National Opinion Research Center showed that LGBs who worked full time had comparable education but lower income than their heterosexual counterparts. More importantly, she found that gay/bisexual status was a significant and negative determinant of income among the men, such that gay and bisexual men who worked earned from 11% to 27% less than their heterosexual counterparts with the same experience, education, occupation, marital status, and regional residence. Although Badgett did not find a consistently statistically significant effect for lesbian/bisexual status among the women, we might speculate, given the 65% gender wage gap, that coupled lesbian households would have lower income than married or coupled heterosexual households. Because these effects were based on behavioral definitions and not workplace disclosure or identity, Badgett argues that they underestimate labor discrimination effects.

Reliable data on Black LGB populations are even more rare. Battle et al. (2002) conducted one of the largest, though venue-based, studies of Black LGBs in the country. Interviewing more than 2000 Black LGBs in nine cities at LGB-related events, Battle and his colleagues profiled a highly educated but relatively low-income Black LGB population. Compared to the national Black population, for example, Black LGBs in this study were three times more likely to have a college degree. Although this higher educational achievement did seem to result in lower poverty rates, it did not translate into higher income. That is, compared to the national Black population, Black LGBs were much less likely to be earning less than $15,000 annually; yet only 10% earned more than $75,000 annually, compared to 13% of the Black population at large. In the case of Battle et al.'s work, the explanation for higher education and lower income may be a result of sampling a younger population in urban areas.

Black LGBs are likely to be affected by socioeconomic determinants affecting both Black and LGB communities, but we do not understand enough about the socioeconomic determinants of health in the LGB community to even speculate on the implications of the structural "intersection" of race and sexual orientation. Furthermore, work on structural pathways has tended to focus almost exclusively on socio-economic factors and on differential access to material conditions. As Jones (2000) has conceptualized institutionalized racism, health disparities can also flow from differential access to power, including a "voice" in voting, governmental representation, the media, and indeed one's own history. How the lack of visibility and representation of Black LGBs in the public sphere (e.g., government and mainstream media) might affect the health and well-being of Black LGBs is completely uncharted territory.

2.2 Psychosocial Pathways

The other broad category of pathways leading from stigma to ill health is psychosocial processes involving stigma-related stressors and individual-level responses to them. These psychosocial processes—including both perceived discrimination and internalization of stigma—are generally seen as distinct from the more structural pathways just discussed. In the psychosocial stress paradigm, coping processes, such as social support and social identity, are often theorized as "buffers" that intervene between stigma-related stressors and their negative health effects. Crocker and Major (1989) and Miller and Kaiser (2001) have provided important elaborations of coping mechanisms. Miller and Kaiser, in particular, provide a schematic of possible voluntary and involuntary coping responses to stigma-related stressors, differentiating between health-inducing and health-reducing coping strategies.

This "social stress" framework has tended to generate research emphasizing psychiatric morbidity as an outcome. For example, the literature clearly indicates that stigma-related stressors, including perceived unfair treatment or discrimination, are risk factors for psychiatric morbidity among LGBs (Meyer, 1995; Mays & Cochran, 2001). Meyer (1995) found that gay-related stressors such as internalized homophobia, stigma, and gay-related discrimination were associated with a two- to threefold increase in risk for high levels of psychological distress among gay men. Mays and Cochran (2001) found a positive association between perceived discrimination and psychiatric morbidity and a negative association between perceived discrimination and quality of life in the population at large, with a homosexual or bisexual orientation more than doubling the risk of perceiving day-to-day discriminatory behaviors, such as perceiving that others think you are inferior, being treated with less respect or courtesy, or being insulted, threatened, or harassed. These stigma-related stressors are thought to help explain the higher prevalence of psychiatric morbidity in the LGB population, as sexual orientation continues to predict morbidity even after controlling for other demographic characteristics (Cochran & Mays, 2000; Cochran, 2001; Gilman et al., 2001; Cochran et al., 2003).[2]

Meyer (2003) conducted a meta-analysis to document the excess prevalence of psychiatric morbidity among LGBs and elaborated a minority stress model to help explain it. The model describes how prejudice and discrimination create a hostile social environment, leading to stigma-related stressors such as experience of prejudice events, internalized homophobia, hiding and concealing, and expectations of rejection, which then manifest in reduced mental health. His conceptual framework also includes minority identity characteristics as an intervening variable in the minority stressors/mental health outcomes pathway.

The picture is more complicated with respect to stigma-related stressors and psychiatric morbidity in the Black population. Some studies have found a link between perceived discrimination or a generalized perception of racism and psychological distress. Jackson et al. (1996), for example, found an association between a negative perception of Whites' intentions and psychological distress among a national sample of Black Americans. Landrine and Klonoff (1996) found associations between perceived racism and psychiatric distress among Black university-based populations. Williams et al. (1997) found a relation between discrimination and psychological distress among Black adults in Detroit, and Sellers et al. (2003) found direct and indirect links between perceived discrimination and psychological distress in a longitudinal study of Black "at-risk" youth in Michigan. Yet, by and large, population level studies have *not* shown excess risk of psychiatric disorders or psychological distress among Black Americans once other factors, including socioeconomic status, are controlled for (Vega & Rumbaut, 1991; CDC, 2004).

Why have these links between perceived discrimination and psychological distress not manifested in population-level disparities in psychiatric morbidity? One possible explanation, discussed more fully

---

[2]Studies consistently show higher risk for psychiatric morbidity among LGBs, although specific patterns vary by sex and there are some inconsistencies in terms of specific disorders. For a review of this research, see Susan Cochran's address at the 2001 APA annual convention, published in the November 2001 issue of *American Psychologist*.

in the section on identity, is that identity-related coping resources may moderate the effects of stigma-related stressors. Although the mechanisms were relatively unexplored, Schultz and colleagues (2000) found that being Black was actually a protective factor for psychological distress among Detroit residents living in high poverty areas once such factors as everyday and acute unfair treatment, acute life events, and role-related and financial stress were accounted for. Among residents of less impoverished communities, race was not a significant predictor of psychological distress.

Another possible explanation lies in the relative size of the "within group" segments driving the group rates of psychiatric morbidity. For example, Williams (2003) argues that middle class Black men have more exposure to individually directed discrimination than lower class Black men. He cites sources of evidence that show positive associations between perceived discrimination and education (Forman et al., 1997), between stress and socioeconomic status (James et al., 1992; Strogatz et al., 1997), and between suicide and socioeconomic status (Lester, 1998; Stack, 1998; Fernquist, 2001) among Black men. Some of these associations are the opposite of what is found among Black women or among Whites. If the stress–mental health relation worked similarly for both Blacks and Whites and was most evident among lower income households, we would definitely expect to see a higher level of psychiatric morbidity in the Black population to the extent that stress is causally related.[3] However, the different patterns of stress among Blacks (particularly males) combined with the different distribution of socioeconomic status characteristics could effectively "wash out" any differential effects. Another theory to consider, though not yet published, has been put forth by James Jackson at the University of Michigan. In short, he argues that some Black people, compared to their White counterparts, have purchased good mental health with bad physical health. In other words, given all of the pressures of life and poverty, "I'm going to find joy even in the midst of the storm."

More recently, studies on discrimination effects have begun to explore the link between perceived discrimination and physical health using the chronic stress model postulated in the medical literature (Sapolsky, 1994; McEwen, 1998; Solarz, 1999). According to this paradigm, stress evokes the "fight or flight" response that involves release of additional hormones. Pulse acceleration, respiratory increases, and slowing of the digestive process are all physical responses to the higher hormone levels. These changes can be adaptive when facing short-lived but immediate danger. However, chronic stress can lead to overexposure to stress hormones, resulting in high blood pressure/hypertension, accelerated arteriosclerosis, calcium loss from bone (among those with depression), and cognitive impairment (McEwen, 1998). The health effects of stress are thought to be so pervasive that some scholars argue that stress is causally implicated in virtually all chronic illness, including diabetes, HIV/AIDS, and asthma (Sapolsky, 1994).

---

[3]About 43% of Black households earn less than $25,000 annually compared to 26% of White households (U.S. Census Bureau, 1998).

Using this paradigm, a number of researchers have found associations between perceived discrimination (stigma-related stressors) and physical health. Pavalko and colleagues (2003), for example, recently established that women at midlife who perceived themselves to be the object of job discrimination were 50% more likely to develop physical limitations several years down the road. Their research was longitudinal to rule out the possibility that the limitations were actually causing the perceived discrimination.

Kreiger and Sidney (1996) found that systolic blood pressure was independently associated with both self-reported racial discrimination and coping strategies among Black young adults. In an earlier study, Kreiger (1990) found a similar relation between self-reported discrimination and self-reported hypertension among Black adults in Oakland, California.

Given the positive association between education and perceived discrimination among Black Americans and the positive association between socioeconomic status and stress among Black men, stigma-related stress could explain the reversal of the socioeconomic gradient on the health of Black men compared to broader population studies (Adler & Boyce, 1994; Williams, 2003). Williams (2003) has shown that middle class Black men are an anomaly in that they do not show the expected advantages in health status that middle class White men show vis-à-vis their lower socioeconomic counterparts. Black men with a college degree, for example, have higher levels of hypertension than those with only some college education (Hypertension Detection and Follow Up Program, 1977). Although income is inversely associated with hypertension among Black women, there is no association between income and hypertension among Black men (Pamuk et al., 1998) despite findings that suggest that college-educated Black men have lower hypertension behavioral risk factors (cigarette smoking, physical inactivity, excess weight) compared to Black men with only a high school degree (Diez-Roux et al., 1999). Suburban residence is associated with higher mortality risks for Black men but lower mortality risks for White men and women (House et al., 2000). In his review of these data, Williams (2003) identified three potential sources of stress that may help explain the excess health burden of higher socioeconomic status Black men: their increased exposure to racial discrimination, the "recent, tenuous and marginal" nature of middle class status, and unfilled expectations due to the lower-than-expected socioeconomic status "returns" they receive for their educational investment (p. 725).

To our knowledge, no work has been done on the relation between physical morbidity and perceived discrimination among the LGB or the Black LGB population. In fact, there is little research even documenting the extent and type of health disparities affecting Black LGBs. In one of the few studies to compare health between a Black homosexually active population and the Black population at large, Mays et al. (2002) found that Black lesbians in Los Angeles county were more likely to rate their health as poor or fair, to be overweight or obese, or to smoke or be heavy drinkers than a racially and demographically matched sample of women in the same area. They were also less likely to be insured, to have a regular source of health care, and to have been checked for high cholesterol (past 5 years) or had a Pap test (past 2 years) or a clinical breast examination (past 2 years). On the other hand, there were no statistically significant differences in prevalence rates for hypertension, asthma, arthritis, cardiovascular problems, or diabetes (though these conditions may be more likely to go undiagnosed among the uninsured). The lesbians were more likely to have had their blood pressure checked during the past year and to be taking medication if they had hypertension. Thus, despite higher risk factors and lower access to care, Black lesbians did not seem to be in appreciably worse health, suggesting the possibility of protective mechanisms. This possibility is worth investigation. However, if indeed Black lesbians, on average, have learned to navigate oppression more successfully, this should in no way displace efforts to challenge the structures that oppress Black lesbians and others in the first place.

Thus, it seems clear that perceived discrimination among both LGBs and Blacks has negative health consequences. Black lesbians face the additional challenge of coping with gender-related discrimination and stress. This leads to a number of research questions. Does multiple marginalization have a multiplicative effect on experiencing stigma-related stress? Do multiple "sources" of stigma-related stressors lead to compromised mental or physical health faster or with more intensity? Or, do multiple forms of marginalization bring additional coping mechanisms that can be adapted to deal with different types of stigma?

Kreiger (2000a) notes that studies on discrimination and health need to address a number of persistent methodologic problems. Such problems include the lack of a standardized, validated instrument for measuring discrimination (which she argues should include the time period, domain, intensity, and frequency of exposure), measurement issues related to susceptibility, and investigation of likely effect modifications (Kreiger, 2000a).

Internalization of stigma has not necessarily worked in the ways that social psychologists originally envisioned, and here Goffman's (1963) distinctions between the "discredited" (those whose stigma is observable) and the "discreditable" (those whose stigma is not immediately apparent) may be germane. For those with discreditable stigma (same-sex sexual preferences, for example), the task of managing stigma, according to Goffman, is one of managing information. Thus, "hiding" an LGB identity, in this framework, is a strategy for managing the homosexual stigma. For the discredited (race), the task is managing tension in social interactions. For example, a casually dressed Black man may feel compelled to "prove" he is not a threat when entering a predominantly White environment, or a professional Black woman might feel she needs to manage others' embarrassment or discomfort when they realize that she is the attorney, not the secretary they assumed.

These differences may affect stress, coping ability, and the likelihood of internalizing the stigma. For decades, social psychologists chased the holy grail of "proving" that the stigmatized suffered from lower self-esteem. Taking their cue from symbolic interactionists (Mead, 1934;

Cooley, 1956), they argued that members of stigmatized groups must have lower self-esteem because their sense of identity was at least in part constructed from their perspective of how the "generalized other" evaluated them. Erikson (1956) and Allport (1954/1979) argued that through internalization of stereotypes the stigmatized were plagued with feelings of worthlessness and self-hate. In their review of studies on self-esteem and stigma, however, Crocker and Major (1989) found that prejudice does not generally lead to lower self-esteem among those from stigmatized groups. Their review covered more than 20 years of research and a wide range of stigmatized groups. With respect to Blacks, they found that levels of self-esteem were equal to and in some cases higher than levels of self-esteem among Whites.[4] Studies among homosexuals showed that self-esteem was "not consistently lower" (Crocker & Major, 1989, p. 611).

Although stigma may not result in lower global self-esteem among Black Americans, the protective mechanisms through which they maintain their self-esteem in the face of persistent discrimination appear to have their own costs. For example, Crocker et al. (1998a) theorized that Black students "disengage" their self-esteem from achievement in a particular domain if they suspect that the domain is "biased." Major and colleagues (1998) were able to show in a series of studies that when Black students perceived that intellectual tests might be biased their self-esteem was "immune" to test performance feedback, compared to White students, whose self-esteem fluctuated with feedback on their test performance. Crocker et al. (1998) call the short-term severing of self-esteem and achievement in a particular domain "disengagement." Over time it can lead to "disidentification" or a longer-term adaptation of removing a particular domain from their personal identity. They point out that disidentification in a particular domain suppresses motivation, regardless of talent, and leads to "systematic group differences in aspirations, skills and achievements, even when individual capabilities do not warrant these differences" (p. 530).

In another study, Steele and Aronson (1995) demonstrated the pernicious effects of a stigma stressor they call "stereotype threat." When given an intellectual test that both Black and White students were told was "just a laboratory exercise," Black and White students scored equally well (controlling for other factors such as socioeconomic status). Black students performed lower than White students, however, when given the same test and told that the test measured intellectual ability. Steele and Aronson argue that Blacks know they are stereotyped in the domain of intellectual achievement and that the threat of being evaluated stereotypically or of having their own behavior reinforce the stereotype was enough, in the absence of any overt discrimination, to raise self-doubt and jeopardize academic performance. The process

---

[4]Marketers are beginning to ponder the implications of differential self-esteem among youth. The *Wall Street Journal* recently reported on a large-scale study, released by Viacom, Inc.'s Nickelodeon, in which researchers found that Black children had the highest levels of self-esteem and perceived efficacy of the ethnic groups studied. (*Wall Street Journal*, Marketplace page, June 18, 2004.)

through which their performance was jeopardized was elucidated through part of the experiment. Students completed word fragments and were asked to indicate their race on an optional questionnaire. Black students who were told the test was diagnostic completed a higher number of word fragments with race-related and self-doubt related words than Black students in the nondiagnostic and control groups. They also were less likely to volunteer race information. White students' responses were unaffected by the test description. Thus, although stigma may not result in reduced global self-esteem, it is clear that it can affect self-doubt and efficacy in specific contexts. Furthermore, the costs of maintaining self-esteem are high. In commenting on Steele and Aronson's work, Link and Phelan (2001) noted how the psychosocial process of stereotype threat contributes to structural discrimination. They argued that the mere existence of a stereotype calls into question the "objective" nature of the test. Because a perceived stereotype undermines the validity of the test results for Black students, use of the test as "objective" in fact systematically discriminates against Black students.

How these dynamics affect the Black LGB population is an area for investigation. For example, Black LGBs may have race identity strategies that prevent the harmful internalization of race-related stigma, although, as we have seen, this can be a double-edged sword, as strategies that offer strong psychic benefits in one domain can, through stereotype threat, "bleed over" into structural disadvantage. As same-gender-loving people, have Black lesbians and gay men learned these same "protective identity strategies"? Or, does racism in the gay/lesbian community prevent them from drawing upon that community's social support? At the same time, are they more likely to internalize the stigma of homosexuality and "hide" their identity to prevent alienating themselves from the Black community? We now consider how identity management among Black LGBs helps or hinders their health and well-being.

3 Stigma, Identity, and Black LGB Well-Being

"Identity" is conceptualized as an important "buffer" that can mitigate the negative consequences flowing from stigmatization. Whereas in modern societies identities generally serve important functions in people's self-definition, self-expression, social affiliations, and sense of well-being (Lewin, 1948; Tajfel & Turner, 1979; Howard, 2000), strong identities are theorized to be especially important for members of stigmatized groups, serving as psychological, social, and political resources for coping with the stresses related to their stigmatized social status (Cass, 1979; Troiden, 1989; Icard, 1996; Lemert, 1997; Cross et al., 1998; Sellers et al., 1998b). Most of this literature focuses on psychosocial rather than structural pathways. Despite "self-acceptance" and "commitment" to the stigmatized group being frequently conceptualized as one of the highest stages of minority (race or sexual orientation) identity development, the relation between strong identities, social change, and structural discrimination is largely unexplored territory.

Although strong identities are seen as an asset, their salubrious effect is interfering with and "neutralizing" an otherwise negative process. In recent research, Ryff et al. (2003) found that minority status (race and ethnicity) was associated with stronger existential aspects of well-being, including the struggle for meaning and purpose in life and a sense of personal growth, autonomy, and mastery, thus establishing a positive and independent realm of mental health that is seemingly more available to members of stigmatized racial/ethnic communities than to those of White/majority status. Sexual orientation was not explored in this study.

How do these streams of research on stigma, discrimination, and identity management inform our understanding of the Black LGB community? Unfortunately, not as well as they should.

Research on identity management has also focused on one "identity" element at a time, failing to explore how those with multiple minority statuses manage to integrate elements of their various stigmatized identities. Thus, research on identity has been conducted on largely heterosexual Black populations and largely White gay populations, with only a handful of studies looking at the intersection of the two. Those who have written about the stresses associated with managing multiple stigmatized identities have done so largely from experience as clinicians or in qualitative research (Icard, 1986, 1996; Loiacano, 1989; Greene, 1994, 2000; Wilson & Miller, 2002). A number of themes have surfaced, including the experiencing of ethnic communities as heterosexist and of gay/lesbian communities as racist. Some have highlighted the pressure Black LGBs experience to "choose" between their identities and to negotiate different identities based on social context. Other themes are the conflict they encounter with their families and churches, the guilt they sometimes harbor due to normative judgments about homosexuality being a "White problem," and the historical, political, and cultural context for the Black community's marginalization of its own gay and lesbian members.

The omission of Black LGBs from the larger literature on identity and on stigma leaves a number of questions unexplored. To what extent, for example, do Black LGBs employ similar or different strategies for coping with racism and with heterosexism? If discrimination's effect is physically "embodied" in its victims, can strong identities provide protection from physical disease, even while larger efforts to eradicate discrimination continue? If being gay, lesbian, or bisexual *and* Black puts one in double jeopardy, is it possible that developing a strong "integrated" identity can be especially beneficial, providing individuals with a stronger sense of purpose and meaning in life? If so, what can the Black LGB community as well as the larger society learn from that experience?

3.1 Identity Management Among Black Americans

There are numerous identity models for race/ethnicity (see reviews by Phinney, 1990; Cross et al., 1991; Sellers et al., 1998b). W.E.B. Du Bois recognized as early as 1903, in the *Souls of Black Folk*, that Blacks could and did draw upon uniquely Black American cultural strengths to reconcile the "double consciousness" born of being Black in a White society that preaches freedom and practices slavery. One of the earliest racial/ethnic identity models (conceptualized as such) was Cross's Nigrescence model (1971). According to this model, the individual begins with low race salience. Then, as a result of some type of "encounter," the individual confronts the stigmatized nature of his/her race and begins to reevaluate his/her racial identity. During the immersion/emersion phase that follows the encounter phase, race identity is typically heightened, and out-group (White) evaluations tend to be negative. The final stage in Cross's Nigrescence model, called internalization/commitment, is a synthesized identity in which race is integrated with other aspects of an individual's identity, such as family, religious affiliation, profession, and avocation, among others (Cross, 2001).

Cross and others have asserted that there is a direct relation between an internalized Black identity and psychological health among Blacks (Parham, 1989; White & Parham, 1996; Cross et al., 1998). Empirical research using the Racial Identity Attitudes Scale (RIAS) has provided some support for this hypothesized link (Parham & Helms, 1985; Pyant & Yanico, 1991; Munford, 1994). Munford (1994), for example, found a relationship between "stage" variables and depressive symptoms, with internalization scores inversely correlated to depressive symptoms and earlier stages (preencounter, encounter, immersion-emersion) associated with elevated depressive symptoms.

The Cross model has been critiqued, however, for failing to explicate the pathway through which the link between identity and psychological functioning occurs and for the analytic inflexibility of a model that assumes a uniformity of attitudes in development stages and thus hampers the ability to explore such potential pathways (Caldwell et al., 2002). For example, as evidence of an inverse relation between stress and mental health mounted, researchers began to conceptualize discrimination as a type of stress and hypothesized how various coping mechanisms could mediate the relation between stress and psychological distress (Landrine & Klonoff, 1996; Miller & Kaiser, 2001; Sellers et al., 2001). Much of this work relied on the conceptual "stress and coping" framework provided earlier by Lazarus and Folkman (1984). As this framework was contextual rather than developmental, new and developmentally fluid models of racial identity emerged in which identity was conceptualized as multidimensional rather than progressive (Phinney, 1992; Sellers et al., 1998b). Sellers and his colleagues (1997, 1998b) proposed The Multidimensional Model of Racial Identity (MMRI), comprised of four dimensions, to explain the personal significance and meaning of being Black. In developing this model, Sellers drew upon two traditions of racial identity models: the mainstream tradition, which focuses primarily on the universal aspects of group identity, and the underground tradition, which focuses on the unique oppression and cultural experiences of Black Americans (Sellers et al., 1998b). The model's dimensions are race salience, centrality, regard, and ideology. Some of these dimensions are conceived as more enduring (e.g., ideology), whereas others are conceived as contextual (e.g., race centrality) (Shelton & Sellers, 2000). "Regard" incorporates both a sense of collective self-esteem, or how the individual evaluates his or her own race (private regard) as well as the "generalized other" perspective from the symbolic interactionist tradition; that is, how one thinks others regard one's race (public regard).

With the more flexible MMRI, researchers began to test the relation between specific dimensions of racial identity and mental health and the role of perceived stress as a potential mediator. In samples of Black high school and college students, for example, Rowley et al. (1998) found that high private regard was associated with high self-esteem, mediated by race centrality. That is, among those who had high race centrality there was an association between private regard and self-esteem, but no such association existed when race centrality was low. Caldwell et al. (2002) found that private regard and race centrality both influenced anxiety and depression among Black adolescents but indirectly through perceived stress. In their research, private regard was inversely related to perceived stress, as one might expect, but race centrality was positively related to perceived stress. Thus, the more central race was to the adolescent's identity, the more stress he or she perceived. Caldwell and her colleagues also found a positive relation between maternal support—the extent to which adolescents perceived that their mothers provided emotional, problem-solving, and moral support—and centrality and private regard. This finding led the authors to hypothesize that "an important part of African American mothers' social support relationships with their children implicitly [may include] transmissions about the significance and meaning of race, in efforts to enhance self-esteem and other competencies in their children" (p. 1331).

Finally, Sellers and his colleagues (2003), in one of the most direct tests of the "buffering" effects of identity, found that high race centrality, although indeed increasing the likelihood of experiencing race discrimination and therefore stress, also reduced the impact that discrimination had on psychological distress among Black youth. In other words, only among those for whom race was a *less* central part of identity was there a relation between perceived discrimination and psychological distress. Among those with *high* race centrality, the link between discrimination and distress was attenuated. Thus, the authors concluded that "the moderating effect of centrality can be interpreted as a protective effect in resilience theory," and that "young adults whose racial identity is central to their self-concept appear to be resilient in the face of risks posed for racial discrimination" (p. 312).

3.2 Sexual Orientation Models of Identity

Many sexual orientation models ignore bisexual identities, either explicitly or implicitly, and bisexuals are included in research inconsistently. They are more likely to be included in studies using same-gender sexual activity as sampling criteria rather than gay or lesbian identity or labeling. Yet behaviorally oriented samples that do not break out bisexuals from gays and lesbians may mask important differences in identity that could be insightful in terms of coping strategies.

Gay/lesbian identity models tend to be stage models that move from sexual identity confusion as the individual grapples with conflicting personal feelings, social norms, and internalized homophobia through identification of same-sex feelings/attractions and acceptance (self labeling), to identity pride/commitment for same-sex sexual orientation identity (see Eliason's review, 1996). Troiden (1993), building on the work of others, conceptualized the final, and presumably healthiest, stage of a same-sex sexual orientation identity as "committed." This stage includes disclosure of one's identity to the public and accepting a gay/lesbian identity as primary. Despite the predominance of the theme that "coming out" is a key process to psychological health and well-being, Cochran (2001) pointed to the lack of an abundance of empirical research to support this hypothesis. Much of the literature on mental health among the LGB population has focused on elevated levels of psychological distress associated with a same-sex sexual identity per se (Rosario et al., 2001; Savin-Williams, 2001; Savin-Williams & Ream, 2003) and not on associations between mental health and specific "stages" implied in the coming out process. Indeed, the latter research is difficult to operationalize as, assuming the model to be a true reflection of sexual orientation identity development, it would be difficult to obtain reliable samples of those exhibiting a same-sex sexual orientation before they have actually come to claim and have some comfort level with that identity.

Sexual orientation is also multidimensional, incorporating elements of same-sex sexual behavior, same-sex attraction, and gay/lesbian/bisexual identity and life-style (Sell 1997). Inconsistent operationalization of "homosexuality," particularly with respect to behavioral versus identity-based definitions, and difficulty using probability-based sampling techniques in this population have inhibited research that would lead to a clearer picture of how identity functions with respect to LGB psychological health. In a review of sampling methodologies used in 152 public health articles that included gay, lesbian, or bisexual populations from 1990 to 1992, Sell and Petrulio (1996) concluded that the authors "rarely conceptually defined the population they were sampling, used a variety of inconsistent methods to identify and select subjects, sampled from settings representative of dramatically different populations, and rarely used probability sampling" (p. 32).

3.3 Dual Identity Among Black LGBs

As we have seen, the identity development processes are different for race and for sexual orientation. Race identity begins early and Caldwell et al.'s study (2002) suggests that mothers play a deliberate role in cultivating race centrality and positive private regard, perhaps in intuitive recognition of their psychic benefits. This may help account for the high levels of self-esteem found among Black adolescents (Jordan, 2004) and for the lack of a relation between public regard (how one thinks others see their group) and mental health among Black youth (Sellers et al., 2003).

By contrast, the LGB population exhibits higher rates of major depression, generalized anxiety disorder, substance abuse/dependence, and suicide (see Cochran, 2001, for a review of sexual orientation and LGB mental health). It is unlikely that parents of LGBs deliberately try to instill protective aspects of a homosexual identity in their children. Indeed, it is unlikely that heterosexual parents envision their children as anything but hetereosexual until long after individuals have developed a same-sex sexual orientation manifested by attraction, behavior, and/or identity. LGBs, then, are likely to have internalized some of the larger society's homophobic attitudes, whereas Black parents may work to protect their children from internalizing the larger society's racist attitudes. Thus, emerging realization of sexual orientation is more likely to be met with shame or at least confusion initially rather than pride, making adolescence a particularly vulnerable time for LGBs (Cochran, 2001). Indeed, members of sexual orientation minorities may not have the same resources vis-à-vis identity formation that enable ethnic minorities to develop higher rates of existential well-being and purpose, as documented by Ryff et al. (2003).

Despite the importance of the "coming out" process in the LGB identity literature, most gay/lesbian models reflect Anglo/White experiences. The scant research on Black LGBs suggests that the "coming out" process for Black gay men is qualitatively different from that of White gay men. In research conducted by Dube and Savin-Williams (1999), for example, older Black gay men generally came to understand and label themselves as gay much later than would be suggested by the theoretical models. Younger Black gay men were more likely to understand themselves as gay *after* having had same-sex sexual encounters, whereas, in contrast, their White and Asian gay counterparts did so *before*. Furthermore, the young Black gay men were substantially less likely to have disclosed their sexual orientation to their families.

Comparisons of coming-out experiences and sexual practices between Black and White lesbians are even less well researched. Narrative literature among Black lesbians, however, emphasizes the importance of coming out and the indivisibility of their identity as Black and as lesbian (Lorde, 1984; Kitzinger, 1987). Catherine McKinley and L. Joyce Delaney published *Afrekete: An Anthology of Black Lesbian Writing* in 1995, and Lisa C. Moore began a publishing house, RedBone Press, featuring the work of Black lesbians. She has since edited *Does Your Mama Know? An Anthology of Lesbian Coming Out Stories* (1997) and published Sharon Bridgforth's *Bull Jean Stories* (1998). One Black lesbian, interviewed about the tumultuous decades of the 1960s and 1970s on the PBS special "Out!: Audre Lorde: A Litany for Survival," commented on the impact Audre Lorde's coming out had on her own identity. She said it made her realize that coming out was not just a rebellious reaction but was integral to survival itself.

For many Black LGBs, however, maintaining the "indivisibility" of identity is difficult. Black LGBs often feel the pressure to "choose" between what are perceived as conflicting identities: their "Black self" or their "LGB self." Experiencing gay/lesbian culture as White and hegemonic, ethnic minority gay men and lesbians feel a strong need for continued ties to their cultural communities (Icard 1986; Loiacano, 1989; Morales, 1992; Greene, 1994; Jackson & Brown, 1996). Psychologically, they cannot "afford" the rejection of the homophobic heterosexual world that is often posited as a "stage" in LGB identity development (Eliason, 1996) because the "homosexual world" does not deliver the same social and psychological benefits for them as it does to the White gay and lesbian community. This is reflected in a propensity for Black lesbians to maintain connections to the heterosexual community (including relationships with men) and to rely more heavily on their families for support than do White lesbians (Bass-Hass, 1968; Bell & Weinberg, 1978; Mays & Cochran, 1988; Greene, 1994; Jackson & Brown, 1996). This may also help explain the rejection of the "gay identity" among many Black men (Icard, 1996). Indeed, experiencing the LGB community as racist, gay Black men in particular may "disengage" from that community (Battle et al., 2003).

Although rarely documented empirically, assertions of racism in the LGB community are supported qualitatively by the experiences of many of the authors as practicing clinicians (Icard, 1986; Greene, 1994), by personal testimonials (Lorde, 1984; Asanti, 1997, 1998, 1999; Burstin, 1999; Herren 2001), and by depth interviews (Lociano, 1989; Mays et al., 1993; Jackson & Brown, 1996). Like racism in the larger culture, racism in gay/lesbian communities takes many forms, including prejudiced treatment (DeMarco, 1983; Icard 1986); invisibility, lack of acknowledgement, distortion, marginalization, and tokenism (Jackson & Brown, 1996); White standards of beauty (Loiacano, 1989); and sexual objectification or perceptions of exoticism (Burstin, 1999; Diaz et al., 2001). In one of the few large-scale empirical studies in the literature (Diaz et al., 2001), 62% of gay or bisexual Latino men reported feeling that they had been sexually objectified due to their race or ethnicity, and one in four (26%) reported feeling uncomfortable in spaces primarily attended by White gays.

3.4 Homophobia in Black and Ethnic Communities

The impact of racism in the gay and lesbian community on Black Americans and other ethnic minorities is double-edged because ethnic minority gay men and lesbians also face homophobia in their ethnic communities (Mays & Cochran, 1988, Chan, 1989; Greene, 1994; Jackson & Brown, 1996; Diaz et al., 2001).

In the Black community, homophobia is attributed to a variety of factors, many of which involve the legacy of slavery. These include a strong Christian heritage, which tends to view homosexuality as a "sin;" the need for Black women, historically perceived to be "at the bottom of the heap," to have another group relieve them of this dubious status; heightened need for "normalcy," as defined by the dominant culture, due to internalization of racist sexual myths and stereotypes; and a reaction to the perceived shortage of marriageable men in Black communities accompanied by strong pressure to continue the race (Greene, 1994; Blaxton, 1998; Fullilove, 1999).

Although the emphasis in the literature on homophobia in the Black community might lead one to suspect that this homophobia is *more* prevalent there than in the White community, a closer reading shows that this is unfounded. In-depth interviews revealed that Black lesbians and gay men who saw the Black community as "extremely homophobic" did not see it as any *more* homophobic than the White community (Loiacano, 1989). In Battle et al.'s (2002) study, Black LGBs rated their experiences with Black heterosexuals in straight Black organizations significantly more favorably than their experiences with White gays/lesbians in White gay organizations, yet expressed higher "agreement" with the statement that "homophobia is a problem within the Black community," than with the statement that "racism is a problem for GLBT Blacks dealing with the GLBT community." In that same study, Black LGBs were also more likely to say they had personally experienced discrimination or harassment as a result of their racial/ethnic identity than as a result of their sexual orientation. Thus, although respondents' personal experiences suggested that racism in the gay community was the more widespread problem, homophobia in the Black community was considered more problematic. Black homophobia is problematic not because of its *magnitude* but because of its *relevance*. Black LGBs cannot risk loss of the Black community's social support or of their racial identity because, as we have seen, these factors play too great a role in helping individuals deal with racism and discrimination in the dominant culture. Black LGBs have been prepared for racism. They have experienced managing the tension. They have strategies for reducing the stress of racial discrimination. They are not prepared, however, for facing the rejection and alienation that flow from the stigma of homosexuality, especially in the Black community. Yet managing the information to protect knowledge of their "discreditable status" in the Black community, to return to Goffman's lexicon, may create its own internalized tension, with consequences for health and well-being. Thus, some have suggested that Black gay men and lesbians may have a difficult time reaching a healthy gay or lesbian identity without harm to their ethnic identity (Akerlund & Cheung, 2000).

In reviewing literature on minority gay and lesbian issues from 1989 to 1998, Akerlund and Cheung (2000) found that discrimination, oppression, assimilation, rejection, and social support were key themes contributing to the challenge of identity formation. These themes are also echoed in Loiacano's (1989) earlier exploratory research on Black gay/lesbian identity development. His interviews with a sample of Black lesbians and gay men revealed three themes: the need to find validation in the gay and lesbian communities; the need to find validation in the Black community; the need to integrate identities.

One study of Black gay men has provided some empirical support for the healthful impact of a strong, integrated racial *and* sexual orientation. Crawford et al. (2002) measured both sexual orientation identity and racial identity among a group of Black gay men to test the hypotheses related to the healthful impact of strong identities on both dimensions. They found that men with strong "dual" identities (that is, men who scored high on both measures of ethnic identity and measures of sexual orientation identity) enjoyed a variety of mental health benefits compared to the other gay men in the sample. These benefits included less psychological stress, less gender role stress, higher life satisfaction and self-esteem, higher perceived social support, and higher confidence in preventing HIV infection. Vis-à-vis the men who had successfully developed and integrated strong identities across race and sexual orientation, those with strong race/ethnicity identities but weak sexual orientation identities suffered from increased gender role stress and reported fewer people in their social support system. Those who had strong sexual orientation identities and weak race/ethnic identities had lower life satisfaction, self-esteem, and HIV prevention self-efficacy compared to the those with strong dual identities. Those who were weak on both race/ethnic and sexual orientation identities were the most vulnerable, with significantly higher levels of psychological distress than those with strong dual identities.

Crawford and his colleagues (2002) also found that a strong identification with the cultural heritage of Black Americans was a far more powerful predictor of life satisfaction than attachment to a gay identity. They concluded that "sexual identity must be integrated with and accepted within the context of one's racial-ethnic identity" and that "current theories and interventions to facilitate African-American manhood and social development do not adequately address sexual orientation" (p. 187).

Crawford et al. (2002) demonstrated the benefits of a strong integrated identity, at least among Black men, but there is little research or guidance on how Black LGBs are to develop this strong integrated identity, as following either the sexual orientation identity model or the race/ethnicity identity model appears to have some risk to the other identity component in need of integration. In one of the few studies in which Black gay men's coping strategies for dealing with heterosexism was explored, Wilson and Miller (2002) identified six strategies, the contexts in which they were used, and the functions they fulfilled. "Role flexing" and "changing sexual behavior" were used to avoid stigma in nongay environments. Role flexing involved changing behaviors, mannerisms, and dress and sometimes using deceit to conceal one's sexual identity and blend in with the heterosexual culture. Another strategy used to avoid stigma in potentially homophobic environments was literally to change sexual behavior and abstain from homosexual sex. Although most of the respondents engaged in some type of role flexing, none was "gay abstinent" at the time of the research, although some had avoided sex with men earlier in their lives to avoid gay-related discrimination and stigma.

Wilson and Miller (2002) identified "keeping the faith" and "creating gay-only spaces" as strategies Black gay men used to "buffer" themselves against what they perceived to be inevitable discrimination. "Keeping the faith" helped respondents protect themselves from their own internalized homophobia. Spirituality offered grace and redemption, despite the church being experienced as homophobic. Creating gay spaces, on the other hand, allowed men to safely and openly express their affection and interest in other men, thereby providing some relief from having to "pass" in the heterosexual world. Some respondents were able to create Black gay spaces, sharing a bond with other Black gay men, whom they felt had a "special sort of identity" that "distinguish[ed them] from other gay men" (p. 384).

"Standing your ground," a strategy identified by Wilson and Miller (2002), involved speaking up and out against homophobia or using silence strategically but refusing to accept the need for identity concealment. Wilson and Miller (2002) argued that this strategy holds potential for fighting homophobia within the Black community.

Finally, "self-acceptance" was a strategy that cut across both gay-friendly and gay-unfriendly environments. Men who used this strategy refused to "accept" the oppression of heterosexism. They deliberately focused on developing positive attitudes about themselves as sexual minorities and were committed to "being themselves" regardless of context. They talked about the significance of age in coming to this self-affirming place in their identity. Wilson and Miller (2002) argued that this strategy can promote social change in gay-friendly and gay-unfriendly environments.

3.5 Being On the "Down-Low" in Context

Recently, there has been a growing controversy over the phenomenon known as being on the "down low." This has come to refer to (primarily Black) men who have gay or bisexual sexual practices but who do not disclose their behavior and/or do not identify as "gay." This topic has been recently explored most sensationally in J.L. King's (2004) partly autobiographic *On the Down Low: A Journey Into the Lives of "Straight" Black Men Who Sleep With Men*. This is hotly-contested terrain with few data to support the widespread pathologizing of Black men it has encouraged. For example, media images leave the impression that undercover bisexual activity is widespread in the Black community and responsible for the high rates of HIV infection among Black women, displacing the focus on poverty, which according to the Centers for Disease Control (CDC) is a far more significant driver of elevated HIV infection rates. Reliable, population-level data on Black gay men are scarce and somewhat inconsistent. However, in an effort to address this gap, we conducted analyses from findings published elsewhere.

For example, NHANES, a large-scale nationally representative, population-based survey conducted periodically by the National Center for Health Statistics of the CDC, collected information about the gender of men's lifetime sexual partners in its third wave (1988–1994). In NHANES III, a slightly elevated proportion of Black men claimed to have had sex with men at some point in their lives compared to White men (3.82% vs. 2.29%, $p = 0.06$) (Cochran & Mays, 2000).

In their analysis of data from the National AIDS Behavioral Survey (NABS), a random digit dialing (RDD) survey of 20 major metropolitan areas, Binson et al. (1995) found a significantly *lower* incidence of past 5-year same-sex behavior among Black men aged 18 to 49 compared to White men in the same age group (3.1 % vs. 9.1%; $p < 0.001$). Among men engaged in same-sex sexual behavior, however, there is evidence of a higher "prevalence" of bisexual behavior among Black men compared to White men (57% vs. 29%, $p = 0.02$) (Binson et al. 1995).

In MIDUS, a large, nationally representative study of the social and psychological determinants of health among Americans at midlife (25–74 years of age), respondents were asked to report their sexual orientation as heterosexual, homosexual, or bisexual—arguably a more "identity"-influenced measure than asking about specific sexual encounters with people of the same sex. These results indicate that 3.19% of White males identified as either homosexual or bisexual compared to only 1.31% of the males who were not White ($p = 0.03$) (Cochran et al., 2003). Unlike the NHANES study, MIDUS included information on sexual orientation for women as well as for men, and there is a striking gender difference in the relation between sexual orientation identity and race. Heterosexually identified men were much more likely to be "not White" (15.7%) compared to gay or bisexually identified men (of whom only 7% were "not White"). Among women, however, there was virtually no difference in how heterosexually identified women and gay or bisexually identified women profiled by race. For example, 16.2% of the heterosexual women were classified as "not White" compared to 17.5% of the gay/bisexual women.

Although these results need to be confirmed with larger base sizes for Black LGBs and with behavioral and identity questions in the same survey, the pattern suggests that comparable or perhaps even lower proportions of Black men (given a recent history, rather than a lifetime history) engage in same-sex sexual behavior compared to White men but that fewer minority men, generally, *identify* as gay. Because these studies did not include definitions of identity and behavior among the same respondents, it is not clear if a higher proportion of Black men who were engaged in same-sex sexual behavior did not *identify* as gay compared to White men engaged in same-sex sexual behavior. In other words, the data are somewhat opaque in terms of the relation between identity and behavior in the Black LGB community and thus to what extent and how different operational definitions of LGB affect measurement.

Despite their limitations, these data do suggest that in the homosexually active Black male community a somewhat higher prevalence of bisexual activity prevails. One hypothesis is, of course, that the higher rates of bisexual activity among Black men who have sex with men is the result of the "role flexing" strategies discussed by Black gay men in Wilson and Miller's study (2002). This implies that the bisexual activity is not "genuine" in terms of a dual sexual orientation but is the result of a weak sexual orientation identity. Whether role flexing among Black men who have sex with other men is associated with the elevated HIV/AIDS rates among Black women is an open question. It would be premature to focus on Black male bisexual activity as the primary causal explanation for the elevated HIV/AIDS rates among Black women. First, the overall population of Black men engaging in bisexual behavior is relatively small. Additionally, these data speak neither to the HIV/AIDS prevention practices nor to identity. Thus, within the small segment of bisexually active Black men, some undoubtedly practice safe sex. Furthermore, and equally important—though all too often ignored—most bisexually active men are not HIV-positive. There is clearly a need for sound social epidemiologic research in this area. However, Black men generally and Black gay men specifically are easy targets for pathologizing. Black women have the highest price to pay if we misallocate our focus and resources on Black male bisexual activity as the sole or primary "cause" of the HIV/AIDS disparity, missing potentially more fundamental causes. Furthermore, any risk associated with bisexual activity underscores how important it is, not just for Black gay men but also for the larger Black community, to create a more accepting and affirming environment for Black gay men, thereby eliminating the need for role flexing. As Crawford, et al. (2002) have shown, development of a strong cultural identity but a weak sexual orientation identity among Black men who have sex with other men results in high gender role stress and weak social support, whereas those with high sexual orientation identity but weak cultural identity have low perceived HIV prevention efficacy.

Most important to this discussion of the "down low" and HIV/AIDS, as eloquently articulated by Keith Boykin (2005) in his recent book, *Beyond The Down Low: Sex, Lies, and Denial in Black America*:

We cannot limit our concern to the surface issues that lead to HIV infection. We—the government, the church, the community, the family—have to deal with deeper socioeconomic conditions . . . we have to deal with jobs, health care, education, homelessness, poverty, drugs, and the disproportionate incarceration of minorities. We have to deal with racism, sexism, classism, misogyny, homophobia, heterosexism, and cultural imperialism [p. 179].

4 Black LGB Health and Well-Being: An Agenda

In terms of the overall health and well-being of the Black LGB community, several overarching issues remain.

First, what are the health and mental health disparities affecting the Black LGB population? Much groundwork is needed just to document and map the issues, and we need to go beyond HIV/AIDS as the only disease of concern. Certainly, areas where Blacks or LGBs are known to be affected by disparities in health outcomes are prime areas for investigation (e.g., hypertension, diabetes, depression, anxiety).

Second, what are the socioeconomic, environmental, and psychosocial pathways through which elevated (or reduced) risk is generated among Black LGBs, and how do they differ as a function of dual marginalization? Compared to the Black population, how much of any health disparity is "explained" by sexual orientation? Similarly, compared to the LGB population, how much of any health disparity can be "explained" by race, above and beyond good socioeconomic status controls? Good socioeconomic status controls may explain less of health disparities than other social disparities (e.g., education, employment) because of the reversal in the socioeconomic status gradient and health among Black men. It would be ironic indeed if by improving material conditions for Black men we *reduced* health owing to increased exposure to interpersonal discrimination and other stigma-related stressors. Such a finding would underscore the need to address racism in both its structural and psychosocial manifestations.

Third, what are the processes through which Black LGBs develop strong identities that integrate their race/cultural heritage and their sexual orientation? What coping mechanisms are facilitated by a strong integrated identity? Do they help attenuate the psychosocial or the more structural effects of discrimination? What are the risks of more situational identity strategies or of disidentification with either LGB, Black, or other cultural communities? Can a self-acceptance strategy—a conscious refusal of the stigma of homosexuality—help Black LGBs access the same eudemonia or sense of well-being, purpose, and growth that Ryff et al. (2003) found to be associated with ethnic minority status? Can such a strategy result in social change, thereby helping to improve the health and well-being of the larger Black LGB community beyond individual effects?

It is critical that research among Black LGBs treat men and women independently. As we have seen, in the race-related health disparities literature, there is considerable heterogeneity of effects by gender. These disparities relate not only to differences in the relation between socioeconomic status and stress (Williams, 2003) but also to gendered differences in response to chronic discriminatory experiences among ethnic minorities (Ryff et al., 2003). Additionally, the marked differences in how Black men and women self-identify as gay, lesbian, or bisexual may reflect different dynamics in how they construct their personal identities as they relate to sexual preference.

Finally, although coping mechanisms and resiliency are important, we can not lose sight, as Kreiger (2001) warns, of who is throwing whom into the water. Research and action needs to be directed against racism (both structural and interpersonal) and homophobia. Greater visibility of LGBs in the Black community, particularly in Black churches, might help build tolerance while at the same time making a Black LGB "network" more accessible as a means of social support, thereby facilitating self-acceptance strategies.

5 Freedom Struggles, Health, and Beyond Black LGBs

Having assessed the significance of the literature for the health and well-being of Black LGBs, we now return to the issue of how the experiences of Black LGBs can inform larger struggles for freedom.

Black American LGBs are at an intersection of two very important struggles: the Civil Rights movement and the Gay Rights movement.

The worldwide impact and import of these movements in liberating millions cannot be understated. For example, in 1977 at the first federally funded national women's conference, drawing on the spirit of the Civil Rights movement, women from all walks of life joined hands and sang "We Shall Overcome." In 1989, during their rebellion, the students in Tiananmen Square, China made constant references to Black America's struggle during the 1950s and 1960s. Later that same year when the Berlin wall fell in Germany, posters were carried signifying "I AM A MAN," a slogan used during the Civil Rights era. Several months later when Nelson Mandela was released, South African supporters gathered around him and sang "Aint Gonna Let Nobody Turn Me Around." During East Timor's independence celebrations on May 20, 2002, former President Bill Clinton participated as their citizens sang "Freedom . . . before I'll be a slave, I'll be buried in my grave," yet another song cadenced during the Civil Right movement.

In 1969, for any number of reasons a group of gay men and lesbian women (including people of color) stood their ground and said no to police and state-sanctioned oppression and discrimination. This began what many have called the beginning of the Gay Rights movement in the United States. The Stonewall rebellion is now legendary and has served as inspiration for sexual minorities the world over in their struggles for independence and freedom, including those in South Africa, the only country in the world where same-gender loving rights are protected in a national constitution.

We have seen the many pathways through which stigma destroys the health and well-being of individuals and results in population-level health disparities. In this context, these freedom movements are important, not only from political and economic perspectives but from a basic health perspective as well, underscoring the breadth and power of basic human rights issues. It is our contention that freedom movements are essential to eliminating stigma and its pernicious health effects and that, conversely, understanding the causal role of stigma in the ill health of populations can also provide powerful impetus to these movements. Again, taking the standpoint theorist point of view, we are convinced that whatever can be done to empower and strengthen the physical, mental, and political (though the political is beyond the scope of this chapter) health of Black LGBs will also prove instrumental in empowering and strengthening *all* people, regardless of social, geographic, cultural, or political location.

References

Adler, N., and Boyce, T.W. (1994) Socioeconomic status and health: the challenge of the gradient. *American Psychologist* 49:15–24.

Akerlund, M., and Cheung, M. (2000) Teaching beyond the deficit model: gay and lesbian issues among African Americans, Latino, and Asian Americans. *Journal of Social Work Education* 36:279–293.

Allport, G.W. (1954/1979) *The Nature of Prejudice*. Addison-Wesley, Reading, MA.

Asanti, T. (1997) Black lesbians and interracial love. *Lesbian News* 23(2):32.

Asanti, T. (1998) Black lesbians: why can't we be friends? *Lesbian News* 23(7):24.

Asanti, T. (1999) Racism in the 21st century: how will the lesbian and gay community respond? *Lesbian News* 24(9):24.

Badgett, M.V.L. (1995) The wage effects of sexual orientation discrimination. *Industrial and Labor Relations Review* 48:726–739.

Badgett, M.V.L. (2000) The myth of gay and lesbian affluence. *Gay and Lesbian Review Worldwide* 7(2):22–25.

Bass-Hass, R. (1968) The lesbian dyad: basic issues and value systems. *Journal of Sex Research* 4:126.

Battle, J., Cohen, C., Warren, D., Fergerson, G., and Audam, S. (2002) *Say it loud: I'm Black and I'm proud; Black pride survey 2000*. The Policy Institute of the National Gay and Lesbian Task Force, New York.

Battle, J., Cohen, C., Harris, A., and Richie, B. (2003) We really are family: embracing our lesbian, gay, bisexual, and transgender (LGBT) family members. In: *The State of Black America*. National Urban League, Washington, DC, pp. 93–106.

Bell, A., and Weinberg, M. (1978) *Homosexualities: a study of human diversity among men and women*. Simon & Schuster, New York.

Binson, D., Michaels, S., Stall, R., and Coates, T.J. (1995) Prevalence and social distribution of men who have sex with men: United States and its urban centers. *Journal of Sex Research* 32:245–254.

Blaxton, R.G. (1998) "Jesus wept": Black churches and HIV. *Harvard Gay and Lesbian Review* 4:13–16.

Boykin, K. (2005) *Beyond the down low: sex, lies, and denial in Black America*. Carroll & Graf, New York.

Bridgforth, S. (1998) *The bull-Jean stories*. RedBone Press, Washington, DC.

Burstin, H.E. (1999) Looking out, looking in: anti-Semitism and racism in lesbian communities. *Journal of Homosexuality* 36:143–157.

Business Week. (2003) Black progress: two ways to look at it. July 14, 2003, issue 3841.

Caldwell, C., Zimmerman, M., Bernat, D., Sellers, R., and Notaro, P. (2002) Racial identity, maternal support and psychological distress among African American adolescents. *Child Development* 73:1322–1336.

Cass, V.C. (1979) Homosexual identity formation: a theoretical model. *Journal of Homosexuality* 4:219–235.

Cassel, J. (1976) The contribution of the social environment to host resistance. *American Journal of Epidemiology* 104:107–123.

CDC (Centers for Disease Control and Prevention). (2004) Self-reported frequent mental distress among adults—United States, 1993–2001. *MMWR Morbidity and Mortality Weekly Report* 53(41).

Chan, C. (1989) Issues of identity development among Asian-American lesbians and gay men. *Journal of Counseling and Development* 68:16–20.

Clark, R., Anderson, N.B., Clark, V.R., and Williams, D.R. (1999) Racism as a stressor for African Americans: a biopsychosocial model. *American Psychologist* 54:805–816.

Cochran, S.D. (2001) Emerging issues in research on lesbians and gay men's mental health: does sexual orientation really matter? *American Psychology* 56:931–947.

Cochran, S.D., and Mays, V.M. (2000) Lifetime prevalence of suicide symptoms and affective disorders among men reporting same-sex sexual partners: results from NHANES III. *American Journal of Public Health* 90:573–578.

Cochran, S.D., Sullivan, J.G., and Mays, V.M. (2003) Prevalence of mental disorders, psychological distress, and mental health services use among lesbian, gay, and bisexual adults in the United States. *Journal of Consulting and Clinical Psychology* 71:53–61.

Collins, C.A., and Williams, D.R. (1999) Segregation and mortality: the deadly effects of racism? *Sociological Forum* 14:495–523.

Collins, P.H. (2003) Some group matters: intersectionality, situated standpoints, and black feminist thought. In: Lott, T.L., and Pittman, J.P. (eds) Blackwell companion to African American philosophy. Blackwell, Oxford, pp. 205–229.

Conley, D. (1999). *Being Black, living in the red: race, wealth and social policy in America.* University of California Press, Berkeley.

Cooley, C.H. (1956) *Human nature and the social order.* Free Press, New York.

Council of Economic Advisers for the President's Initiative on Race. (1998) *Changing America: indicators of social and economic well-being by race and Hispanic origin.* CEAPIR, Washington, DC.

Crawford, I., Allison, K., Zamboni, B., and Soto, T. (2002) The influence of dual-identity development on the psychosocial functioning of African American gay and bisexual men. *The Journal of Sex Research* 39:179–189.

Crocker, J., and Major, B. (1989) Social stigma and self-esteem: the self-protective properties of stigma. *Psychological Review* 96:608–630.

Crocker, J., Major, B., and Steele, C. (1998) Social stigma. In: Gilbert, D., Fiske, S.T., and Lindzey, G. (eds) *The handbook of social psychology,* 4th ed. McGraw-Hill, Boston, pp. 504–553.

Cross, W.E. (1971) The Negro-to-Black conversion experience. *Black World* 20(9):13–27.

Cross, W.E. (2001) The psychology of Nigrescence. In: Ponterotto, J.G., Casas, J.M., Suzuki, L.A., and Alexander, C.M. (eds) *Handbook of multicultural counseling.* Sage, London, pp. 93–122.

Cross, W.E., Parham, T.A., and Helms, J.E. (1991) The stages of Black identity development: nigrescence models. In: Jones, R. (ed) *Black psychology.* Cobb & Henry, Oakland, pp. 319–338.

Cross, W.E., Parham, T.A., and Helms, J.E. (1998) Nigrescence revisited: theory and research. In: Jones, R.L. (ed) *African American identity development: theory, research, and intervention.* Cobb & Henry, Hampton, VA.

Darity, W.A., Jr. (1998) Intergroup disparity: economic theory and social science evidence. *Southern Economic Journal* 64:805–826.

Darity, W., and Myers, S. (1998) *Persistent disparity: race and economic inequality in the United States since 1945.* Edward Elgar, Northhampton, MA.

Darity, W.A., Jr., Guilkey, D.K., and Winfrey, W. (1996) Explaining differences in economic performance among racial and ethnic groups in the USA: the data examined. *American Journal of Economics and Sociology* 55:411–425.

DeMarco, J. (1983) Gay racism. In: Smith, M.J. (ed) *Black men/white men: a gay anthology.* Gay Sunshine Press, San Francisco, pp. 109–118.

Diaz, R., Ayala, G., Bein, E., Henne, J., and Marin, B. (2001) The impact on homophobia, poverty, and racism on the mental health of gay and bisexual Latino men: findings from 3 US cities. *American Journal of Public Health* 91:927–933.

Diez-Roux, A.V., Northbridge, M.E., Morabia, A., Bassett, M.T., and Shea, S. (1999) Prevalence and social correlates of cardiovascular disease risk factors in Harlem. *American Journal of Public Health* 89:302–307.

DiPlacido, J. (1998) Minority stress among lesbians, gay men, and bisexuals: a consequence of heterosexism, homophobia, and stigmatization. In: Herek, G.M. (ed) *Stigma and sexual orientation: understanding prejudice against lesbians, gay men, and bisexuals.* Sage, Thousand Oaks, CA, pp. 138–159.

Dube, E.M., and Savin-Williams, R.C. (1999) Sexual identity development among ethnic sexual-minority male youths. *Developmental Psychology* 35:1389–1398.

Eliason, M.J. (1996) Identity formation for lesbian, bisexual and gay persons: beyond a "minoritizing" view. *Journal of Homosexuality* 30(3):31–58.

Epstein, H. (2003) There's a killer haunting America's inner cities: not drugs, not handguns, but . . . stress? The new ghetto miasma. *The New York Times Magazine* October 12, 2003.

Erikson, E. (1956) The problem of ego-identity. *Journal of the American Psychoanalytic Association* 4:56–121.

Fernquist, R.M. (2001) Education, race/ethnicity, age, sex and suicide: individual-level data in the United States. *Current Research in Social Psychology* 3:277–290.

Forman, T.A., Williams, D.R., and Jackson, J.S. (1997) Race, place, and discrimination. In: Gardner, C. (ed) *Perspectives on social problems*, Vol. 9. JAI Press, New York, pp. 231–261.

Fullilove, M.T. (1999) Stigma as an obstacle to AIDS action: the case of the Black community. *American Behavioral Scientist* 42:1117–1129.

Gilman, S.E., Cochran, S.D., Mays, V.M., Hughes, M., Ostrow, D., and Kessler, R. (2001) Risk of psychiatric disorders among individuals reporting same sex sexual partners in the national comorbidity survey. *American Journal of Public Health* 91:933–939.

Goffman, E. (1963) *Stigma: notes on the management of spoiled identity.* Touchstone, New York.

Greene, B. (1994) Ethnic-minority lesbians and gay men: mental health and treatment issues. *Journal of Consulting and Clinical Psychology* 62:243–251.

Greene, B. (2000) African American lesbian and bisexual women. *Journal of Social Issues* 56:239–249.

Hacker, A. (2003) *Two nations: black and white, separate, hostile, unequal.* Scribner, New York.

Herek, G., and Glunt, E. (1995) Identity and community among gay and bisexual men in the AIDS era: preliminary findings from the Sacramento Men's Health Study. In: Herek, G., and Greene, B. (eds) *AIDS, identity, and community: the HIV epidemic and lesbians and gay men.* Sage, Thousand Oaks, CA, pp. 55–84.

Herren, G. (2001) I don't discuss myself in halves: frank words from James Earl Hardy about racism, homophobia, Hip-Hop and shopping at Macy's. *Lambda Book Report* 10(2):7–9.

House, J.S., Lepkowski, J.M., Williams, D.R., Moro, R.P., Lantz, P.M., Robert, S.A., and Chaw, J. (2000) Excess mortality among urban residents: how much, for whom, and why? *American Journal of Public Health* 90:1898–1904.

Howard, J.A. (2000) Social psychology of identities. *Annual Review of Sociology* 26:267–393.

Hypertension Detection and Follow-Up Program Cooperative Group. (1977) Race, education and prevalence of hypertension. *American Journal of Epidemiology* 106:351–361.

Icard, L. (1986) Black gay men and conflicting social identities: sexual orientation versus racial identity. In: Gripton, J., and Valentich, M. (eds) *Journal of Social Work & Human Sexuality* 4(112):83–93 [special issue].

Icard, L. (1996) Assessing the psychosocial well being of African American gays: a multidimensional perspective. *Journal of Gay and Lesbian Social Services* 5(2/3):25–49.

Jackson, J.S., Brown, T.N., Williams, D.R., Torres, M., Sellers, R.L., and Brown, K. (1996) Racism and the physical and mental health status of African Americans: a thirteen year national panel study. *Ethnicity and Disease* 6:132–147.

Jackson, K., and Brown, L. (1996) Lesbians of African heritage: coming out in the straight community. *Journal of Gay and Lesbian Social Services* 5(4):53–61.

James, S.A., Keenan, N.L., Strogatz, D.S., Browning, S.R., and Garrett, J.M. (1992) Socioeconomic status, John Henryism, and blood pressure in Black adults: the Pitt County study. *American Journal of Epidemiology* 135:59–67.

Jones, C.P. (2000) Levels of racism: a theoretic framework and a gardener's tale. *American Journal of Public Health* 90:1212–1215.

Jordan, M. (2004) Ethnic diversity doesn't blend in kids' lives. *Wall Street Journal* Marketplace page, June 18.

Kaufman, J.S., Cooper, R.S., and McGee, D.L. (1997) Socioeconomic status and health in blacks and whites: the problem of residual confounding and the resiliency of race. *Epidemiology* 8:621–628.

King, J.L. (2004) *On the down low: a journey into the lives of "straight" Black men who sleep with men.* Broadway Books, New York.

Kitzinger, C. (1987) *The social construction of lesbianism.* Sage, London.

Krieger, N. (1990) Racial and gender discrimination: risk factors for high blood pressure? *Social Science Medicine* 12:1273–1281.

Kreiger, N. (2000a) Discrimination and health. In: Berkman, L.F., and Kawachi, I. (eds) *Social epidemiology.* Oxford University Press, New York, pp. 36–75.

Krieger, N. (2000b) Epidemiology and social sciences: towards a critical reengagement in the 21st century. *Epidemiologic Reviews* 22:155–163.

Krieger, N. (2001) Theories for social epidemiology in the 21st century: an ecosocial perspective. *International Journal of Epidemiology* 30:668–677.

Krieger, N., and Sidney, S. (1996) Racial discrimination and blood pressure: the CARDIA study of young Black and White adults. *American Journal of Public Health* 86:1370–1378.

Krieger, N., Rowley, D.L., Herman, A.A., Avery, B., and Philip, M.T. (1993) Racism, sexism, and social class: implications for studies of health, disease, and well-being. *American Journal of Preventive Medicine* 9:82–122.

Landrine, H., and Klonoff, E.A. (1996) The schedule of racist events: a measure of racial discrimination and a study of its negative physical and mental health consequences. *Journal of Black Psychology* 22:144–168.

Lazarus, R.S., and Folkman, S. (1984) *Stress, appraisal, and coping.* Springer, New York.

Lemert, C. (1997) *Postmodernism is not what you think.* Blackwell, Malden, MA.

Lester, D. (1998) *Suicide in African Americans.* Nova Science, Commack, NY.

Lewin, K. (1948) *Resolving social conflicts.* Harper, New York.

Link, B.G., and Phelan, J.C. (2001) Conceptualizing stigma. *Annual Review of Sociology* 27:363–385.

Loiacano, D. (1989) Gay identity issues among black Americans: racism, homophobia and the need for validation. *Journal of Counseling and Development* 68:21–25.

Lorde, A. (1984) *Sister outsider.* The Crossing Press Feminist Series. Crossing Press, Trumansburg, NY.

Major, B., Spencer, S., and Schmader, T. (1998) Coping with negative stereotypes about intellectual performance: the role of psychological disengagement. *Personality & Social Psychology Bulletin* 24:34–50.

Mays, V., and Cochran, S. (1988) The Black women's relationship project: a national survey of Black lesbians. In: Shernoff, M., and Scott, W. (eds) *The sourcebook on lesbian/gay health care,* 2nd ed. National Lesbian and Gay Health Foundation, Washington, DC, pp. 54–62.

Mays, V.M., and Cochran, S.D. (2001) Mental health correlates of perceived discrimination among lesbian, gay, and bisexual adults in the United States. *American Journal of Public Health* 91:1869–1876.

Mays, V.M., Cochran, S.D., and Rhue, S. (1993) The impact of perceived discrimination on the intimate relationships of black lesbians. *Journal of Homosexuality* 25:1–14.

Mays, V.M., Yancey, A.K., Cochran, S.D., Weber, M., and Fielding, J.E. (2002) Heterogeneity of health disparities among African American, Hispanic, and Asian American women: unrecognized influences of sexual orientation. *American Journal of Public Health* 92:632–639.

McEwen, B. (1998) Protective and damaging effects of stress mediators: allostatis and allostatic load. *New England Journal of Medicine* 338:171–179.

McKeown, T. (1976) *The modern rise of population.* Academic, Saw Diego.

McKinley, C.E., and DeLaney, L.J. (eds) (1995) *Afrekete: an anthology of Black lesbian writing.* Anchor Books, New York.

Mead, G.H. (1934) *Mind, self and society.* University of Chicago Press, Chicago.

Meyer, I.H. (1995) Minority stress and mental health in gay men. *Journal of Health and Social Behavior* 7:9–25.

Meyer, I.H. (2003) Prejudice, social stress, and mental health in lesbian, gay and bisexual populations: conceptual issues and research evidence. *Psychological Bulletin* 129:674–697.

Miller, C., and Kaiser, C. (2001) A theoretical perspective on coping with stigma. *Journal of Social Issues* 57:73–92.

Moore, L.C. (ed) (1998) *Does your mama know? An anthology of Black lesbian coming out stores.* Redbone, Washington, DC.

Morales, E. (1992) Latino gays and Latina lesbians. In: Dworkin, S., and Gutierrez, F. (eds) *Counseling gay men and lesbians: journey to the end of the rainbow.* American Association for Counseling and Development, Alexandria, VA, pp. 125–139.

Munford, M.B. (1994) Relationship of gender, self-esteem, social class, and racial identity to depression in blacks. *Journal of Black Psychology* 20:157–174.

Oliver, M.L., and Shapiro, T.M. (1997) *Black wealth/White wealth: a new perspective on racial inequality.* Routledge, New York.

Pamuk, E., Makuk, D. Heck, K., and Reuben, C. (1998) *Health, United States, 1998: with socioeconomic status and health chartbook.* National Center for Health Statistics, Hyattsville, MD.

Parham, T.A. (1989) Cycles of psychological nigrescence. *Counseling Psychologist* 17:187–226.

Parham, T.A., and Helms, J.E. (1985) Relation of racial identity attitudes to self-actualization and affective states of black students. *Journal of Counseling Psychology* 32:431–440.

Pavalko, E.K., Mossakowski, K.N., and Hamilton, V.J. (2003) Does perceived discrimination affect health? Longitudinal relationships between work discrimination and women's physical and emotional health. *Journal of Health and Social Behavior* 44:18–33.

Pearce, N. (1996) Traditional epidemiology, modern epidemiology, and public health. *American Journal of Public Health* 86:678–683.

Phinney, J.S. (1990) Ethnic identity in adolescence and adulthood: a review and integration. *Psychological Bulletin* 108:499–514.

Phinney, J.S. (1992) The multigroup ethnic identity measure: a new scale for use with diverse groups. *Journal of Adolescent Research* 7:156–176.

Pyant, C.T., and Yanico, B.J. (1991) Relationship of racial identity and gender-role attitudes to Black women's psychological well-being. *Journal of Counseling Psychology* 38:315–322.

Rosario, M., Hunter, J., Maguen, S., Gwadz, M., and Smith, R. (2001) The coming-out process and its adaptational and health-related associations among gay, lesbian and bisexual youths: stipulation and exploration of a model. *American Journal of Community Psychology* 29:133–160.

Rowley, S.J., Sellers, R.M., Chavous, T.M., and Smith, M.A. (1998) The relationship between racial identity and self-esteem in African American college and high school students. *Journal of Personality and Social Psychology* 74:715–724.

Ryff, C.D., Keyes, C.L.M., and Hughes, D.L. (2003) Status inequalities, perceived discrimination, and eudaimonic well-being: do the challenges of minority life hone purpose and growth?" *Journal of Health and Social Behavior* 44:275–291.

Sapolsky, R. (1994) *Why zebras don't get ulcers: a guide to stress, stress-related diseases and coping.* W.H. Freeman, New York.

Savin-Williams, R.C. (2001) Suicide attempts among sexual-minority youths: population and measurement issues. *Journal of Consulting and Clinical Psychology* 69:983–991.

Savin-Williams, R.C., and Ream, G.L. (2003) Suicide attempts among sexual-minority male youth. *Journal of Clinical Child and Adolescent Psychology* 32:509–522.

Schultz, A., Williams, D., Israel, B., Becker, A., Parker, E., James, S.A., and Jackson, J. (2000) Unfair treatment, neighborhood effects, and mental health in the Detroit metropolitan area. *Journal of Health and Social Behavior* 41:314–332.

Sell, R.L. (1997) Defining and measuring sexual orientation: a review. *Archives of Sexual Behavior* 26:643–658.

Sell, R.L., and Petrulio, C. (1996) Sampling homosexuals, bisexuals, gays, and lesbians for public health research: a review of the literature from 1990 to 1992. *Journal of Homosexuality* 30:31–47.

Sellers, R.M., Rowley, S.A.J., Chavous, T.M., Shelton, J., and Smith, M.A. (1997) Multidimensional inventory of black identity: a preliminary investigation of reliability and construct validity. *Journal of Personality and Social Psychology* 73:805–815.

Sellers, R.M., Chavous, T.M., and Cooke, D.Y. (1998a) Racial ideology and racial centrality as predictors of African American college students' academic performance. *Journal of Black Psychology* 24:8–27.

Sellers, R.M., Smith, M.A., Shelton, J.N., Rowley, S.A.J., and Chavous, T.M. (1998b) Multidimensional model of racial identity: a reconceptualization of African American racial identity. *Personality and Social Psychology Review* 2:18–39.

Sellers, R.M., Morgan, L., and Brown, T.N. (2001) A multidimensional approach to racial identity: implications for African American children. In: Neal-Barnett, A., Contreras, J., and Kerns, K. (eds) *Forging links: African American children: clinical developmental perspectives.* Praeger, Westport, CT, pp. 23–56.

Sellers, R.M., Caldwell, C.H., Schmeelk-Cone, K., and Zimmerman, M.A. (2003) Racial identity, racial discrimination, perceived stress, and psychological distress among African American young adults. *Journal of Health and Social Behavior* 44:302–317.

Shelton, J.N., and Sellers, R.M. (2000) Situational stability and variability in African American racial identity. *Journal of Black Psychology* 1:27–50.

Sigelman, L., and Welch, S. (1991) *Black Americans' views of racial inequality: the dream deferred.* Cambridge University Press, New York.

Solarz, A. (1999) *Committee on lesbian health research priorities, I. O. M. lesbian health: current assessment and direction for the future.* National Academy Press, Washington, DC.

Stack, S. (1998) Education and risk of suicide: an analysis of African Americans. *Sociological Focus* 31:295–302.

Steele, C.M., and Aronson, J. (1995) Stereotype vulnerability and the intellectual test performance of African Americans. *Journal of Personality and Social Psychology* 69:797–811.

Strogatz, D.S., Croft, J.B., James, S.A., Keenan, N.L., Browning, S.R., Garrett, J.M., and Curtis, A.B. (1997) Social support, stress, and blood pressure in Black adults. *Epidemiology* 8:482–487.

Susser, M., and Susser, E. (1996) Choosing a future for epidemiology. I. Eras and paradigms. *American Journal of Public Health* 86:668–673.

Tajfel, H., and Turner, J. (1979) An integrative theory of intergroup conflict. In: Austin, W.G., and Worchel, S. (eds) *The social psychology of intergroup relations.* Brooks/Cole, Monterey, CA, pp. 33–47.

The President's Initiative on Race. (1998) One America in the 21st century. Accessed at: Clinton2.nara.gov/Initiatives/OneAmerica/PIR_main.pdf.

Troiden, R.R. (1989) The formation of homosexual identities. *Journal of Homosexuality* 17:43–73.

Troiden, R.R. (1993) The formation of homosexual identities. In: Garnets, L., and Kimmel, D. (eds) *Psychological perspectives on lesbian and gay male experiences.* Columbia University Press, New York, pp. 191–217.

U.S. Census Bureau. (1998) Historical income and poverty page: historical income and poverty tables, 1998, Washington DC. Accessed at: http://www.census.gov/hhes/income/histinc/index.html.

Vega, W.A., and Rumbaut, R.G. (1991) Ethnic minorities and mental health. *Annual Review of Sociology* 17:351–383.

White, J.L., and Parham, T.A. (1996) The struggle for identity congruence in African Americans. In: Jennings, G-H. (ed) *Passages beyond the gate: a Jungian approach to understanding the nature of American psychology at the dawn of the new millennium.* Simon & Schuster Custom Publishing, Needham Heights, MA, pp. 246–253.

Williams, D.R. (2003) The health of men: structured inequalities and opportunities. *American Journal of Public Health* 93:724–731.

Williams, D.R., Yu, Y., Jackson, J., and Anderson, N. (1997) Racial differences in physical and mental heatlh: socioeconomic status, stress, and discrimination. *Journal of Health Psychology* 2:335–351.

Wilson, B.D.M., and Miller, R.L. (2002) Strategies for managing heterosexism used among African American gay and bisexual men. *Journal of Black Psychology* 4:371–391.

Part IV
Research Methodologies

Defining and Measuring Sexual Orientation for Research

Randall L. Sell

1 Introduction

Conceptually defining populations, such as those defined by race and ethnicity, and developing methods to identify members of those populations operationally have continually challenged researchers (LaVeist, 2002). Today, as scientists begin to treat sexual orientation as a demographic variable like race and ethnicity, it is important to examine critically and clarify our conceptualizations of sexual orientation as well as critically examine measures used for operationally identifying the sexual orientation of research subjects.

There is much evidence that researchers are often confused as to what they are studying when they assess sexual orientation in their research. Several literature reviews have found that researchers' conceptual definitions of these populations are rarely included in reports of their research, and when they are included they often differ theoretically. Furthermore, the methods used to measure sexual orientation in these studies do not always correspond with the most common conceptualizations of sexual orientation (Shively et al., 1985; Sell & Petrulio, 1995; Chung & Katayama, 1996). Sell and Petrulio recommended that researchers work to develop uniform conceptual definitions of terms used to label sexual orientation and that uniform methods of operationally identifying sexual orientation be agreed upon for use in research studies. They believe it is imperative that researchers who claim to be studying these populations begin to clarify what it is they are actually studying and recognize more explicitly the effect their research methods have on their findings. Sell and Petrulio's recommendation's echo the much earlier work of Henry (1941), who conducted one of the most detailed studies of homosexuality ever produced. Henry concluded that: "Unless the word homosexual is

This chapter has been adapted from Sell, R.L. Defining and measuring sexual orientation: a review. *Archives of Sexual Behavior* 1997;26:643–58.

clearly defined, objective discussion regarding it is futile, and misunderstanding and erroneous conclusions are inevitable" (Henry, 1955).

To clear up some of this confusion, this chapter reviews and critiques conceptual definitions of sexual orientations and the measures used to identify and classify subjects' sexual orientations that have been proposed and used by scientists and laypersons since the 1860s in Europe and the United States. It was during the 1860s that the formal study of sexual orientation was founded by Ulrichs. It is hoped that this review will encourage researchers to be more critical of the methods they use to identify and label the sexual orientation of research subjects.

2 Conceptual Definitions of Sexual Orientation

Many terms and definitions have been proposed over the last 140 years to describe the sexual orientation of study subjects. One of the earliest and most important sexual orientation classification schemes was proposed by Ulrichs in a series of pamphlets he privately published in the 1860s (Carpenter, 1908; Ulrichs, 1994). Ulrichs' scheme, which was only intended to describe males, separated them into three basic categories: *dionings*, *urnings*, and *uranodionings* (see Fig. 14.1). These terms were derived from a speech by Pausanias in Plato's Symposium in which Pausanias refers to Uranus (heaven) (Plato, 1993). Arguably these categories directly correspond with the categories used today: heterosexual, homosexual, and bisexual (Cory, 1951). Homosexual women, who were largely ignored by early researchers, were referred to as urningins and heterosexual women as dioningins by Ulrichs (Bullough, 1990).

The Human Male: A. Dioning[1]

                                                       B. Urning[2]
                                                             1. Mannling[3]
      2. Weibling[4]
      3. Zwischen[5]
      4. Virilised[6]

                                                      C. Urano-Dioning[7]

Notes:

1 – Comparable to the modern term "heterosexual." A Dioning that sexually behaves like a Urning is termed an "Uraniaster."
2 – Comparable to the modern term "homosexual."
3 – A manly Urning.
4 – An effeminate Urning.
5 – A somewhat manly and somewhat effeminate Urning.
6 – An Urning that sexually behaves like a Dioning.
7 – Comparable to the modern term "bisexual."

(for additional information see Ulrichs, K. H. *The Riddle of Man-Manly Love*, Prometheus Books, Buffalo, NY, 1994.; Carpenter, E. *The Intermediate Sex*, Allen and Unwin, London, 1908.)

Figure 14.1 Male sexual orientation classification scheme of Karl Ulrichs.

Mayne, a follower of Ulrichs, provided a definition of an urning in the first major work on homosexuality to be written by an American. He defined an urning as "a human being that is more or less perfectly, even distinctly, masculine in physique; often a virile type of fine intellectual, oral and aesthetic sensibilities: but who, through an inborn or later-developed preference feels sexual passion for the male human species. His sexual preference may quite exclude any desire for the female sex: or may exist concurrently with that instinct" (Mayne, 1908). Mayne's definition also encompasses male uranodionings by stating that desire for the female sex may exist concurrently.

In addition to his effect on Mayne, Ulrichs had a profound influence on the works of many early researchers including Westphal (1869), Symonds (1883, 1891), Krafft-Ebing (1886), Moll (1891), Carpenter (1894, 1908), Ellis and Symonds (1898), and Hirschfeld (1914). Furthermore, through the works of these researchers, Ulrichs is credited with influencing Freud and Jung (Bullough, 1994). Although they may differ significantly, the conceptualizations of sexual orientation most often cited today generally have their root in the work of Ulrichs.

Even the terms "homosexuality" and "heterosexuality," which Ulrichs did not prefer, have direct links to him. The term homosexual is an inappropriate combination of Greek and Latin that disturbed many early researchers who wanted it replaced but recognized that it was too deeply rooted in the literature by the time they arrived on the scene (Robinson, 1936; Kinsey et al., 1948). The term homosexual may have been introduced into English by Symonds in his first edition of *A Problem of Modern Ethics* in 1891 (Boswell, 1980). The terms homosexuality and heterosexuality first appeared in a letter to Ulrichs drafted on May 6, 1868, from Benkert, a German-Hungarian physician and writer (Ulrichs, 1994). Later, Benkert (cited in Robinson, 1936) outlined his definition of homosexuality in a pamphlet published in 1869. His definition read:

In addition to the normal sexual urge in man and woman, Nature in her sovereign mood has endowed at birth certain male and female individuals with the homosexual urge, thus placing them in a sexual bondage which renders them physically and psychically incapable—even with the best intention—of normal erection. This urge creates in advance a direct horror of the opposite sexual [sic] and the victim of this passion finds it impossible to suppress the feeling which individuals of his own sex exercise upon him.

Today, "heterosexual" (straight), "homosexual" (gay and lesbian), and "bisexual" are the most commonly used terms by researchers to describe sexual orientation (Shively et al., 1985; Sell & Petrulio, 1995). Although not many other terms have been proposed to describe heterosexuality or bisexuality, an overabundance of terms have been used by researchers to describe homosexuality: uranianism, homogenic love, contrasexuality, homoerotism, similsexualism, tribadism, sexual inversion, intersexuality, transexuality, third sex, and psychosexual hermaphroditism (Moll, 1891; Carpenter, 1894, 1908; Ellis & Symonds, 1898; Mayne, 1908; Kinsey et al., 1948, 1953; Ulrichs, 1994). Even today, terms take on new meaning and importance for describing sexual orientations. The term "queer," for example, was defined by Legman in 1941 as: "Homosexual; more often used of male homosexuals than of Lesbians. As an adjective it is the most common in use in America." At the time Legman wrote this, the term was slang and used pejoratively. Currently, the term still means "homosexual" but is frequently used nonpejoratively in scholarly works (e.g., Signorile, 1993; Brett et al., 1994; Feinberg, 1994; Goldberg, 1994; Packard & Packard, 2005). Today's preferred terms and the term "sexual orientation" itself have a wide variety of definitions in the literature, but they generally comprise one or both of two components: a "psychological" component and a "behavioral" component. Not all definitions include both of these components; and as is discussed in detail below, definitions that include both components use either "and" or "or" to join them.

Mayne's (1908) definition of urning and Benkert's definition of homosexual (Robinson, 1936) included descriptions of only the psychological state. Mayne discussed how the individual's feelings of sexual passion determine his or her sexual orientation, whereas Benkert talked of an "urge." Ellis, one of the most important writers on sexuality during the late nineteenth and early twentieth century England also talked only of a psychological entity, which he described as "sexual instinct." Ellis defined homosexuality as "sexual instinct turned by inborn constitutional abnormality toward persons of the same sex" (Ellis & Symonds, 1898). Ellis used the term "sexual inversion" at the time this definition was provided; but in later versions of his work he substituted the term "homosexuality" (Ellis & Symonds, 1898; Ellis, 1942). Two of the earliest medical journal articles about homosexuality to appear in the English language provided a definition that, like the other early definitions, does not discuss sexual behavior. Their definitions, which in both cases is a translation of Westphal's German definition, describes homosexuals as persons who: "as a result of their inborn nature felt themselves drawn by sexual desire to male individuals exclusively" (Blumer, 1882; Shaw & Ferris, 1883).

These definitions and other early ones generally omitted any discussion of behavior (and in particular sexual behavior), except to say that the thought of it with the other sex is repulsive or horrifying to the homosexual. Another definition of this type was provided by Forel (1924) in his popular book *The Sexual Question*. Forel stated,

However shocking or absurd the aberrations of the sexual appetite and its irradiations may be, of which we have spoken hitherto, they are at any rate derived from originally normal intercourse with adults of the opposite sex. Those we have now to deal with are distinguished by the fact that not only the appetite itself, but all its psychic irradiations are directed to the same sex as the perverted individual, the latter being horrified at the idea of genital contact with the opposite sex, quite as much as a normal man is horrified at the idea of homosexual union.

Krafft-Ebing, like his contemporaries, even made the point to exclude behavior from the diagnosis of homosexuality. Krafft-Ebing

(1886) stated that "the determining factor here is the demonstration of perverse feelings for the same sex; not the proof of sexual acts with the same sex. These two phenomena must not be confounded with each other."

More recent definitions often include both components. For example LeVay (1993) defined sexual orientation as "the direction of sexual feelings or behavior, toward individuals of the opposite sex (heterosexuality), the same sex (homosexuality), or some combination of the two (bisexuality)." Weinrich (1994) defined homosexuality "either (1) as a genital act or (2) as a long-term sexuoerotic status." Here the psychological states referred to are "sexual feelings" and "sexuoerotic status"; and the behavioral outcome is "sexual behavior" as referred to by LeVay or a "genital act" as referred to by Weinrich. The psychological and behavioral components in both definitions are joined by "or" signifying that either one can be used to assess sexual orientation.

In *A Descriptive Dictionary and Atlas of Sexology* (Francoeur et al., 1991), homosexuality is broadly defined as "the occurrence or existence of sexual attraction, interest and genitally intimate activity between an individual and other members of the same gender." Here (the psychological components are "sexual attraction" and "interest," and the behavioral outcome is described as "genitally intimate activity." Unlike the definitions of LeVay (1993) and Weinrich (1994), this definition joins the two components with the conjunction "and." Using the conjunction "and" makes it unclear as to whether both components are necessary for the assignment of sexual orientation classification.

At the other extreme from the early definitions provided by Mayne and Benkert are definitions that include only discussions of the behavioral component. For example, *Stedman's Medical Dictionary* (1982) defined homosexuality as "sexual behavior, including sexual congress, between individuals of the same sex, especially past puberty." Here the psychological component does not seem to hold much, if any, importance for the assessment of sexual orientation. Beach (1950) was emphatic about including only sexual behavior in the definition of sexual orientation in his critique of the first English-language translation of Gide's defense of homosexuality, Corydon. Beach (1950) stated that

the term (homosexuality) means different things to different people . . . it is preferable to set forth the significance of the term as used in this discussion. Homosexuality refers exclusively to overt behavior between two individuals of the same sex. The behavior must be patently sexual, involving erotic arousal and, in most instances at least, resulting in the satisfaction of the sexual urge.

According to Diamond (1993), it is this type of definition that is favored by researchers determining the size of the "homosexual" population in various countries. In the studies reviewed by Diamond, although all used some assessment of sexual behavior to determine the prevalence of sexual orientations, none used any assessment of a psychological state (such as sexual attraction).

Thus far, I have discussed the two definitional components of sexual orientation as if the components themselves were uniform across definitions; but as is evident in the examples already provided, there are important variations. Psychological components of definitions may include the terms "sexual passion," "sexual urge . . . sexual feelings," "sexual attraction," "sexual interest," "sexual arousal," "sexual desire," "affectional preference," "sexual instinct," "sexual orientation identity," and "sexual preference." "Sexual preference" has been used as a substitute for the term "sexual orientation," but Gonsiorek and Weinrich (1991) believe it "is misleading as it assumes conscious or deliberate choice and may trivialize the depth of the psychological processes involved." They therefore recommend the term "sexual orientation" because most research findings indicate that homosexual feelings are a basic part of an individual's psyche and are established much earlier than conscious choice would indicate. Each of these terms may have a distinct meaning and not necessarily be indicative of the same phenomenon. That is, different terms in definitions may be describing slightly different phenomena despite the similar label for that phenomenon.

Similarly, the behavioral component varies among definitions. Behavior can be stated simply as "sexual behavior," or it can be described, for example, as "genital activity," "sexual intercourse," "sexual contact," or "sexual contact that achieves orgasm." Each one of these presents further challenges for researchers. That is, how do we define each of these terms within the definition itself, and how would we operationalize them for measurement?

Obviously, definitions and preferred terms vary significantly from one researcher to another and across time. Although it is not possible from this review to say one definition or set of terms is "better" than another, it is possible to make a few modest recommendations. First, all researchers who intend to collect sexual orientation data should dedicate time to choosing one of the definitions described here or developing their own definition before they begin their research. Second, researchers should make the terms and definitions they are using explicit when discussing research studies and findings.

3 Measures of Sexual Orientation

As was demonstrated above, conceptualizations of sexual orientation vary dramatically among researchers. Measures of sexual orientation, as is shown below, vary widely as well. However, this variation, like the variation in definitions, provides important insight to modern researchers.

Some of the earliest reports of assessing sexual orientation are found in the documents of the Western Church, which encouraged individuals to confess their sins. In particular, religious documents show the Church's concern with asking sensitive questions about such topics as sodomy. These documents instructed priests during the 1500s "not to show amazement; exhibit a contorted face; show revulsion (no matter what enormities are confessed) rebuke the penitent; or exclaim 'Oh, what vile sins!'" when discussing sensitive subjects (Tentler, 1977; Lee, 1993).

De Pareja, who went to Florida as a missionary to the Timucua Indians in 1595, outlined specific questions to identify sodomites in his book *Confessionario* (Katz, 1992). These questions included the following (Katz, 1992).

1. Have you had intercourse with another man?
2. Or have you gone around trying out or making fun in order to do that?

Pareja further provided questions to be asked of boys who may have committed sodomy (Katz, 1992).

3. Has someone been investigating you from behind?
4. Did you consummate the act?

Several centuries later, Ulrichs, in his series of pamphlets during the 1860s, outlined a set of questions that could be asked to determine if a man was an Urning (Ulrichs, 1994).

1. Does he feel for males and only for males a passionate yearning of love, be it gushing and gentle, or fiery and sensual?
2. Does he feel horror at sexual contact with women? This horror may not always be found; but when it is found, it is decisive.
3. Does he experience a beneficial magnetic current when making contact with a male body in its prime?
4. Does the excitement of attraction find its apex in the male sexual organs?

Mayne (1908) also outlined a series of several hundred questions for the personal diagnosis of urnings and urningins.

1. At what age did your sexual desire show itself distinctly?
2. Did it direct itself at first most to the male or to the female sex? Or did it hesitate awhile between both?
3. Is the instinct unvaryingly toward the male or female sex now? Or do you take pleasure (or would you experience it) with now a man, now a woman?
4. Do you give way to it rather mentally or physically? Or are both in equal measure?
5. Is the similsexual desire constant, periodic or irregularly felt?
6. In dreams, do you have visions of sexual relations with men or women, the more frequently and ardently?

The respondents to Pareja's, Ulrichs', and Mayne's questions were expected to be able to provide a yes or no answer. That is, the person was either categorized as a "sodomite," "urning," or "urningin"—or not. This simple categorical scheme for the classification of sexual orientations remains the dominant one used by researchers today. That is, subjects are classified as homosexual or heterosexual based on their sexual orientation identity or sexual behavior (Sell & Petrulio, 1995). In major health surveys, the state of the art question to assess sexual orientation, when only one question can be asked, is the following (Miller, 2002).

Which of the following best describes how you think of yourself? (1) straight or heterosexual; (2) gay or lesbian; (3) bisexual; (4) don't know/not sure.

Despite this focus on single question measures, more sophisticated measures of sexual orientation have been proposed over the last 50 years as researchers have encountered or discovered the limitations of simple categorical measures. The most important of these measures are reviewed below.

The most influential scale to be proposed during these years was put forth by Kinsey et al. (1948, 1953) in their reports on sexual behavior in the human male and female. Kinsey et al. proposed (see Fig. 14.2) a bipolar scale that allowed a continuum between "exclusive heterosexuality" and "exclusive homosexuality." Kinsey et al. provided the following important justifications for their decision to depart from the dichotomous measures of his predecessors:

---

0   **Exclusively heterosexual-** Individuals who make no physicial contacts which result in erotic arousal or orgasm, and make no psychic responses to individuals of their own sex.

1   **Predominantly heterosexual/only incidentally homosexual-** Individuals which have only incidental homosexual contacts which have involved physical or psychic response, or incidental psychic response without physical contact.

2   **Predominantly heterosexual but more than incidentally homosexual-** individuals who have more than incidental homosexual experience, and/or if they respond rather definitely to homosexual stimuli.

3   **Equally heterosexual and homosexual-** individuals who are about equally homosexual and heterosexual in their overt experience and/or the their psychic reactions.

4   **Predominantly homosexual but more than incidentally heterosexual-** individuals who have more overt activity and/or psychic reactions in the homosexual, while still maintaining a fair amount of heterosexual activity and/or responding rather definitive to heterosexual contact.

5   **Predominantly homosexual/only incidentally heterosexual-** individuals who are almost entirely homosexual in their overt activities and/or reactions.

6   **Exclusively homosexual-** individuals who are exclusively homosexual, both in regard to their overt experience and in regard to their psychic reactions.

(for additional information see Kinsey, A. C, Pomeroy, W. B., and Martin, C. E. *Sexual Behavior in the Human Male*, W. B. Saunders, Philadelphia, PA, 1948; Kinsey, A. C., Pomeroy, W. B., Martin. C. E., and Gebhard, P. H. *Sexual Behavior in the Human Female*, W. B. Saunders, Philadelphia, PA, 1953.)

Figure 14.2 Kinsey scale.

The world is not to be divided into sheep and goats. Not all things are black nor all things white. It is a fundamental of taxonomy that nature rarely deals with discrete categories. Only the human mind invents categories and tries to force facts into separated pigeon-holes. The living world is a continuum in each and every one of its aspects. The sooner we learn this concerning human sexual behavior the sooner we shall reach a sound understanding of the realities of sex [Kinsey et al., 1948].

It is characteristic of the human mind that it tries to dichotomize in its classification of phenomena. Things are either so, or they are not so. Sexual behavior is either normal or abnormal, socially acceptable or unacceptable, heterosexual or homosexual; and many persons do not want to believe that there are gradations in these matters from one to the other extreme [Kinsey et al., 1953].

One of the more striking facts about these statements is that Kinsey had been trained as a taxonomist (Weinrich, 1990). It had been much of his life work to develop such dichotomous, yes or no, classifications as he so easily dismissed here. By dismissing dichotomous classifications and developing a bipolar continuous model, a new way of measuring sexual orientation, providing a new perspective on sexuality, was created. However, as it forces subjects into one of seven categories, the Kinsey Scale is not a true continuum. This is fortunate in some ways because the seven points are difficult to assign; and if there were an infinite number of points, the task would be that much more difficult.

Masters and Johnson (1979), in a major study of homosexuality, provided the following discussion about the difficulty of assigning Kinsey ratings.

There was also concern in arbitrarily selecting the specific classification of Kinsey grades 2 through 4 for any individual who had had a large number of both homosexual and heterosexual experiences. The ratings were assigned by the research team after detailed history-taking, but it is difficult for any individual to be fully objective in assessing the amount of his or her eterosexual versus homosexual experience when there has been a considerable amount of both types of interaction. Some of these preferences ratings might well be subject to different interpretation by other health-care professionals.

Masters and Johnson further stated that:

Kinsey 3 classification was the most difficult to assign of the ratings. Relative equality in any form of diverse physical activity is hard to establish. Particularly was this so when the interviewer, in attempting to separate mature sexual experience into its homosexual and heterosexual components, was faced with a history of a multiplicity of partners of either sex. The problem was augmented by the subjects' frequently vague recall of the average number of sexual interactions with each partner.

It is evident from these reports that it is difficult to determine the relative importance of the heterosexual and homosexual in a person's history when using the Kinsey Scale, but this is only one of several concerns often expressed by researchers about this scale. A second concern with the Kinsey Scale is that it lumps individuals who are significantly different based on different aspects or dimensions of sexuality into the same categories (Weinrich et al., 1993; Weinberg et al., 1994). In fact, Kinsey himself took two dimensions of sexual orientation, "overt sexual experience" and "psychosexual reactions," into account when applying his scale. Kinsey el al. (1948) provided the following discussion of these two dimensions and how they were used in the assessment of sexual orientation.

It will be observed that the rating which an individual receives has a dual basis. It takes into account his overt sexual experience and/or his psychosexual reactions. In the majority of instances the two aspects of the history parallel but sometimes they are not in accord. In the latter case, the rating of an individual must be based upon an evaluation of the relative importance of the overt and the psychic in his history [Kinsey et al., 1948].

It can be argued that valuable information was lost by collapsing these two values into one final score. A common solution that avoids the loss of information is to assess dimensions of sexual orientation separately and report the scores independently as Kinsey could have easily done. When this approach is taken, the two most commonly assessed aspects of sexual orientation are sexual behavior and sexual fantasies. These two dimensions are most likely chosen because they correspond with the two dimensions "overt sexual experience" and "psychosexual reaction" proposed by Kinsey (Kinsey et al., 1948; Sell & Petrulio, 1995). They may also be chosen because they reflect the behavioral and psychological components of definitions as discussed in the previous section. However, sexual behavior and sexual fantasies are not the only dimensions that may be considered. For example, Klein et al. (1985) proposed in the Klein Sexual Orientation Grid (KSOG) the assessment of seven dimensions including sexual attraction, sexual behavior, sexual fantasies, emotional preference, social preference, self-identification, and heterosexual/homosexual life-style (see Fig. 14.3). A concern with assessing multiple dimensions is that as each is added the overall scale becomes more burdensome and less practical for many research purposes. Researchers therefore tend to limit the number of assessed dimensions.

Diamond (1993) reviewed several research studies in which sexual behavior and sexual fantasies were assessed on the Kinsey Scale. He reported that this is somewhat common in studies of specific gay populations. In the studies reviewed, there appears to be a high but not perfect correlation between reported sexual behavior and fantasy. The value of measuring these two dimensions for the assessment of sexual orientation or any other dimension has not been well determined (Ross et al., 2003).

Only a few published studies have explicitly examined the value of studying more than one dimension of sexual orientation. Weinrich et al. (1993) found, using factor analysis, that all of the dimensions of

Variable	PAST	PRESENT	IDEAL
A. Sexual Attraction			
B. Sexual Behavior			
C. Sexual Fantasies			
D. Emotional Preferences			
E. Social Preference			
F. Self-Identification			
G. Heterosexual/ Homosexual Lifestyle			

I. Scale to Measure Dimensions A, B, C, D and E of the Klein Sexual Orientation Grid

0	1	2	3	4	5	6
other sex only	other sex mostly	other sex somewhat	both sexes equally	same sex somewhat	same sex mostly	same sex only

II. Scale to Measure Dimension E and F of the Klein Sexual Orientation Grid

0	1	2	3	4	5	6
heterosexual only	heterosexual mostly	heterosexual more	hetero/homo equally	homosexual more	homosexual somewhat	homosexual only

(for additional information see Klein, F., Sepekoff, B., and Wolf, T. J. Sexual orientation: A multi-variable dynamic process. *J. Homosexuality.* 1985;11: 35-49.)

Figure 14.3 Klein sexual orientation grid.

sexual orientation proposed by Klein in the KSOG seem to be measuring the same construct. That is, all of the dimensions load on a first factor, which accounts for most of the variance. However, they further found in the two samples that were studied that a second factor emerged containing time dimensions of social and emotional preferences, suggesting that the social and emotional preference dimensions may have also been measuring something other than sexual orientation.

Another study, The National Health and Social Life Survey, demonstrated that sexual attraction, sexual behavior, and sexual orientation identity measures of sexual orientation identify different (albeit overlapping) populations. Laumann et al. (1994) found that of the 8.6% of women reporting some same-gender sexuality, 88% reported same-gender sexual desire, 41% reported some same-gender sexual behavior, and 16% reported a lesbian or gay identity. Of the 10.1% of men reporting some same-gender sexuality, 75% reported same-gender sexual desire, 52% reported some same-gender sexual behavior, and 27% reported a gay identity.

In another study, Ross et al. (2003) showed that there was a discrepancy between self-reported sexual orientation identity and sexual behavior in a street outreach sample in Houston. In their study, which was focused on human immunodeficiency virus/acquired immunodeficiency syndrome (HIV/AIDS) prevention, they concluded that it was critical to assess sexual behavior rather than identity when conducting research to inform HIV-risk interventions and clinical screening programs.

A third concern with the Kinsey Scale is that it inappropriately measures homosexuality and heterosexuality on the same scale, making one the trade-off of the other. This concern arises out of research during the

1970s on masculinity and femininity which found that the concepts of masculinity and femininity are more appropriately measured as independent concepts on separate scales rather than as a single continuum, with each representing opposite extremes (Bem, 1981). Measured on the same scale, masculinity and femininity acted as trade-offs in which to be more feminine one had to be less masculine or to be more masculine one had to be less feminine. Considered as separate dimensions one could be simultaneously very masculine and very feminine (androgynous) or not very much of either (undifferentiated). Similarly, considering homosexuality and heterosexuality on separate scales allows for one to be both very heterosexual and homosexual (bisexual) or not very much of either (asexual). Bullough (1990) echoed this concern with the Kinsey scale in the following statement.

> I am, however, at this point in my research, convinced that the Kinsey scale has outlived its political usefulness and we need a more effective scholarly measuring tool. In fact, the Kinsey scale offers the same kind of difficulty that the traditional masculine-feminine scale did until it was realized that women could have masculine traits and still be feminine and vice versa.

When homosexuality and heterosexuality are measured independently rather than as a continuum, the degree of homosexuality and heterosexuality can be independently determined, rather than simply the balance between homosexuality and heterosexuality as determined using the Kinsey Scale. This idea was first put forth by Shively and DeCecco (1977), who proposed a five-point scale on which heterosexuality and homosexuality would be independently measured (see Fig. 14.4). Using this scale they proposed the assessment of two dimensions of sexual orientation: physical and affectional preference.

Unfortunately, studies using or examining Shively and DeCecco's (1977) proposed measure of sexual orientation could not be found in the published literature, although a study that briefly examined this issue was found using a different scale. In this study, Storms (1980) measured the extent of sexual fantasies with the other sex on one scale and the extent of sexual fantasies with the same sex on another scale. He found that bisexuals in his sample were as likely to report homosexual fantasies as homosexuals were to report homosexual fantasies, and his bisexuals were as likely to report heterosexual fantasies as heterosexuals were to report heterosexual fantasies. Using the logic that

1	2	3	4	5
Not at all Heterosexual		Somewhat Heterosexual		Very Heterosexual

1	2	3	4	5
Not at all Homosexual		Somewhat Homosexual		Very Homosexual

(for additional information see Shively, M. G., and DeCecco, J. P. Components of sexual identity. *J. Homosexuality.* 1977;3:41-48.)

Figure 14.4 Shively scale of sexual orientation.

bisexuals should be less likely to report homosexual fantasies than homosexuals and less likely to report heterosexual fantasies than heterosexuals, he concluded that homosexuality and heterosexuality should be measured independently (at least in relation to fantasies).

The Sell Assessment of Sexual Orientation was developed in light of the major concerns with existing sexual orientation measures as discussed above (Fig. 14.5) (Gonsiorek et al., 1995; Sell, 1996). That is, the

I. Sexual Attractions- The following six questions are asked to assess how frequently and intensely you are sexually attracted to men and women. Consider times you had sexual fantasies, daydreams, or dreams about a man or woman, or have been sexually aroused by a man or woman.

1. During the past year, how many different men were you sexually attracted to (choose one answer):
   - a. None.
   - b. 1.
   - c. 2.
   - d. 3-5.
   - e. 6-10.
   - f. 11-49.
   - g. 50-99
   - h. 100 or more.

2. During the past year, on average, how often were you sexually attracted to a man (choose one answer):
   - a. Never.
   - b. Less than 1 time per month.
   - c. 1-3 times per month.
   - d. 1 time per week
   - e. 2-3 times per week.
   - f. 4-6 times per week.
   - g. Daily.

3. During the past year, the most I was sexually attracted to a man was (choose one answer):
   - a. Not at all sexually attracted.
   - b. Slightly sexually attracted.
   - c. Mildly sexually attracted.
   - d. Moderately sexually attracted.
   - e. Significantly sexually attracted.
   - f. Very sexually attracted.
   - g. Extremely sexually attracted.

4. During the past year, how many different women were you sexually attracted to (choose one answer):
   - a. None.
   - b. 1.
   - c. 2.
   - d. 3-5.
   - e. 6-10.
   - f. 11-49.
   - g. 50-99.
   - h. 100 or more.

5. During the past year, on average, how often were you sexually attracted to a woman (choose one answer):
   - a. Never.
   - b. Less than 1 time per month.
   - c. 1-3 times per month.
   - d. 1 time per week
   - e. 2-3 times per week.
   - f. 4-6 times per week.
   - g. Daily.

6. During the past year, the most I was sexually attracted to a woman was (choose one answer):
   - a. Not at all sexually attracted.
   - b. Slightly sexually attracted.
   - c. Mildly sexually attracted.
   - d. Moderately sexually attracted.
   - e. Significantly sexually attracted.
   - f. Very sexually attracted.
   - g. Extremely sexually attracted.

Figure 14.5 Sell assessment of sexual orientation.

II. Sexual Contact – The following four questions are asked to assess your sexual contacts. Consider times when you had contact between your body and another man or woman's body for the purpose of sexual arousal or gratification.

7. During the past year, how many <u>different men</u> did you have sexual contact with (choose one answer):
   a. None.
   b. 1.
   c. 2.
   d. 3-5.
   e. 6-10.
   f. 11-49.
   g. 50-99.
   h. 100 or more.

8. During the past year, on average, how often did you have sexual contact with a <u>man</u> (choose one answer):
   a. Never.
   b. Less than 1 time per month.
   c. 1-3 times per month
   d. 1 time per week.
   e. 2-3 times per week.
   f. 4-6 times per week.
   g. Daily.

9. During the past year, how many <u>different women</u> did you have sexual contact with (choose one answer):
   a. None.
   b. 1.
   c. 2.
   d. 3-5.
   e. 6-10.
   f. 11-49.
   g. 50-99.
   h. 100 or more.

10. During the past year, on average, how often did you have sexual contact with a woman (choose one answer):
   a. Never.
   b. Less than 1 time per month.
   c. 1-3 times per month
   d. 1 time per week.
   e. 2-3 times per week.
   f. 4-6 times per week.
   g. Daily.

III. Sexual Orientation Identity- The following two questions are asked to assess your sexual orientation identity.

11. I consider myself (choose one answer):
   a. Not at all homosexual.
   b. Slightly homosexual.
   c. Mildly homosexual.
   d. Moderately homosexual.
   e. Significantly homosexual.
   f. Very homosexual.
   g. Extremely homosexual.

12. I consider myself (choose one answer):
   a. Not at all heterosexual.
   b. Slightly heterosexual.
   c. Mildly heterosexual.
   d. Moderately heterosexual.
   e. Significantly heterosexual.
   f. Very heterosexual.
   g. Extremely heterosexual.

(for additional information see Sell, R.L. (1996) The Sell assessment of sexual orientation: background and scoring. *Journal of Lesbian, Gay and Bisexual Identity* 1(4):295–310.

Figure 14.5 *Continued*

Sell Assessment measures sexual orientation on a continuum, considers various dimensions of sexual orientation, and considers homosexuality and heterosexuality separately. The Sell Assessment contains 12 questions, 6 of which assess sexual attractions, 4 of which assess sexual behavior, and 2 of which assess sexual orientation identity. Among them, Sell considered the questions assessing sexual attractions to be the most important when the intent of the study is to measure sexual orientation, as he defined sexual orientation as the "extent of sexual attractions toward members of the other, same, both sexes, or neither." Therefore, sexual attractions more closely reflect this conceptualization of sexual orientation than other attributes, such as sexual behavior or sexual orientation identity, and therefore are a better measure of sexual orientation.

Sexual behaviors and sexual orientation identity are measured in addition to sexual attractions in the Sell Assessment to provide supplemental information. Sexual behaviors are measured because they are often the result of sexual attractions and therefore provide a reflection of them. However, as a result of social and cultural influences, sexual attractions and behaviors do not always correspond. Sexual orientation identity is measured because it should also be closely linked to sexual attractions. That is, a person should/may identify as homosexual if attracted to the same sex, as heterosexual if attracted to the other sex, and as bisexual if attracted to both sexes. Once again, however, as a result of social and cultural influences, sexual attractions and sexual orientation identity do not always correspond.

Questions concerning sexual attraction, sexual behavior, and sexual orientation identity are not equally important in all studies and must be considered in the context of the study. For example, a study examining the spread of HIV among homosexual men would want to measure sexual attraction to identify the total population of homosexuals and measure sexual behavior to identify individuals most at risk for the spread of HIV. The same study may want to measure sexual orientation identity if the results are to be used for prevention efforts. That is, individuals who identify as homosexual may be different from and easier to target with prevention efforts than homosexual men (identified as homosexual based on reported sexual attractions and/or behavior) who do not identify as homosexual.

Unmodified, the six pairs of questions and responses to the Sell Assessment provide a profile of a subject's sexual orientation. This is, however, more information than many researchers find necessary to assess a subject's sexual orientation. There are, therefore, four sets of "summaries" of the Sell Assessment that can be used to simplify data analysis. The biggest concern with the Sell Assessment is that its reliability and validity, like previous measures, remains largely unexamined (Gonsiorek et al., 1995; Sell, 1996).

The Sell Assessment of sexual orientation is intended to provoke debate about the measurement of sexual orientations, not necessarily provide a final solution to the question of how best to measure this construct. Researchers are encouraged to use it as a foundation of or beginning for the creation of better measures. One researcher who has attempted to do this is Friedman who is developing an adolescent measure of sexual orientation (Friedman et al., 2004).

4 Choosing a Measure of Sexual Orientation

Researchers are ever more frequently recognizing the need to include a sexual orientation variable in their research studies. Although problems assessing other demographic variables such as race and ethnicity have been examined and debated extensively in the literature, this process is only beginning for sexual orientation. With the review provided here, this chapter informs and hopefully advances this important process. However, definitive recommendations of one measure over another cannot legitimately be offered at this time. Rather, as with other recent reports, further research on the measurement of sexual orientation is recommended here (Solarz, 1999; Gay and Lesbian Medical Association, 2001).

Researchers wanting to measure sexual orientation today have a number of measurement tools from which to choose. They include simple categorical measures such as the one proposed by Miller (2002), the Kinsey Scale (Kinsey et al., 1948), the Klein Scale (Klein et al., 1985), the Shively and DeCecco Scale (Shively & DeCecco, 1977), the Sell Assessment (Sell, 1996), and the Friedman Measure of Adolescent Sexual Orientation (Friedman et al., 2004).[1] None of these is completely satisfactory. First, simple categorical scales are unsatisfactory for the reasons outlined by Kinsey but also because they have rarely had their validity and reliability thoroughly examined. Second, the Kinsey Scale is unsatisfactory because it forces the artificial combination of psychological and behavioral components and perhaps incorrectly requires individuals to make trade-offs between homosexuality and heterosexuality. Third, the Klein Scale is unsatisfactory because the relative importance of each dimension for measuring sexual orientation has not been thoroughly investigated or grounded in theory; and like Kinsey, Klein required subjects to make trade-offs between heterosexuality and homosexuality. Fourth, the Shively and DeCecco scale is unsatisfactory because its properties have not been thoroughly investigated, and its consideration of physical and affectional preference may be oversimplified or even inappropriate. Finally, the Sell Assessment and Friedman Measure of Adolescent Sexual Orientation, while firmly grounded in current theoretical thinking about the measurement of sexual orientations, remain largely untested and are perhaps too complicated and burdensome for average research requirements.

In reality, most research studies that want to assess sexual orientations can add only a single question to do so. The problems inherent

---

[1]Other proposed scales that do not advance the field of sexual orientation measurement theoretically but are of some interest include those of Sambrooks and MacCulloch (1973), Berkey et al. (1990), and Coleman (1990).

in this approach should be particularly evident from this review. However, if one must be chosen, there are resources available to assist with making such choices. One such resources is www.gaydata.org, which attempts to track all such measures and makes recommendations concerning them. Currently, www.gaydata.org makes the following recommendations concerning individual questions to assess sexual orientation:

Sexual orientation identity (from Massachusetts 2003 Youth Risk Behavior Survey)
• Which of the following best describes you? (1) heterosexual (straight); (2) gay or lesbian; (3) bisexual; (4) not sure

Sexual behavior (from Vermont and Massachusetts Behavioral Risk Factor Surveillance Surveys)
• During the past 12 months, have you had sex with only males, only females, or both males and females?

Sexual attraction (from the National Survey of Family Growth)
• People are different in their sexual attraction to other people. Which best describes your feelings? Are you: only attracted to females; mostly attracted to females; equally attracted to females and males; mostly attracted to males; only attracted to males; not sure.

These questions were taken from surveys that have collected sexual orientation data. They are good questions but may not be perfect for every need. For example, the identity question was used on a self-completed questionnaire and may not work well over the telephone because it requires the respondent to repeat the response categories out loud in their home. The sexual behavior question also may not suit every need because it does not assess how many male or female partners with whom the respondent has had sex or the frequency of that sex; moreover, it limits the time period to the past 12 months. When selecting questions, one must therefore carefully think about what the data will be used for as well as how it will be collected.

References

Beach, F. (1950) Comments on the second dialogue. In: Gide, A. *Corydon*. Farrar Straus, New York.

Berkey, B.R., Perelman-Ifall, T., and Kurdek, L.A. (1990) The multidimensional scale of sexuality. *Journal of Homosexuality* 19(4):67–87.

Bem, S.L. (1981) *Bem sex-role inventory professional manual*. Consulting Psychologists Press, Palo Alto, CA.

Blumer, O.A. (1882) A case of perverted sexual instinct (contrare sexualempfindung). *Journal of Insanity* 39:22–35.

Boswell, J. (1980) *Christianity, social tolerance, and homosexuality*. University of Chicago Press, Chicago.

Bullough, V. (1990) The Kinsey scale in historical perspective. In: McWhirter, D.P., Sanders, S.A., and Reinisch, J.M. (eds) *Homosexuality/heterosexuality: concepts of sexual orientation*. Oxford University Press, New York.

Bullough, V. (1994) Introduction. In: *The riddle of man-manly love*. Prometheus Books, Buffalo, NY.

Carpenter, E. (1894) *Homogenic love and its place in a free society*. Labour Press, Manchester, UK.

Carpenter, E. (1908) *The intermediate sex*. Allen & Unwin, London.

Chung, Y.B., and Katayama, M. (1996) Assessment of sexual orientation in lesbian/gay/bisexual studies. *Journal of Homosexuality* 30(4):49–62.

Coleman, E. (1990) Toward a synthetic understanding of sexual orientation. In: McWhirter, D.P., Sanders, S.A., and Reinisch, J.M. (eds) *Homosexuality/heterosextiality: concepts of sexual orientation*. Oxford University Press, New York.

Cory, D.W. (1951) *The homosexual in America*. Greenberg, New York.

Diamond, M. (1993) Homosexuality and bisexuality in different populations. *Archives of Sexual Behavior* 22:291–310.

Ellis, H. (1942) *Studies in the Psychology of Sex*. Random House, New York.

Ellis, I., and Symonds, J.A. (1898) *Sexual Inversion*. Wilson & Macmillan, London.

Feinberg, D.B. (1994) *Queer and loathing: rants and raves of a raging AIDS clone*. Viking, New York.

Forel, A. (1924) *The sexual question: a scientific psychological hygienic and sociological study*. Physicians & Surgeons Book Company, New York.

Francoeur, R.T., Perper, T., and Scherzer, N.A. (eds) (1991) *A descriptive dictionary and atlas of sexology*. Greenwood, New York.

Friedman, M.S., Silvestre, A.J., Gold, M.A., Markovic, N., Savin-Williams, R.C., Huggins, J., and Sell, R.L. (2004) Adolescents define sexual orientation and suggest ways to measure it. *Journal of Adolescence* 27:303–317.

Gay and Lesbian Medical Association and LGBT Health Experts. (2001) *Healthy people 2010 companion document for lesbian, gay, bisexual and transgender health*. Gay and Lesbian Medical Association, San Francisco.

Goldberg, J. (ed). (1994) *Queering the Renaissance*. Duke University Press, Durham, NC.

Gonsiorek, J.C., and Weinrich, J.D. (1991) The definition and scope of sexual orientation. In: *Homosexuality: research implications for public policy*. Sage, Newbury Park, CA.

Gonsiorek, J.C., Sell, R.L., and Weinrich, J.D. (1995) Definition and measurement of sexual orientation. *Suicide and Life-Threatening Behavior* 25(Suppl.): 40–51.

Henry, G.W. (1941) *Sex variants: a study of homosexual patterns*, Vols. 1 and 2. Hoeber, New York.

Henry, G.W. (1955) *All the sexes: a study of masculinity and femininity*. Rinehart, New York.

Hirschfeld, M. (1914) *Die Homosexualitat des Mannes und des Weibes*. Louis Marcus, Berlin.

Katz, N. (1992) *Gay American history: lesbians and gay men in the United States*. Meridian, New York.

Kinsey, A.C, Pomeroy, W.B., and Martin, C.E. (1948) *Sexual behavior in the human male*. Saunders, Philadelphia.

Kinsey, A.C., Pomeroy, W.B., Martin, C.E., and Gebhard, P.H. (1953) *Sexual behavior in the human female*. Saunders, Philadelphia.

Klein, F., Sepekoff, B., and Wolf, T.J. (1985) Sexual orientation: a multi-variable dynamic process. *Journal of Homosexuality* 11:35–49.

Kraft-Ebing, R.V. (1886) *Psychopathia Sexualis: eine Klinisch-Forensische Studie*. Enke, Stuttgart.

Laumann, E., Gagnon, J., Michael, R., and Michaels, S. (1994) *The social organization of sexuality: sexual practices in the United States*. University of Chicago Press, Chicago.

LaVeist, T.A. (2002) Beyond dummy variables and sample selection: what health services researchers ought to know about race as a variable. In: LaVeist, T.A. (ed) *Race, ethnicity, and health: a public health reader*, Jossey-Bass, San Francisco.

Lee, R.M. (1993) *Doing research on sensitive topics*. Sage, London.

Legman, O. (1941) The language of homosexuality; an American glossary. In: Henry, O.W. (ed) *Sex variants: a study of homosexual patterns*. Hoeber, New York.

LeVay, S. (1993) *The sexual brain*. MIT Press, Cambridge, MA.

Masters, W.I., and Johnson, V.E. (1979) *Homosexuality in perspective*. Little, Brown, Boston.

Mayne, X. (1908) *The intersexes: a history of similsexualism at a problem in social life*. Privately printed, Paris.

Mercer, J.D. (1959) *They walk in shadow: a study of sexual variations with emphasis on the ambisexual and homosexual components and our contemporary set laws*. Comet, New York.

Miller, K. (2002) *Cognitive Analysis of Sexual Identity, Attraction and Behavior Questions*. National Center for Health Statistics Working Paper No. 32. NCHS, Washington, DC.

Moll, A. (1891) *Die Kontrare Geschlechtsempfindung*. Fischer's Medicin, Berlin.

Packard, E., and Packard, C. (2005) *Queer cowboys and other erotic male friend-ships in nineteenth-century American literature*. Palgrave Macmillan, New York.

Plato. (1993) *The Symposium and the Phaedrus*. State of New York Press, Albany, NY.

Robinson, V. (ed). (1936) *Encyclopedia sexualis*. Dingwall-Rock, New York.

Ross, M.W., Essien, E.J., Williams, M.L., and Fernandez-Esquer, M.E. (2003) Concordance between sexual behavior and sexul identity in street outreach samples of four racial/ethnic groups. *Sexually Transmitted Diseases* 30:110–113.

Sambrooks, J.E., and MacCulloch, M.J. (1973) A modification of the sexual ori-entation method and automated technique for presentation and scoring. *British Journal of Social and Clinical Psychology* 12:163–174.

Sell, R.L. (1996) The Sell assessment of sexual orientation: background and scoring. *Journal of Lesbian, Gay and Bisexual Identity* 1(4):295–310.

Sell, R.L., and Petrulio, C. (1995) Sampling homosexuals, bisexuals, gay, and lesbians for public health research: a review of the literature from 1990–1992. *Journal of Homosexuality* 30:31–47.

Shaw, T.C., and Ferris, G.N. (1883) Perverted sexual instinct. *Journal of Nervous Mental Disease* 10:185–204.

Shively, M.G., and DeCecco, J.P. (1977) Components of sexual identity. *Journal of Homosexuality* 3:41–48.

Shively, M.G., Jones, C., and DeCecco, J.P. (1985) Research on sexual orienta-tion: definitions and methods. In: DeCecco, J.P., and Find Shively, M.G. (eds) *Origins of sexuality and homosexuality*. Harrington Park Press, New York.

Signorle, Pvt. (1993) *Queer in America*. Random House, New York.

Solarz, A.L. (ed). (1999) *Lesbian health: current assessment and directions for the future*. Institute of Medicine, National Academy Press, Washington, DC.

Stedman's Medical Dictionary. (1982) Williams & Wilkins, Baltimore.

Storms, M.D. (1980) Theories of sexual orientation. *Journal of Personality and Social Psychology* 38:783–792.

Symonds, I.A. (1883) *A problem in Greek ethics*. Privately printed, London.

Symonds, I.A. (1891) *A problem in modem ethics*. Privately printed, London.

Tentler, T.N. (1977) *Sin and confession on the eve of the Reformation*. Princeton University Press, Princeton.

Ulrichs, K.H. (1994) *The Riddle of Man-Manly Love*, Prometheus Books, Buffalo, NY.

Weinberg, M.S., Williams, C.J., and Pryor, D.W. (1994) *Dual attraction*. Oxford University Press, New York.

Weinrich, J.D. (1990) The Kinsey Scale in biology, with a note on Kinsey as a biologist. In: McWhirter, D.P., Sander-, S.A., and Reinisch, J.M. (eds) *Homosexuality: concepts of sexual orientation*. Oxford University Press, New York.

Weinrich, J.D. (1994) Homosexuality. In: Bullough, V.L., and Bullough, B. (eds) *Human sexuality: an encyclopedia*. Garland, New York.

Weinrich, J.D., Snyder, P.J., Pillard, R.C., Grant, I., Jacobson, D.L., Robinson, S.R., and McCutchan, I.A. (1993) A factor analysis of the Klein Sexual Orientation Grid in two disparate samples. *Archives of Sexual Behavior* 22:157–168.

Westphal, K. (1869) Die Kontrare Sexualempfindung: Symptom eines neuro-pathologischen (psychopalhischen) Zustandes. *Archiv for Psychiatrie und Nervenkrankheiten* 2:73–108.

Sampling in Surveys of Lesbian, Gay, and Bisexual People

Diane Binson, Johnny Blair, David M. Huebner, and William J. Woods

1 Introduction

One purpose of this volume is to provide methodological tools for conducting public health research for lesbian, gay, and bisexual (LGB) populations. Among the most fundamental methodological considerations in any kind of research is how best to sample the population of interest. The importance of sampling in health research among LGB people can be seen in how the medical profession initially came to consider homosexuality a mental disorder. The "evidence" supporting such judgments came from studies of psychiatrists' patients and inmates in mental hospitals and prisons. The possibility that such samples might be biased—that is, that these individuals might not be representative of homosexuals who were not in treatment or institutionalized—was not considered seriously, in large part due to prevailing attitudes about homosexuality. Nevertheless, the historical lesson of how poor sampling can create significant problems for the health and well-being of LGB people should be enough to make all of us ardent promoters of the use of sound sampling procedures in public health research.

This chapter addresses sampling broadly but focuses primarily on procedures for probability sampling used in survey research. Although nonprobability sampling is discussed and has proved useful in particular circumstances, it should be stated clearly that the lack of representativeness, as one has no basis for knowing if they are representative, makes them significantly less useful when describing the larger LGB population. Public health has been seriously underserved by the lack of statistically defensible information describing the health behaviors and needs of the various LGB populations.

This lack of information on LGB health is not due to an absence of population studies. National government agencies have conducted health-related studies of the U.S. population using sophisticated sample designs for decades. The National Health Interview Survey (NHIS), which monitors the "health of the nation," has been conducted since 1957. Without asking even basic questions about sexual behavior, identification, or partnership on such population surveys, it was not possible to estimate accurately the number of LGB persons in the U.S. population or to identify their unique health care needs.

Kinsey and colleagues (1948, 1953) conducted extensive studies of human sexual behavior, but it is well known that there were fundamental problems with the sample of men and women on whom Kinsey and colleagues reported. For example, we know that the participants were made up of volunteers; as volunteers, one would expect that they would be somewhat more comfortable discussing and disclosing aspects of their sexuality and might well be more sexually experienced. Additionally, we know that the sample in the Kinsey group's 1948 volume on men included respondents drawn from sources that would have increased their likelihood of having had homosexual experiences, in particular, men from all-male institutions such as reform schools, jails, and prisons as well as men drawn from homosexual social networks. This has been discussed at some length by one of Kinsey's major collaborators (Gebhard, 1972; Gebhard & Johnson, 1979). Gebhard made a reasoned estimate on the prevalence of male homosexuality based on a cleaned-up sample and using somewhat different criteria. He concluded that "about 4% of the white college-educated males are predominately homosexual" over the course of their lives (Gebhard, 1972, p. 27).

Sadly, it took a health crisis among gay men to acknowledge the need for basic population data on LGB communities. When circumstances of the acquired immunodeficiency syndrome (AIDS) epidemic called for information on the patterns of sexual behavior of the U.S. population—information needed to design, implement, and evaluate programs to curb the spread of the epidemic—the public health archive of suitable data was virtually empty. In the context of the AIDS epidemic, however, funding was finally made available to draw samples of the general population that would allow prevalence estimates of same-gender sexual contact, as was later funding to draw representative samples of gay men. It was only recently that large federal- and state-level health surveys included questions related to sexual behavior and same-gender sexuality that facilitate analysis of health issues of LGB populations. Without continued resources, both financial and scientific, LGB health studies would be limited to small, nonprobability samples that limit the generalizability of findings (Solarz, 1999). Probability samples can provide reliable estimates and descriptions of health behavior and risks among LGB communities, thereby creating opportunities to design and target more accurately health education and disease prevention efforts that are relevant to the behavioral risks and needs of LGB people.

The rest of the chapter is divided into several parts. First, we provide a rationale for choosing to use probability sample designs and then define basic concepts used for probability sampling. The middle sections describe available probability sampling designs. These are followed by examples of uses of probability sampling in the literature on LGB health. The next section deals with nonprobability sampling, and the circumstances when such sampling is appropriate, the kinds of nonprobability sampling used, and examples of studies using such procedures. Finally, we provide a short discussion of two areas of sampling that are attracting a lot of attention among researchers: respondent-driven sampling and web-based sampling.

2 Drawing a Probability Sample

Careful sampling begins with the ability to enumerate (i.e., identify and count) the population of interest. If a population can be easily enumerated, it can be sampled in a fairly straightforward manner; to the extent that enumeration is difficult, the sampling is similarly difficult. Many circumstances may make a population difficult to enumerate. Samples of LGB populations or other groups defined by behaviors or self-identification are typically difficult to enumerate for two reasons. First, the population is not identifiable from the sampling frame (as, for example, are residential households in the telephone directory); therefore potential sample members have to be screened and asked to provide information to indicate whether they should be counted as population members. Second, the nature of the information may be considered, by some or most population members, to be sensitive and/or socially undesirable or to entail possible societal risks should it become known. LGB populations are what sampling statisticians would describe as "rare and elusive populations" (Sudman et al., 1988; Solarz, 1999). Although sampling these various rare and elusive populations may present several similar obstacles, each population has unique characteristics that need to be taken into consideration when designing a sample.

2.1 Sampling Rare Populations: Unknown Screening Rates and Costs

Conducting a general population survey of LGB individuals in the U.S. population is a daunting task. In the absence of detailed population information to be used when designing an efficient sample, such a survey would rely mainly or entirely on screening a general-purpose household sample. A massive screening effort would be needed to locate eligible respondents among the general population. Hundreds of thousands of households would have to be contacted before locating potentially eligible persons. Even then, how likely would the potentially eligible persons be to identify as a member of the target population? If they did report eligibility, would they be willing to participate in the survey? Because there are total geographic areas in which the prevalence of the targeted population is unknown and because the screening costs would undoubtedly be expensive, one strategy has been to focus research in cities that tend to have large concentrations of LGB populations and then to screen only households in certain neighborhoods in those cities. In the Urban Men's Health Study (UMHS) (Catania et al., 2001), for example, telephone numbers in selected ZIP codes were screened for eligibility. Nevertheless, while limiting the geographic area reduced the time and effort needed to screen households, the process still resulted in a large number of dialed phone numbers. For example, in one city in the UMHS study, 53,050 phone numbers in selected areas of the city were dialed to complete 915 interviews (Pollack, 1999, personal communication). Added to screening costs is the issue that screening rates are unknown and can vary across areas where sampling is being done. Generally when a sample is drawn, the number of households that must be screened to result in a desired number of completed interviews can be estimated using census data or other estimates of the population residing in particular areas. Given the lack of reliable prevalence data of LGB households, how large a sample one needs to start with to end up with "X" number of interviews involves significant guesswork. Starting with too small a sample typically poses a larger problem than beginning with too large a sample, as underestimating the initial sample requires selecting a second sample, which means a serious increase in effort. Hence starting with a larger sample, and then working a subsample from the larger sample to learn the actual screening rates, and using as many subsamples as needed to end up with the projected number of completed interviews is a less costly, more prudent procedure.

2.2 Sampling Elusive Populations: Identification and Response Rate

Another obstacle in sampling LGB populations involves the willingness of potential eligible respondents to be interviewed. Although successfully convincing individuals to participate in an interview is a common problem for most surveys, sampling LGB individuals may also present another difficulty. Some individuals are comfortable telling anyone, strangers and friends alike, that they are gay. However, there may be good reasons (e.g., fear of stigmatization or discrimination) why other individuals would not be willing to tell strangers on the phone that they identify as gay and/or engage in the particular behaviors that would make them eligible to participate in the study. Sampling is further complicated by how researchers may approach defining eligibility and who then is eligible to be in the sample. Sometimes eligibility is defined as how one wants to self-identify; other times it is behavioral, as is the case for most human immunodeficiency virus (HIV)-related studies. To complicate eligibility even further, behavioral definitions may include time boundaries. These challenges make it difficult to compute response rates, as there is so little information on which to base population estimates. Hence, computation of response rates in such situations relies on making certain assumptions about sample members whose eligibility is unknown. For example, when there is less information available than might be wished to estimate the prevalence of the targeted population among "noncontacts" (i.e., households that were selected to be in the sample but when contacted were never home during the entire data collection period of a study), information about these noncontacts remains unknown.

3 Basic Sampling Concepts

Many of the sample designs necessary to sample LGB populations efficiently are specialized and complex. However, all of them depend on understanding a few basic sampling principles and designs. This section provides a brief overview of some fundamental concepts of probability sampling. It is necessary to understand the logic of these common sampling approaches before confronting the more complex issues involved in sampling rare or elusive populations or populations that cannot be easily sampled via household selection. With this background, the next section describes variations and combinations of the basic sample designs to adapt them to LGB populations and includes specialized designs such as network sampling and site or time/location sampling.

3.1 Defining the Population of Interest

Defining the population is the starting point in survey sample design. Survey populations should always be precisely defined. The essence of the population definition has to do with the boundaries set on the group of interest. Whatever definition is settled on, it must be operationalized; that is, there must be a clear set of rules that can be applied to a sampling frame or to individuals who are potential sample members to determine their eligibility for inclusion uniformly. This operationalization sometimes requires compromises that create a slight divergence between the survey population and the (target) population for which the researchers wish to make inferences.

It is important to recognize that a population definition is a construct of the researcher, formulated to meet a particular survey purpose. For one survey, a gay 20-year-old Latino is simply a member of the "general population of adults." For another survey that person may be part of a target population, "Latino males." Still another survey may "define" him as part of the target population because he is gay. The survey construct may or may not be how that person thinks of himself. The terms "gay" or "homosexual" in screening questions do not necessarily identify the entire population of "men who have sex with men." It captures only those sample members who use those terms themselves or are willing to be labeled with them for the purposes of a survey.

The process of defining the population begins to suggest some sampling issues that need to be addressed. If the population is defined as visitors to some venue, questions of access, available lists (frames), or on-site enumeration need to be answered. If the population is defined more generally as a subset of the general population, questions of overall prevalence, differential prevalence by location, and screening response rates must be addressed before a sample design and sample size can be finalized.

3.2 Representative Sample

The goal of a probability sample is to select samples from populations of interest for the purpose of describing characteristics of those populations, testing models about how their members behave, or assessing the impact of programs and interventions, among other possible analyses. These objectives all involve statistical procedures that assume certain characteristics of the sample, such as randomness and independence of observations. Although a formal consideration of the assumptions of different statistical procedures is beyond the scope of this chapter, it is essential to keep in mind that statistical procedures and results are valid only if the assumptions on which they are based are not seriously violated. Careful analysis of a haphazardly selected sample is pointless.

In an everyday sense, any group of population members, however selected, is a sample of the population. Selection could be by way of volunteer respondents (as when people call a 1-900 telephone number to register their opinion on some issue), people selected by the interviewers' discretion on the street or in a retail establishment, even people selected haphazardly from a telephone book or other list. Such samples *may*, on some level, reflect characteristics of the populations from which they were selected, but we cannot be sure this is true; we have no scientific basis for asserting that samples drawn in these ways are at all "representative" of the target population from which they were taken.

What does *representative* mean? As with many survey terms, representative has multiple everyday meanings. It also has been noted that even in the scientific literature the term has been used in quite different ways. In a review and examination of those uses, Kruskal and Mosteller (1979) took a definition from a sampling text by Stephan and McCarthy (1958) as being closest to what we mean by representative in survey research. The central criterion of this definition is that representative samples are those permitting good estimation.

A *representative sample* is a sample which, for a specified set of variables, resembles the population . . . [in that] certain specified analyses . . . (computation of means, standard deviations etc.) yield results. . . . within acceptable limits set about the corresponding population values, except that . . . [rarely] the results will fall outside the limits [Stephan & McCarthy, 1958, pp. 31–32].

A couple of aspects of this definition are worth pointing out. First, the "representation" is linked to "specific analyses." Specific analyses imply particular variables (population parameters) of interest. This means that one wants the sample statistic, such as the proportion of people with health insurance coverage, to resemble the same statistic for the population. The researcher has a list of such variables that are operationalized (i.e., defined) by the survey questions corresponding to each variable. The objective is that the survey be representative with respect to this list of variables and their associated analyses.

Second, the definition requires that these sample statistics be close to the corresponding population values "within acceptable limits." This implies that each sample statistic is an "estimate" of the corresponding population statistic (i.e., population parameter). An estimate is not expected to be 100% accurate. It is important to be able to describe how accurate is a sample estimate. That is, the sample estimates *resemble* the population to an extent that can be quantitatively specified.

It is a common misunderstanding to envision a sample as being either representative or not. Frequently, in discussions of sample size, one hears the criterion that the sample should be large enough that it is "representative of the population." The matter is more complicated than that. The notion of representativeness is realistically viewed only as a continuum of precision in the context of the survey's needs.

To have a statistical basis for projecting from a sample back to the population from which it was selected, the sample must be one in which population members are chosen by some random mechanism in such a way that every member has a known, nonzero chance or probability to be included. When these conditions hold, there are laws of statistics that provide a basis for saying that the sample represents the population from which it was chosen. Such a sample is called a *probability sample*. Probability samples are representative of their populations in the Stephan-McCarthy sense. Probability samples also permit estimates of their precision, or *sampling error*.

3.3 Locate or Construct Frames

The *sampling frame* is a set of elements from which a subset is selected during each stage of the process of sampling population members. Ideally, the sampling frame is simply a list that includes all the eligible population members and no nonpopulation members. But a sampling frame may be one or more steps away from the actual sample members. For example, in a telephone survey of the adult population, the primary sampling frame is a list of telephone numbers. These telephone numbers are not themselves sample members. Telephone numbers are the first set of elements sampled *during the process* of reaching population members. The first stage of that process is sampling households. Some of the telephone numbers are residences in which one or more adults reside. Typically, the adults in the household are enumerated. That list is a second sampling frame from which the household (target population) members are selected.

To take one more example, suppose one is sampling visitors to a retail establishment. Ignoring the sample design details for now, one way this might be done is to sample times of day when the establishment is open for business and for each of the selected times sample customers who are present. The primary sampling frame is some list of all the possible times of day, perhaps in 1-hour intervals. A subset of these times is selected. Then, within each selected time, the customers are enumerated. The secondary frame is this list of customers. It is from this frame that target population members (customers) are selected.

The idealized sample frame as a list of all population members and only those population members is rarely achieved, but it is nonetheless important to keep in mind. Actual sample selection begins at this conceptual starting point. The need to have a suitable frame at each stage of selection is also important. Each frame should be a complete listing of that stage's sample elements; when it is not, the whole design is weakened.

Care must be taken when making use of available frames. First, the frame may have problems in terms of coverage of the population, including some eligibles, omitting others, and including some ineligibles as well. For example, a list of club members may include some who are no longer active and omitting recent registrants. Second, the information in the frame, such as addresses and telephone numbers, may be incorrect. Almost no frame is perfectly accurate.

There are four general problems one typically encounters with frames: eligible population members not on the list, ineligible members included in it, some eligibles appearing multiple times (duplication), and the reverse: some group of two or more eligibles having only one representation on the list. The first two problems are of concern because they create a mismatch (i.e., undercoverage or overcoverage) between the population of interest and the frame population. If those people who are omitted in error differ (in terms of the study variables) from those included, it clearly represents a source of error in the resulting sample estimates. Inadvertently including nonpopulation members in the sample means that the sample estimates do not fully correspond to the target population.

The next two problems concern effects on the chances of selection. Selection is typically made from entries on the list (i.e., the frame elements). If some population members appear multiple times in the frame, they have a greater likelihood of selection than those who appear only once. Similarly, individuals in a group of population members combined into one listing have a lower chance of selection than the population members who each have his or her own separate listing. There are procedures for dealing with each of these problems. The point is that failure to deal with them has consequences, sometimes quite serious, for the quality of the sample estimates.

3.4 Sampling Error

One source of variation in a sample estimate is due solely to the fact that a sample, not the entire population, is selected. This source of variation is called the *sampling error*. In the process we have been describing, a sample (n) selected from a population and interviewed producing a set of responses (R) from the n respondents (assuming for the moment perfect survey cooperation). From this set R, the corresponding set of sample estimates (E) of the population values is computed.

There are many samples of size n that *could have been selected* from the population. Only one of those samples, $n1$, was actually chosen; and its set of responses, $R1$, gave us one set of estimates $E1$ of the population parameters.

Suppose another sample (of the same size) is independently selected from this same population using exactly the same sample design, sampling frame, questionnaire, and data collection techniques (and that each survey obtains perfect cooperation). Now we have sample $n2$, the set of responses, R2, and a second set of sample estimates, E2. Because everything else in the process is unchanged, any difference between the sets E1 and E2 is due solely to the fact that each collected data from a somewhat different set of respondents.

Sampling error is defined (conceptually) as the average variation on a particular statistic between all possible samples of size n selected from the same population in the same manner. Sampling error depends on (i.e., is a function of) the sample size, the sample design, and the amount of variation in the target population on the variable being measured.

First consider the sample size: With large sample sizes one expects less variation from one to the other. There are simply fewer possible large samples that can be selected from the fixed population. In addition, the sampling error depends on the sample design and is computed differently for different designs. A common error is to compute the sampling error without taking the design into account; another is to run statistical tests that assume a simple random sample (discussed below) without taking into account that the survey sample was selected using another design. Finally, regardless of sample size or design, variation exists in the sample simply because individuals in the population differ from one another. Although this is not technically a sampling *error* (it is a reflection of true population variation), it is included in standard measures of the sample error.

In summary, the general sampling procedure outlined so far requires that the researcher define the target population, obtain a suitable sampling, determine the necessary sample size, select a probability sample, and compute sample estimates of population parameters. The next sections outline both simple and more complex sample designs.

4 Available Sample Designs

4.1 Simple Random Sampling

The objective of many, but by no means all, sample designs is to give every population member the same chance of selection as every other population member. One sample design that accomplishes this is simple random sampling.

With simple random sampling, each member of the sampling frame is numbered 1 through N (i.e., $1,2,3 \ldots N$), where N is the total number of listings. If a sample of size n is desired, then n random numbers are selected (in the range 1 to N) from a table of random numbers or a random number generator. Each random number that corresponds to a number 1–N identifies a selected sample member (numbers selected more than once are ignored after their first occurrence). There are more details, but this gives the general conception. A simple random sample gives each member of the sampling frame the same chance of selection, and that chance is n/N. Moreover, with simple random sampling *every possible sample* of size n has the same chance of being selected. This implies that every member of the population, N, has the same chance of selection, which is what we are usually interested in.

Simple random sampling has several practical shortcomings. We focus here on just two. First, it can be a rather cumbersome procedure to implement partly because most lists used for surveys were not created for sampling purposes. Unless the sampling operation is computerized, numbering a list is time-consuming and tedious. If the sample is even moderately large, many random numbers must be selected (generated) and duplicates recorded. Second, although unlikely, it is possible that a simple random sample now and then produces a sample with a distribution quite unlike that of the population from which is was selected. This is more likely when the sample is small. Such "odd" distributions rarely occur, but it would be good to avoid them altogether. Depending on the order of the list, systematic sampling can reduce the chances of such distributions; stratified sampling can eliminate them altogether.

4.2 Systematic Random Sampling

Simple random sampling gives each possible sample the same chance of selection; this is more than we require for most survey sampling purposes. It is the individual's chance of inclusion that concerns us; this is a goal that can be attained in a simpler fashion. Systematic random sampling is a more common method used to sample a list by selecting every k^{th} person on the list (sampling interval). This is clearly a simpler procedure, especially when the population list is large. This technique differs from simple random sampling in that every possible sample of size n no longer has a chance of being selected (e.g., using this method there is no way that two population members next to each other on the list can be in the same sample). The number of possible samples has been greatly reduced. In fact, the number of possible samples is exactly equal to the sampling interval, but each individual list member has an equal chance of inclusion, and that is the primary goal.

In a sense, this approach will produce perfectly acceptable samples that meet the requirement of "representativeness" as defined earlier. However, many times there are practical obstacles to using this method; for example, it may be that no satisfactory single frame is available. More importantly, however, there are often ways we can improve the effectiveness and efficiency of the design. By *effectiveness* we mean the precision of the sample estimates for a given sample size, and by *efficiency* we mean the cost of implementing the sample in an actual survey. These are important issues when sampling easily enumerable populations; they become critical when the population is rare or elusive.

4.3 Stratified Sampling

Assume that a population contains sets of individuals similar to each other on some variable, such as education, neighborhood of residence, or some other demographic characteristic. If that variable is also related to the survey's substantive measures, such as health-related behavior or leisure activities, it may be possible to improve the sample design efficiency by grouping similar individuals together into *strata* and then sampling each stratum independently. This assumes that information about the stratification variable is available in the sampling frame. (There are methods for stratification that can sometimes be used when the variable is not in the sampling frame, but this discussion does not address those complications.)

There are two general types of stratification: proportional and disproportional. Both begin with defining the strata of interest and then follow with dividing the population/frame into strata and selecting a portion of the total sample from each stratum. With proportional stratification, the percentage of the sample allocated to each stratum equals that stratum's proportion of the total target population. With disproportional stratification, some (perhaps all) strata receive sample allocations that are either more or less than their percentage of the total target population.

4.3.1 Proportional Stratification
Proportional allocation of the sample is used to improve the precision of the sample's representativeness of certain important characteristics. For example, assume one was to sample female clinic patients from a list that contained each woman's age, and age was thought to be correlated with some outcome variable. Before sampling, the list could be rearranged into age strata: 18 to 29, 30 to 39, 40 to 49, 50 and older. A sample would be selected from each age stratum proportional to that stratum's percentage of the total female patient population. If no stratification was done, these are still the proportions that would be expected on average over repeated independent samples. However, any one particular simple random sample might, by chance, underrepresent or overrepresent a particular stratum, even by a large amount. If the stratum variable is related to the dependent variables, it would be good to avoid the possibility of such a sample. This is what proportional stratification does. It is not a very powerful technique, meaning that it usually produces only modest improvements in the precision of sample estimates. If proportional allocation can be done inexpensively (e.g., by reordering a computerized list before sampling from it), it can be useful. It is generally not worth a large investment of study resources.

4.3.2 Disproportional Stratification
Disproportional stratification is a much more versatile and powerful design. With disproportional stratification, the proportion of the sample allocated to a stratum is not the same as that stratum's proportion of the population. There are several broad reasons to use disproportional stratification that are relevant to and summarized in this chapter.

The first general reason for using disproportional stratification is because the strata are of interest in themselves. In many surveys, in addition to estimates for the total target population, the researchers may be interested in either separate analysis of certain subgroups or comparing some subgroups to others. Often the natural proportions do not produce enough cases for these objectives.

Assume that in a survey of lesbians the main objective is to compare lesbians who live in the inner city of a metropolitan area to those who live in the suburbs. The most efficient sample allocation *for this objective* is to take half the sample from the city and half from the suburbs, even though the actual distribution of the total lesbian population may differ considerably from a 50:50 sampling distribution. This allocation minimizes the sampling error of differences found between the two strata, the main type of analysis for a study comparing subgroups (strata).

Another common objective is to ensure that enough of a population subgroup is sampled to permit separate analysis. Assume, in the same survey of lesbians, that 80% of the target population are expected to reside in the suburbs and 20% in the inner city. If the total sample were 400 interviews, only about 80 would be expected to fall in the city if no stratification was used. If 80 were considered too few for the planned analysis, one might, for example, take a double sample from the city to produce 160 interviews. It is useful to keep in mind that even within a targeted subgroup further subgroups may be of interest. So, even if 80 cases were considered marginally acceptable for examining inner-city lesbians in total, if further analysis by age or education was also planned at that level the 80 cases would likely be insufficient. Once again, it is seen how the sample design depends on the planned analysis.

A second reason to use disproportional stratification is that costs differ by stratum (i.e., certain sample members may be more expensive to survey than others). When surveying a population that is not evenly distributed geographically (e.g., Hispanic adults), it may be much more costly to locate sample members in some areas (in this case, the northwestern United States) than in others (e.g., the southwestern United States).

Sample designs for rare populations may have widely varying costs for the same reason (i.e., the distribution of the population). Even small absolute differences can have major effects. Consider sampling for a population that has 5% prevalence in one stratum and 12% prevalence in a second stratum. Although the difference is only 7%, more than twice as much screening is needed in the first stratum than in the second one to locate each sample member.

The usefulness of disproportionate stratified sampling for rare groups depends on the extent to which the prevalence of the target group varies across strata (e.g., geographic areas). For the procedure to be effective, some geographic areas need to have *both* a higher prevalence of the target group *and* include a large proportion of the total target population. This may be best illustrated with a simple example.

Assume that for a citywide, household survey of gay males three strata are identified. Stratum one consists of a set of neighborhoods known to have a high prevalence of gay males, say 60% of all households. Stratum two is a set of more "mixed" neighborhoods also known to have a high prevalence of, say, 15% of households. Stratum three is the remainder of the city, where the prevalence is expected to be 3%. Clearly, the cost per case, which depends largely on the screening costs to locate eligible households, varies greatly from one stratum to another. A sensible sample design oversamples *to some extent* strata one and two. Consider two possible situations, keeping in mind that people who reside in certain neighborhoods may very well differ both demographically (e.g., age, income, education) and in terms of the substantive variables being measured from those who choose to reside outside those neighborhoods.

In the first situation, assume that *of the total gay male population of the city* 50% reside in stratum one, 25% in stratum two, and the remaining 25% in stratum three, the rest of the city. This population distribution is fortunate for sampling purposes. The strata that have high prevalence rates (percentages of stratum households that are eligible) also contain a large proportion (75%) of the target population. So it is statistically logical to heavily oversample those strata.

Now consider a second situation in which stratum one contains 15% of all the city's gay males, stratum two has an additional 15%, and the remaining 70% are in stratum three, which happens to have the lowest within-stratum prevalence. Although strata one and two can still be oversampled to some extent, the sample cannot be heavily concentrated there because even though the density of eligibles is high *most of the city's gay males do not reside in those neighborhoods.* Although the technical details of computing the correct sample allocations is beyond the scope of this chapter (see Kalton, 1993, for those procedures), the reasoning behind disproportional stratification is that one has to consider each stratum's prevalence *and* the percentage of the entire population it includes to design an efficient sample. This is analogous to a national survey of Hispanics in which it is known that New Mexico has a high prevalence of Hispanics (i.e., most of New Mexico's population is Hispanic), but New Mexico contains a very small proportion of all the nation's Hispanics. It would be unwise to concentrate a national sample in New Mexico. It would be cost-effective, but the final sample would not accurately reflect the nation's Hispanic population.

Finally, in regard to costs differing by strata, if multiple methods of data collection are used, such as telephone and face-to-face interviews (for those without telephones), the face-to-face sample may be considered a separate stratum for which the cost per interview is greatly increased. In each of these cases, an allocation of the sample that is disproportional to the population distribution may be necessary.

When each sample member has the same probability of selection, we describe the sample design as "self weighting." Each sample member represents the same number of population members; put another way, each population member is equally represented. When (and this can come about in various ways) sample members have different probabilities of selection, some population members are overrepresented relative to others. This needs to be accounted for to produce unbiased sample estimates of population parameters.

Recall an earlier example. In a disproportionally stratified sample of lesbians, those living in the city were oversampled relative to those in the suburbs. In one instance, this was to compare the two groups optimally; in another, it was to have sufficient cases for separate analysis.

Both uses of stratification were justified for those analytic purposes. Usually, however, one would also want to combine the two samples for total target population estimates (i.e., for the whole metro area). If city and suburban residents differed on substantive variables, the city residents would be overrepresented and the resulting sample estimates biased in their direction. To produce unbiased total estimates, these different probabilities of selection (for those particular analyses) must be corrected. This is accomplished with weighting. The details of weight construction are beyond the scope of this discussion, but the effect is that, in this example, suburban residents are assigned a greater weight to make up for the fact that there are fewer of them in the sample than their portion of the population requires.

With weighting, each sample member's response to a substantive question is multiplied by that sample member's "weight." The *weight* is a number that can be greater than 1, meaning that the response is counted more heavily in the estimate (as if there were more of that "type" of sample member in the sample). This type of weight makes up for underrepresentation (having a lower probability of selection than equal representation would require). Similarly, a case can have a weight of less than 1, achieving the opposite effect of reducing the impact of that case's answer on the estimate.

4.4 Cluster Sampling

With the sample designs discussed to this point, respondents have been selected essentially one by one. There are many instances where considerable cost savings can be realized by selecting groups or clusters of respondents. Clusters are *naturally occurring* groups of potential respondents. Often costs can be reduced by sampling clusters, but there is a statistical *cost*. There are often similarities between people in a natural cluster. That is, people who live on the same city block, those treated at the same clinic, or those who are in the same school classroom may be alike in some way, perhaps by age or income. People are not grouped into clusters at random. Put another way, the interview measures within a cluster may be correlated; that is, they are not completely independent observations. This means that a sample of size n selected by way of clusters is almost always inferior to a sample of the same size selected by a simple (or systematic) random sample; that is, the sampling error is larger for the same size sample).

Recall that the sampling error is partly a function of sample size; thus, as sample size increases, sampling error decreases. The way around the problem of within-cluster homogeneity is to increase the total sample size to offset its effects. The cost per case is often so much lower with cluster sampling that, for the fixed cost that constrains real-world surveys, a larger sample can be selected to offset the effects of within-cluster correlation.

Although the main rationale for cluster sampling is lower sampling errors for the available fixed costs, there are other reasons as well. A common reason is the unavailability of sampling frames for many populations.

An important application of cluster sampling for rare populations is telephone cluster sampling (TCS). TCS is a variant of Mitofsky-Waksberg (Waksberg, 1978, 1983) sampling applicable to rare groups and was described by Blair and Czaja (1982). With TCS, a random telephone number is dialed in a bank of telephone numbers (a bank is 100 numbers generated by randomizing the last two digits of telephone numbers). This number can be selected via list-assisted random digit dialing or any other procedure.[1] If the number is found to be a working household number, the household (or person) is screened for membership in the target group. If the household is not a member of the target group or if the number is not a working household number, no further sampling is done within that bank. However, if a group member is found, further sampling is done within the bank until a pre-specified number of group members are identified.[2] This procedure has the effect of rapidly dropping telephone banks with no target group members.

The usefulness of TCS for sampling a rare group generally depends on the extent to which the group is geographically clustered. If the group is spread evenly across telephone exchanges, and there are few phone banks in which it does not occur, then TCS increases the operational complexity of the research without improving its efficiency.

An alternative perspective to geographic clustering for deciding whether TCS will be efficient is to consider the effectiveness of TCS using ρ, the intracluster coefficient of homogeneity, as an indicator of the rare group's tendency to cluster within telephone banks (ρ is the conventional measure of tendency for similar elements to co-occur within clusters (i.e., the correlation between elements within clusters with regard to the characteristic of interest) (cf. Sudman, 1976)).

Assume we use the TCS method described earlier, in which subsequent calls in a telephone bank are made if and only if the first call produces a member of the rare group. Let π be the proportion of the general population who fall into the target group and thus the expected screening rate for "first calls" into random telephone banks (ignoring, for the moment, the effects of nonworking numbers, business numbers, noncontacts, and refusals to participate). Let π' represent a comparable screening rate for second and subsequent calls into telephone banks

---

[1]The original purpose for Waksberg sampling was to find working household telephone numbers and eliminate banks of nonworking numbers. For this purpose, list-assisted RDD competes with Waksberg sampling (list-assisted methods eliminate nonworking banks by restricting the sampling to banks that are known to have at least one listed household). However, when the goal is to find members of a rare group, the two procedures are complementary. List-assisted methods can eliminate banks of completely nonworking numbers, and Waksberg sampling can eliminate working banks in which the target group does not occur.

[2]The cluster size is defined as identified, not cooperating, eligible households or individuals. If the cluster size is k, calling in the bank stops after k group members are identified by screening, regardless of whether they consent to the main interview.

where the first call has produced a member of the rare group; in other words, π' represents the conditional probability of drawing a member of the group given that one has already been drawn. Finally, assume that ρ is the intratelephone bank coefficient of homogeneity for the defining characteristic(s) of the target group, defined as the correlation in incidence between successive elements within banks (e.g., "first call" and "second call"). It can be shown (Blair & Blair, 2004) that the relationship between π and π' is as follows:

$$\pi' = \pi + \rho(1 - \pi)$$

Essentially, this expression indicates that if the first number called in a bank is eligible, the prevalence of eligibles in that bank π' is greater than the overall eligibility rate π. The actual screening rates experienced in a research project are lower than indicated because of nonworking numbers, business numbers, noncontacts, and refusals.

The details of the analysis of the efficiency of TCS are beyond the scope of this chapter, but the conclusion of that analysis is that the rareness of the target group was found to be at least as important as the level of geographic clustering (and arguably more important) for determining the relative efficiency of TCS. The intuition is that as first-stage respondents become more difficult to find it becomes increasingly beneficial to look near those respondents for others like them if there is even a mild tendency for respondents to cluster. On the other hand, if first-stage respondents are easy to find, there is little to gain from clustered sampling, even given a strong tendency to cluster.

This design has been incorporated into an "adaptive sampling" approach to produce an efficient two-phase approach for locating a population of men who have sex with men (MSM) in a multicity survey (Blair, 1999).

5 Complex Sample Designs

5.1 Adaptive Designs

With all the designs described to this point, the sample design is "fixed." That is, using the best information available at the outset of the study, a sample design is selected, sample size determined, sample allocated to strata, and so on; and the survey proceeds. In short, the sample is selected and its procedures followed to select and interview sample members. Another class of sample designs are termed adaptive samples. "Adaptive sampling refers to sampling designs in which the procedures for selecting sites or units to be included in the sample may depend on values of the variable of interest observed during the survey" (Thompson & Collins, 2002). This is an appealing approach for some LGB surveys, although it is easy to underestimate the complications involved in its careful implementation.

Sample designs rely to varying degrees on prior information about the target population. In the case of rare or elusive populations, the estimate of prevalence of the target population within the larger population is one such piece of information that is especially important—even more so if the prevalence varies significantly by geography or other sample units (as was the case with TCS). In some situations this prior information about prevalence may be suspect for various reasons. The prevalence information may not exactly match the survey's population definition, or it may be dated. Different sources of information may produce different prevalence estimates. The data source may be from the census, from some type of administrative records, or from a survey that did not involve screening for the particular population. In many such instances the degree of underreporting may differ markedly from what would be found in a screening survey. Finally, data from multiple sources may be combined into one "best value" estimate of prevalence. The procedure for combining the data has error properties that may be difficult to specify. All these possibilities produce situations in which crucial design decisions are based on imperfect data.

Adaptive sample designs may permit a quantitative assessment of the prevalence data before all the sampling is completed. Consider, for example, a stratification design in which costs differ by stratum. As noted earlier, disproportionate stratification may be an efficient design when costs differ substantially by stratum. Following Hansen et al. (1953), Sudman (1976) produced a simplified formula relating the cost per interview to the sample allocation to strata. Essentially, a disproportionally larger percentage of the sample is allocated to strata in which the cost per case is lower and less of the sample to the strata with higher cost per case. When the target population's prevalence is the only factor that differs by stratum, the cost per interview is directly proportional to the prevalence. The estimated cost per interview, and hence the strata allocations, depend on knowing the target population prevalence in each stratum.

An adaptive design using disproportional stratification owing to differential costs would release a small portion of the sample, based on the estimated prevalence, in each stratum for surveying. The screening rate for each stratum would be determined based on contacting the released sample. That is, the estimate of prevalence would be corrected based on actual screening. To the extent that the screening rates differ from the expectations, the remaining (unreleased) sample would be allocated based on this new information. Even though the screening rates are themselves estimates, subject to sampling error, it is possible to detect major differences between the expected and actual prevalence. This approach was used to improve the sampling efficiency of a survey of gay urban males in multiple citywide surveys (Blair, 1999).

5.2 Network Sampling

In a survey to locate a target population with a particular characteristic, the most direct procedure is, as we have seen, to screen a random sample of households and for each one determine whether someone with the characteristic of interest resides there. If the target population is rare, this procedure requires screening many households. The *reporting rule*, in such a conventional survey, asks a household to report about all of its members and only those members.

Network sampling uses a different reporting rule. Households in the selected sample are conceptually linked to other households (which almost always are not in the sample). Some of those other households contain a member of the target population. The reporting rule asks a sample household to report about its own residents *and* about the residents of households to which is it linked. The screening rate is increased to the extent that target population households are linked to households in the sample.

Birnbaum and Sirken (1965) first described this sampling approach as a method for estimating the prevalence of rare diseases. The method has been used or tested as a technique to identify cancer patients (Czaja et al., 1986), crime victims (Czaja & Blair, 1990), and other rare populations (Sudman et al., 1988).

There are various possible applications of network sampling to LGB surveys when the objective is to identify these target groups within the general population. The first and intuitively most appealing application is to use network sampling to identify and interview target population members. With this approach, respondents are asked whether the members of some prespecified social network (e.g., their brothers and sisters) have the characteristic(s) of interest. If any member of the network belongs to the group, the respondent is asked for contact information, and the researcher attempts to interview those network members.

Network sampling is effective only if the defining characteristic of the group, in this case sexual orientation, is known to other members of a measurable network. Also, if network members are to be interviewed, the initial respondents must be, in the main, willing to provide referrals to other network members. Even then, the benefits of the procedure are offset by the difficulty of having to find networked respondents, the difficulty of developing reliable weights to correct the differential inclusion probabilities resulting from varying numbers of people who might have nominated them, and design effects from weighting. Even if all these conditions are met, if the researcher's target population is limited to a specified geographic area, then identified network members who reside outside that area are ineligible for the survey. Because of these limitations and difficulties, network sampling is rarely used to locate and interview target population members.

There are two other contexts where the procedure might be effective. First, when the purpose of the research, or some phase of it, is to estimate the prevalence of the target group rather than contacting its members, the researchers might choose network sampling. If all one needs is prevalence data, then network sampling has the potential to expand the effective sample size without imposing the difficulty of obtaining referrals and finding networked respondents. This, in fact, is how the procedure was used in its early days (cf. Sirken, 1970), but that application has faded.

The second possible application is related to the first. Network sampling might prove useful when adaptive procedures are employed to guide disproportionate stratified sampling, and prevalence data are needed to guide the strata definitions and allocations. Here, one is in the position of estimating prevalence based on relatively few data in any given geographic area, and the increase in effective sample size associated with network sampling might be helpful.

In both contexts, it is still necessary that group membership is identifiable by other network members, and it is still necessary to estimate or control the number of people who might nominate any given network member. Also, in the latter context, because network measures are used to inform a geographically based stratification scheme, it must be possible to link network identifications to that scheme (i.e., determine in which stratum a nominee lives). This might be done, for example, by obtaining the ZIP code or the first four digits of each network member's telephone number. These requirements continue to limit the use of network sampling; but considering the value of prevalence information in studies of rare groups, the possibility of using network sampling should not be overlooked.

5.3 Site or Time/Location Sampling

With site sampling, visitors to a well defined location are sampled at that location. The sample may be selected at one point in time, multiple discrete points in time, or over some continuous period of days or weeks. Locations can be single retail establishments, groups of such establishments (e.g., a retail chain or a mall), and recreational locations such as parks or theaters; even temporary settings such as street fairs can, under certain conditions, be sampled. Sampled respondents usually answer questions about themselves but can be asked about the particular establishment instead of, or in addition to, personal information.

Site or time/location sampling, properly executed, is a probability design applied to a limited, nonhousehold population. Site sample designs are used when the particular site or location is of interest in itself, or when the site is a gathering place for a population of interest. The population may be sampled on site because the site is part of the population definition (e.g., patrons of lesbian bars) or simply because the site is convenient to find members of a more broadly defined population (e.g., all lesbians in a particular geographic area). All visitors to the site may be eligible sample members or only those with particular characteristics.

Although such samples may be appealing for a number of reasons, two cautions should be noted. First, typically the population of inference is severely restricted, often representing only visitors to the particular location(s). Second, if inappropriate sampling procedures are used, the probability design can quickly degenerate into a sample of convenience.

A limited definition may or may not be useful. If for example, the site is one gay bar that happens to be accessible, for whatever reason, to the researcher, the sample represents only patrons of that bar. It does not represent all bar patrons and certainly not all gays in a city or neighborhood. For some purposes, that definition boundary might be acceptable.

It is possible to expand the scope of the definition by selecting a probability sample of establishments and then sampling patrons within each one. For example, if a list of all gay bars (assuming that "gay bar" can be rigorously defined) in a town is available, a sample of bars could be selected using probability sampling, and site sampling could be done at the sampled bars. The population definition is thus expanded to cover patrons to bars (of the selected type) in that town.

The bars could either be chosen with equal probabilities and the sample allocated across them in proportion to an estimate of each bar's size (total patrons per week or some other measure related to the size of the target population the bar's patrons includes). If the entire census of bars were included, proportional allocation of the sample would also be the simplest legitimate approach. Alternatively, a sample of bars could be selected with probabilities proportional to size. In that case, a fixed number (cluster size) of sample members would be selected at each bar. The latter approach would be useful for practical reasons (i.e., to equalize the burden on each bar); or the same allocation might be an efficient way to ensure enough sample of all size (or other characteristic of) bars for subgroup analysis.

Assume a site has been selected by whatever means: How does site sampling work? Most often, a two-stage, cluster sample design is used. In the first stage, time slots are selected; in the second stage, respondents visiting the establishment during those time slots are sampled. If the time slots are selected with probabilities proportional to size (where the measure of size is number of expected visitors or some correlate of that, such as sales), then a fixed cluster size of respondents is chosen. The two stages taken together produce an equal probability sample of visits. It is important to note that the sample is of visits, not visitors. The probability of an individual visitor is proportional to the number of times he visits the establishment during the data collection period. The sample of visits may be weighted to convert it to a sample of individual visitors, as shown below.

The two-stage cluster approach was used to select a sample of patrons for an exit survey of patrons at a gay bathhouse. We are including this example because a time/location design is often used for sampling LGB populations, and detailed examples of how it is used are not easily available elsewhere, unlike examples of other, more conventional sample designs. The following description focuses on the estimation procedure, which is essentially a process of constructing weights to produce unbiased sample estimates. This detailed description also illustrates some general principles of sample weighting for nonresponse and for differential probabilities of selection. The general procedure is to construct individual weights, including (1) a "base weight" to account for the overall probability of selection (this base weight, which theoretically is a simple inverse of the probability of selection, has to be constructed taking into account some practical steps in sample selection); (2) a weight to convert the sample of visits into a sample of individuals, the units of analysis; and (3) a weight to adjust for differential nonresponse. These individual weights are then combined into one overall weight for data analysis.

The participating bathhouse was open 24 hours a day, 7 days a week. A time probability sample was selected over a 5-week period. Using data on the number of customers per employee work shift, a probability sample of shifts was selected during week 1, with probabilities proportional to the number of customers expected (i.e., busy shifts were selected more often). Within each selected shift, a systematic sample of customers was selected with equal probabilities. During the subsequent weeks, the expected number of customers per shift was updated based on counts in the sampled shifts. Using this sampling design, we sampled 708 patrons exiting the bathhouse, with 440 (62.1%) agreeing to participate in the survey. Those declining to participate were not significantly different from participants by age ($p = 0.38$) or race ($p = 0.73$). There was a significant difference in refusals during the 3 to 6 PM shifts ($p < 0.003$), where we averaged 57% of the men refusing compared to all other shifts, which ranged as low as 23.5% (3 to 6 AM) to as high as 48.7% (9 AM to noon). There was also a significant improvement in acceptance as the weeks passed, with the highest rate of refusals occurring in week 1 (48.2%) and the lowest in week 5 (25.3%).

This time-probability sampling design did not produce a self-weighting sample of either visits or of individuals. A series of weights were necessary to produce unbiased, or nearly unbiased, estimates. Strictly speaking, each week, k, has a base weight

$$\text{WB}_k = 1/P_{vk}$$

the inverse of probability of selection in week k, where

$$P_{vk} = P_{sk} \times P_{(s)k}$$

Hence, the probability of a visit P_{vk} during a given week k is the probability of a shift being chosen

$$P_{sk} = N_{sk}\Big/\sum N_k$$

times the probability of selection within the shift.

$$P_{(s)k} = n_{sk}/N_{sk}$$

The complication in computing this weight is that we have only an estimate of the total number of visits for a week:

$$\sum N_k$$

Counts of visits are available only for the shifts that were sampled. For the nonsampled shifts, the counts are either the previous weeks' counts or the initial count provided by the establishment.

To simplify this computation, we have assumed a fixed mean of 600 visits each week, for a total of 3000 visits for the 5-week period. The probability of selection of a visit is then modeled as the ratio of the total sample selected over this estimate of total visits.

The sample size for a shift was modeled as the target number of completed interviews, 6, adjusted for the mean expected response rate 50%, $6/0.5 = 12$. The selected sample varies when the actual number of visits for a shift differs from the expected measure of size for the shift. The probability of a visit over the entire data collection period is estimated as

$$P_v = \sum_k \hat{n}_k \Big/ \sum_k \hat{N}_k$$

where $\sum_k \hat{N}_k = 3000$ and

$$\sum_k \hat{n}_k = 12 \sum_i s$$

or 12 times the number of shifts selected over the 5 weeks.

5.3.1 Visits Weight

A respondent visits weight (WV) is necessary to adjust for differential numbers of visits by different respondents during the 5-week data collection period. This weight essentially changes the sample from a sample of visits to a sample of individuals.

The probability of person j being selected is proportional to that person's total visits during the data collection period (obtained from survey questions).

$$P_{vj} \propto \sum_i v_{ij}$$

The "visits" weight is the inverse of the estimated total visits for a person.

$$WV_j = 1 \Big/ \sum_i v_{ij}$$

5.3.2 Nonresponse Weight

The shift nonresponse weight is used to adjust for situations when the actual number of completed interviews for a shift (c_a) falls short of the target cluster size (c_t) (of completed interviews) for that sampled shift.

$$W_{nr} = c_t/c_a$$

This weight adjusts both for shortfalls due to nonresponse and due to an inadequate number of visits in the shift to reach the target c_t.

5.3.3 *Total Weight*

The total weight (*WT*) is obtained by combining all three weights into one weight variable.

$$WT = WB \times WV \times W_{nr}$$

This total weight (*WT*) then weights the sample back to the estimated total population.

5.4 Cautions When Using Complex Designs

These complex sample designs have been developed to handle the special problems of cost-effectively sampling rare or elusive populations. Some of these approaches are extensions of basic designs such as disproportional stratification; others, such as network sampling, differ radically from conventional sample designs.

Some points of caution are relevant here. Complex designs typically require more specialized expertise to select the sample and may also rely on difficult procedures being properly executed as part of the data collection. Even when the idea underlying a design is fairly simple, its implementation may not be. A second caution flows from the first. When a design is badly implemented, its advantages may be lost or may be attained at an unacceptable price, such as when cost savings are realized in return for major increases in sampling variance or high nonresponse rates. Such unfortunate consequences may be present, even if they are overlooked by the researcher. An even more serious consequence of poor execution is that the sample may cease to be a probability sample at all, such as when incorrect sampling procedures make it impossible to specify probabilities of selection or to produce valid sample estimates. Additionally, some of these designs are based on assumptions or conditions, such as that respondents can provide certain information or perform particular response tasks. Some of these required conditions can be easily met, whereas for others it is quite problematic, even dubious, that they can be realized. If a design rests on strong assumptions, they must be carefully assessed, perhaps by conducting a pilot study, before proceeding.

Finally, when using complex sample designs, it is important to note that although for many designs there are formulas to compute sampling errors directly, in many instances such formulas do not exist. It is standard practice today to use one of several software packages that have been made available in recent years for the correct computation of sampling errors for complex surveys. SUDAAN and WesVar are two of the most popular and statistically sound. A common error of novice researchers is to apply the formula for simple random sampling errors to other designs, leading to often severe underestimation of sampling errors. Even though a complex design may produce equal probabilities of selection for individual sample members after many steps and statistical weighting adjustments, it by no means constitutes a simple random sample.

6 Research of LGB Populations Using Probability Samples

As we have discussed in this chapter, probability sampling allows researchers interested in LGB topics to generalize their findings to a larger population (i.e., beyond the sample itself). This might involve estimating the size of a particular population or the prevalence of a specific phenomenon.

Approaches to probability sampling in LGB research have fallen into three broad categories. The first category includes designs where investigators draw a probability sample of the general population (gay and nongay) and then conduct analyses on the subsample of LGB respondents within the larger sample. In this case, the LGB individuals are a subpopulation of the larger population, and research findings from the subsample of LGB respondents can be generalized or projected back to that subpopulation. In the second category, researchers may employ techniques to increase the size of the sample with desired characteristics (e.g., homosexual identity or HIV infection). These techniques typically involve focusing on preselected ZIP codes, census tracts, or social settings thought to have a greater concentration of the desired characteristic and then drawing a probability sample of all or a segment of the population only from within that focused area. The primary benefit of such techniques is that the subsample of interest (e.g., LGB persons) is larger than what could be sampled in general population studies. However, such techniques also limit the ability of investigators to generalize to the LGB population beyond the selected ZIP code or setting. The third category of designs is similar to the second, except that investigators draw a probability sample by screening for *LGB individuals only*, again generally in selected ZIP codes or settings. In these cases, generalizations are made from the LGB probability sample to the LGB population in the selected ZIP code or setting and generally result in larger samples than the previous categories, which allow for more extensive analyses.

Table 15.1 lists several examples of studies in each of these categories of research. For each of the studies cited in Table 15.1, we list the population the researchers were interested in studying, the substantive research interest, the sample design, the actual population that was sampled, and the mode of data collection. Our goal was to cite studies that displayed a range of population interest, type of probability design, and mode of data collection. When possible, we selected studies that described the sample design in some detail to provide the reader with more information than is generally provided in journal articles. For some studies the same design is described in the substantive article or book chapter listed; for others additional articles or chapters that provide extensive discussion of the sample design are cited for more detailed descriptions.

Not surprisingly, most of the LGB-related studies using probability sample designs are quite recent. The funding that provides researchers with sufficient resources to draw probability samples of populations reporting same-gender sexuality is a recent phenomenon (last 15 years)

Table 15.1. Examples of Probability Sample Designs in Studies of Lesbian, Gay, Bisexual Adults, and Adolescents

Population of interest	Research interest	Sample design and [mode of data collection]	Population sampled	Reference
Subpopulation of LGB in a general population				
Lesbian, bisexual women	Patterns of cigarette smoking and alcohol use among lesbians and bisexual women	Stratified random sample from membership list [self-administered questionnaire (SAQ); mail]	Kaiser Permanente members residing in northern California region at least 20 years of age and members at least 3 months	Gruskin et al. (2001)
Men reporting same-sex sexual contact	Prevalence of men who have sex with men (MSM)	Multistage area probability samples from five samples [personal, SAQ]	U.S. adult population (ages varied by sample); also sampled residents of Dallas County, Texas aged 18–54)	Rogers & Turner (1991)
Women and men reporting same-gender sex, desire, attraction	Comparison of men/women same-gender sexuality	Multistage area probability using multiple samples [personal, SAQ]	U.S. adult population contiguous states (ages 18–59)	Michaels (1994) Description of methods: Laumann et al. (1994, Chapter 2 and Appendix A)
Men reporting same-sex sexual contact	Prevalence of MSM nationally, and in urban, suburban, and rural areas of the USA	Multistage area probability sample and random digit dialing (RDD) sample [personal, SAQ, phone]	U.S. adult population (ages 18–49)	Binson et al. (1995)
Women and men reporting same gender sexuality	Prevalence of homosexual behavior/attraction in USA, UK, and France	Multistage area probability sample [personal/SAQ]	Adult populations of USA, UK, and France (ages 16–50)	Sell et al. (1995)
Same-sex and opposite-sex cohabiting couples	Comparison of partner selection among same-sex and opposite-sex couples	Multistage design [SAQ]	Cohabiting couples/households (ages 19–65) from 5% sample of 1990 Public Use Microdata Set (PUMS) of 1990 U.S. census	Jepsen & Jepsen (2002)
Black same-sex cohabiting couples	Comparison of demographic characteristics of Black and White same-sex and opposite-sex couples	Multistage design [SAQ]	Cohabiting couples/households from the 5% PUMS of 2000 U.S. census	Dang & Frazer (2004)

Table 15.1. *Continued*

Population of interest	Research interest	Sample design and [mode of data collection]	Population sampled	Reference
Adults with same-sex sexual partners	Prevalence of psychiatric syndromes	Multistage probability sample [personal]	U.S. noninstitutionalized adult population (surveyed through 1996 National Household Survey of Drug Abuse)	Cochran & Mays (2000)
Gay, lesbian, and bisexual (GLB) adolescents	Relationship between gay-sensitive HIV instruction and risk behaviors of GLB youth	Multistage probability sample of schools, classes [SAQ]	Students enrolled in grades 9–12 in public high schools in Massachusetts	Blake et al. (2001)
Men reporting same-sex sexual orientation	Prevalence of homosexual and bisexual men	RDD sample [phone]	U.S. adult population from all 50 states from ABC-Washington Post poll	Harry (1990)
Youth with same-sex attractions	Relationship between same-sex attraction and experiences of violence	Multistage sample of USA feeder and high schools [Audio Computer assisted self-interview (ACASI)]	Students enrolled in grades 7–12 in sampled high schools and feeder schools in USA	Russell et al. (2001)

Subpopulation of LGB in selected settings or ZIP codes

Population of interest	Research interest	Sample design and [mode of data collection]	Population sampled	Reference
Homosexual, bisexual men	Prevalence of HIV-related risk and HIV status	Multistage area probability sample [personal]	Single men (ages 25–54) residing in 19 selected census tracts of San Francisco	Winkelstein et al. (1987)
Young homosexual and bisexual men	Prevalence of HIV status	Multistage area probability sample [personal]	Single men (ages 18–29) residing in 21 census tracts in San Francisco	Osmond et al. (1994)
Lesbian and bisexual women	Feasibility of assessing sexual orientation among an RDD sample of women	RDD sample [phone]	Women (ages 18–59) residing in Boston's Jamaica Plain neighborhood	Meyer et al. (2002)

Table 15.1. *Continued*

Population of interest	Research interest	Sample design and [mode of data collection]	Population sampled	Reference
Adolescent and young adult MSM in USA	Prevalence of HIV status and HIV-related risk behavior	Time/location probability design (multiple sites) [personal]	Men (ages 15–22) in public venues frequented by young MSM (e.g., urban shopping blocks, dance clubs, bars, social organizations, bathhouses, parks, beaches) in seven U.S. cities	Valleroy et al. (2000) Description of methods: MacKellar et al. (1996)
Population of LGB in selected settings or ZIP codes				
Homosexual, bisexual men	Prevalence of HIV-related risk	RDD sample [phone]	Adult MSM residing in 24 ZIP code areas of Los Angeles County (ages 18–75)	Kanouse et al. (1991)
MSM	Characterize AIDS epidemic among urban MSM	RDD sample [phone]	Adult MSM residing in selected ZIP code areas in four urban centers (ages 18 and older)	Catania et al. (2001) Description of sample design: Binson et al. (1996); Blair (1999)
Self-identified gay and bisexual Latinos men	Impact of discrimination and poverty on mental health	Time/location probability design (multiple sites) [personal]	Men entering bars, clubs, and weeknight events primarily attended by Latinos and gay men in three U.S. cities	Diaz et al. (2001)
Young African American MSM	Social determinants of youth accessing HIV testing	Time/location probability design (multiple sites) [personal]	African American Youth (ages 16–25) entering venues frequented by young MSM (clubs, coffee houses, public parks, gay-pride events) in Atlanta, GA; Birmingham, AL; and Chicago, IL	Mashburn et al. (2004)

HIV, human immunodeficiency virus.

and, in the context of the AIDS epidemic, has been confined mainly to gay men. General population studies conducted by government agencies have only recently included questions related to same-gender sexual behavior. These data have provided opportunities for researchers to conduct analyses of health issues of populations reporting same-gender sexuality, particularly lesbian and bisexual women and adolescent populations.

The first and fourth columns of Table 15.1 describe the "population of interest" and "population sampled" of each of the studies. The "population of interest" is the group the researchers are interested in describing in some way (i.e., the group to which they want to generalize the results of their study). The "population sampled" provides the reader with information as to what population had some possibility or probability of being included in the sample (including geographic boundaries and age eligibility) and is an important factor to consider when thinking about who the sample represents. For example, in the Gruskin et al. (2001) study, the sample was Kaiser Permanente members residing in northern California who were at least 20 years of age. Hence, the population of lesbian and bisexual women to which one can generalize are those who have Kaiser Permanente health care, are residing in northern California, and are at least 20 years of age. Other examples of limited generalizability can be noted in the Centers for Disease Control and Prevention (CDC) study of young gay men (Valleroy et al., 2000) and the Urban Men's Health Study (UMHS) (Catania et al., 2001). The sample frames for these studies are quite different, and it is important to recognize that the sample represents a particular stratum of men. In the CDC study the sample frame was public venues frequented by young men who have sex with men (MSM), and in the UMHS it was telephone numbers assigned to households in selected ZIP codes. In the case of the CDC study the sample reflected men who are comfortable going to public venues that cater to young gay men, and in the UMHS the sample reflects men who are comfortable residing in city neighborhoods that are likely to have high concentrations of gay men. In both studies (and in most studies of LGB populations), resulting samples tend to be more sensitive to populations who are comfortable identifying as gay or bisexual or frequenting gay venues (as in the CDC study) or living in gay neighborhoods (as in UMHS). The seriousness of such biases is unknown. One can only speculate about whether the differences between MSM, for example, who live in areas of the city with high concentrations of gay men and those who live in other neighborhoods are significant. One important concern is the research question being posed (i.e., how the data are to be used). Nevertheless, in all cases, the potential bias must be acknowledged and taken into consideration when reporting findings.

The focus of most of these studies is on individuals residing in the United States, although one study compares populations in the United States, the United Kingdom, and France. Two of the studies focus on couples rather than individuals.

6.1 Subpopulation of LGB Within a General Population

The first group of studies in Table 15.1 represents sampling strategies in which the general population is sampled (both heterosexual and LGB), and analyses are conducted on the subsample of LGB respondents. Random sampling from a list is a simple yet elegant design that allows the researcher to generalize the results to the larger population that was contained on the list. It is a relatively easy sample design if a suitable list is available, yet the Gruskin et al. (2001) study was the only one we could locate that used a list sample, in this case a membership list of Kaiser Permanente members in northern California. The research goal was to determine lesbian and bisexual women's cigarette smoking and alcohol use patterns.

In general, the population from which a LGB subpopulation is analyzed is geographically bounded, sometimes including the entire country or sometimes a smaller area, such as a state, a city, or even just a neighborhood. Studies that project back to subgroups or LGB subpopulations of larger populations involve drawing large sample sizes. One research interest is to analyze only the LGB portion of the sample. The Rogers and Turner (1991), Michaels (1994), and Binson et al. (1995) studies used various types of complex sample designs (multistage area probability design and random digit dialing) and various modes of data collection (personal, self-administered questionnaire, phone) to determine the prevalence of MSM in the United States and in large cities, suburbs, and rural counties. There is an excellent discussion in Laumann et al. (1994) of the multistage area probability sample design and the sampling procedures used for drawing the national sample for the National Health and Social Life Study (NHSLS) that was used in Michaels' (1994) work on the prevalence of same-sex attraction, desire, and sexual behavior among adult women and men in the United States. A similar sample design was used in Sell et al. (1995) in their study to determine the prevalence of same-gender attraction and sexual behavior in the United States, the United Kingdom, and France.

Several additional studies in this section are examples of innovative use of preexisting data from large probability samples to study LGB adults and adolescents. Only during the last 10 to 15 years have government and even private (e.g., Gallup or Harris) agencies included questions on their surveys that would allow researchers to select subsamples of LGB populations. The studies of same-sex couples (Jepsen & Jepsen, 2002; Dang & Franzer, 2004) used data collected as part of the U.S. census. Beginning with the 1990 census, individuals were allowed to select "unmarried partner" (bypassing the choice of "roommate") for the category "relationship to head of household." The Harry (1990) study used data from the ABC-Washington Post Poll to examine the prevalence of men reporting same-sex sexual orientation in the United States. Determining the prevalence of homosexuality is not particularly sensitive to the sample size (drawn from the general population) because the intended purpose is to determine the proportion of same-sex sexual orientation among sampled respondents. Cochran has published a number of papers examining the prevalence of various psychiatric disorders among LGB adults (e.g., Cochran & Mays, 2000) using existing probability samples collected in large national studies of health (e.g., the National Household Survey of Drug Abuse, the National Survey of Midlife Development). In the two studies of lesbian, gay, and bisexual adolescents listed in Table 15.1 (Blake et al., 2001; Russell et al., 2001), respondents were sampled from in-school youth using a multistage design of first selecting schools and then classes in the selected schools. For some types of research, the small samples of LGB adolescents in the school samples can limit more complex analysis.

6.2 Subpopulation of LGB Within Selected Settings or ZIP Codes

The next group of studies in Table 15.1 are examples of sampling in geographic areas or in particular social settings in which LGB populations reside or socialize. In all four of the studies in this section, selecting census tracts, neighborhoods, or social settings based on the likelihood of high concentrations of the population of interest allowed investigators to recruit samples that included sufficient LGB subsamples efficiently, sparing valuable resources, time, and study personnel. The Winkelstein et al. (1987) classic study of young gay and bisexual men and the follow-up study by Osmond et al. (1994) both used multistage area probability designs. The sample for both studies was confined to a geographic area of the city that was defined by census tracts with the largest numbers of AIDS cases. The research interest was to determine the prevalence of HIV risk and HIV-related risk behavior of men residing in selected census tracts in San Francisco. Meyer et al. (2002) applied similar techniques in a random digit dialing (RDD) study to determine the feasibility of assessing sexual orientation among women residing in a selected ZIP code in an urban neighborhood in which there was an expectation of a high concentration of lesbians. Valleroy and her colleagues' (2000) study of HIV seroprevalence in young MSM is also technically an example of this type of study because once the researchers selected settings where young MSM were likely to be found, they conducted a time/location probability sample of all young men in those settings, independent of their sexual histories or identities.

6.3 Population of LGB Within Selected Settings or ZIP Codes

One limit to the population-based surveys described above is the relatively small size of the lesbian, gay, or bisexual sample that is generated, even sometimes when selected ZIP codes or settings are emphasized. Often these small numbers preclude more complex analyses of the interrelationship of relational, individual, and/or social behavioral variables. Only in general population surveys with large samples (e.g., 50,000) would there be adequate numbers for complex analysis. Conducting interviews with such a large number of respondents would be expensive. To overcome the small samples of LGB individuals generated in general population studies, researchers have designed probability studies that ensure the sample includes only respondents from the intended population. The Kanouse et al. (1991) study of gay and bisexual men in Los Angeles County was one of the early studies that screened potential respondents in an attempt to confine the sampled population to gay and bisexual men and to draw a large enough sample so more complex analyses could be achieved. Catania et al. (2001) extended the design to include three additional cities: San Francisco, New York, and Chicago. In both studies, the sample was drawn from ZIP codes that were selected based on their projected higher concentrations of gay and bisexual men. Data were collected by telephone using an RDD sample design. Because telephone number area codes and telephone prefixes are unique within ZIP codes in some cities, using ZIP codes to define the geographic boundaries in cities is a feasible, efficient sample design. However, because the overlay of telephone prefixes and ZIP codes are not always exact, researchers also query potential respondents regarding their residential ZIP code to ensure that the telephone number dialed was within the selected ZIP code. References (Kanouse et al., 1991; Binson et al., 1996; Blair, 1999) cited for both studies provide extensive details of the methods and sample designs used in these studies. The Diaz et al. (2001) and Mashburn et al. (2004) projects used a time/location probability design drawing, screening their samples of ethnic minority MSM from multiple sites where these men were known to congregate.

7 Suitable Use of Nonprobability Sample

Although only a probability sample allows us to make generalizations from the sample to the population, it was an experiment with a nonprobability sample that first challenged the medical model of homosexuality as psychopathology. In her revolutionary study, Evelyn Hooker (1957) acknowledged that her work was necessary because of years of bad sampling practice among researchers who sampled psychiatric and correctional institutions for their studies, resulting in skewed pictures of homosexuals as necessarily abnormal individuals with significant personality disorders. Hooker stated clearly why a probability sample was not necessary to address her research question: "for the present investigation the question is whether homosexuality is necessarily a symptom of pathology. All we need is a single case in which the answer is negative" (p. 30). By having expert judges evaluate responses to projective tests (Rorschach, TAT, MAPS) for 30 pairs of homosexual and heterosexual men (matched for age, IQ, and years of education), she could answer her question. Most of the men were viewed as functioning normally, and the judges could not do better than chance in identifying the homosexual men from their heterosexual counterparts. This is an example of an experimental design where the intention was to compare two samples that differ on (presumably) only one characteristic, not to project to some other population.

The health care literature is replete with numerous other examples of important studies conducted with nonprobability samples.

The reasons for this have to do with the scientific questions under investigation and the relative challenges of identifying the population to be sampled coupled with the high cost of probability designs. There can be good reasons not to recruit a probability sample but, rather, to draw a specific sample appropriate to the research question. For example, when studying a disease or a condition, researchers often have access to a limited number of patients who are all eligible for the study but who are not necessarily representative of the population. In such uses of nonprobability designs, the researcher is typically doing two things. First, the researcher is defining a population of interest for a particular project. That research population is usually representative of a larger population only in a limited way necessary for the research, perhaps on just one dimension. That is part of the reason one cannot generalize back to that larger population. The second thing the researcher is doing is using some low-cost method to obtain some members of the research population. With inappropriate use of non-probability designs, step one is omitted or not recognized, leading to unsupportable claims of generalization. In addition to an acknowledgment that a given study has sample design limitations, a more difficult but useful extension of that recognition would involve a discussion of the ensuing biases and how the study results are affected.

Although there are various nonprobability sampling designs, there is no standard language for describing and categorizing nonprobability sampling, as terms become widely used in one field of research and not in others. For our purposes, we talk broadly about nonprobability samples as "convenience samples," which is to say that the researcher samples individuals from the population who are easily available. The least systematic would be taking whoever comes along in whatever order they happen along until the desired number of individuals are selected. Each variation adds some level of systematic exclusion and inclusion criteria, such as seeking participants of the population of interest who provide a rich source of information that addresses the research question (purposive sampling) or selecting a set number of participants according to demographic and/or other categories to increase the variability in the sample, as Kinsey did (quota sampling), or having participants refer others they know to the study (snowball sampling). Obviously, these sample types are fluid, and researchers sometimes use combinations of approaches to achieve a sample that best suits their interests in achieving the research goals. Although in general more systematic recruitment appears to result in more diversity in the sample, it is nevertheless important to be aware of the significant limitations to generalizability from any convenience sample to the population of interest.

Determining the best approach requires thorough consideration of the research question and how the biases associated with a given convenience sampling strategy affect the interpretation of results. An often-cited example is the case of recruiting from gay bars for studies of alcohol use. If the research question involves understanding the subgroup of gay men at high risk for substance abuse or alcoholism, seeking out subjects from gay bars can be a purposive approach that might yield a large number of individuals at higher risk than the general population of gay men. However, if the goal of the research is to determine the prevalence of substance use in the population of gay men, the bias present in a sample taken from bars would render the results useless.

In an example of purposive convenience sampling, Dilley et al. (2002) were interested in determining the efficacy of an experimental cognitive counseling intervention for high-risk men testing for HIV. Their sample, obviously, was purposive in that they had to select only high-risk men (defined as men who reported a previous testing history and high-risk sex with another man who was HIV-positive or of unknown status in the past 6 months). Although they asked every high-risk man in their program to participate—and in that sense they technically used a census sample of the program—it was still treated as a nonprobability sample because they could not generalize to the population beyond the testing program. Men who agreed to participate were randomly assigned to one of several groups, half of whom underwent the cognitive counseling intervention. Those who had the intervention were more likely than men who did not have it to reduce their risk behavior during the 12 months following testing. Although the study successfully measured the effect of the intervention, it would be inappropriate to take the descriptive data about levels of risk and characteristics of the highest risk men in the study and generalize from the study sample to high-risk men or to gay and bisexual men in general. The sample design was not constructed to answer such research questions. On the other hand, given that the sample was in effect a census, the characteristics and reported risk behavior can be generalized to high-risk men who seek HIV testing in this particular program. Even with this design, however, it would be prudent to determine if there were significant differences between those who participated and those who did not. In addition, further discussion of the ways in which the participants differ from other high-risk men, as best as can be determined, would help deepen the readers' assessment of the intervention.

7.1 Nonprobability Sampling for Pilot or Exploratory Studies

Nonprobability samples also can be appropriately utilized in pilot or exploratory studies. A conventional pilot study to test an instrument or interview protocol on a small number of participants usually provides enough variation in interviewing experiences and participant comments needed to improve the instrument. The only critical factor is that the participants in the pilot study have characteristics similar to those who will be interviewed in the main study; otherwise problematic questions may be missed. The same can be said for more formal pilots studies (e.g., those in which the interaction between interviewer and respondent is monitored and/or coded or those that explore respondent cognitive processes to determine participant comprehension and strategies used when responding to survey questions) (Presser & Blair, 1994). In the UMHS (Catania et al., 2001), several pilots were conducted to determine potential problems in item wording. In one of these pilot studies, a convenience sample of respondents was asked questions about what the researchers thought might be potentially problematic question items. Each respondent was asked a survey question and then asked what the question meant to him, what difficulties he might have had in responding, and other comments he had about his perception of the intent of the question.

Sometimes the urgency of a public health crisis creates a need for rapid data collection that outweighs the limitations inherent in nonprobability samples. During the early period of the AIDS epidemic, as more and more gay men began coming down with various rare infections and immune problems it became critical to determine how gay men were responding to this epidemic. There was little time, as well as few financial or scientific resources, to consider drawing a random sample. The Multi-Center AIDS Cohort (MAC) study began recruiting as many gay men as were willing to complete a comprehensive set of questions every 6 months. This exploratory study was one of the first studies that tried to understand the relationship between psychosocial factors and gay men's attempt to change their sexual behavior in response to the epidemic (Emmons et al., 1986).

7.2 Nonprobability Sampling in Qualitative Research

Another broad area of research that uses nonprobability sampling to great advantage is qualitative research. Although qualitative studies cannot be generalized to the larger population, they allow researchers to explore the depth and richness of the LGB experience in ways that surveys often cannot. Frequently, the variables explored in surveys are first identified and developed through qualitative studies. Nevertheless, the sampling strategies for qualitative studies are often systematic, such as using purposive or theoretical sampling (i.e., selecting particular cases of the targeted population from which one can learn a great deal about issues of central importance to the purpose of the research).

Gartrell and colleagues provide an excellent example of using various convenience-sampling techniques to acquire a sample for a qualitative study of lesbian mothers (Gartrell et al., 1996, 1999, 2000). From 1986 to 1992, they recruited study participants who were either pregnant or in the process of inseminating, using "informal networking and word of mouth referrals . . . announcements at lesbian events, in women's bookstores and in lesbian newspapers" (p. 274) in the three cities where the investigators were located (i.e., Boston, Washington, DC, and San Francisco). Although they did not report a preset quota for numbers of women of color to include, they distributed "flyers at events for women of color" to ensure diversity of racial/ethnic background within the sample (p. 274). Using these techniques, the study team recruited 84 families (39 from San Francisco, 37 from Boston, 8 from Washington); 14 of the families were headed by single mothers, and the remaining families were headed by two mothers. This is an excellent example of applying purposive, snowball, and quota sampling procedures to ensure a large and diverse sample from which to identify and understand important issues of lesbian motherhood.

The above examples are not meant to be exhaustive, as the possibilities for useful studies with nonprobability samples are virtually endless. It is also worth noting, however, that for some populations nonprobability sampling may be inadequate and probability sampling actually more efficient for identifying otherwise difficult to reach populations or recruiting individuals of interest. For instance, we have proposed studying men at exceptionally high-risk for HIV; that is, from a public health perspective, the "core" members of sexual networks who are at significant risk both of acquiring and spreading HIV and other sexually transmitted diseases. The reason that probability sampling can be useful for identifying these core members is that we know from other studies that core members do not respond to standard nonprobability recruitment efforts. Martin et al. (2003) looked at sampling effects comparing a probability sample to a snowball sample. They found that high-risk men recruited into a probability sample were less likely than low-risk men to refer other men into the snowball sample, and that high-risk men who did refer men into the snowball sample were less likely to refer other high-risk men. Therefore, it is likely that we would have difficulty recruiting these "core" men through convenience sampling. Fortunately, core men can be and have been recruited reliably through probability sampling. Thus, probability sampling appears to be a good method for recruiting the target population.

8 Emerging Sampling Designs

8.1 Respondent-Driven Sampling

Thompson and Collins (2002) identified a category of sampling designs they termed "link-tracing" designs, which they defined as "Any design in which links or connections between units are used in obtaining the sample." Of recent interest is a link-tracing design called respondent-driven sampling (Heckathorn, 1997), which if its assumptions hold can produce a probability sample.

In respondent-driven sampling, a sample is collected using a chain-referral procedure. That is, respondents are not selected from a sampling frame, but are selected from the social network of existing members of the sample . . . the sample is used to make estimates about the social network connecting the population. Then, this information about the social network is used to derive the proportion of the population in different groups (for example, HIV+ or HIV–) [Salganik & Heckathorn, 2004].

This design has been proposed primarily as a method of sampling "hidden" populations.

For the estimation procedure to be unbiased, several assumptions must be met. It is assumed that the "seeds," who are the first wave of respondents, are drawn with probabilities proportional to their network size (i.e., the number of other people in the network to whom they are linked), although this condition is sometimes relaxed. It also is assumed that respondents recruit randomly from the other people in their network to whom they are linked. Finally, it is assumed that respondents know the number of people in the target population to whom they are linked (i.e., the number of people they might possibly have referred into the study, or their "degree").

Whether these conditions hold in a particular application is an empirical question. Certainly, it is not difficult to suggest factors that might undermine them. Because there are no rules for selecting the seeds, it is possible that their chance of selection is not proportional to the size of their network or degree. For example, if seeds are selected because they are somehow known previously to the researcher or through an advertising mechanism such as flyers, their chance of selection is no longer proportional to the size of their degree. Even if the chance of their selection is *related* to degree (i.e., that people with larger degree in general are more likely to be selected than those with smaller degree), this is still not the same as "proportional to degree." That is, a person with degree 10 may be more likely than someone with degree 2 to be selected as a seed, but perhaps not five times as likely.

Recruitment involves, in the main example given in the Salganik and Heckathorn article (2004), passing a coupon to those who are recruited and receiving payment for recruitment of participants. It does seem likely that respondents might favor recruiting those network members they think are more willing to participate in the study, rather than selecting them at random. That is, one rational recruitment strategy would be to achieve the highest (or quickest) payoff for the least effort. When this occurs, it violates the assumption that participants will recruit randomly from the other people in their networks.

One final concern is whether participants would really know the number of people in the target population to whom they are linked. Of course, some may know, whereas others may not. A reasonable scenario would be that those with small personal networks could report the number more accurately than those with large networks. The counting task is simply easier for those with tiny personal networks. If this were the case, a systematic reporting bias would result.

This is a complex design (only partially described here) that depends on a number of assumptions. The key point is that for some studies the assumptions may hold well, whereas in other situations they do not. Prior to deciding whether to use this sampling strategy, investigators should attempt to make some assessment of the extent to which the circumstances of their study would result in significant departures from these assumptions. This possibility too, however, would vary in difficulty from case to case.

In contrast to more basic designs, respondent-driven sampling, such as network sampling, relies to a greater degree on certain conditions and respondent behaviors. As such, they carry greater risks of the type noted for complex sampling designs—most seriously the loss of a statistical basis on which to make sample estimates of population parameters. However, if future work shows that the assumptions of respondent-driven sampling are not as easily violated as they might seem, or that the estimates produced are robust to violations of those assumptions, respondent-driven sampling may provide a more economical way of drawing probability samples with difficult-to-sreach populations. The use of pilot studies, if feasible, may be the wisest course.

8.2 Web-Based Surveys

The web (Internet) is an attractive data collection mode for a variety of reasons, cost being a primary one. It permits a level of administrative control, such as skip patterns and edit checks, that are not possible in noncomputerized modes, such as conventional mail. There are many possibilities for incorporating multimedia technologies in web surveys, although they are not yet widely used in survey research applications. It is important, however, not to allow the utility of web technologies as a *survey administration mode* to eclipse the limitations inherent in its use as a *sampling strategy*.

Although the web is essentially an alternative means of data collection and not a sampling procedure, its effective use (outside of list samples or nonprobability samples) often requires dealing with multimode designs, which do have special sampling issues. Although multimode designs in general are beyond the scope of this chapter, we believe it useful to address some of the specific sampling issues that may, under some circumstances, permit effective use of the web. The major drawbacks to web surveys involve sampling and response rates. These obstacles are often sufficiently severe to render proposed research impractical. However, there are some circumstances under which the web, alone or in conjunction with another mode, may produce acceptable results.

One might consider several broad categories of web surveys. First, a population may be defined by virtue of web access (e.g., members of a listserv or some other type of online group). Second, the web may simply be a convenient mode for reaching a narrowly defined, special population, such as members of a professional association or subscribers to a magazine for whom e-mail contact lists are available. Third, the target population may be simply a subgroup of the general population.

The first two types of survey are relatively straightforward. Assuming that the e-mail list is available, they present no special problems beyond those that apply to sampling from any other list. The use of the web for conducting general population surveys, and by extension subgroups within the general population, is far more problematic.

First, only about 40% of the U.S. population is currently on the Internet (Newburger, 2001). Even if a list of this population were available, which it is not, the degree of undercoverage would make the web inappropriate for serious research (though it might be acceptable for some types of instrument testing, developing hypotheses, and other applications where either nonprobability samples or seriously flawed probability samples are useful).

At present, utilizing the web for general population surveys seems feasible only as part of a dual-frame design. It is worth considering the savings that might be available from dual-frame designs in which web-based data collection is used for web-accessible members of the target group, and telephone data collection is used for those who are not in the web frame. Web-phone designs might be particularly cost-effective for reaching rare groups; and if so, we need to understand those circumstances.

Screening costs on the web should be lower than on the phone because no incremental labor is needed to contact potential respondents. This reduction in cost is not dependent on geographic clustering in the target group; therefore, web-based data collection may offer savings where TCS cannot. Also, the inherently lower cost of web-based screening should be increasingly important as the group becomes more rare, so web-based sampling may be useful for very rare groups even if they are geographically clustered and hence amenable to TCS and/or stratification.

For telephone interviewing, if the target group has zero tendency to cluster geographically, RDD with no clustering is the best option. If the target group has a nonzero tendency to cluster geographically, TCS is preferable (e.g., with list-assisted RDD at the first stage and a cluster size of 3).

The question now becomes how can web sampling be combined with one of these telephone alternatives to improve the cost efficiency of the sampling plan?

Web-based data collection can be accomplished in three main ways. First the questionnaire may be posted on some web site for any and all who might want to participate. Obviously, this method generates a pure sample of volunteers and is not acceptable if our goal is to achieve a probability sample. There is no way to know the inclusion probabilities of a sample obtained in this manner.

With the second method a sample is drawn from a panel of web users who have agreed to participate in research projects: Examples include the panels maintained by Harris Interactive, Ipsos Research, and more recently Survey Sampling. Because the members have explicitly agreed to participate in research, usually with some system of incentives, panel vendors are often able to estimate the level of response—30% or so is not uncommon.

The third method utilizes a sample drawn from a list of "opt-in" users. These sample members are people who, in the process of using the Internet, have agreed to receive e-mail communications. Such lists are constructed from multiple sources, and their quality is far less clear than a panel. Because opt-in list members have agreed to receive communications, solicitation to participate in a survey does not violate anti-"spam" restrictions. However, they did not explicitly agree to respond to survey solicitations, and their response rate is correspondingly low, often in the single digits. However, it is important to note that this frame is generally much larger and provides greater population coverage than does a panel. Both of these characteristics are important issues when sampling rare populations.

Essentially, implementing this design becomes a problem of optimal allocation between a telephone stratum (where coverage is high, but the costs of screening are as well) and a web stratum (which has poorer coverage but very low costs for screening). The detailed calculations to determine optimum allocation are beyond the intent of this chapter (see Blair & Blair, 2005, for a full treatment). However, even though the correct use of the dual frame approach would require consulting with a sampling statistician, it is useful to understand the general issues involved.

Blair and Blair (2006) conclude that cost savings may be available from dual-frame web-phone designs (versus all phone), but the situation is complex and is not entirely free of some of the basic drawbacks noted at the outset of this discussion. The main finding was that web-based data collection with web panels might offer substantial savings for rare groups even when there is some clustering in the population.

Given the cost benefits that might be available from web-based data collection for rare groups, should it be used? The answer, of course, depends on one's willingness to treat a sample of opt-in users or a sample of panel members, knowing the potential for coverage bias, as representative of the larger online population. This decision sometimes must be made in the context of being able to do the survey or not, given a fixed budget.

A theoretical solution to this problem is to stratify the general population on the basis of "in frame vs. not in frame" rather than "online vs. not online." However, there is the practical difficulty of getting telephone respondents to give an accurate indication of whether they appear in any given online frame so they can be sorted out. Overall, there are two practical responses to the issue of coverage bias in the online frame. One is to use the biggest possible frame, actively draw the sample, and take a leap of faith that the result is representative (and do likewise regarding the issue of nonresponse bias). Second, one may try to estimate the bias by comparing the telephone and online results. If the bias can be estimated, one has the possibility of correcting for it while retaining the cost savings that led the researcher down this design path originally.

For some research goals, the possible cost advantages of web-based data collection in reaching rare groups may be sufficient to overcome its theoretical drawbacks; in other cases it may not. What is important is that the decision be informed and that the potential implications for the accuracy of the survey results be understood.

In conclusion, even if web-based data collection is cheaper than telephone interviewing, it is not desirable to rely exclusively on web-based data unless the target group is limited to Internet users because of the potential for coverage bias in the sample. The more defensible approach is a dual-frame design in which web-based data collection is used to gather data from web-accessible members of the target group, and telephone interviewing is used to reach the others.

9 Summary

Having faced the AIDS epidemic more than 20 years ago with few reliable data about the prevalence and sexual practices of gay men in the United States, it is exciting to see so much growth in the health research area where probability sample designs are used to describe the LGB populations. Clearly these studies (and others like them not presented here) provide far more reliable information about these rare and elusive groups than had been known in all the years of research on homosexuality that preceded them.

The detailed discussions included in this chapter provide only a basic introduction to probability sampling. The information presented is intended only to provide a description of the principles underlying probability sampling, why they are important when designing reliable surveys, and some sense of the range of available designs. Additional knowledge is required to develop appropriate sample designs for specific applications. Quite a bit more training and experience is necessary, and someone with sufficient expertise and experience should be sought out to provide consultation or to collaborate in the development and implementation of a study's sample design. It is important to keep in mind how much sampling interfaces with the data collection operation in many of the more complex sample designs. If a research question is worth asking, it is certainly worth generating an appropriate sample so the time, effort, and resources involved in collecting and analyzing the research data can provide reliable answers to the research questions proposed. Certainly more studies using well thought-out sample designs will do much to improve our knowledge of, and efforts to improve, the health and well-being of LGB populations.

Finally, the understandable pressures to conduct studies that produce useful substantive results have made it difficult to also conduct the survey methodological research needed to improve the design of LGB surveys. Until more methodological research is done, large uncertainties will remain about how well different designs will perform in particular circumstances. These uncertainties underlie this chapter's emphasis on expert consultation, careful planning, and the use of pilot studies as the bases for successful sample design.

References

Binson, D., Michaels, S., Stall, R., Coates, T.J., Gagnon, J.H., and Catania, J.A. (1995) Prevalence and social distribution of men who have sex with men: United States and its urban centers. *Journal of Sex Research* 32:245–254.

Binson, D., Moskowitz, J., Mills, T., Anderson, K., Paul, J., Stall, R., and Catania, J. (1996) Sampling men who have sex with men: strategies for a telephone survey in urban areas in the United States. In: *Proceedings of the Section on Survey Research Methods, American Statistical* Association, pp. 68–72.

Birnbaum, Z.W., and Sirken, M.G. (1965) Design of sample surveys to estimate the prevalence of rare diseases: three unbiased estimates. *Vital and Health Statistics*, Series 2, No. 11. Washington, DC: US Government Printing Office.

Blair, E., and Blair, J. (2004) On telephone sampling for rare groups. Unpublished observation.

Blair, E., and Blair, J. (2006) Dual frame web-telephone sampling for rare groups. *Journal of Official Statistics* 22(2):1–10.

Blair, J. (1999) A probability sample of gay urban males: the use of two-phase adaptive sampling. *Journal of Sex Research* 36(1):39–44.

Blair, J., and Czaja, R. (1982) Locating a special population using random digit dialing. *Public Opinion Quarterly* 46:585–590.

Blake, S.M., Ledsky, R., Lehman, T., Goodenow, C., Sawyer, R., and Hack, T. (2001) Preventing sexual risk behaviors among gay, lesbian, and bisexual adolescents: the benefits of gay-sensitive HIV instruction in schools. *American Journal of Public Health* 91:940–946.

Catania, J.A., Osmond, D., Stall, R.D., Pollack, L., Paul, J.P., Blower, S., Binson, D., Canchola, J.A., Mills, T.C., Fisher, L., Choi, K.H., Porco, T., Turner, C., Blair, J., Henne, J., Bye, L.L., and Coates, T. (2001) The continuing HIV epidemic among men who have sex with men. *American Journal of Public Health* 91:907–914.

Cochran, S.D., and Mays, V.M. (2000) Relation between psychiatric syndromes and behaviorally defined sexual orientation in a sample of the US population. *American Journal of Epidemiology* 151:516–523.

Czaja, R., and Blair, J. (1990) Using network sampling in crime victimization surveys. *Journal of Quantitative Criminology* 6:185–206.

Czaja, R.F., Snowden, C.B., and Casady, R.J. (1986) Reporting bias and sampling errors in a survey of a rare population using multiplicity counting rules. *Journal of the American Statistical Association* 81:411–419.

Dang, A., and Frazer, S. (2004) Black same-sex households in the United States: a report from the 2000 census. National Gay & Lesbian Task Force Policy Institute and National Black Justice Coalition, New York.

Diaz, R.M., Ayala, G., Bein, E., Henne, J., and Marin, B.V. (2001) The impact of homophobia, poverty and racism on the mental health of gay and bisexual latino men: findings from 3 US cities. *American Journal of Public Health* 91:927–932.

Dilley, J.W., Woods, W. J., Sabatino, J., Lihatsh, T., Adler, B., Casey, S., Rinaldi, J., Brand, R., and McFarland, W. (2002) Changing sexual behavior among gay male repeat testers for HIV: a randomized, controlled trial of a single session intervention. *J AIDS* 30:177–186.

Emmons, C.A., Joseph, J.G., Kessler, R.C., Wortman, C.B., Montgomery, S.B., and Ostrow, D.G. (1986) Psychosocial predictors of reported behavior change in homosexual men at risk for AIDS. *Health Education Quarterly* 13:331–345.

Gartrell, N., Hamilton, J., Banks, A., Mosbacher, D., Reed, N., Sparks, C., and Bishop, H. (1996) The national lesbian family study. 1. Interviews with prospective mothers. *American Journal of Orthopsychiatry* 66:272–281.

Gartrell, N., Banks, A., Hamilton, J., Reed, N., Bishop, H., and Rodas, C. (1999) The National Lesbian Family Study. 2. Interviews with mothers of toddlers. *American Journal of Orthopsychiatry* 69:362–369.

Gartrell, N., Banks, A., Reed, N., Hamilton, J., Rodas, C., and Deck, A. (2000) The national lesbian family study. 3. Interviews with mothers of five-year-olds. *American Journal of Orthopsychiatry* 70:542–548.

Gebhard, P. (1972) Incidence of overt homosexuality in the United States and western Europe. In Livingwood, L.M. (ed) National Institute of Mental Health Task Force on Homosexuality. National Institute of Mental Health, Washington, DC.

Gebhard, P.H., and Johnson, A.B. (1979) The Kinsey data: marginal tabulations of the 1938–1963 interviews conducted by the Institute of Sex Research. Saunders, Philadelphia.

Gruskin, E.P., Hart, S., Gordon, N., and Ackerson, L. (2001) Patterns of cigarette smoking and alcohol use among lesbians and bisexual women enrolled in a large health maintenance organization. *American Journal of Public Health* 91:976–979.

Hansen, M.H., Hurwitz, W.N., and Madow, W.G. (1953) *Sample survey methods and theory*. Wiley, New York.

Harry, J. (1990) A probability sample of gay males. *Journal of Homosexuality* 19:89–104.

Heckathorn, D.D. (1997) Respondent-driven sampling: a new approach to the study of hidden populations. *Social Problems* 44:174–199.

Hooker, E. (1957) The adjustment of the male overt homosexual. *Journal of Projective Techniques* 21:18–31.

Jepsen, L.K., and Jepsen, C.A. (2002) An empirical analysis of the matching patterns of same-sex and opposite-sex couples. *Demography* 39:435–453.

Kalton, G. (1993) *Sampling rare and elusive populations*. United Nations Statistical Division, National Household Survey Capability Programme. Technical Studies Series. United Nations, New York.

Kanouse, D.E., Berry, S.H., Gorman, E.M., Yano, E.M., and Carson, S. (1991) *Response to the AIDS epidemic*. RAND, Santa Monica, R-4031-LACH.

Kinsey, A., Pomeroy, W., and Martin, C. (1948) *Sexual behavior in the human male*. Saunders, Philadelphia.

Kinsey, A., Pomeroy, W., Martin, C., and Gebhard, P. (1953) *Sexual behavior in the human female*. Saunders, Philadelphia.

Kruskal, W.H., and Mosteller, F. (1979) Representative sampling. III. The current statistical literature. *International Statistical Review* 47:245–265.

Laumann, E.O., Gagnon, G.H., Michael, R.T., and Michaels, S. (1994) *The social organization of sexuality*. University of Chicago Press, Chicago.

MacKellar, D., Valleroy, L., Karon, J., Lemp, G., and Janssen, R. (1996) The young men's survey: methods for estimating HIV seroprevalence and risk factors among young men who have sex with men. *Public Health Reports* 3(Suppl):138–144.

Martin, J.L., Wiley, J., and Osmond, D. (2003) Social networks and unobserved heterogeneity in risk for AIDS. *Population Research and Policy Review* 22:65–90.

Mashburn, A.J., Peterson, J.L., Bakeman, R., Miller, R.L., Clark, L. The Community Intervention Trial for Youth Study Team. (2004) Influences on HIV testing among African American men who have sex with men and the moderating effect of geographic setting. *Journal of Community Psychology* 32:45–60.

Meyer, I.H., Rossano, L., Ellis, J.M., and Brandford, J. (2002) A brief telephone interview to identify lesbian and bisexual women in random digit dialing sampling. *Journal of Sex Research* 39:139–144.

Michaels, S. (1994) Homosexuality. In: Laumann, E.O., Gagnon, J.H., Michael, R.T., and Michaels, S. *The social organization of sexuality*. University of Chicago Press, Chicago.

Newburger, E. (2001) *Home computers and Internet use in the United States: August 2000. Current Population Reports*. U.S. Bureau of the Census, September, Washington, DC.

Osmond, D.H., Page, K., Wiley, J., Garrett, K., Sheppard, H.W., Moss, A.R., Schrager, L., and Winkelstein, W. (1994) HIV infection in homosexual and bisexual men 18 to 29 years of age: the San Francisco young men's health study. *American Journal of Public Health* 84:1933–1937.

Presser, S., and Blair, J. (1994) Survey pretesting: do different methods produce different results? In: Marsden, P.V., (ed) *Sociological methodology*, Vol. 24. Blackwell, Cambridge, MA.

Rogers, S.M., and Turner, C.F. (1991) Male-male sexual contact in the USA: findings from five sample surveys, 1970–1990. *Journal of Sex Research* 28:491–519.

Russell, S.T., Franz, B.T., and Driscoll, A.K. (2001) Same-sex romantic attraction and experiences of violence in adolescence. *American Journal of Public Health* 91:903–906.

Salganik, M.J., and Heckathorn, D.D. (2004) Sampling and estimation in hidden populations using respondent-driven sampling. In: Stolzenberg, R. (ed) *Sociological methodology*, Vol. 34. Blackwell, Oxford.

Sell, R.L., Wells, J.A., and Wypij, D. (1995) The prevalence of homosexual behavior and attraction in the United States, the United Kingdom and France: results of national population-based samples. *Archives of Sexual Behavior* 24:235–248.

Sirken, M.G. (1970) Household surveys with multiplicity. *Journal of American Statistical Association* 67:257–266.

Solarz, A.L., (ed). (1999) *Lesbian health: current assessment and directions for the future*. National Academy Press, Washington, DC.

Stephan, F.F., and McCarthy, P.J. (1958) Sampling opinions: *an analysis of survey procedure*. Wiley, New York.

Sudman, S. (1976) *Applied sampling*. Academic, San Diego.

Sudman, S., Sirken, M.G., and Cowan, C.D. (1988) Sampling rare and elusive populations. *Science* 240:991–996.

Thompson, S.K., Collins, L.M. (2002) Adaptive sampling in research on risk-related behaviors. *Drug and Alcohol Dependence* 68:S57–S67.

Valleroy, L.A., MacKellar, D.A., Karon, J.M., Rosen, D.H., McFarland, W., Shehan, D.A., Stoyanoff, S.R., LaLota, M., Celentano, D.D., Koblin, B.A., Thiede, H., Katz, M.H., Torian, L.V., and Janssen, R.S. (2000) HIV prevalence and associated risks in young men who have sex with men. *JAMA* 284:198–204.

Waksberg, J. (1978) Sampling methods for random digit dialing. *Journal of the American Statistical Association* 73(March):40–46.

Waksberg, J. (1983) A note on "locating a special population using random digit dialing." *Public Opinion Quarterly* 47:576–578.

Winkelstein, W. Jr., Lyman, D.M., Padian, N., Grant, R., Samuel, M., Wiley, J.A., Anderson, R.E., Lang, W., Riggs, J., and Levy, J.A. (1987) Sexual practices and risk of infection by the human immunodeficiency virus. *JAMA* 257(3):321–325.

Further Reading Related to Sampling Methods

Berry, S.H., Duan, N., and Kanouse, D. (1996) Use of probability versus convenience samples of street prostitutes for research on sexually transmitted diseases and HIV risk behaviors: how much does it matter? In: Warnecke, R. (ed) *Health survey research methods conference proceedings DHHS*, pp. 93–97. *One of the few articles that compares probability sampling and convenience sampling in a carefully designed and executed study.*

Czaja, R., and Blair, J. (1996, 2005) *Designing surveys: a guide to decisions and procedures*. Pine Forge Press, Thousand Oaks, CA. *Book includes an extensive discussion on survey sampling for readers' reference (chapters 7 and 8).*

Frankel, M.R., and Frankel, L.R. (1987) Fifty years of survey sampling in the United States. *Public Opinion Quarterly* 51:S127–S138. *This article is included in a special issue of* Public Opinion Quarterly *celebrating 50 years of survey research. The article provides an excellent overview of the history of survey sampling in the United States.*

Kalton, G. (1983) *Introduction to survey sampling.* Sage, Newbury Park, CA. *One of the Little Green Sage series and an excellent resource for someone interested in learning about probability sampling.*

Kalton, G. (1993) Sampling considerations in research on HIV risk and illness. In: Ostrow, D.G., and Kessler, R.C. (eds) *Methodological issues in AIDS behavioral research.* Plenum, New York. *Chapter covers many basic sampling issues for surveys related to HIV risk and illness.*

Sudman, S. (1983) Applied sampling. In: Rossi, P.H., Wright, J.D., and Anderson, A.B., (eds) *Handbook of survey research.* Academic, San Diego, pp. 145–194. *An overview and practical guide to survey sampling taking into consideration limited resources. It includes many interesting and useful real world examples. Material for this chapter was obtained from the book* Applied Sampling Academic, San Diego, 1976.

Sudman, S., Sirken, M.G., and Cowan, C.D. (1988) Sampling rare and elusive populations. *Science* 240:991–996. *An excellent overview to sampling hard to reach populations.*

National Professional Associations of Survey Research and Sampling

American Association for Public Opinion Research. Website: http://www.aapor.org/.

American Statistical Association, Section on Survey Research Methods. Website: http://www.amstat.org/sections/SRMS/index.html.

National Survey Research Centers

Abt Associates, Cambridge, MA

Mathematica, Princeton, NJ

National Opinion Research Center (NORC), University of Chicago, Chicago, IL

Rand, Survey Research Group, Santa Monica, CA

Research Triangle Institute (RTI), Research Triangle Park, NC

Survey Research Center, Institute for Social Research, University of Michigan, Ann Arbor, MI

Westat, Rockville, MD

Researching Gay Men's Health: The Promise of Qualitative Methodology

Gary W. Dowsett

1 Introduction

Public health research has always been dominated by the cross-sectional population survey as the most frequently used technique, and it frames much thinking about how social and behavioral research is conducted on public health issues (Kavanagh et al., 2002). It has become the dominant and default research methodology. Nevertheless, in recent years there has been a growing interest in developing new research techniques to investigate public health in the humanities, social science, and even in clinical research in medicine. One area of growing interest lies in qualitative methodology.

Although qualitative methodology is not new in other research fields, it would not be untrue to say that there has, at times, been a suspicion in public health that qualitative methodology is "soft," unrigorous, and therefore unable to answer key questions that public health seeks to clarify or answer. The irony is that qualitative data-gathering techniques have long been part of health: The clinical case study is a good example of an important research technique that has yielded valuable information and insight into health issues. Field observation and other ethnographic techniques used in medical anthropology have also proven their worth over the course of the twentieth century in investigating other cultures (and sometimes our own) and the relation of social practices and processes to health experiences and outcomes. Also, for quite some time there has been effective use of qualitative methodology as a rapid appraisal or pilot data-gathering technique to ground a later survey in appropriate languages or to flesh out the list of options available to use in structured questionnaires.

The distinction made between experimental and observational studies in health research, with the former seen as truly scientific and the latter as producing less-rigorous evidence, has tended to cluster many qualitative data-gathering techniques into a single category (at the observational end) artificially contrasted to quantitative methodology and assuming some substantive differences. More recent experience has softened this contrast considerably as complex public health problems seem to require new and varied approaches to information gathering and more sophisticated understanding of persons and context. For gay men's health—the focus of this chapter—the advent of the human immunodeficiency virus (HIV) epidemics in many parts of the world proved a significant stimulus in calling forth qualitative methodology to assist in comprehending one of the most complicated public health problems of the modern period. Yet it is important to remember that gay men have health issues other than HIV infection and acquired immunodeficiency syndrome (AIDS), and the discussion below, although referring to HIV/AIDS at times, aims to be applicable to gay men's other health issues as well. Indeed, much of what follows might well apply to lesbian health (or even to transgender or bisexually active people); but the examples used and the argument mounted are most directly focused on gay men (for a critical framework for these issues, see Wilton, 2002).

1.1 Sexuality and Health Research

There is no moment more important in the conceptualization of sexuality as a field of scientific study than the invention of the *homosexual*. This categorization by Benkert in 1868 of a wide range of sexual activity and interests into a single common category (to be joined by its alter ego *heterosexual* some 10 years later) signaled the first significant step in subjecting human sexual activity to a new form of scrutiny and investigation (Foucault, 1978; Weeks, 1985). These scientific research endeavors, their epistemological bases in positivism, and its belief in the facticity of natural science converged with a parallel development in the human and social sciences. Within this framework, the invention of sexuality as an object of study was to produce more than a century of scientific work in health, psychology, and biology, in particular, that attempted to categorize, classify, investigate the causes of, and seek to reform and cure the homosexual—men as well as women. The term homosexual (or *homosexuality*) is used here to name that scientific and discursive invention; the common term *gay men* is very much a construct of the late twentieth century and originated in the West. Its growing usage as a common "hold-all" term should not mask the fact that this term does not describe all the various cultural understandings and forms in which male-to-male eroticism occurs globally (this is elaborated later). Moreover, until only recently, the major frame of reference for thinking about gay men (and lesbians) was primarily as a category of the *sexual*—and a deviant and "sick" one at that; and the deeper and various cultural understandings just referred to were often neglected or unrecognized by science.

Defining gay men's (and lesbians') health as a field that includes but goes beyond sexual matters has been a long struggle—ironically, one that HIV/AIDS both hindered and stimulated. The definitional frameworks through which the HIV pandemic has been seen have changed, progressing from an sexually transmissible infection to a disease defined by certain sexual and cultural practices and meanings (e.g., men's sexual privilege or risks present in commercial sex work), then to a disease of development and socioeconomic factors (e.g., in relation to poverty), and now increasingly to one involving human rights. Yet, for some reason, HIV/AIDS is often still thought of as a gay disease first and foremost.

1.2 The Rise of Critical Sexuality Studies

The post-World War II period witnessed a rise in new scientific approaches to studying sexuality, particularly after in/famous Kinsey reports (Kinsey et al., 1948, 1953) revealed, *inter alia*, widespread same-sex sexual interests and practice among men and to a lesser extent among women. This research stimulated the last 50 years of sex research, in the United States in particular, which continues to reveal a diverse sexual culture in this country and in many other Western developed countries. That research eventually provided evidence for, and argument on, the nature of human sexuality, which supported the rise of the sexual liberation movements (mainly among women and among homosexual people) from the late 1960s onward. These new social movements fostered new forms of research on sexuality in general and homosexuality in particular that began to utilize qualitative methodology more. Historians, psychologists, sociologists, anthropologists, and cultural and media studies intellectuals began to investigate homosexuality in what came to be called *gay and lesbian studies*, which later merged, in the United States mainly, into *queer studies. Sex research* and *sexology* (as the traditional twentieth-century fields of study were known) themselves became the object of a new *critical sexuality studies,* which continues to question these older formulations. Gay and lesbian studies, queer theory, and the new critical sexuality studies not only challenged the prevailing understanding of human sexuality, its origins, and elaboration in science but also raised the possibility of studying sexuality with new methods.

1.3 What Does This Mean for Gay Men's Health?

Raising these issues here is important for gay men's (and lesbians') health because the presuppositions that are prevalent in our culture about homosexuality often formulate research questions in ways that are either *heterosexist* (i.e., based on, and working with, models, assumptions, and ideas that mostly apply to opposite-sex-attracted people and their activities and see them as normal because of a larger prevalence of those sexual interests) or *homophobic* (i.e., directly growing from frameworks and predispositions that render homosexuality as bad, sad, or abject and include ideas that demonstrate considerable negative affect in relation to homosexual people and engender support for punishment, violence, marginalization, and stigmatization). Beyond these formulations, seeing gay men and lesbians first and foremost as sexual beings in a world that has distinct and often contradictory values concerning sex and sexuality makes it important—and often complex and difficult—to understand what and how social issues such as health are shaped for and by gay people.

Sexual health as a field suffers in particular from this assumption about gay people primarily as a sexual category. Yet it may also be that the historical effects of such categorization and its stigmatization do produce real, adverse health consequences: for example, how might we seek to understand the evidence on late presentation by lesbian women for breast cancer screening or on the growing concern about gay men's approaches to recreational drug use and sex, as just two examples (Leonard, 2002). The issue for anyone concerned with gay men's and lesbians' health is to recognize the convergence of, and clash between, these historical and scientific paradigms and their influence not only on determining what health is for homosexual people but also on how homosexuality and health have ridden in tandem throughout the development of modern medicine and public health as fields of major scientific scrutiny and social endeavor. It behooves any social researchers working in public health to familiarize themselves with this history and with its residual effects in shaping current research approaches to gay men's health and to assess in our own research ways in which this history of the homosexual in biomedicine and public health still shapes the prevailing ideas about gay people and our health needs and concerns.

2 Gay Men as Subjects of Research

This background begs an important question. Just what is a *gay man*? The same question could be asked about lesbians even though that term has been in common usage longer. How do we recognize a gay man as such for our research, and where or what is the boundary between him and other men? These are not silly or simple questions; they recognize both the modernity of gay and its uncertainty. By this is meant that gay as a category of human beings recognizing themselves and defined as such by others—who, by default, must be nongay—is a very recent event in human history and not a fully achieved or stable one. In pointing to the invention of the modern homosexual (noted earlier), British gay historian Jeffrey Weeks and homosexual French philosopher Michael Foucault alerted us to the historical and discursive contingency residing in the category gay. Their work reveals, in Western thought, the unfolding delineation of human beings (usually men) into categories defined by sexual interests and activities (one might call them *sexual preferences*) over the previous two centuries. This resulted in the eventual transfer of interests in certain sexual practices (iconically, sodomy, defined mostly by that time as anal intercourse between men) from an occasional or regular act into a kind or person (one might call it a *sexual orientation*). This, in turn, became the defining characteristic of the self (one might call it a *sexual identity*). To paraphrase Foucault: sodomy, the act, became homosexuality, a category of persons (i.e., a *sexuality*).

This achievement in Western thought, though exported imperially to the rest of the world ever since, has yet to consolidate its global domination, even if it has gained a hegemonic position in medical and health research with the onset of the HIV pandemic. Many other cultures have other meaning-making systems of action and thought to understand same-sex attraction and activity. Indeed, many postcolonial legal and moral systems reflect the contradictions between the Western-derived and Western-imposed categories of sexuality and the lived experience of local, historical sexual cultures (Altman, 2001).

Less well known are analyses in our own Western culture that reveal the same uncertainty about sexuality categories and their applicability in describing sexual interests exercised by men (and women) in New York, London, Sydney, San Francisco, Amsterdam, and other such major Western cities. We often think we know what gay is and who gay men are in such cities where *gay community* is a valid concept, a geographic precinct or neighborhood, a political mobilization, or an infrastructure that provides goods, services, public validation, and sex to those who inhabit it. Much of the mid-to-late twentieth century saw concerted scientific and political efforts to develop those very communities, those very categories, and those sexual practices as not *un*-normal, as worthy of civil equality before the law, and deserving fair treatment as human beings just like you and me. In partly achieving those ends (full civil equality has not been achieved anywhere yet), this concerted action had the effect of "hardening" the very categories with which it was forced to work. To use the social scientific term, gay was reified.

That historically contingent moment that invented the homosexual operated largely unquestioned, even in science, for most of the twentieth century and generated a much warranted critique only with the advent of the gay liberation movement during the late 1960s. Ironically, it was that movement—whose ideas were by the late 1970s questioning all sexuality categories as historically contingent and to be eventually supplanted or discarded—that needed the very terms it eschewed to mobilize its forces, consolidate its "membership," and demand social and civic space. The more that gay liberation claimed gay as a standpoint from which to mount a critical appraisal of sexuality itself, the more gay as a category of persons became firm.

Soon, during the early 1980s, the liberationists' deconstructive urgings ("everyone can be bisexual") were seriously weakened—and the countervailing convergence toward the category gay was strongly bolstered—by the need to mobilize to fight HIV/AIDS in those very gay communities that had been consolidating by the end of the twentieth century as one consequence of the gay civil rights struggle. Gay men were soundly nominalized and the gay community also reified into definitive social categories more so than ever before. The social research in public health that pursued gay men and gay communities to help us find out how HIV was spread and how sexual acts between men might be transformed to prevent transmission of the virus was itself an important contributor to this nominalization and reification. Science was productive here, not simply reflective, of the very sexuality categories it researched.

2.1 Gay Men as Study Populations and Samples

This history and science's part in it still have important implications for researching gay men (and lesbians, bisexual, transgender, and intersex people). The first important issue here is the definition of gay men as the "population" for our research. *Population* in this usage is the totality of persons who are known to form a bounded or whole cluster of like people and who constitute the focus of, or are constituted by, the research questions in our studies. For example, if we are keen to study the experience of a flood that affected a whole small town, the population for our study might be all the people in that town. If we are keen to understand how households manage having a member living with a particular disability, the population might be all households living with that disability. It is from the potential population of any study we plan that we select a sample (a smaller group representing the larger) for our studies when the population is too large to study in its entirety. Therefore, in the case of the flooded town the whole population might be small enough to constitute the sample; in the case of the disability study, there may be too many such households in the United States, so we might take every one in one hundred such families across the country, or we might sample all those in one city in the hope that the sample represents the whole population well enough to allow us to speak from our findings about and to the whole population. Sampling techniques and issues concerning them are discussed technically elsewhere in this volume and in many research methodology textbooks. Here, and first, I want to canvass some of the population definition issues and sampling consequences for us when we are researching gay men's health.

The main dilemma when sampling gay men is that we do not have much of an idea, anywhere, of the boundaries to populations of gay men; nor might we ever find real boundaries. This is partly due to gay men being quite a new social category, not simply evolving from the earlier homosexual but actually brought into being from its collision with left liberationist ideas during the 1960s, as noted above. This category now is evolving in its own right; but it has not supplanted earlier categories, nor has it incorporated all other forms, meanings, and cultural understandings of same-sex desire and activity still operative in our culture. It is also a category of persons who appear to be growing a sexual identity that many men with same-sex interests (but not all) take on to describe themselves. Gay men appear to be visible everywhere and therefore are easily knowable.

The rise of modern gay communities and quite a few places, neighborhoods, or precincts that are understood to coincide with gay community life, such as Chelsea and the West Village in New York City or the Castro in San Francisco, make the identification of gay men as study respondents seem fairly easy. The use of gay community resources, such as social and commercial businesses, clubs and advocacy groups, gay media, and sex venues (bathhouses and sex clubs) has featured prominently in health research, particularly regarding HIV/AIDS for the last 20 years. This has been less used or useful where such precincts are more hidden or dispersed. In these cases, social networks of respondents are often used to recruit respondents for studies. These communities, precincts, or networks have certainly allowed a great deal of research on gay men to be undertaken in recent years and have offered valid research findings for public health purposes in most instances. The attraction of this kind of research recruitment and its underlying assumption of who gay men are is that it finds in such men all the convergence that science seeks in terms of sexual behavior, sexual orientation, sexual attraction, and a socially identified density of like men.

Yet, a great deal of sex between men takes place outside the identity-category gay man; indeed, the term *men who have sex with men* (commonly, MSM), coined during the HIV pandemic, came into being precisely because men in studies of male-to-male sexual behavior and HIV transmission risk did not use the term gay or see any sense in that term to describe themselves. Framed as an identity/practice dissonance or as some sort of social paradox, it is often incorrectly assumed that MSM are *really* gay but do not admit it or have not fully realized it yet. This dissonance or paradox is evidence that sex between men does not always find meaning or cultural definition for the men practicing it as gay sex. Such men do not live among "gay-identified" men in gay communities, do not want to do so, have other ways of living lives (e.g., marriages, male and/or female partners), are subject to other social forces that shape their choices of how to live their lives, and find the idea and practice of gay life unsuitable.

In the United States, recent discussions of African American men on the "down low" and growing awareness about institutionally produced sexual cultures (e.g., in prisons, the military, sporting teams, schools, fraternities) indicate that a great deal of sex between men finds no relevance in the constructs of gay men and gay communities at all. Indeed, Kinsey et al. (1948) found more than 50 years ago that only a small percentage of men were exclusively homosexual throughout their lives (4%), and the sexual interests of other men change over time. Their various percentages for homosexual sex between men are mostly measures over a 3-year period precisely because of the variability of sexual practice over a lifetime.

2.2 Population Definition in Qualitative Research

Our first problem in gay men's health, then, might be wrestling with the uncertainty of the population we are seeking to investigate. This is an issue for any research methodology, quantitative or qualitative; but it becomes even more pressing because of the smaller sample sizes and the different sampling frames used in qualitative studies. There is a blurred boundary between gay and "straight" (i.e., between homosexual and heterosexual), and we must make important definitional compromises and assume population boundaries that are often arbitrary and not indigenous to the population itself (i.e., defined by a research project's needs rather than the population itself). Therefore, when we sample from populations of gay men for qualitative research, we must be explicit about decisions made on population definition.

We must also be critical of any underlying assumptions about that population ("we recruited them at gay bars, therefore they must be gay men"; "all gay men live in Chelsea, New York, or the 'Castro', San Francisco—let's recruit there"). Also, we must be clear that our samples have limitations in "standing in" for gay men at large or all gay men because of the difficulty inherent in defining the boundaries of gay. This population definition issue has become more crucial as younger generations of homosexually active people resist and refuse the category of gay man (or lesbian) and use *queer* or *bisexual* or *undecided* and *questioning* (Hillier & Rosenthal, 2001) both in their daily lives and in response to researchers' requests for sexual identity choices. We need, then, to find other ways to define our populations. One way to establish more clarity on population definition and boundary in qualitative research is related to clarifying each particular study's research object.

2.3 Defining a Research Object

Even if the uncertainties of study populations are bypassed, for example by selecting to study only gay-identified men and/or those who live distinctly gay life-styles (e.g., in male domestic partnerships or members of gay community organizations), we still cannot guarantee that our sample will be gay men, clean and simple. The reason for this lies in the selection of the *research object* for qualitative studies. A research object can be defined as the "place" where the research questions will be best answered by providing data and information or materials for analysis; this has to be clarified before the population definition and sampling can be established. For example, in the study of the flooded small town mentioned earlier, the research object is the town's experience of the flood itself. There might be a number of sources of information and data in the town documenting that experience, such as affected inhabitants, emergency workers, local community leaders; and we can obtain official accounts, newspaper reports, television footage, and so on. In this example, the people in the study are not the research object as such but, rather, one of the sources of data about the research object—the town's experience. In other words, that object offers a number of potential populations to investigate. This is similar to classical anthropology, where whole villages or exotic cultures are studied; people and practices are in the study but are not the research object as such. In qualitative research, even in public health, people may not at all be the research object of a study, even if they are included in an investigation in some way.

The research objects in many qualitative studies on gay men's health can be quite varied; and although gay men might assist as research respondents, they may not always be the principal focus. For example, we might be evaluating a home care program for aged gay men or assessing the training needs of youth workers who work with young gay men. Here the care program and the training needs are the research objects. Similarly, we might see value in understanding how the "choreography of drug taking" affects gay men's drug use (Southgate & Hopwood, 2001); that is, how the ebb and flow of recreational drug taking over an evening of partying takes place and how it generates any related sexual activity during such events. In such a study, we would not necessarily assess the amount of drugs taken or the frequency of sex practices engaged in for the purpose of generalizing about the amounts of drugs gay men use on average or how much sex they had when "high." Useful as it might be to find out, we would leave that to the quantitative researchers. Rather, qualitative research would seek to understand how the sensations of drug-taking are regarded by gay men and are pursued throughout the night. We might want to know what expectations gay men have of such drug-facilitated partying and sexual activity and how they plan for and execute that choreography of drug-taking. In such a study, we are seeking a complex and deep understanding of how, why, and in what ways drugs, sex, and gay men produce these events and what is possible at, and unique to, such events in relation to a broader notion of gay men's culture (Dowsett et al., 2005). Such a study might have a goal of providing findings that can inform the design of appropriate health promotion messages about safer drug use and sexual activity; the amount of drug use and sex occurring are less relevant here than the meanings of, and expectations associated with, such activity for contextualizing, specifying, and tailoring health promotion messages for such events.

An important thing to recognize about the many uses of qualitative methodology in health research, and one of its central strengths, is that we are not necessarily constrained to focus only on individual people and their knowledge, attitudes, and behaviors; we can actually formulate quite different questions that might throw light on health issues using the strengths of quite different theories—theories of culture, theories of practice, theories of language, social learning theories, theories of communication and media—focusing on groups of people, institutions and their processes, the role and effects of policy, program activities, value systems, the effects of powerful discourses and ideas, and many others. This is health seen as a social process, a product, a resource, an ideal, an effect, a focus for broader social issues (e.g., health inequalities or disparities), a way identity is lived and assessed, and so on.

This type and variety of research objects utilizes the strengths of qualitative methodology. With such issues, processes, experiences, and ideas as our potential research objects when studying gay men's health using qualitative methodology, defining the research object comes first. Identifying the population of gay men and how to determine its boundary then becomes primarily an issue of establishing and clarifying how such men relate to the research object and for which aspect of it they offer information or evidence. Here lies the crucial importance of problematizing the definition of gay men in any study and seeking to define which men in what groups, networks, or clusters of potential research participants whose same-sex sexual interests relate best to the research questions of any project. That is the starting point of defining the population and thereafter any sampling technique to employ. The research

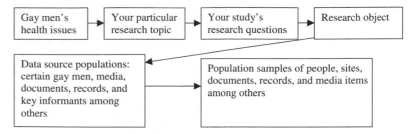

Figure 16.1 Research design sequence.

design and decision-making sequence of these issues are shown in Figure 16.1.

2.4 A Case Study in Qualitative Research Design

As a research design example, here is a brief description of my own recent study of how Australian gay community HIV/AIDS educators understand, utilize, and deploy the idea of gay community as part of their HIV prevention messages and in support for people living with HIV/AIDS. In terms of the design sequence in Figure 16.1, the general social problem was clearly the broader issue of *gay men's health education*, and this study's particular *research topic* (or focus) was the discourse of gay community itself (the full methodology of this study can be found in Dowsett et al., 2001). The *research questions* were as follows:

1. How are constructs of gay community deployed in HIV/AIDS health education and among gay and other homosexually active men? What is the role of, and meanings attached to, the construct gay community in HIV/AIDS health education as a result?
2. What are the educational practices and professional paradigms of gay community-based HIV/AIDS educators? How do the activities of HIV/AIDS health education engage their meanings and experiences of gay community?
3. What are the forms of sociality (i.e., the structuring of human relationships) emerging among gay and other homosexually active men in current "post-AIDS" contexts (Dowsett, 1996a)? How do gay and other homosexually active men experience "community" in their everyday lives and sexual practices?

The *research object* was the "discourse of gay community" in operation and/or practice.

This study, of course, involved gay men; but it also involved investigating how the idea of gay community played out in community events and venues, in documents (e.g., educational program protocols, resources, and in the gay media), how it was assumed in other research findings being used in the community, and how it was deployed by and among community leaders. These then comprised the *data source populations* available for the study and from which to sample. In this study, there were a number of *population samples*, both human and nonhuman. For some populations, the definition was relatively simple. For the nonhuman populations of documents, venues and events, and other research findings, we bounded data collection by site (there were three identified gay communities), the fieldwork time period (6 months), and by community mapping or audits undertaken with the guidance of key informants and the project's community advisory committees in each site.

Defining the human populations to be involved (i.e., gay men) was more complex in light of the earlier discussion of population definition. The key lay in the study's research questions listed above. We theorized that a certain population of gay men was more likely to utilize and deploy ideas of gay community in HIV/AIDS work. Therefore, the gay men involved were quite specifically chosen: gay community HIV educators who work with the idea and instance of community every day; gay community "performers" (defined as those whose cultural and political work utilizes notions of gay community); and gay men actively involved in HIV/AIDS programs as "consumers" (not just gay men as some generic or ubiquitous group out there passively exposed to HIV/AIDS efforts). The sampling was done from these specific groups. These men were clearly important to the study, yet formed just one part of the research population to be sampled and investigated.

It can sometimes be difficult for traditional public health researchers to grasp the fact that qualitative research does not always have people and their knowledge, attitudes, practices, and behaviors as the primary focus of its attention. This is not new for anyone in program evaluation research, in some health education research, in ethnographic studies of contemporary subcultures, or when undertaking rapid assessment research in developing countries. In these kinds of studies, sampling decisions are made not just concerning nonhuman populations of data sources but also in human subjects sampling based on criteria that can look quite strange to classic public health researchers.

2.5 Sampling Gay Men

Sampling in classic public health research usually relies on frame sampling, using social descriptors (sometimes called demographic variables or factors) such as sex, age, race/ethnicity, occupation, income, educational level, residence, family role (mother, father, child), faith, and so on. For qualitative studies, such sampling criteria should only operate *if* and *when* they relate directly to the research questions. So, in the example above of researching gay men's sex and drug-taking activities at dance parties, the population might be all those who attend certain events or venues within a certain time frame (e.g., in the United States, over the summer on Fire Island or during annual gay celebrations such as Gay Pride). Depending on the research questions, race/ethnicity, relationship status (single, involved, married), occupation, education level, and so on may not necessarily be the central population and sample-defining attributes in such studies. Sex (male) certainly is, and age might be, as such partying tends to attract younger people; but sexual identity may not be, as we are not necessarily sure that all such men participating in such events are gay, and we cannot assume that all participants can stand in for gay men in general. If there are too many participants at such events to include them all as study respondents, it might be far more pertinent, for example, to frame the sample by drug of choice (e.g., alcohol, marijuana, "speed," crystal methamphetamine, heroin). Alternatively, or in addition, we might interview dance party organizers, DJs, bar and security workers, even drug dealers to obtain different perspectives on the practice of drug-taking at such events. The researcher observations undertaken at these events might yield different information, and sampling is quite a different issue when this field method is employed. This is just one illustration of the kind of possible sampling frameworks that mark one of the key distinguishing features of qualitative methodology.

When examining gay men's sexual health, sex practices are often the focus—in part a legacy of sexually transmissible infection (STI) epidemiology—and seeing sex practices in terms other than as behaviors of people to be measured (instead of, say, rituals or rites of passage, as cultural affirmation and group membership, as identification with collective activity, as enactments of mutuality or interpersonal relations, or merely as codified pleasure) is unexpected and not well understood in much of the public health arena. Yet it is when examining these formulations of sexuality that qualitative research comes into its own, as it helps us understand what drives sexual interests and the cultures they create. That can mean quite hard thinking is needed again on how we understand the practice of sex between men beyond the notion of gay men as a sexual identity category. This could mean seeking different kinds of men: men who engage in unprotected sex; gay men with substance use problems; young men or older men; men of particular racial or ethnic origin; men from various social origins and classes; men in certain geographic locations, precincts, or sites (such as gay bathhouses) or homeless gay men; men with various health-related concerns (disabilities, aging, other illnesses); and, important often for HIV/AIDS, men who are HIV-positive, HIV-negative, or untested.

Beyond the specific health-related activities and practices we are researching, when determining who are gay men and whom shall we select for our research, we may need to define that population differently each time based on the men's own *sexual subjectivity* (Dowsett, 1996b) as: gay identified men; homosexually active men; men who occasionally have sex with men; bisexually identified men; men who have sex with men but would never admit to doing so; men who once had sex with men but do not do so now; men who have sex in men only in institutional settings (prisons, schools); men who have sex with men but do not understand those acts as sex; men who see themselves as female when having sex with other men; men who claim a gay identity or membership of a gay community irrespective of life-style or sex practices; those who refuse gay as an identity and choose queer instead; and so on. There are so many potential subsets of gay men, each relating to the specificities of each research project. When in doubt, we must return to our research questions; if these do not tell us how to decide, there is something amiss with the questions themselves.

3 Importance of Social Theory in Qualitative Methodology

Note in the argument above that a sample in qualitative studies is not necessarily and always constituted by individual people. One can sample households, institutions and processes, programs, places, practices, language, interactions, meanings, cultural objects such as art images used in health promotion for gay men, and so on. Yet seeing gay men as individual men with individual health problems is the predominant way of understanding health. The emphasis on the individual (as patient, as research respondent, as *the* unit of analysis) masks the origins and processes of many social determinants of health for gay men. Today, new theories—for example, social network theory and its simple versions used in contact tracing among gay men for STI detection—help us understand that individuals alone are not always sufficient as a research focus, particularly in infectious disease control. Collective cultures are as much part of the issue as other social and contextual influences, such as institutional policies and practices (e.g., condom provision in gay bath houses or in prisons), community expectations (e.g., growing a safe sex culture, or regularly providing risk reduction measures in drug-facilitated events, such as needle exchange), political and legislative action (e.g., the illegality of male-to-male sex driving men away from services, or providing a national health scheme for the uninsured), and subcultural forms (e.g., initiation rituals, gang membership rules). In other words, in public health today we are not just concerned with behaviors alone and do not see them as lying only within the locus of individual choice and control but, rather, understand them *socially* as *practices* embedded in complex forces that facilitate and constrain individuals and groups in relation to health-related decisions and actions.

This becomes particularly important when gay men are seen not just as sexual beings first and foremost, and other health issues come into focus, such as oppression and violence, homophobia and stigmatization (particularly related to mental health), alcohol and drug use, dilemmas of body image (steroid use, excessive dieting), aging, relationships, and social circumstances (health-care insurance, old age provision), ownership of resources (the gay marriage debate deals with much of this), and other health-related issues. These all affect the health and well-being of gay men. Therefore, there is a need to develop ways of understanding and investigating the situatedness of gay men's health issues, as embedded in social process and relations and contextualized by circumstance. Part of the reason qualitative methodology is useful is that it can more readily focus beyond the individual on more complex social determinants of health that cannot be easily quantified or are understood best when measured. Complexity in social and sexual life often requires more detail and subtlety.

Indeed, sometimes social processes do not lend themselves readily to measurement, for example in understanding how trust works during sexual negotiation of condom use. Even if a survey found that a certain percentage of unprotected sex acts among gay men in regular partnerships involves trust as the main factor in decision-making, we would still not know how this actually operates, particularly if we were to develop health promotion initiatives that seek to utilize that dynamic and ensure that sexual safety is always maximized. Even if we can define trust as "confidence in or reliance on some quality or attribute of a person or thing, or the truth of a statement" (*Oxford English Dictionary* online), we still do not know how gay men determine that they trust each other, how it operates from situation to situation, in what contexts, or how HIV/AIDS might have forced new versions of trust to be developed and operate.

Hence, the importance of those new theories of sexuality discussed earlier, as they have grown not from and with a legacy of a pathologized homosexuality but as ways of seeing sexuality as a creative field of human practice, socially as well as individually generated, historically and culturally contingent and specific, and mutable. These ways of seeing sexuality offer real research resources that can be utilized well by qualitative research, particularly with its multiple and various typical methodologies and data-gathering techniques, and in ways that can make best use of the flexibility that qualitative methodology provides the researcher.

4 Choosing a Qualitative Methodolgy

Although qualitative methodology is often contrasted with quantitative methodology as if they are two singular, competing frameworks, in fact there are a number of qualitative methodologies. This does not refer to the many field methods available in qualitative research; rather, it refers to different epistemological frameworks that may use different or similar combinations of those field methods but seek different ends and pursue different intellectual purposes—hence the importance of social theory. For example, anthropologists undertaking ethnographic description (e.g., using interviews, observations) of diets and nutritional understanding of other cultures are using *ethnography* in a quite different way from that of urban sociologists using similar field methods to investigate urban homophobic violence by gangs of young men. The various social theories underpinning such research efforts form the key to these differences in the application of qualitative methodology and the knowledge it generates (May, 2001). That said, these different frameworks and their differential uses of field methods all register one important common characteristic in their application in qualitative research design and research practice: flexibility.

4.1 Flexibility

One of the beauties of qualitative research is that we do not have to settle completely the details of the operation of our methodology during the research design phase (beyond what research funders require), and we can adopt a flexible approach to field work. This means that, in practice, if the field work and the data gathered during one phase of the research suggest changing interview guides or sampling techniques, for example, we can change them to achieve a better study. We are not trapped with an inapposite question or an unreliable measure (as might happen with a predesigned, structured questionnaire); if a question does not elicit useful responses, we can dispense with, change, or even replace it. Also, if the fieldwork suggests that the phenomenon being researched is manifesting differently than at first envisaged with a slightly different group of gay men than anticipated (e.g., recreational drug injection is occurring with an older age group than originally thought), the sample can be reshaped to fit better with the research questions. Similarly, if community stakeholders or gatekeepers decide to hamper a study for any reason, attention can be shifted to other related populations as sources of information. Rarely in qualitative research are data-gathering techniques structured on rigid operational lines, such as asking each question in the same way in the same order; instead, we prefer more conversational ways of engaging with respondents, and most field methods are conceived in broad outline rather than specified line-by-line or minute-by-minute, and they do not need to be tightly replicable.

This flexibility is important when working with gay men and gay communities because, as discussed earlier, these men and communities are new phenomena, indeed newly created and still in the process of creation. Study populations are fluid and difficult to define *a priori*. Previous theories about community or sexuality might be seriously contradicted by newly emerging sexual and community formations, and in-depth investigation might reveal that our precepts when designing a study are wrong, inadequate, or just ill-informed. We may have to change approaches, ideas, theories, and the fieldwork in midstream, and qualitative methodology allows this. Yet this is not a haphazard or accidental process. Using such flexibility to advantage takes experience and is guided by a long history of methodological debate and exemplification; it is also encoded within a set of typical qualitative methodologies and trusted field methods that bring security and rigor to this flexibility.

4.2 Typical Qualitative Methodologies

Those not experienced in qualitative methodology may puzzle about the best way to investigate such complex framings of sexuality noted above, particularly when there seems to be an ever-enlarging set of field methods (or data-gathering techniques) available to be used. However, there are *typical methodologies* used in qualitative research that have been tried and tested in the health arena over the years and that form the starting point when designing research. There are many textbooks that can provide detailed descriptions of, and rationales for, such methodologies—particularly good is the *Handbook of Qualitative Research* (Denzin & Lincoln, 2000)—so these methodologies are not fully discussed here. Some examples can suffice.

Table 1. Examples of Typical Methodologies

Research focus	Typical methodologies
Specifics of individual experience	Phenomenology
	Oral history or biography
Culture, language, and society	Ethnography
	Descriptive
	Critical
	Comparative
Politics/patterns of practice	Action research, evaluation studies
Theory building	Grounded theory
	Theorized life history
Elucidation, description	Case study
	Individual
	Institutional

In Table 1 are examples in which studies with certain research focuses typically suggest certain methodologies. Note that for quantitative research—the most common type of public health research—the cross-sectional population study typically uses a survey method fully structured with various types of question, established (reliable) measures, and preformed answers to be selected (forced-choice). In qualitative research, if we are interested in individual experience (i.e., not as part of aggregated population studies but in its own right), we might approach this *phenomenologically* (as a descriptive study of experience) or as an *oral history* or *biography*, including using various data sources [see Plummer (2001) for a rich account of this kind of research]. *Ethnography* is particularly useful when we are focused on the study of cultures or unities of forms (e.g., studying a gay community, as if it were a separate small society, in its responses to HIV/AIDS; e.g., Dowsett, 1996a). *Case studies* are useful in clinical settings but can also be done in institutions (research in a prison, for example; e.g., Wacquant & Willis, 2002), or on particular controversies (research on gay and lesbian parenting; e.g., Dempsey, 2004).

There are other typical methodologies in qualitative research, each with its own logic and assumptions about knowledge production, so the field is not just a catalogue of field methods (e.g., interviewing, group techniques, document analysis) that we choose at random. We can rely on these typical methodologies as frameworks to guide our research design; and each prefers various data-gathering techniques that then constitute an individual study's approach.

4.3 Data-Gathering Techniques in Qualitative Research

One of dilemmas for new researchers starting qualitative inquiry is choosing data-gathering techniques or field methods. Often a choice of methods can drive a study; for example, using focus groups because it seems a popular method nowadays or other studies using in-depth interviews may seem to achieve the goals. Unfortunately, this is the wrong approach to choosing data-gathering techniques; the research project and its research questions should determine the field methods used, not the other way round. Thus, a health policy analysis might include individual interviews (maybe with policymakers) but would clearly need to review policy documents as well, thereby calling also for a method of systematically collecting documents and reviewing and analyzing them. This kind of connection between research question and field methods is epistemological at heart (i.e., it is about understanding knowledge building) and a key decision-making task in qualitative research because there are so many methods, each with strengths and limitations. We often use a combination of complementary methods in qualitative research, depending on the project (as we saw in the gay community discourse study discussed earlier). Also, new methods are being invented all the time. For example, research on the Internet has called for new ways to understand that phenomenon and investigate it, particularly as the certainties in other human subject research are less so in this medium (Hine, 2000).

That said, there are some often-used and central field methods that can guide the choice for any particular project: the individual interview, often called an in-depth interview and one capable of a variety of formats and processes; various group techniques such as in-depth group interviews, less-intensive focus group discussions, memory work groups (Haug, 1992), and group observations; participant observations of many kinds; and document or textual analysis. Documenting personal experience through these methods is a vital tool of qualitative research: For example, we have learned much about early sex research and its misplaced efforts to cure homosexuality through personal accounts of aversion therapy, institutional confinement, and chemical interventions (e.g., hormone therapy). Personal papers, photographs, and documents are also wonderful sources of material for health research, as are newspaper reports, electronic media resources, and other public records (Plummer, 2001). Those undertaking public health history research are expert users of such materials.

The field methods just listed are the main types, but each can take many and varied forms. Indeed, as public health research questions proliferate and postindustrial society becomes ever more complex, field methods are always being refined and adjusted, and innovative methods are being developed. Again, as one example, the Internet and its resources, the potential for communication, and technical reach has called for and already developed a plethora of new field methods (e.g., Carballo-Diéguez et al., 2004, and their use of *cybercartography*). Gay men are major users of the Internet and have become a testing ground for, and one of the first populations to be involved in, research using this medium. There are some interesting studies underway in the United States and elsewhere; but we are still unsure how to judge the validity of such research findings given the unresolved issues of population definition and sampling discussed earlier and a great deal of uncertainty about the reliability of instruments developed for the Internet. The most difficult question of all is: How do you really know who is on the end of the computer your research is reaching?

The key issues concerning typical methodologies and their field methods concerning gay men's health research relate to the earlier discussion of research objects. Gay men's lives and histories of engagement with public health have much to teach us about modern medicine, its health systems, and its professional practice. Many minorities or marginalized populations have similar stories to tell and an understandable reluctance at times to participate in research that comes from the very sources that were so hurtful and damaging in the first place. The selection of a typical methodology and its field methods must recognize that marginalized, oppressed, or stigmatized populations are mildly skeptical or deeply distrustful of researchers in the light of these histories. Thus, when choosing methods we must take that into account as well as simply relying on the technical strengths of the methodology itself—or the field method preferences of the researcher for that matter.

That said, the experience of researchers working in HIV/AIDS has been one that reveals just how generous gay men have been in participating in research about themselves, their lives and communities, their histories, and *inter alia* their sexuality by keeping diaries, being guinea pigs for prevention intervention research, and undergoing a relentless battery of questioning about their sex activities regularly over the last two decades. Perhaps it is the ease with which gay men talk to each other about bodies and sex that enables their ready participation in such a public (and publicly funded) scrutiny of their intimate lives. Perhaps it is a collective commitment to ending this terrible HIV pandemic that supports such research participation by those who, less than a generation ago, were forced to hide their sexuality from view. The good will gay men show public health research is to be neither squandered nor taken for granted. Methodology becomes, therefore, not just the preferred mode of operation of a researcher but something that engages the consideration of the researched. Gay men are no longer passive research subjects, and that demands something from the researcher that qualitative methodology uniquely enhances: reflexivity.

5 The Reflexive Researcher

Whatever methods we utilize in qualitative research and what methodological frameworks they constitute, there is a central and overriding principle that applies to understanding the way qualitative research works. The key idea here is *reflexivity*. There is a major ongoing debate in qualitative methodology (see Denzin and Lincoln, 2000, for a full discussion) about qualitative research and its presumptions concerning the nature of scientific inquiry and the nature of knowledge itself. Mostly, in qualitative work we do not seek to distance the researcher from the researched in pursuit of some specious kind of objectivity; rather, we embrace the situatedness of the researcher as actively contributing to the research, and we see the dialogic nature of the interactions between the researcher and the researched as a major and positive component of the research process at every stage—indeed, the dialogue is itself data. This becomes clear when embarking on community-based or action research; working with gay communities during the HIV epidemic has stimulated a great deal of innovation in such typical research methodologies, partly at the insistence of gay men critical of the legacy of earlier scientific research, particularly biomedical research, that mistreated homosexual people in the name of science.

This movement toward more collaborative and participatory forms of research did not occur merely as a political maneuver but was required to find ways to investigate aspects of gay men's lives that did not readily lend themselves to scrutiny through standardized survey techniques and other classic public health methods. A second contribution to the shift in approaches derived support from earlier feminist critiques of the scientific method and its assumptions about knowledge, the researched, and objectivity itself (May, 2001). These critiques noted the domination of (heterosexual) men in research and the domination of findings based on research conducted by men on men (excluding and sometimes inaccurately describing women). Far from being objective, such research often deployed sexist assumptions and understanding of women and their situation. This critique had significant effect in the humanities and in certain social science disciplines, mainly social psychology, comparative anthropology, and critical sociology but less so or to a lesser effect in other places. The critique came to occupy a central place among those engaged in critical sexuality studies and queer theory and has provided a solid basis for a serious and sophisticated reappraisal of the way gay men (and lesbian, transgender, and more recently intersex people) have been and are researched.

The researcher's familiarity with, and understanding of, these quite significant and sophisticated critiques becomes an important part of any research done on gay men. The researcher must be situated within these debates as well as within his or her own disciplinary traditions and experience. In HIV/AIDS work, it is not surprising to find many qualified and experienced social researchers who also happen to be gay men (as am I) and some are HIV-positive gay men as well (e.g., Willis, 2002). Does this mean we are likely to be biased in our approach or better situated to research gay men? These are not the right questions: The key question is how do we understand, explain, and work with the situatedness of researchers no matter what their relation to the issue at the core of the research questions, the populations being studied, or the paradigm within whichever academic disciplines framed the research in the first place. In qualitative research, these are central issues being constantly debated, refined, and rehearsed. Such issues become quite important in participatory and collaborative research projects where the interaction between the researched and the researcher is an explicit and prominent part of the process; but these issues are not irrelevant to even the most classic kinds of research.

In qualitative research, the researcher is seen as a partner with the researched in the production of knowledge, not just the technical means of its discovery or retrieval. This places the burden of reflexivity on the researcher. She or he must become part of what is examined and scrutinized; there is no place outside the research object for the researcher to stand, to find objectivity—we are always part of the world we study. There is only involvement, implication, and intervention. Reflexivity is the concept that captures the active participation of the researcher in the qualitative research process and is central to making the most of what qualitative research has to offer science and human knowledge. Ironically, gay men, by virtue of having to come to grips with sexual interests that are themselves the central object of the study of human sexuality, are reflexive by definition: Being gay in a straight world is perforce a reflexive place to reside. That makes researching gay men and their health issues using qualitative methodology decidedly queer for us all.

6 Limitations to Qualitative Methodology

All research methodologies have strengths and weaknesses, insight and blind sports, specialties and limitations. It is difficult to outline these factors as they pertain to qualitative methodology as, has been shown, this is not one methodology but multiple approaches to social research, influenced by the academic discipline involved, the epistemological standpoint of the project, the field methods employed, the researchers' experience, and ultimately the purpose underpinning the research project. So, for example, research investigating popular cultural representations of mental illness might involve a cultural studies disciplinary perspective, a standpoint on the part played by cultural representations in producing common prejudice about mental health sufferers; it might utilize content analysis of popular media forms; and it might be undertaken by a graduate student for the purpose of fulfilling course requirements for predoctoral training. This greatly affects the kind of research done and the way in which it is able to offer new insight into a complex social phenomenon.

This example reveals how specific the findings of qualitative research are to the research design and why qualitative researchers must be careful about how to present their findings in research reports. One of the major areas of difficulty for qualitative research concerns *generalizability* (i.e., the drawing of broadly applicable conclusions about common experiences or events on the basis of evidence from particular or specific ones). This capacity is generally regarded as one of the strengths of *quantitative* research because of its large sample sizes and their capacity to stand in for, or speak about, a population at large (e.g., a study of 5000 high-school students carefully structured to mirror the demographic makeup of such students in general or the sampling frames utilized that try to obtain representative samples of specific subpopulations that share characteristics (e.g., gay men) and therefore allow findings from the study to be reasonably applicable to the rest of that subpopulation).

In qualitative research, we can speak about our findings only in terms related to the specific sampling models used. If we have done a study of 20 young gay men attending a local coming-out support group and found that 10 had experienced bullying at school, we cannot conclude that half of all young gay men had such experiences. The apportionment of findings in qualitative research's usually small samples is a trap many inexperienced researchers fall into because this is how the much larger numbers in quantitative research are reported, but it is usually wrong and misleading.

What qualitative research is good at providing at a generalizable level is an account of social processes at work. In the case study in research design presented earlier, we found that most of the gay HIV prevention educators we interviewed reported that they had increasing difficulty is being safe all the time in their own sexual behavior, even though they were undertaking prevention education in their gay communities. We cannot conclude from this that all HIV educators as a population are engaged in unsafe sexual acts or even that many of them are. This is the type of generalization that incorrect apportionment produces and is based in misunderstanding how sampling is understood in qualitative research. We can say that it is clear that gay HIV prevention educators struggle with sexual practice and safety issues even though it is central to their jobs because they are also part of the sexual cultures they serve. Clearly, also some of these educators are taking sexual risks, for they are gay men too and not outside the personal pressures the epidemic has produced. This is generalization at the level of social process and might be a finding applicable to other gay communities. It certainly warrants further research. From this example, we see that great care has to be taken in understanding how qualitative studies reveal larger social process and more depth about experience. The key to understanding how any qualitative research project can offer generalizable findings is to return to the research questions of each project and to review again that project's research object. Rarely are apportionment and measurement statements about qualitative research likely to be valid. Those not familiar with qualitative research may see this as a lack or a weakness, and it is if that is the only way the social world can be understood; but once the real strengths of qualitative research are grasped, its particular type of generalizability can become a powerful, efficient way to understand many social worlds.

7 Summary

Qualitative methodology offers public health research a remarkable resource for investigating pressing and difficult issues. Its flexibility, its own form of rigor, its theoretical underpinnings, its technical diversity, and its multidisciplinary approaches constitute a rich store of ideas, methods, tools, and frameworks for investigating pressing public health problems. The methodology is undergoing rapid development and change, driven largely by the experience of research itself and the inbuilt reflexivity mentioned earlier. No two projects are the same in qualitative methodology because what is learned during the process of doing one inevitably changes what happens next. More importantly, the researcher is changed and can never simply repeat a project: Replication is not an option in this methodology.

Just as important is an increasing interest in using participatory-action research and community-based research approaches using qualitative methodology as a more respondent-friendly research style. These developments take seriously the ethical and social values concerns that have long produced complaints by respondents that researchers simply treat them as objects. People living with HIV/AIDS, often drawing on a critical activism derived from gay men's sexual politics, have been particularly forceful in challenging the lack of democracy in medical and health research. Such a challenge is more than a technical issue about field methods and community consultation processes; it concerns the way human experience is conceptualized, understood, and made available for scientific scrutiny. Such issues are at the core of the philosophy of science debates occurring among qualitative researchers the world over.

Increasingly, academic journals specializing in qualitative research are available, and more conventional health journals are opening their pages to research using qualitative methodology. This has not an easy process of change, particularly when traditional journal formats (e.g., organizing the article into background, methodology, findings, discussion) do not readily lend themselves to the ways in which knowledge is understood to be produced and assembled in qualitative methodology. It becomes important not only that qualitative researchers develop new and more appropriate ways to report our research; it is also incumbent upon us to be clearer, more explicit, and extremely careful when explaining how we do our research and what it offers.

Finally, in gay men's health issues (and this also applies to lesbians), the population with whom we are working has significant resources to bring to the research process as well in terms of ideas, experience, theories, good will, a research agenda, and research needs, to name just a few. This offers qualitative researchers in particular a real opportunity to engage in new and exciting research strategies with a willing, if occasionally skeptical, population of respondents. This is an opportunity to be embraced.

References

Altman, D. (2001) *Global sex.* Allen & Unwin, Sydney.

Carballo-Diéguez, A., Shedlin, M., Dowsett, G., Remien, R., Lin, P., Dolezal, C., Balan, I., and Ventuneac, A. (2004) Ethnography of "bareback" Internet services. Presented at the International Academy of Sex Research Annual Meeting, Helsinki.

Dempsey, D. (2004) Donor, father or parent? Conceiving paternity in the Australian Family Court. *International Journal of Law, Policy and the Family* 18:76–102.

Denzin, N.K., and Lincoln, Y.S. (2000) *Handbook of qualitative research,* 2nd ed. Sage, Thousand Oaks, CA.

Dowsett, G.W. (1996a) Perspectives in Australian HIV/AIDS health promotion. In: NSW AIDS/Infectious Diseases Branch (comp.) *NSW HIV/AIDS Health*

Promotion Conference: keynote addresses, selected papers and future directions. New South Wales Health Publication (AIDS) 96–0067, Sydney, pp. 19–31.

Dowsett, G.W. (1996b) *Practicing desire: homosexual sex in the era of AIDS.* Stanford University Press, Stanford, CA.

Dowsett, G.W., Bollen, J., McInnes, D., Couch, M., and Edwards, B. (2001) HIV/AIDS and constructs of gay community: researching educational practice within community-based health promotion for gay men. *International Journal of Social Research Methodology* 4:205–223.

Dowsett, G.W., Keys, D., and Wain, D. (2005) Good gay men don't get "messy": injecting drug use and gay community. *Sexuality Research and Social Policy: Journal of the National Sexuality Resource Center* 2(1):23–29.

Foucault, M. (1978) *The history of sexuality.* Vol. 1. *An introduction* (Hurley, R., trans). Penguin, Harmondsworth.

Haug, F. (1992) *Beyond female masochism: memory-work and politics* (Livingstone, R., trans). Verso, London.

Hillier, L., and Rosenthal, D. (eds). (2001) *Journal of Adolescence* 24(1) [special issue on gay lesbian and bisexual youth].

Hine, C. (2000) *Virtual ethnography.* Sage, London.

Kavanagh, A., Daly, J., and Jolley, D. (2002) Research methods, evidence and public health. *Australian and New Zealand Journal of Public Health* 26:337–342.

Kinsey, A.C., Pomeroy, W.D., and Martin, C.E. (1948) *Sexual behavior in the human male.* Saunders, Philadelphia.

Kinsey, A.C., Pomeroy, W.D., Martin, C.E., and Gebhard, P.H. (1953) *Sexual behavior in the human female.* Saunders, Philadelphia.

Leonard, W. (ed). (2002). *What's the difference?* Research paper by the Victorian Ministerial Advisory on Gay and Lesbian Health. Victorian Government Department of Human Services, Melbourne.

May, T. (2001) *Social research: issues, methods, process,* 3rd ed. Open University Press, Buckingham, UK.

Plummer, K. (2001) *Documents of life 2: an invitation to a critical humanism,* 2nd ed. Sage, London.

Southgate, E., and Hopwood, M. (2001) The role of folk pharmacology and lay experts in harm reduction: Sydney gay drug using networks. *The International Journal of Drug Policy* 12:321–335.

Wacquant, L., and Willis, P. (eds). (2002) *Ethnography* 3(4). Special issue on "In and Out of the Belly of the Beast": Dissecting the Prison.

Weeks, J. (1985) *Sexuality and its discontents: meanings, myths and modern sexualities.* Routledge & Kegan Paul, London.

Willis, J. (2002) *It's Disturbing.* Presented at the Bridging Session—from Basic Science to Real Life: Disturbing Metabolic Disturbances, XIV International AIDS Conference, Barcelona. Available at: http://www.prous.com/aids2002/disturbances/index.asp.

Wilton, T. (2002) Lesbian and gay health: power, paradigms and bodies. In: Richardson, D., and Seidmann, S. (eds) *Handbook of gay and lesbian studies.* Sage, London, pp. 253–270.

17

From Science Fiction to Computer-Generated Technology: Sampling Lesbian, Gay, and Bisexual Individuals

Esther D. Rothblum

1 Science Fiction: Role of Clinical Samples up to the 1970s

Imagine that you have interviewed eight extraterrestrials and submitted the results for publication in a mental health journal. When you eventually receive the editor's decision letter, it is likely to take one of several forms. The editor may state that the topic area is outside the purview of the journal. Reading between the lines, you may wonder if the editor questions your sanity—What is wrong with you to be studying *them*? The editor may question your results—either because you have presented extraterrestrials as so similar to humans that it defies credibility or else the factors that set them apart are so bizarre the editor does not believe them. If the editor knows you personally, you may be advised to pursue more mainstream research, especially if you are junior in your career. In short, you may be criticized for your choice of topic or your results, but no one is going to be concerned with sampling issues. Eight extraterrestrials are sensational enough—there is no need to explain whether your selection was representative.

This scenario describes research on sexual minorities up through the 1970s. Once in a while, an article appeared in a mental health journal based on a small sample of gay men and sometimes an even smaller sample of lesbians (there was little research on bisexuals). At first, the author was likely to be a mental health professional at a clinic or psychiatric hospital that treated people with severe mental health problems. Given that homosexuality was classified as a mental health problem, articles about this topic focused on psychopathology. Even after homosexuality was removed as a diagnosis from the *Diagnostic and Statistical Manual of Mental Disorders* in 1973, the new edition of the DSM omitting this diagnosis did not appear in print until 1980 (American Psychiatric Association, 1968, 1980). Articles about homosexuality usually emphasized the participants' masculine versus feminine appearance and gender roles, parental child-rearing behaviors that "caused" the abnormal behavior, current "sexual deviations," and associated mental health problems (depression, anxiety, substance abuse, suicidality).

Today, we are quick to identify sources of sampling error in these articles. We know that many people "passed" as heterosexual in those days, including some of our own friends and colleagues who lied to their therapists about the gender of their lovers or the source of their sexual attractions. Thus, the lesbians and gay men who came to the attention of mental health professionals were those least able to pass owing to their gender-nonconforming appearance or those who were caught during police raids of gay bars or public restrooms. Lesbians and gay men who disclosed their sexual orientation to a therapist had a lot to lose if word got out but often had already lost a lot (e.g., custody of their children, their job, respect of their family) and were desperate to try to become heterosexual to regain societal privileges.

Given the homophobic views and practices of mainstream therapists, it would not be surprising if lesbians, gay men, and bisexuals (LGBs) avoided therapists altogether. In fact, the converse seems to have occurred. Beginning in the 1970s (see Silverstein, 1991, for a review), LGB newspapers and community resources advertised the services of affirmative therapists. Practicing without degrees from mainstream mental health institutions and usually LGBs themselves, these therapists often served as important role models for closeted and isolated individuals who did not know anyone else like them. Among "out" LGBs who lived in urban settings, it was acceptable to talk about one's individual or couples therapy in social settings. Silverstein recalls this period (1991, p. 5): "While gays flocked to our services, established professionals, who earned their living by 'curing' gay men and women, saw us as a cabal of reckless incompetents who, when successful, doomed our clients to a life of misery."

This generation of therapists knew more about the LGB communities, based on issues arising within their clients' lives, than did any researchers at the time. These therapists too began publishing articles about LGB issues but from an affirmative rather than a pathologic perspective. In the early feminist and social issue journals, they described such normative processes in the LGB communities as the coming-out process, sex and relationships, adolescence, aging, race and ethnicity, stress and social support, workplace issues, and friendships. They introduced the general mental health professionals reading these articles to concepts such as lesbian "merger," gay bathhouses, bi-phobia, fluid gender identity among Native Americans, and heteronormativity.

Here too there was little thought about sampling. Just as in the earlier articles written about "homosexuals" from a pathologizing perspective, these affirmative articles were based on clients in therapy. These clients were thus affluent (and also middle-class, highly educated, young, and European American), open about their own sexual orientation, and knowledgeable about LGB communities. For traditionally trained mental health professionals who treated the occasional lesbian or gay man, these clinical studies defied credibility (gay men coming out in the workplace, lesbians having children). For LGBs who came across these publications while closeted or isolated in rural or conservative settings, the content was an ideal of what could be possible if they moved to urban areas or "came out." In short, the first wave of LGB samples was not so much science as science fiction.

Is there a place for anecdotal articles about LGBs today? Yes, indeed. Before researchers embark on a topic that has been understudied with LGB populations, it is extremely useful to conduct interviews with just a handful of LGBs. This allows researchers to understand some basic themes and perhaps modify their research measures before surveying hundreds of participants. Publishing the results of these preliminary interviews is still a useful way of disseminating information on new topics; it might be a year or two before the results of the larger study, with standardized measures, is completed.

2 Tips of the Icebergs: Role of Convenience Samples During the 1980s and Beyond

The lesbian publication *The Ladder* contained the following quote in 1958 (p. 9):

There has been much bitter comment that all the published data on Lesbians comes either from badly maladjusted women who have sought psychiatric help or from women in prison. It is high time information was collected and published covering all Lesbians, not just a few. And apparently the only way to make sure this is done is to do it ourselves.

The Ladder went on to do just that in 1959, publishing the results of a survey of 157 lesbians that focused on demographic and mental health information. This survey has rarely been cited in the academic literature, although it was larger and more lesbian-affirmative than the many published studies of 10 or 20 participants that were the norm during the 1970s.

The 1980s was the decade of the lesbian and gay convenience survey. A few LGB researchers were "out" enough in graduate school or as faculty to conduct studies about sexual minorities. At the same time, the LGB communities were expanding to include not only gay bars and social groups but religious organizations, land collectives, campus student groups, bookstores, and subscribers of periodicals (Rothblum, 1994). This gave researchers the opportunity to locate research participants in their geographic region with relative ease. Furthermore, annual events such as gay pride parades and women's music festivals enabled researchers to distribute and collect hundreds of questionnaires in one day. Participants were also encouraged to take extra copies of questionnaires for their friends and acquaintances, a process called snowball sampling. Perhaps the largest and best known of these convenience studies was the National Lesbian Health Care Survey

(Bradford et al., 1994) conducted in the mid-1980s that resulted in 1917 completed questionnaires. The recruitment procedure included women's centers, lesbian and gay organizations, personal networks, social and organizational contacts, bookstores, prisons, and gay newspapers. Furthermore, researchers could focus on subcommunities, such as African American lesbians (Mays & Cochran, 1988), older gay men (Pope & Schultz, 1991), and adolescent lesbians (Schneider, 1989).

From the outset, convenience surveys were considered nonrepresentative because they were limited to LGBs who were "out" or open enough about their sexual orientation to attend community events or subscribe to periodicals. Even with all of these recruitment methods, researchers acknowledged that many LGBs are so closeted, isolated, or mistrustful of researchers that they cannot be reached with these methods. The results were thus not generalizable to LGBs in the general population, and researchers tended to apologize for this weakness. For example, in the National Lesbian Health Care Survey, Bradford and Ryan stated (1987, p. v): "results of the survey, therefore, cannot be generalized to represent all lesbians in the United States."

There is a tendency to assume that those LGBs who are out are only the very tip of the iceberg. This is partly due to the not-so-distant past when homosexuality was a mental illness and LGBs had much to lose by coming out. The general public may assume that the spokespeople for LGB rights they see on television live in gay enclaves (San Francisco, Provincetown, Northampton), have nontraditional jobs (e.g., work for a gay bar or lesbian magazine), and lead a certain kind of "life-style" (e.g., without children or stable relationships). Meanwhile, it is assumed that many LGBs live more "mainstream" but hidden lives (constituting the major part of the iceberg, which is concealed). Consequently, there is pressure for researchers to find more closeted LGBs who are presumed to live in smaller towns or rural areas, have more traditional jobs, have children, and so on. Thus, researchers who study only LGB communities or individuals who are "out" are using samples that cannot be generalized to more hidden, rural, or closeted LGB individuals.

It is interesting that no one has studied similarities and differences between LGBs who are "out" and those who are closeted. This would seem possible because some researchers have included items or scales of "outness" in their questionnaires (e.g., Bradford et al., 1994; Morris & Rothblum, 1999; Solomon et al., 2004) and consequently could compare characteristics of LGBs who differ in levels of outness. The results of such comparisons would justify whether focusing on LGBs who are "out" bears any resemblance to those who are closeted.

Convenience samples with LGB samples are still heavily used today, and there are two other challenges facing researchers who use this method. First, LGBs recruited via convenience sampling tend to have high levels of education, earn incomes that are low relative to their educational level, and do not belong to religious organizations (e.g., Bradford et al., 1994; Morris & Rothblum, 1999; Badgett, 2001). In addition, gay men tend to live in large cities (Laumann et al., 1994). Thus, convenience studies have been criticized for focusing on members of a middle-class lesbian and gay subculture, ignoring participants who lived in rural settings, did not have a college education, or were more closeted. Yet these demographic data may in fact be an accurate general profile of LGBs. For example, LGBs may have had more educational opportunities due to not being married and/or not having children at a young age. Gay men may move to large cities for greater anonymity and to find supportive LGB communities. Given the homophobic positions of most major religions, it is not surprising that LGBs would be less religious.

The second challenge for researchers who utilize LGB convenience samples is the lack of a heterosexual comparison group. This is not an issue when the focus is on factors unique to LGBs, such as the coming-out process. However, this issue becomes more important for researchers who want to study factors such as health and mental health, where there is an enormous literature on the population at large. Recruiting participants via LGB community organizations, events, and periodicals is going to yield few heterosexuals (and *they* are probably quite atypical of the general heterosexual population). One clever solution to this dilemma was a study by Kris Morgan (1992) who distributed questionnaires at a college women's basketball game, knowing how popular women's sports were in the lesbian community. Sure enough, she found high percentages of both lesbian and heterosexual women from the community among the spectators. Researchers can also recruit heterosexuals via different sources (e.g., feminist periodicals, counterculture events) than those from which they recruit LGBs, but they would most likely find that the LGB and heterosexual samples differ on a number of demographic variables, which then have to be covaried. Finally, they can compare results of LGBs to published norms of the general population, but such norms are often collected on homogeneous samples, such as college students or psychiatric populations, making comparisons difficult.

Despite the sampling constraints of convenience studies, this method yielded an enormous amount of data about lesbians and gay men (though less about bisexuals). I have argued previously (Rothblum, 1994) that convenience samples of members of the LGB communities *are* important for understanding LGBs who are "out" and integrated into community activities and organizations. Trends and issues in the gay/lesbian communities also influence people who are more closeted or just coming out. Finally, historians will search this literature in the future, when LGB communities as we currently know them may be quite different or obsolete.

3 Reaching John and Jane Doe via Computer-Generated Technology: Role of Population-Based Samples in the 1990s and Beyond

By the end of the 1980s, large-scale health and mental health community surveys were beginning to include an item or two about same-sex behavior, mostly due to the fact that the HIV/AIDS epidemic was becoming widespread. Researchers who would not have considered items about same-sex sexual orientation in the past now realized that they needed to determine the gender of the sexual partner to assess sexual behavior. Even today it is difficult to persuade epidemiologic research teams to include more than one or two items about sexual orientation; their concern is that participants will be offended and refuse to answer the rest of the questionnaire. For example, the U.S. census in 2000 added an item about gender of partners who were cohabiting—a significant improvement (see Gates & Ost, 2004 for data collected by the latest census). However, this leaves out information about LGBs who are single and those who are not living with their partner.

A number of technologic advances made large-scale community surveys more feasible near the end of the twentieth century. First, random digit telephone dialing, whereby computers randomly dialed a number and interviewers then posed questions to the person who answered the telephone, ensured greater anonymity and also had the potential to reach anyone who owned a phone. Second, some researchers allowed respondents to fill out questionnaires directly on a portable laptop, bypassing the need to tell a stranger about personal information. Finally, the Internet became a source of reaching respondents and having them complete information on line.

Needless to say, population-based sampling has several advantages over convenient studies. The researcher is not limited to friends of friends of his or her networks or social groups. The heterosexual comparison group is usually part of the same population, especially in the case of national surveys. Any differences between LGBs and heterosexuals can be attributed to sexual orientation, not sampling biases.

There are three problems, however, with population-based surveys, no matter how technologically sophisticated. First, the numbers of men and (especially) women who identify as being nonheterosexual in population-based surveys are extremely small. For example, Laumann et al. (1994) interviewed close to 3500 individuals using representative sampling. Only 24 women and 49 men in this sample identified as lesbian, bisexual, or "other." Sandfort and his colleagues (Sandfort et al., 2001, 2003) conducted a stratified, random-sampling household survey of 7046 people in The Netherlands, who answered a question about sexual behavior during the past year. Altogether, 82 (2.8%) men and 43 (1.4%) women reported being sexually active with a member of the same sex during the past year (some of these individuals had been sexually active with opposite-sex partners as well). Using data from the second (questionnaire) phase of the National Survey of Midlife Development in the United States (Mays & Cochran, 2001; Cochran et al., 2003), data for 2917 respondents were examined who answered the single question about sexual orientation. Only 41 respondents identified as homosexual and 32 as bisexual; these two groups were combined to increase power. The second part of the National Comorbidity Survey included two items about the number of men and women with whom respondents had had "sexual intercourse" during the past 5 years (Gilman et al., 2001, p. 934). The sample included 4785 respondents with exclusively opposite-sex partners, 48 with exclusively same-sex partners (33 men and 15 women), 77 with both same-sex and opposite-sex partners (41 men and 36 women), and 967 who reported no intercourse. Respondents with exclusively same-sex partners and those with same-sex and opposite-sex partners were combined and compared with respondents who had only opposite-sex partners. Using the VET Registry of 4774 male twin-pairs who had both served in the military, Herrell and his colleagues (1999) compared 103 twin pairs in which one member of the pair reported having had male sexual partners since age 18 and the other member did not.

Why do large, national surveys find so few LGBs? It is possible that few people in the general population identify as LGBs. On the other hand, it is also possible that LGB individuals are reluctant to "come out" to mainstream survey researchers (including the U.S. census) through standardized sampling methods. This has resulted in a large and somewhat paradoxical discrepancy between convenience surveys that yield hundreds and even thousands of participants and population-based samples that yield, at most, a few dozen.

A second problem with national survey research is that owing to the small number of LGBs national survey researchers have had to combine gay with bisexual men and lesbians with bisexual women. Evidence from community surveys has shown that bisexuals may be at especially high risk for mental health disorders (Jorm et al., 2001). Thus, combining data in this way may yield higher rates of mental health problems than convenience samples that focus only on lesbians and gay men. This also means that we continue to know little about bisexual women and men, a group that may have different experiences than lesbians and gay men.

The third problem with population-based surveys has been the way in which sexual orientation is defined or obtained. Looking at the examples above, national survey researchers have used self-identity, sexual activity, and cohabiting status as ways to find nonheterosexual respondents. Yet these dimensions are not highly intercorrelated. Research during the 1990s began to identify dimensions of sexual orientation, such as self-identity (I am a lesbian), sexual behavior (I have sex with women), sexual fantasies and attraction (I imagine having sex with women), and participation in LGBT communities (I belong to a lesbian softball league) (see Laumann et al., 1994; Morris & Rothblum, 1999, for reviews of this literature). In the National Comorbidity Study (Gilman et al., 2001) and in The Netherlands study (Sandfort et al., 2001, 2003), there were seven to eight times as many respondents who reported no sexual behavior as there were who reported some same-sex behavior. This means that some of the respondents who indicated no sexual behavior may have identified as LGB but were not included as such by the researchers, who used same-sex sexual behavior as the defining variable. Community surveys have shown lesbians to have sex less often than gay men or heterosexuals (e.g., Blumstein & Schwartz, 1983; Loulan, 1988; Peplau et al., 2004), so defining sexual orientation via sexual behavior may underrepresent lesbians in particular. Furthermore, research on lesbians (Morris & Rothblum, 1999) found Native American, Asian American, and European American lesbians to have particularly low interrelationships among dimensions of lesbianism (such as self-identity, outness/disclosure to others, number of years being out, proportion of sexual relationships with women, and participation in lesbian community events). Even for African American and Latina lesbians, these interrelationships were only moderately correlated.

Population-based studies are viewed as representative in their sampling methods. Yet one can question how representative a sample of 30 to 40 LGBs can be, even if recruited via highly sophisticated sampling methods. Laumann et al. (1994), for example, chose not to interpret the results they found for the 24 nonheterosexual women and 49 nonheterosexual men of their total 3500 participants. They decided that this group was too small to be meaningful as a representation of LGBs in the society at large.

4 Methods for the Future: New Methods for the New Century?

Just as community groups may not be typical of the general LGB population, population-based studies may not be typical of LGB communities. As this chapter has shown, LGB convenience samples lack a heterosexual comparison group, whereas national population-based samples lack a large enough subsample of LGBs. What are some future directions for sampling sexual minorities?

4.1 Siblings as a Comparison Group

I have argued in the past (Rothblum, 1994) that siblings of LGBs could serve as an appropriate comparison group. Unlike members of other oppressed groups (e.g., immigrants, Asian Americans), LGBs often have siblings who are members of the dominant group (heterosexuals). Comparable in race, ethnicity, age cohort, and parental socioeconomic status, siblings who differ in adult sexual orientation illustrate some of the ways that coming out as lesbian or gay is associated with demographic factors. This method allows convenience sampling (and thus obtaining large LGB sample sizes) at the same time that heterosexual siblings provide a comparison group.

My colleagues and I have conducted studies on lesbians and their heterosexual and bisexual sisters (Rothblum & Factor, 1999), LGBs and heterosexual siblings (Rothblum et al., 2004; Balsam et al., 2005a,b) and same-sex couples who had civil unions in Vermont compared with heterosexual siblings and spouses (Solomon et al., 2004). The sibling recruitment and comparison method has some advantages. First, it is possible to include LGBs who are not out to their heterosexual siblings. In our first study of lesbians and their sisters, the questionnaire we sent to all participants did not indicate that we were focusing on sexual orientation and contained only two items about sexual orientation among many demographic items. In the second study of LGBs and heterosexual siblings, LGBs were sent an additional lavender questionnaire with extra questions about sexual orientation.

Second, many LGBs have multiple siblings, and we sent question-naires to all instead of making decisions about which sibling to include. In hindsight, this had a major benefit: the response rate of the index participants (the original participants who contacted us) was much higher than those of their siblings. With multiple siblings, however, we ended up with nearly identical numbers of lesbians and heterosexual women and with gay and heterosexual men.

The number of self-identified bisexuals was much smaller than par-ticipants who identified as lesbian, gay, or heterosexual. Nevertheless, we found a number of statistically significant differences between bisexuals and other groups, indicating that even small numbers of bisexuals yield important information.

Furthermore, some index participants had siblings who were them-selves LGB. This allowed us to compare index participants with sib-lings who were similar in sexual orientation to see if the recruitment method (e.g., bisexual women who actively sought us out versus those dragged into the study by their sisters) made a difference (it did not).

The results of all three studies show many differences between LGBs and heterosexuals recruited from siblings. Lesbians are more highly educated, have occupations with greater status, are less religious, and are more geographically mobile than heterosexual women. Heterosex-ual women are more similar to census data in terms of marriage, chil-dren, religion, and homemaker status. Gay men have moved to large cities and are more highly educated than heterosexual men. In general, bisexual women are most comparable demographically to lesbians, whereas bisexual men are most similar to heterosexual men. These results have two important implications. First, given that LGBs have heterosexual siblings who are demographically similar to the census data indicates that convenience samples may not be reaching biased samples of LGBs. Instead, LGBs probably are more highly educated, less religious, and more urban than heterosexuals. Second, all of the heterosexuals in these studies were siblings of LGBs, so one could spec-ulate that these heterosexuals might also come from less traditional families. Yet they were quite traditional demographically and thus present a feasible comparison group.

Our first study (Rothblum & Factor, 1999) performed matched com-parisons of lesbians with their heterosexual sisters. In the second study (Rothblum et al., 2004), some of the heterosexual women were sisters of lesbians and others were sisters of gay men, for example. Yet we achieved similar results whether we compared lesbians with their het-erosexual sisters or when we compared all women who identified as lesbians with all women who identified as heterosexual (and similarly for gay and heterosexual men). This means that researchers can include both same-gender and opposite-gender siblings of LGBs for a larger sample size without affecting the results.

It is also possible to use a nested design (siblings nested within fam-ilies) and calculate the effect of family variance. For example, when studies examine mental health problems among LGBs, this design makes it possible to determine whether mental health problems are the result of being part of a high-risk family (i.e., siblings have similar mental health problems) or sexual orientation (LGBs have more mental health problems than their siblings). Researchers have used siblings to investigate the genetics of sexual orientation (e.g., Bailey et al., 2000) but rarely to investigate sexual orientation differences in mental health and other psychological variables. In fact, our research did not find differences between LGBs and heterosexuals when sibling variance was taken into account (Balsam et al., 2005a) although LGBs had higher rates of traumatic victimization even when sibling variance was accounted for (Balsam et al., 2005b).

Obviously, the sibling methodology has some limitations. It excludes LGB respondents without siblings as well as those who are not in contact with their siblings. It cannot be used under all circumstances. For example, lesbians tend to have children much later, on average, than their sisters (because of the high cost of ways in which lesbians become pregnant, such as adoption and reproductive technologies). Thus, comparing lesbian and heterosexual sisters on child rearing compares mothers who differ in age by as much as a decade and is not a useful method.

The sibling methodology does not constitute representative sampling. It can answer the question of how LGBs in a particular sample are similar to or different from their heterosexual siblings, but it cannot determine, for example, how many people in the general population have LGB siblings.

4.2 Accessing an Entire Population of LGBs

In our research on same-sex couples who had civil unions in Vermont (Solomon et al., 2004), we were able to compare basic information about survey respondents to the civil union population as a whole because civil unions, like marriage certificates, are a matter of public record. Thus, this study had access to a population, not just a sample, and represents methodologic improvement over previous research in this area. It was not possible in the past to compare LGB respondents with nonrespondents; even population-based surveys do not know how many people who refused to participate were in fact LGBs. As U.S. states and other countries legalize same-sex relationships, including same-sex marriage, this kind of information will become increasingly possible.

4.3 Changes in Definition of Sexual Orientation

Language about sexual orientation has changed over time and across cultures. Thus, old terms such as "invert" and new terms such as "queer" complicate research on sexual orientation because inclusion criteria differ across place and time. People who are bisexual are less inclined to use labels for self-identity (Rust, 2000), possibly explaining the relatively small numbers of bisexuals we found in our siblings research. New theory and writing from the transgender movement will increase our understanding about the intersection of gender identity with sexual orientation.

5 Summary

What are the costs and benefits of various research methodologies when used with LGB samples? First, I encourage researchers to write about (and journal editors to accept for publication) theoretical issues regarding the application of research methodologies for use with LGB samples. Too often researchers are forced into a specific methodology (by their graduate thesis advisor, granting agencies, and manuscript reviewers) simply because such methods are the status quo among the general population. As I have argued earlier, an ideal method such as population-based sampling may not work with LGBs if it yields only a handful of respondents.

Similarly, publishing anecdotal articles, pilot studies, or results of a few interviews with LGBs on new topic areas can be extremely useful in generating discussion among mental health practitioners, policy-makers, and researchers. Sometimes the most interesting parts of large, standardized, questionnaire studies are to be found in the comments written in by participants at the end of the questionnaire. Such qualitative impressions should be written up, and luckily there are now a number of LGBT journals across academic disciplines for submission of such qualitative content.

The advantage of convenience studies lies in the large number of LGBs who are eager to participate in research. The disadvantage, however, is the inability to find heterosexuals via the same sources. Thus, it is not possible to know if any differences between LGBs and published norms of the general population are the result of sexual orientation or sampling bias. As I argued above, incorporating siblings of LGBs controls for a number of variables that are often similar among siblings. This method allows researchers to examine the effect of sexual orientation among participants recruited via the same sample.

Obviously, population-based sampling is an ideal method in theory. However, this chapter has described some of the problems when this method is used to examine sexual orientation. Large samples are needed to find even tiny numbers of LGBs, and researchers may need to combine anyone who is not heterosexual (in either identity or sexual behavior) to increase the statistical power. Thus, this method may end up being too cost-ineffective for most researchers studying LGBs.

Finally, a time may come when LGBs are so assimilated into mainstream society that it will be difficult to conceptualize sexual orientation as separate categories. This will necessitate new methods for a new age. All of these challenges will affect sampling.

References

American Psychiatric Association. (1968) *The diagnostic and statistical manual of mental disorders*, 2nd ed. American Psychiatric Association, Washington, DC.

American Psychiatric Association. (1980) *The diagnostic and statistical manual of mental disorders*, 3rd ed. American Psychiatric Association, Washington, DC.

Badgett, M.V.L. (2001) *Money, myths, and change: the economic lives of lesbians and gay men*. University of Chicago Press, Chicago.

Bailey, J.M., Dunne, M.P., and Martin, N.G. (2000) Genetic and environmental influences on sexual orientation and its correlates in an Australian twin sample. *Journal of Personality and Social Psychology* 78:524–536.

Balsam, K.F., Beauchaine, T.P., Mickey, R.M., and Rothblum, E.D. (2005a) Mental health of lesbian, gay, bisexual, and heterosexual siblings: Effects of gender, sexual orientation, and family. *Journal of Abnormal Psychology* 114:471–476.

Balsam, K.F., Rothblum, E.D., and Beauchaine, T.P. (2005b) Victimization over the life span: a comparison of lesbian, gay, bisexual, and heterosexual siblings. *Journal of Consulting and Clinical Psychology* 73:477–487.

Bradford, J.B., and Ryan, C. (1987) *National lesbian health care survey: mental health implications for lesbians*. PB88-201496/AS. National Institute of Mental Health, National Technical Information Service, Bethesda, MD.

Bradford, J., Ryan, C., and Rothblum, E.D. (1994) National lesbian health care survey: implications for mental health. *Journal of Consulting and Clinical Psychology* 62:228–242.

Cochran, S.D., Sullivan, J.G., and Mays, V.M. (2003) Prevalence of mental disorders, psychological distress, and mental health services use among lesbian, gay, and bisexual adults in the United States. *Journal of Consulting and Clinical Psychology* 71:53–61.

Gates, G.J., and Ost, J. (2004) *The gay and lesbian atlas*. Urban Institute Press, Washington, DC.

Gilman, S.E., Cochran, S.D., Mays, V.M., Hughes, M., Ostrow, D., and Kessler, R.C. (2001) Prevalences of DSM-III-R disorders among individuals reporting same-gender sexual partners in the National Comorbidity Survey. *American Journal of Public Health* 91:933–939.

Herrell, R., Goldberg, J., True, W.R., Ramakrishnan, V., Lyons, M., Eisen, S., and Tsuang, M.T. (1999) Sexual orientation and suicidality: a co-twin control study in adult men. *Archives of General Psychiatry* 56:867–874.

Jorm, A.F., Korten, A.E., Rodgers, B., Jacomb, P.A., and Christensen, H. (2001) Sexual orientation and mental health: results from a community survey of young and middle-aged adults. *British Journal of Psychiatry* 180:423–427.

Laumann, E.O., Gagnon, J.H., Michael, R.T., and Michaels, S. (1994) *The social organization of sexuality: sexual practices in the United States*. University of Chicago Press, Chicago.

Loulan, J. (1988) Research on the sex practices of 1566 lesbians and the clinical implications. *Women & Therapy* 7:221–234.

Mays, V.M., and Cochran, S.D. (1988) The black women's relationship project: a national survey of Black lesbians. In: Shernoff, M., and Scott, W.A. (eds) *A sourcebook of gay/lesbian health care*, 2nd ed. National Gay and Lesbian Health Foundation, Washington, DC, pp. 54–62.

Mays, V.M., and Cochran, S.D. (2001) Mental health correlates of perceived discrimination among lesbian, gay, and bisexual adults in the United States. *American Journal of Public Health* 91:1869–1876.

Morgan, K.S. (1992) Caucasian lesbians' use of psychotherapy. *Psychology of Women Quarterly* 16:127–130.

Morris, J.F., and Rothblum, E.D. (1999) Who fills out a "lesbian" questionnaire? The interrelationship of sexual orientation, years "out," disclosure of sexual orientation, sexual experience with women, and participation in the lesbian community. *Psychology of Women Quarterly* 23:537–557.

Peplau, L.A., Fingerhut, A., and Beals, K.P. (2004) Sexuality in the relationships of lesbians and gay men. In: Harvey, J., Wenzel, A., and Sprecher, S. (eds)

Handbook of sexuality in close relationships. Erlbaum, Mahway, NJ, pp. 349–369.

Pope, M., and Schulz, R. (1991) Sexual attitudes and behavior in midlife and aging homosexual males. *Journal of Homosexuality* 21:169–177.

Rothblum, E.D. (1994) "I only read about myself on bathroom walls": the need for research on the mental health of lesbians and gay men. *Journal of Consulting and Clinical Psychology* 62:213–220.

Rothblum, E.D., and Factor, R. (2001) Lesbians and their sisters as a control group: demographic and mental health factors. *Psychological Science* 12:63–69.

Rothblum, E.D., Balsam, K.F., and Mickey, R.M. (2004) Brothers and sisters of lesbians, gay men, and bisexuals as a demographic comparison group: an innovative research methodology to examine social change. *Journal of Applied Behavioral Science* 40:283–301.

Rust, P.R. (2000) *Bisexuality in the United States.* Columbia University Press, New York.

Sandfort, T.G.M., de Graaf, R., and Bijl, R.V. (2003) Same-sex sexuality and quality of life: findings from The Netherlands Mental Health Survey and Incidence Study. *Archives of Sexual Behavior* 32:15–22.

Sandfort, T.G.M., de Graaf, R., Bijl, R.V., and Schnabel, P. (2001) Same-sex sexual behavior and psychiatric disorders: findings from The Netherlands mental health survey and incidence study (NEMESIS). *Archives of General Psychiatry* 58:85–91.

Schneider, M. (1989) Sappho was a right-on adolescent: growing up lesbian. *Journal of Homosexuality* 17:111–130.

Silverstein, C. (1991) *Gays, lesbians, and their therapists.* Norton, New York.

Solomon, S.E., Rothblum, E.D., and Balsam, K.F. (2004) Pioneers in partnership: lesbian and gay male couples in civil unions compared with those not in civil unions, and heterosexual married siblings. *Journal of Family Psychology* 18:275–286.

The Ladder (1958) Letter to editor. May, p. 9.

Using Community-Based Participatory Research to Understand and Eliminate Social Disparities in Health for Lesbian, Gay, Bisexual, and Transgender Populations

Mary E. Northridge, Brian P. McGrath, and Sam Quan Krueger

1 Introduction

In the United States, public health developed to a large degree as a voluntary movement—or, more accurately, a set of different voluntary movements—each campaigning for some particular health reform. As these movements became professionalized, as the first health departments were created, and as the first schools of public health were developed, scientific education was seen as the necessary basis of rational social and health reform. Over time, and especially after World War II, pressures on schools of public health led to an ever greater emphasis on research than on practice, a tendency fueled by the funding mechanisms of the National Institutes of Health. By the 1980s it had become clear that the schools of public health and their research productivity had become ever more clearly divorced from the activities of public health departments. The movement to community-based participatory research (CBPR) was, then, an attempt to reconnect the research enterprise with the actual needs of public health as defined by the people whose health was to be affected.

In this, the final methodologic chapter of this volume, we build on the foundation presented in earlier chapters and introduce a research approach that we have found useful for confronting social disparities in health for disadvantaged communities. The credit (blame?) for including this chapter goes to our devoted colleague, Ilan H. Meyer, who has been encouraging us for years to apply participatory research approaches to issues of concern in lesbian, gay, bisexual, and transgender (LGBT) communities and finally succeeded in cajoling (pushing?) us to give it a go. Hence, we draw heavily on our experiences in designing and conducting participatory research, practice, and advocacy work in population health initiatives, urban design projects, and Asian and Pacific Islander (API) coalitions. Our hope is that by writing this interdisciplinary chapter together, we can clarify our own thinking and perhaps motivate future research and interventions by our group and others that address egregious social disparities in health for LBGT populations.

We begin with a brief history of participatory research and why we believe it has the potential to contribute meaningfully to the scientific basis for both understanding and eliminating social disparities in health for LGBT populations. Second, we draw apt examples from the peer-reviewed public health literature of studies that have explicitly used participatory research to understand and/or address social disparities in health for LGBT communities. Third, we present a conceptual framework entitled Social Determinants of LGBT Health to trace pathways whereby factors at various levels [e.g., heterosexism, workplace policies, human immunodeficiency virus (HIV) screening] may lead to inequalities in health and well-being for LGBT individuals and communities. In doing so, we include examples drawn from our own participatory research, practice, and education initiatives that were explicitly designed to intervene to eliminate social disparities in health for LGBT populations. In closing, we emphasize the importance of extracting the core issues from the context in which they are researched and practiced to derive *best principles* and *best processes* that may be transferable to other settings (Green, 2001; Sclar et al., 2005). This is essential if public health research and practice in LGBT populations is to benefit from the seminal participatory work conducted in other politically and socially oppressed communities.

It is important to note that CBPR has a long history. During the 1940s, social psychologist Kurt Lewin (1946) developed the action research school, which emphasized active involvement in the research of those affected by the problem through a cyclical process of fact finding, action, and reflection. During the 1970s, more revolutionary approaches to research emerged—often independently of one another—from work in oppressed communities throughout the developing world (Minkler, 2005). In particular, Brazilian educator Paulo Friere (1970) provided critical grounding for CBPR in his dialogic method accenting co-learning and action based on critical reflection. Scholars in the developing countries of South America, Asia, and Africa fostered their alternative approaches to scientific inquiry as a direct counter to the colonizing nature of research to which oppressed communities were routinely subjected. More recent efforts by feminists and racial/ethnic minorities have added further conceptual richness to CBPR approaches (Maguire, 1987; Duran & Duran, 1995).

Although these historical efforts around participatory research vary, they share the same impulse and commitment: to make health research and public health services responsive to the expressed needs of people in communities. Although many of the individual efforts were short-lived, their legacy is impressive, and their examples serve as models today. One continuing structural problem is that the most successful of such participatory experiments tend to provoke political opposition—they are vulnerable to being closed down (e.g., by the imprisonment of their leaders) or slowly starved of energy (e.g., by the withdrawal of funds). Indeed, one historical lesson is that such pioneering efforts need continued support and energetic political pressure to keep the doors of opportunity open. Next we provide examples from the public health literature of the use of participatory research approaches to address needs and concerns in LGBT communities.

2 Use of Participatory Research Approaches to Examine Social Disparities in LGBT Health

It is essential when discussing CBPR and LGBT health to stress the critical role that ACT UP (AIDS Coalition to Unleash Power) and other LGBT groups have played in bringing vital government attention and resources to HIV-acquired immunodeficiency syndrome (HIV/AIDS) and other health research focused on LGBT concerns (ACT UP, 2005). Indeed, ACT UP is credited with fostering revolutionary changes in research procedures, including those involved in clinical trials. LGBT individuals, through ACT UP and other organized efforts, responded to the HIV/AIDS crisis by starting their own community-based research projects inside and outside the academic world. They raised funds to advance their agendas in the face of governmental inaction and pushed a collection of activist organizations into a national civil rights movement that challenged some of the most powerful U.S. institutions (Andriote, 1999).

Other sections of this volume are devoted to *health services* for LGBT populations (see especially Chapter 28 on the Fenway Community Health model, previously described by Mayer et al., 2001). In this chapter, we deliberately focus attention instead on the *social determinants of health* of special concern for LGBT individuals and populations to ensure vital coverage of this emerging public health research area.

We make no claim of being comprehensive. Rather, we have selected from the peer-reviewed public health literature those studies we believe are illustrative of an assortment of health issues addressed by a variety of participatory approaches. According to Minkler (2005, p. ii5), "CBPR is not a method per se but an orientation to research that may employ any of a number of qualitative and quantitative methodologies." Cornwall and Jewkes (1995) have argued that what is distinctive about CBPR is the attitudes of the researchers, which in turn determine how, by, and for whom research is conceptualized and conducted, and the corresponding location of power at every stage of the research *process* (italics are our own). Our hope in this section is that by highlighting thoughtful examples of participatory research in LGBT populations across a range of concerns using various methods, the conceptual model and best principles we later invoke might be better grounded in the reality of people's lives and more readily applied to improve their health and well-being.

Photovoice (Wang & Burris, 1997) is a form of participatory action research that uses documentary photography and storytelling. Using this approach, Graziano (2004) examined how Black gay men and lesbians view themselves in relation to White gay men and lesbians in South Africa. Participants included four women and three men from four South African townships who reported being sexually and physically assaulted for challenging the heterosexual status quo. Themes that emerged from this study were that class bias, cultural traditions of visiting African healers, and segregated social spaces are important issues to consider in future efforts to understand and address LGBT health in South Africa. Notably, Graziano (2004) concluded that amidst oppression and despair study participants showed signs of strength, hope, and optimism.

MacQueen et al. (2001) conducted qualitative interviews with 25 African Americans in Durham (North Carolina), 26 gay men in San Francisco, 25 injection drug users in Philadelphia, and 42 HIV vaccine researchers across the United States to identify strategies to support community collaboration in HIV vaccine trials. Verbatim responses to the question, "What does the word community mean to you?" were analyzed. Cluster analysis was used to identify similarities in the way community was described. A common definition of community emerged as a group of people with diverse characteristics who are linked by social ties, share common perspectives, and engage in joint action in geographic locations or settings. The salience of the various elements of community for each of the four participant groups had implications for the ways in which collaborations developed. In particular, for gay men in San Francisco, a strong sense of shared history and perspective was a dominant theme, followed by a sense of identity with a specific location, the creation of strong and lasting social ties, established avenues for joint action, and the role of diversity. This profile is superficially similar to the one elicited from the vaccine researchers; however, particular elements were discussed less frequently than in San Francisco. Significant differences also existed with regard to *how* the elements were discussed. Most of the San Francisco participants had thought about community, and many were struggling to reconcile their need for community with a sense of marginalization from society at large. In contrast, the scientists tended to describe themselves as well grounded in multiple communities.

Griffin (1992) described the experiences of 13 lesbian and gay educators in a participatory research project that aimed to empower the participants through collective reflection and action. Each participant was interviewed and given a copy of her or his audio-tape and transcript. Using these materials, each participant developed a profile of himself or herself to share with the other participants. During a series of group meetings that spanned 15 months, participants discussed their experiences, searched for common themes, and planned two collective actions. Griffin relates the professional experiences of these lesbian and gay educators and the process of empowerment that changed their lives.

Finally, Mulvey et al. (2000) collected stories about community work in New Zealand and Scotland so they could describe and reflect on issues central to feminist community psychology. Organizing a lesbian festival, Ingrid Huygens describes feminist processes used to equalize resources across Maori (Indigenous) and Pakeha (White) groups. Heather Hamerton presents her experiences as a researcher using collective memory work to reflect on adolescent experiences related to gender, ethnicity, and class. Sharon Cahill chronicles dilemmas and insights from focus groups about anger with women living in public housing in Scotland. Each story chronicles experiences related to oppression and privilege and describes the author's emotions and reflections. Individually and collectively, the stories illustrate the potential offered by narrative methods and participatory processes for challenging inequalities and encouraging social justice.

Together, these studies examine a range of health concerns that affect LGBT communities to a larger extent than other communities, namely, sexual and physical violence, HIV/AIDS, and individual and community mental health. To trace the pathways whereby factors operating at various levels (e.g., heterosexism at the societal level in South Africa, collaboration in HIV vaccine trials at the community level, and empowering lesbian and gay educators at the interpersonal level) may lead to or rectify inequalities in health and well-being for LGBT communities, we next present a conceptual model.

3 Social Determinants of LGBT Health: Ecologic Model

The authors of this chapter have previously been involved in efforts to understand how social, political, economic, and historical processes generate the urban built environment and shape population health and well-being. By the built environment, we mean that part of the physical environment made by people for people, including buildings such as houses, schools, and workplaces; transportation systems such as highways and railways; and open spaces such as parks and vacant lots (Northridge & Sclar, 2003). To clarify our thinking, we previously developed an ecologic model entitled Social Determinants of Health and Environmental Health Promotion (Northridge et al., 2003; Schulz & Northridge, 2004) to trace the pathways whereby social factors operating at different levels (societal, community, interpersonal) affect population health and well-being.

In meeting the challenge to adapt this conceptual framework to focus particularly on the research needs of LGBT populations, we drew heavily on the work of Meyer (2003), who had formerly examined minority stress processes in lesbian, gay, and bisexual populations. The result is a combined ecologic model we refer to as Social Determinants of LGBT Health (see Fig. 18.1).

We posit with our new model that the natural environment (including topography, climate, water supply, and air quality), macrosocial factors (including historical conditions, political and economic orders, and human rights doctrines), and inequalities (including those related to the distribution of wealth, employment and educational opportunities, and political influence) are *fundamental factors* operating at the *societal level* that underlie and influence the health and well-being of LGBT individuals and populations via multiple pathways through differential access to power, information, and resources (Link

FUNDAMENTAL (societal level)	INTERMEDIATE (community level)	PROXIMATE (interpersonal level)	HEALTH AND WELL-BEING (individual and population levels)
Natural environment • topography • climate • water supply • air quality	**Built environment** • land use (industrial, residential; mixed use or single use) • transportation systems • services (shopping, banking, health care facilities) • public resources (parks, museums, libraries) • zoning regulations • buildings (housing, schools, workplaces)	**Stressors/Buffers** • environmental, neighborhood, workplace, and housing conditions • violent crime and safety • police response • financial insecurity • environmental toxins (lead, particulates) • unfair treatment (stigma, prejudice, discrimination)	**Health outcomes** • mental health • injury/violence • HIV/AIDS • obesity/overweight • cardiovascular diseases • diabetes • cancers • infectious diseases • sexually transmitted diseases • respiratory health • all-cause mortality
Macrosocial factors • historical conditions • political orders • economic orders • legal codes • human rights doctrines • social and cultural institutions • ideologies (heterosexism, sexism, racism, social justice, democracy) **Inequalities** • distribution of material wealth • distribution of employment opportunities • distribution of educational opportunities • distribution of political influence	**Social context** • minority identity (gay, lesbian, bisexual, transgender) • community investment (economic development, maintenance, police services) • policies (public, fiscal, environmental, workplace) • enforcement of ordinances (public, environmental, workplace) • community capacity • civic participation and political influence • quality of education	**Health behaviors** • health screenings (HIV, cancer, hypertension) • physical activity • dietary practices • substance use (tobacco, alcohol, other) **Social integration** • social participation and integration • shape of social networks • available resources within networks • coping and social support	**Well-being** • hope/despair • life satisfaction • psychosocial distress • happiness • disability • internalized homophobia • concealment of identity • expectations of rejection • body size and body image

Figure 18.1 Social determinants of LGBT health: This ecological framework for thinking about pathways whereby social determinants at various levels (societal, community, and interpersonal) influence LGBT health and well-being for both individuals and populations is adapted from a conceptual model entitled Social Determinants of Health and Environmental Health Promotion that first appeared in Northridge et al. (2003). In keeping with our emphasis here on social determinants of LGBT health, the model has been modified to incorporate insights from the conceptual framework entitled, Minority Stress Processes in Lesbian, Gay, and Bisexual Populations originally reported in Meyer (2003).

& Phelan, 1995). Note that we have added *heterosexism* and *sexism* to the list of ideologies delineated under macrosocial factors that operate to undermine the health and well-being of LGBT individuals and populations.

Fundamental factors, in turn, influence *intermediate factors*. We added minority identity (gay, lesbian, bisexual, transgender) to the factors currently listed under social context that may positively and/or negatively affect the health and well-being of LGBT populations. That is, characteristics of minority identity may be both a source of harm (e.g., when they are associated with discrimination in employment or anti-gay violence) and strength (e.g., when they are associated with opportunities for enhanced social integration and social support).

Intermediate factors comprise both the built environment (including land use, transportation systems, services, public resources, zoning regulations, and buildings) and social context (including community investment, public and fiscal policies, and civic participation, among others). An example of such work is Brian P. McGrath's installation for the 1994 Queer Space exhibition at the Store Front for Art and Architecture in New York City. McGrath's project was entitled There Is No **Queer Space**, Only Different Points of View. This statement ran at eye level along a semicircular plexiglass screen showing computer-generated images of various Manhattan locales (Reed, 1996).

As McGrath et al. (1994) explained:

This project is not about the making of queer space, but it is a representation of the possibilities of individual and minority appropriations of majority space.

My intention is to describe the appropriation of public space, not to define a minority realm which exists separated from *normative* space. We must not make exclusive ghettos or enclaves, queer or straight. *Queer space* exists potentially everywhere in the public realm. Unbounded and ever-present, it is the individual's appropriation of the public realm through their personal, ever-changing points of view. An acoustical guide and navigational chart are provided in this project to describe a space which can barely be perceived by those outside of it, but vividly present to those who *occupy* it. The installation aims to invite others to occupy New York City from many different points of view.

The intention of community-based urban design work is to examine new possibilities for creating aesthetically experimental (i.e., queer) participatory design practices. Queer theory provides tools to mix and hybridize what are now separate and marginalized wings in architectural and urban design practices: aesthetic experimentation and participatory design.

Our challenge is to create opportunities for LGBT populations and other marginalized groups to benefit from great design through their own curiosity and interest, not as a prescription from on high. This is where queer theory might provide some compelling clues and examples with its techniques of irony, camp, theatricality, irreverence, ambiguity, and style. Self-seriousness, self-importance, and aesthetic conservatism in participatory methods can be turned around through humor, humility, and a bit of style. Queer theory knows no, nor respects, any boundaries or margins. Change and invention occur at the margins, not at the center. Queer aesthetic experiments learned in the harsh life and death reality of the HIV/AIDS crisis are not light or frivolous diversions from the seriousness of the design issues we face. We use queer aesthetics to get at truths that are often disguised by the rhetoric and images deployed by power. In the physical design of healthy urban neighborhoods, we must utilize participatory approaches to understand and rebuild vibrant cities from the household up through city blocks and entire neighborhoods, with due respect for individual and group differences and ample time and space for voicing these differences.

Similarly, our colleague Erika S. Svendsen of the USDA Forest Service used participatory research principles to design memorials to the victims of terrorism after September 11, 2001, their families, our communities, and the entire nation (USDA Forest Service, 2005). The Living Memorials Project (Svendsen & Campbell, 2005) invokes the resonating power of trees to bring people together and create lasting, living memorials. Explains Svendsen:

This research goes beyond examining the practice of planting commemorative trees. It looks at the creation and maintenance of living memorials as physical, social, emotional, and spiritual acts, examining these places as intersections of human and natural systems. . . . This study shows a living memorial as any place that over time rises to meet people where they are rather than where they are expected to be. . . . Living memorials can be the physical, mental, and social spaces for thought, reflection, teaching, community action, and resilience. Often, participants comment that the healing aspects of living memorials come not just from the finished site, but also from the *process* of conceptualizing a project, finding a site, creating events, and working with others on the project. These values are both challenging to document and to quantify, but may be an example of how participatory design can create and strengthen community. (Erika S. Svendsen, personal communication, italics added)

There are two important points we wish to emphasize about the intermediate or community level in our model as it pertains to participatory research to advance LGBT health and well-being. First, it is here that we believe interventions may be the most effective in pushing up against the more entrenched factors at the societal level (e.g., heterosexism) to improve the health and well-being of sexual minorities. Such interventions may include providing safe shelters for LGBT youths and enforcing workplace policies that forbid discrimination on the basis of sexual orientation. Second, most of the interventions at the community level necessarily involve organizations and agencies outside the health sector per se. We believe that interdisciplinary and participatory collaboration among urban planners, civic organizers, educators, and public health practitioners holds the greatest promise for devising effective, sustained community-based interventions.

The more *proximate factors* influencing health and well-being at the *interpersonal level* are depicted in our conceptual model as stressors/buffers (including violent crime and safety, financial insecurity, and unfair treatment), health behaviors (including health screenings, physical activity, and dietary practices), and social integration (including the shape of social networks and the resources available within networks). This is the more familiar terrain of public health, although Meyer (2003) warns that relying overly much on, for example, the coping abilities of the oppressed rather than the transgressions of the oppressor, could lead to ignoring the need for important political and structural changes. Nonetheless, individual agency and resilience are no doubt important in affecting the health and well-being of sexual minorities.

For instance, Sexually Liberated Art Activist Asian People! (SLAAAP!), originated by Sam Quan Krueger and seven other queer community organizers of Asian descent living in New York City, is an example of community-originated response to the needs of an under-served LGBT community. SLAAAP! members identified the absence of healthy Asian images in the queer visual environment and joined together to initiate research and an intervention to address it. Members noted that the visual environment in New York City's LGBT communities was largely vacant of constructive images of Asian people. Instead, perverse notions of *Orientals* continued to fill the visual lexicon. Asians were often depicted as kung-fu fighters, sexually servile geishas, turbaned gurus, asocial scientists, or kowtowing foreigners from exotic lands. Historical stereotypes persist and limit the utility of public health interventions aimed at people of Asian descent.

Intuitively, SLAAAP! members understood that a visual environment dominated by White sexuality can lead to low self-esteem, compromised decision-making regarding sexual behaviors, and isolation from Asian-specific resources in sexual health among Asian queers. SLAAAP! sought to address these health risks through a visual campaign in service to its own community.

The initial SLAAAP! team consisted of eight organizers representing various LGBT groups, including the South Asian Lesbian and Gay Association (SALGA), Iban/Queer Koreans of New York (QKNY), the Audrey Lorde Project (ALP), Kilawin Kolektibo, and the Asian Pacific Islander Coalition on HIV and AIDS (APICHA, 2005). Relevant skill sets and knowledge bases within SLAAAP! included community organizing, HIV/AIDS prevention, graphic design, illustration, photography, political art history, fundraising, project management, marketing, and proficiency in English and various Asian languages. APICHA provided umbrella support, which included $500 in production costs, partial financial support for one staff member, and meeting space.

Based on an internal needs assessment, SLAAAP! members developed a 4-month schedule that culminated in social action at the June 1998 Manhattan Gay Pride Parade. The schedule began with an education and training component consisting of workshops on political art history and social action, team building, current themes germane to queer Asians living in New York City, and the process of marketing ideas. Discussions focused the following themes and questions:

- Creativity: using history as imagination; generating a visual vocabulary; managing an equitable, collaborative effort.
- Sexual determination and determinants: the conflict between and hybridization of Asian and U.S. cultures and their effect on sexual determination; the relation between our sexualities and our communities and families.
- What is the "queer Asian community" in New York City? Who are the constituents? What are the productive resources to build and

strengthen the community? What are the opportunities for growth as well as threats to growth? How might social service provision be used as a venue for organizing around or creating identity?

The two primary objectives for the campaign were (1) to promote affirmative images of queer Asians; and (2) to connect individual queer Asians to health-related resources specific to their needs. To reach these objectives, SLAAAP! members designed a comic logo as a consistent identifier of SLAAAP!'s presence and values, which was later popularized through distributed materials. Next, a postcard campaign consisting of four vignettes was created as part of a social action, with a design intended to stand apart from typical nonprofit outreach materials. One of the four original SLAAAP! postcards is presented here as Figure 18.2 (APICHA, 2005).

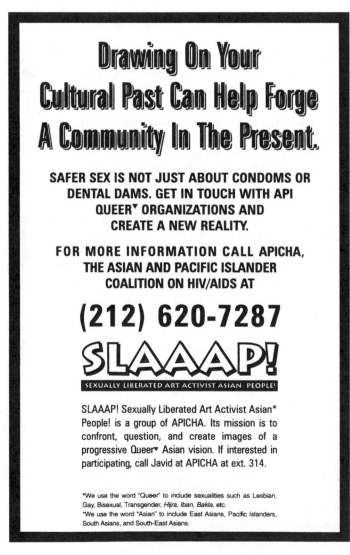

Figure 18.2 Drawing on your cultural past can help forge a community in the present (APICHA, 2005).

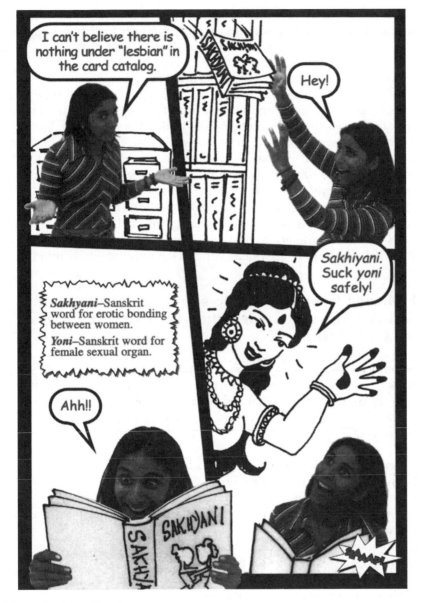

Figure 18.2 *Continued*

During the 1998 Manhattan Pride Parade, SLAAAP! members marched in drag and costumes with members from other queer Asian and HIV/AIDS organizations and handed out postcards to people of Asian descent along the parade route. In sum, nearly 400 postcards were distributed. Moreover, SLAAAP! involvement transformed its members by providing a formal structure where they shared skills, talents, experiences, and friendship.

In 1999, APICHA incorporated SLAAAP! into its ongoing educational programming, thus providing sustainability for the campaign. In its first year, SLAAAP! established a process that could be modified and repeated each year. Subsequent visual campaigns followed the approach of the first season, and word-of-mouth further propagated SLAAAP!'s work throughout the queer Asian community in New York City.

Finally, the last column in the conceptual model represents *health and well-being*, and lists a wide range of health outcomes (including mental health, injury/violence, and obesity/overweight) while also embracing various measures of well-being (including hope/despair, life satisfaction, and psychosocial distress). We expanded the list of well-being measures to include internalized homophobia, concealment of identity, and expectations of rejection in concert with Meyer's (2003) notions of proximal minority stress processes. It is important to emphasize that health and well-being can be measured at both the individual and population levels; that is, societal, community, and interpersonal determinants may affect the health and well-being of individual members of the LGBT community as well as various subpopulations within it.

4 Moving from Best Practices to Best Processes and Best Principles to Guide Future Participatory Research in LGBT Health

Community-based participatory research rarely follows a strict set of guidelines, notwithstanding efforts to identify key principles (Israel et al., 1998). Barbara A. Israel has been at the forefront of CBPR efforts in the United States and has enumerated nine principles of CBPR (Israel, 2000):

1. Recognizes community as unit of identity
2. Builds on strengths and resources
3. Facilitates collaborative partnership
4. Integrates knowledge and intervention for mutual benefit of all partners
5. Promotes co-learning and empowering process
6. Involves a cyclic, iterative process
7. Addresses health from positive and ecologic perspectives
8. Disseminates findings and knowledge gained to all partners
9. Involves a long-term commitment by all partners

Israel and her colleagues in Detroit never intended this set of principles to be static or universal and actively encouraged adaptation depending on needs and contexts. Many if not all of these CBPR principles may be useful to consider in LGBT health issues.

Another central figure in CBPR in the United States and especially in Canada is Lawrence W. Green (e.g., Green et al., 1995). Green (2001) recently argued for replacing *best practices* with *best processes* in health promotion and other applications of health behavioral research, in concert with our focus in this chapter on the *process* involved in CBPR initiatives. His reasoning is that, "[H]ealth promotion needs to be pursued not as a reductionist exercise in changing individual behavior, but as an empowering process of giving people and populations greater control over the determinants of their health" (Green, 2001, p. 165).

In light of the diversity in LGBT populations and the difficulty that exists when attempting to generalize from clinical to community settings, we stress the need to develop new research, practice, and education programs with an emphasis on transferable principles (as per Israel, 2000) and participatory processes (as per Green, 2001) to profit meaningfully from CBPR conducted in other historically oppressed and marginalized populations. The term *best principles* is invoked here rather than the more customary term *best practices* to underscore the need—especially at an early stage of development of new research, practice, and education programs in LGBT health—to extract the core issues from the context in which they are carried out. We are confronting situations in which community and institutional settings vary greatly, even as the ostensible research activities are the same. In such cases, best practices do not always easily transfer across either population or institutional boundaries. Best principles are invoked to remind us that although communities and settings can be critically different the encompassed research questions and practice applications that we are seeking to answer and bring about often have underlying principles that can be readily adapted. The application of best principles requires that we develop a more critical understanding of the goals and constraints of different organizational structures as we develop new programs. Put slightly differently, *process* is as important as *plan* in the creation of innovative research to address the challenges of LGBT health and well-being (Sclar et al., 2005).

5 Summary

In writing this chapter, the authors came together with histories of involvement in participatory research, design, and outreach in other populations as well as those related here that are specific to LGBT health. We maintain that a hopeful promise of CBPR lies in its capacity to promote civil society and help eliminate egregious disparities in health and health care for those without sufficient resources to pay high costs for safe and affordable housing, education across the life course, and adequate and respectful medical care (Northridge et al., 2002, 2005). A contribution of this chapter, we believe, is the extension of our previous CBPR scholarship and applications to embrace the varied yet particular needs of sexual minorities and to address explicitly the pathways whereby heterosexism, sexism, and racism lead to social disparities in health and well-being for LGBT individuals and populations.

Specifically, we began this chapter with a brief history of participatory research in public health and then examined the peer-reviewed literature for evidence of participatory approaches to understand and address social determinants of LGBT health. To motivate future research, we presented a conceptual model entitled Social Determinants of LGBT Health and then traced the pathways whereby factors operating at various levels (societal, community, interpersonal) might effect health and well-being for LGBT individuals and populations. In doing so, we incorporated case studies with an emphasis on participatory processes, rather than research tools and methods per se. Finally, we proposed moving from best practices to best processes and best principles to guide future CBPR intended to advance the health and well-being of LGBT communities.

If we have learned anything from former community-based interventions, including those centered on HIV prevention for young gay men (Kegeles et al., 1996), it is that the active involvement of disadvantaged and oppressed populations in creating health programs embedded in their social activities and community lives are likely to be more effective and sustained than top down approaches. Our own future CBPR initiatives will no doubt aim to intervene on what Meyer (2003) has termed both the subjective and objective views. The subjective view—which highlights individual processes—suggests that interventions should aim to change the appraisal process, that is, the person's way of evaluating her/his condition and coping with stress and adversity. This corresponds to the interpersonal level in our conceptual model and is no doubt effective in helping individuals advance their own health and well-being. The objective view—which highlights the external properties of the stressors—points to remedies that would aim to alter the stress-inducing environment. This corresponds to the community level in our conceptual model and is where we believe that interventions are especially subject to policy manipulation. A corollary is that interventions at the community level may have the greatest potential benefit for improvements in the health and well-being of LGBT populations. Hence, a hopeful promise in writing this chapter is to inspire our team and others to forge collaborations among public health, urban planning, urban design, and social activists united in the commitment to advancing LGBT health and thereby the health of all of us.

Acknowledgments: The authors thank Elizabeth Fee for her contributions to the section on the history of participatory research in public health, Erika S. Svendsen for her analysis of the participatory process involved in the Living Memorials Project, and Elliott D. Sclar for originating the concept of transferable best principles and providing essential foundations for the conceptual model we advanced here entitled Social Determinants of LGBT Health. A special thanks to Ilan H. Meyer for his intellectual inspiration and expert editing, and to Jennifer L. Northridge, Jessica M. Northridge, and John F. Duane for their constant support throughout the long journey of writing this chapter.

References

AIDS Coalition to Unleash Power (ACT UP). (2005) http://www.actupny.org.
Andriote, J-M. (1999) *Victory deferred: how AIDS changed gay life in America*. University of Chicago Press, Chicago.

Asian and Pacific Islander Coalition on HIV/AIDS (APICHA). (2005) http://www.apicha.org/apicha/pages/education/lgbt/slaaap.html.

Cornwall, A., and Jewkes, R. (1995) What is participatory research? *Social Science and Medicine* 41:1667–1676.

Duran, E., and Duran, B. (1995) *Native American postcolonial psychology.* State University of New York Press, Albany, NY.

Friere, P. (1970) *Pedagogy of the oppressed.* Seabury Press, New York.

Graziano, K.J. (2004) Oppression and resiliency in a post-apartheid South Africa: unheard voices of Black gay men and lesbians. *Cultural Diversity & Ethnic Minority Psychology* 10:302–316.

Green, L., George, M.A., Daniel, M., Frankish, C.J., Herbert, C.P., Bowie, W.R., and O'Neill, M. (1995) *Study of participatory research in health promotion: review and recommendations for the development of participatory research in health promotion in Canada.* Royal Society of Canada, Vancouver, BC.

Green, L.W. (2001) From research to "best practices" in other settings and populations. *American Journal of Health Behavior* 25:165–178.

Griffin, P. (1992) From hiding out to coming out: empowering lesbian and gay educators. *Journal of Homosexuality* 22:167–196.

Israel, B.A. (2000) The Detroit community-academic Urban Research Center: principles, rationale, challenges and lessons learned through a community-based participatory research partnership. Presented at the Summer Public Health Research Institute and Videoconference on Minority Health, Chapel Hill, NC, June 16, 2000. Available at: http://minority.unc.edu/institute/2000/materials/slides/BarbaraIsrael-2000–06–12.ppt.

Israel, B.A., Schulz, A.J., Parker, E., and Becker, A.B. (1998) Review of community-based research: assessing partnership approaches to improve public health. *Annual Review of Public Health* 19:173–202.

Kegeles, S.M., Hays, R.B., and Coates, T.J. (1996) The Mpowerment Project: a community-level HIV intervention for young gay men. *American Journal of Public Health* 86:1129–1136.

Lewin, K. (1946) Action research and minority problems. *Journal of Social Issues* 2:34–46.

Link, B.G., and Phelan, J.C. (1995) Social conditions as fundamental causes of disease. *Journal of Health and Social Behavior* 36:80–94 (extra issue).

MacQueen, K.M., McLellan, E., Metzger, D.S., Kegeles, S., Strauss, R.P., Scotti, R., Blanchard, L., and Trotter, R.T. II (2001) What is community? An evidence-based definition for participatory public health. *American Journal of Public Health* 91:1929–1938.

Maguire, P. (1987) *Doing participatory research: a feminist approach.* Center for International Education, Amherst, MA.

Mayer, K., Appelbaum, J., Rogers, T., Lo, W., Bradford, J., and Boswell, S. (2001) The evolution of the Fenway Community Health model. *American Journal of Public Health* 91:892–894.

McGrath, B., Watkins, M., and Lee, M-J. (1994) In *Queer space.* Exhibition pamphlet, Store Front for Art and Architecture, New York, June 1994, unpaginated.

Meyer, I.H. (2001) Why lesbian, gay, bisexual, and transgender public health? *American Journal of Public Health* 91:856–859.

Minkler, M. (2005) Community-based research partnerships: challenges and opportunities. *Journal of Urban Health* 82(Suppl 2):ii3–ii12.

Mulvey, A., Terenzio, M., Hill, J., Bond, M.A., Huygens, I., Hamerton, H.R., and Cahill, S. (2000) Stories of relative privilege: power and social change in feminist community psychology. *American Journal of Community Psychology* 28:883–911.

Northridge, M.E., and Sclar, E. (2003) A joint urban planning and public health framework: contributions to health impact assessment. *American Journal of Public Health* 93:118–121.

Northridge, M.E., Meyer, I.H., and Dunn, L. (2002) Overlooked and under-served in Harlem: a population-based survey of adults with asthma. *Environmental Health Perspectives* 110(Suppl 2):217–220.

Northridge, M.E., Sclar, E.D., and Biswas, P. (2003) Sorting out the connections between the built environment and health: a conceptual framework for navigating pathways and planning healthy cities. *Journal of Urban Health* 80:556–568.

Northridge, M.E., Shoemaker, K., Jean-Louis, B., Ortiz, B., Swaner, R., Vaughan, R.D., Cushman, L.F., Hutchinson, V.E., and Nicholas, S.W. (2005) What matters to communities? Using community-based participatory research to ask and answer questions regarding the environment and health; essays on the future of environmental health research: a tribute to Dr. Kenneth Olden. *Environmental Health Perspectives* 113(Suppl 1):34–41.

Reed, C. (1996) Imminent domain: queer space in the built environment—we're here: gay and lesbian presence in art and art history. *Art Journal* (Winter 1996). Available at: http://www.findarticles.com/p/articles/mi_m0425/is_n4_v55/ai_19101786.

Schulz, A., and Northridge, M.E. (2004) Social determinants of health: implications for environmental health promotion. *Health Education & Behavior* 31:455–471.

Sclar, E.D., Northridge, M.E., and Karpel, E.M. (2005) Promoting interdisciplinary curricula and training in transportation, land use, physical activity, and health. Commissioned by the Transportation Research Board and the Institute of Medicine Committee on Physical Activity, Health, Transportation and Land Use. In: *Does the built environment influence physical activity? Examining the evidence*. Transportation Research Board Special Report 282. Washington, DC (November 20, 2005). Available at: http://www.trb.org/downloads/sr282papers/sr282paperstoc.pdf.

Svendsen, E.S., and Campbell, L.K., (2005) Living Memorials Project—year 1 social and site assessment. General technical report NE-333. Newtown Square, PA. U.S. Department of Agriculture, Forest Service, Northeastern Research Station.

USDA Forest Service, Northeastern Research Station. (2005) Living Memorials Project (November 20, 1995). Available at: http://www.livingmemorialsproject.net/index.htm.

Wang, C., and Burris, M.A. (1997) Photovoice: concept, methodology, and use for participatory needs assessment. *Health Education and Behavior* 24:369–387.

Part V

Health Concerns

19

Transgender Health Concerns

Anne A. Lawrence

1 Introduction

1.1 Overview of Transgender Health Concerns

Transgender persons are those who live full-time or part-time in the gender role of the opposite biologic sex (Lawrence et al., 1996). Transgender persons share the same health concerns as nontransgender persons; as members of a minority group characterized by complex identities and often by visibly gender-variant social presentations, transgender persons also have special health concerns related to the delivery of health services in a manner that recognizes and takes account of their identities and presentations (see Chapter 26).

Transgender persons also have a number of other, more specific health concerns that are the focus of this chapter. Many transgender persons receive cross-sex hormone therapy, which must be managed carefully to maximize the beneficial effects and minimize complications and side effects. Some transgender persons undergo surgical procedures to masculinize or feminize their bodies, especially their genitals and breasts; these procedures can result in complications as well as benefits. Transgender persons who have undergone cross-sex hormone treatment may require screening for neoplasia in organ systems associated with both their birth sex and the sex with which they identify or to which they have been reassigned. Some male-to-female (MtF) transgender persons attempt to modify their bodies using injections of liquid silicone, which can be a source of significant morbidity and mortality. Some transgender persons have a high prevalence of human immunodeficiency virus/acquired immunodeficiency syndrome (HIV/AIDS) and other sexually transmitted infections (STIs). Transgender persons appear to have an elevated prevalence of co-existing mental health problems. A disproportionate number of transgender persons attempt or complete suicide, engage in other forms of self-harm, and are victims of violence.

1.2 Health Concerns in Relation to Transgender Diversity

Transgender is an umbrella term that includes many diverse groups whose health concerns may differ substantially. Only a few categories of transgender persons have been studied with reference to health concerns; these categories are not mutually exclusive and sometimes overlap significantly. *Transsexuals* comprise the most-studied transgender group; they are individuals who express extreme discomfort with their biologic sex, a phenomenon called *gender dysphoria*, and who typically seek hormone therapy and genital surgery to change their bodies to resemble the opposite sex (American Psychiatric Association [APA], 1987). Transsexualism is rare, affecting about 1 in 12,000 males and 1 in 30,000 females in Western countries (Bakker et al., 1993).

Another transgender group that has undergone significant study is MtF transgender sex workers, many of whom use cross-sex hormones; the size of the MtF transgender sex-worker population is unknown. Some MtF transgender sex workers are transsexuals; others are *transgenderists*, persons who usually live full-time in the cross-gender role and may use cross-gender hormones but who have not undergone, or do not wish to undergo, feminizing genital surgery (Docter & Prince, 1997).

Cross-dressers, or transvestites—men who dress in the clothing of the opposite sex for sexual excitement, gender expression, or both—probably comprise the largest transgender group. In one recent survey, 2.8% of adult males reported having experienced sexual arousal in association with cross-dressing (Langstrom & Zucker, 2005). The health concerns of cross-dressers have received little study, although it is recognized that some cross-dressers use cross-sex hormones to feminize their bodies (Docter & Fleming, 1992; Docter & Prince, 1997). Cross-dressers and MtF transsexuals share many characteristics in common (Docter & Fleming, 2001), suggesting that they comprise part of a continuum of MtF transgender expression, rather than representing discrete entities. With the exception of female-to-male (FtM) transsexuals, the spectrum of female transgender expression and the health concerns of female transgender persons have received little attention.

It should be apparent that the health concerns of an 18-year-old MtF transgender sex worker who takes nonprescribed cross-sex hormones and lives full-time in cross-gender role may be quite different from those of a 50-year-old male computer systems analyst who cross-dresses occasionally but does not take cross-sex hormones, even though both can be considered transgender persons. Consequently, when examining research findings relevant to transgender health concerns, it is important to consider the specific transgender populations in which studies were conducted to avoid unwarranted generalizations.

2 Cross-Sex Hormone Therapy in Transgender Persons

2.1 Overview and Criteria for Provision of Cross-Sex Hormone Therapy

Some transgender persons undergo cross-sex hormone treatment to look and feel more like members of the sex as which they present themselves or with which they identify. Cross-sex hormone therapy stimulates the development of secondary sex characteristics of the sex with which the person identifies and suppresses the secondary sex characteristics of the person's birth sex. Several comprehensive reviews address the management of cross-sex hormone therapy in transgender persons (Meyer et al., 1986; Asscheman & Gooren, 1992; Schlatterer et al., 1996; Futterweit, 1998; Gooren, 1999, 2005; Oriel, 2000; Michel et al., 2001; Moore et al., 2003; Tangpricha et al., 2003; Dahl et al., 2006). Eligibility criteria and general guidelines for the conduct of cross-sex hormone therapy are also discussed in the *Standards of Care for Gender Identity Disorders* (*Standards of Care*) (Meyer et al., 2001), promulgated by the Harry Benjamin International Gender Dysphoria Association (HBIGDA), a professional group of transgender care specialists.

Hormone therapy is prescribed primarily for persons who meet criteria for a diagnosis of Gender Identity Disorder (GID) in adolescents or adults in the *Diagnostic and Statistical Manual of Mental Disorders*, Fourth Edition, Text Revision (DSM-IV-TR) (APA, 2000) or Transsexualism in the *Diagnostic and Statistical Manual of Mental Disorders*, Third Edition, Revised (DSM-III-R) (APA, 1987). Prescribing hormones for persons not meeting these criteria was called a "deeply controversial" practice in the 1998 version of the HBIGDA *Standards of Care* (Levine et al., 1998, p. 32), but it is clear that many persons who do not meet these criteria nevertheless seek and undergo hormone therapy (Docter & Fleming, 1992; Docter & Prince, 1997; Hage & Karim, 2000). The most recent version of the *Standards of Care* (Meyer et al., 2001) specifically states that hormone therapy can be appropriate for and "can provide significant comfort to" (p. 21) transgender patients who do not wish to live full-time in cross-gender role or who do not desire feminizing or masculinizing surgical procedures; these criteria seem to apply primarily to male cross-dressers. Nearly half of the male cross-dressers surveyed by Docter and Prince (1997) reported an interest in using feminizing hormones; given the prevalence of cross-dressing in the male population, the number of patients potentially interested in feminizing hormone therapy appears to be large.

According to the HBIGDA *Standards of Care* (Meyer et al., 2001), cross-sex hormone therapy is ideally prescribed only on the recommendation of an experienced mental health professional. However, transgender persons frequently acquire and self-administer hormones without such a recommendation and without medical supervision (McGowan, 1999; Xavier, 2000; Clements-Nolle et al., 2001). In response to this phenomenon, the most recent version of the *Standards of Care* (Meyer et al., 2001) authorized prescription of hormones without the recommendation of a mental health professional in selected cases to persons engaged in unsupervised hormone use to encourage medically monitored therapy. This mode of prescribing has been used for many years by clinics that serve large numbers of transgender clients (e.g., the Tom Waddell Health Center in San Francisco) (Tom Waddell Health Center Transgender Team, 2001).

2.2 Feminizing Hormone Therapy in Adults

2.2.1 Administration and Effects of Feminizing Hormone Therapy
Estrogens are the principal medications used to promote feminization in MtF transsexuals and transgender persons. Estrogens induce femi-

nization by binding to estrogen receptors and promote demasculinization by suppressing the release of pituitary gonadotropins, thereby reducing testicular production of testosterone. Estrogens also directly inhibit testosterone production in the testes (Leinonen et al., 1981; Schulze, 1988). Estrogens can be administered orally, by intramuscular injection, or using transdermal patches.

Progesterone or medications with progesterone-like activity (progestagens) are also sometimes prescribed for MtF transgender persons, either to promote breast development or for their antiandrogenic effects. The most frequently prescribed drugs are progesterone, medroxyprogesterone acetate, and cyproterone acetate (CPA); the last of these medications is not available in the United States. Progesterone and progestagens promote the growth of lobules and acinii in breast tissue by binding to progesterone receptors; Kanhai et al. (2000) demonstrated that the use of medications with progesterone-like activity is necessary for the full development of breast histology similar to that of natal women in MtF transsexuals. However, Meyer et al. (1986) could find no appreciable effect of medroxyprogesterone acetate on breast size in MtF transsexuals. Because of their potential risks and uncertain benefits (Moore et al., 2003), progesterone and progestagens are not routinely prescribed for MtF patients (e.g., Tom Waddell Health Center Transgender Team, 2001; Tangpricha et al., 2003; Dittrich et al., 2005).

Antiandrogens are often prescribed in conjunction with estrogens to reduce the dose of estrogen required. In the United States, spironolactone, a medication originally developed as a diuretic, is probably the most commonly prescribed antiandrogen; it promotes demasculinization by reducing testosterone production, inhibiting the conversion of testosterone to its active metabolite dihydrotestosterone (DHT), and blocking the effects of testosterone and DHT at tissue receptors (Prior et al., 1989). Outside the United States, CPA is often prescribed for its antiandrogenic effects (e.g., Jequier et al., 1989; Asscheman & Gooren, 1992). Gonadotropin-releasing hormone (GnRH) agonists, such as gosserelin, triptorelin, and leuprolide, reduce testosterone levels by suppressing the production of pituitary gonadotropins and are sometimes prescribed for their antiandrogenic effects (Dittrich et al., 2005).

Desirable effects of feminizing hormone therapy include breast growth (Orentreich & Durr, 1974; Kanhai et al., 2000b), redistribution of body fat to a more female-typical pattern (Elbers et al., 1999), increased subcutaneous fat and decreased muscle mass (Elbers et al., 1997, 1999), softening of the skin (Schlatterer et al., 1996), reduction in the rate of growth of facial and body hair (Giltay & Gooren, 2000), reduction or cessation of scalp hair loss, decreased testicular size (Meyer et al., 1986), and reduction or elimination of spontaneous erections (Kwan et al., 1985). Feminizing hormone therapy has no appreciable effect on vocal pitch or penile length (Meyer et al., 1986). Bone mineral density is well preserved and also increases (van Kesteren et al., 1996a, 1998; Reutrakul et al., 1998; Schlatterer et al., 1998a; Sosa et al., 2003; Mueller et al., 2005). Reported side effects of feminizing hormone therapy include weight gain (Elbers et al., 1997, 1999), galactorrhea (fluid discharge from the nipples) (Gooren et al., 1985; Schlatterer et al., 1998b), decreased red cell mass (Rosenmund et al., 1988; Schlatterer et al., 1998b), decreased libido (van Kemenade et al., 1989; van Goozen et al., 1995; Schlatterer et al., 1996), and infertility (Lübbert et al., 1992). Most hormone-induced changes are reversible if feminizing hormones are discontinued, but breast growth must be assumed to be permanent. The time course and permanence of the testicular changes leading to reduced testosterone production and infertility are incompletely understood. Testosterone response to gonadotropin challenge can disappear after a period of estrogen treatment as short as 13 months but has been observed after a period of treatment as long as 25 months (Futterweit et al., 1984). Cessation of feminizing hormone therapy after 140 days of treatment has been observed to result in complete recovery of sperm counts and sperm quality (Lübbert et al., 1992).

Feminizing hormones have emotional and psychological effects in addition to inducing physical changes. Early observers noted that feminizing hormones had a calming effect in MtF transsexuals and seemed to act as a "biotranquilizer" (Block & Tessler, 1971, p. 518). Leavitt et al. (1980) found that a group of MtF transsexuals taking feminizing hormones displayed better psychological adjustment than a comparable group not using hormones and that, in the hormone-using group, greater duration of hormone use was associated with better psychological adjustment. Cohen-Kettenis and Gooren (1992) concluded that in MtF transsexuals "the main effect of estrogen seems to be one of calming down emotional turbulences" (p. 63). Van Kemenade et al. (1989) observed that antiandrogen treatment increased feelings of relaxation and energy in MtF transsexuals. Slabbekoorn et al. (2001) reported that feminizing hormone therapy increased the intensity of positive emotions in MtF transsexuals; nonverbal emotional expressivity also increased. Asscheman et al. (1989) found an increased prevalence of depressive mood changes in association with feminizing hormone therapy, but T'Sjoen et al. (2004) have questioned whether this finding is attributable to hormone therapy.

Medical treatments that result in loss of fertility are usually preceded by a discussion of reproductive consequences and options, and feminizing hormone therapy should be no exception (Lawrence et al., 1996; De Sutter, 2001). The HBIGDA *Standards of Care* (Meyer et al., 2001) state that MtF transsexuals should be counseled about reproductive options, including cryopreservation (freezing and banking) of sperm, before beginning feminizing hormone therapy. In an Internet survey, a significant number of MtF transsexuals expressed an interest in sperm cryopreservation before beginning hormone therapy (De Sutter et al., 2003).

2.2.2 Complications of Feminizing Hormone Therapy

One report from the Netherlands found an increased mortality rate among hormone-treated MtF transsexuals (Asscheman et al., 1989), but this finding was not confirmed in a later study in the same population (van Kesteren et al., 1997). Feminizing hormone therapy is associated with potentially serious medical complications, including an increased risk of developing blood clots (venous thrombosis and pulmonary embolism) (van Kesteren et al., 1997), gallstones (van Kesteren et al.,

1997), liver disease (Meyer et al., 1986; van Kesteren et al., 1997; Tangpricha et al., 2001), pancreatitis (Perego et al., 2004), insulin resistance (Polderman et al., 1994) and glucose intolerance (Feldman, 2002), and elevated prolactin levels (van Kesteren et al., 1997), rarely accompanied by pituitary enlargement or the development of prolactin-secreting pituitary tumors called prolactinomas.

The most significant complications of feminizing hormone therapy are related to the development of venous thrombosis and pulmonary embolism. Van Kesteren et al. (1997) found that in a group of 816 MtF transsexual patients treated with oral CPA and either oral ethinyl estradiol (a potent synthetic estrogen) or transdermal estradiol, 45 patients (5.5%) experienced venous thrombosis or pulmonary embolism, a percentage more than 19 times that observed in the general population. Most thromboembolic events occurred during the first 12 months of treatment, and all but one occurred in persons taking ethinyl estradiol. Oral ethinyl estradiol appears to be significantly more thrombogenic than either oral or transdermal estradiol: Toorians et al. (2003) found that MtF transsexual patients treated with CPA and oral ethinyl estradiol showed significantly greater changes in hemostatic variables, especially resistance to the anticoagulant factor *activated protein C*, than patients treated with CPA and transdermal estradiol, CPA and oral estradiol, or CPA alone. Patients in the last three groups showed similar and relatively minor changes in hemostatic variables. These results suggest that the high prevalence of venous thrombosis and pulmonary embolism observed in MtF patients treated with oral ethinyl estradiol (van Kesteren et al., 1997) was probably related more to the specific chemical structure of ethinyl estradiol than to oral administration of estrogen per se (Toorians et al., 2003). However, data from natal women receiving postmenopausal estrogen replacement therapy suggest that transdermal estrogen is associated with a significantly lower risk of venous thromboembolism than oral estrogen (Scarabin et al., 2003).

The risks of estrogen-induced thrombosis may be increased in men and MtF transgender persons with known cardiovascular disease. In the Coronary Drug Project, conducted during the 1960s in middle-aged men with one or more previous myocardial infarctions, treatment with oral conjugated estrogens in dosages comparable to those used in MtF transsexuals resulted in a significantly increased incidence of venous thrombosis and pulmonary embolism relative to a placebo-treated group (Coronary Drug Project Research Group, 1970).

Postmenopausal estrogen therapy in natal women carries an increased risk of stroke (Women's Health Initiative Steering Committee, 2004) and postmenopausal therapy with an estrogen-progestagen combination carries an increased risk of both coronary heart disease and stroke (Writing Group for the Women's Health Initiative Investigators, 2002). Surprisingly, however, feminizing hormone therapy has not been demonstrated to increase the risk of either stroke or myocardial infarction in MtF transsexuals (van Kesteren et al., 1997). Feminizing hormone therapy appears to offer some cardiovascular benefits to MtF transsexuals, which plausibly may counterbalance the undesirable thrombogenic effects of estrogens and progestagens. For example, in comparison with untreated men, estrogen-treated MtF transsexuals demonstrated greater arterial reactivity following arterial occlusion or nitroglycerine infusion (McCrohon et al., 1997; New et al., 1997), which may confer cardioprotective benefits in persons with atherosclerosis. Estrogen treatment in MtF transsexuals also reduces levels of homocysteine (Giltay et al., 1998), a known risk factor for cardiovascular disease.

Estrogen treatment in MtF transsexuals appears to shift lipid profiles toward a more female-typical pattern, potentially reducing cardiovascular risk. Relative to male controls, estrogen-treated MtF transsexuals have been observed to have significantly lower total cholesterol (TC)/high-density lipoprotein cholesterol (HDL-C) ratios (Damewood et al., 1989), higher levels of HDL-C and lower levels of low-density lipoprotein cholesterol (LDL-C) (New et al., 1997; Elbers et al., 2003), and lower levels of TC and LDL-C (Sosa et al., 2004). McCrohon et al. (1997), however, found no difference in TC or HDL-C between estrogen-treated MtF transsexuals and untreated men. Not all reported effects of feminizing hormones on lipid profiles are positive. Elbers et al. (2003) reported that treatment with estrogen and CPA increased triglyceride levels in MtF transsexuals, and New et al. (1997) found that estrogen-treated MtF transsexuals had somewhat higher triglyceride levels than untreated men.

Elevated prolactin levels are observed in many MtF transsexuals treated with feminizing hormone therapy (van Kesteren et al., 1997). Moderate elevations of prolactin are not of concern, but prolactin levels that persistently exceed about three times the upper limit of normal have occasionally been associated with pituitary enlargement (Asscheman et al., 1988) or rarely with development of prolactin-secreting tumors (prolactinomas) (Gooren et al., 1988; Kovacs et al., 1994; Serri et al., 1996; Futterweit, 1998). Loss of peripheral vision due to compression of the optic nerves, a potential complication of pituitary enlargement or prolactinoma, has apparently never been reported in estrogen-treated MtF transsexuals.

2.3 Masculinizing Hormone Therapy in Adults

2.3.1 Administration and Effects of Masculinizing Hormone Therapy

Testosterone is usually the only medication prescribed to induce masculinization in FtM transsexuals and transgender persons. It is typically administered by intramuscular (IM) injection at a dosage of about 200 mg every 2 weeks. Testosterone induces masculinization by binding to androgen receptors. Theoretically, it should also contribute to defeminization by suppressing the release of pituitary gonadotropins, thereby reducing ovarian production of estrogen and progesterone. However, suppression of gonadotropin production is often incomplete with moderate doses of testosterone (e.g., 300 mg IM per month) (Zwirska-Korczala et al., 1996), although significant suppression is usual with larger doses (e.g., 500 mg IM per month) (Spinder et al., 1989). Because testosterone undergoes peripheral conversion to estradiol, estradiol levels in FtM transsexuals often remain within the normal female range, both before and after ovariectomy (Spinder et al., 1989; Elbers et al., 1997). Although testosterone is usually administered by IM injection, transdermal preparations (patches and gel) are also available.

Transdermal testosterone is more expensive than injectable testosterone, appears to induce masculinization more slowly (Tangpricha et al., 2003), and is probably less effective for suppressing menses; consequently, it is usually prescribed only for persons who seek limited masculinization or for maintenance therapy following initial masculinization with injectable testosterone in persons who have undergone hysterectomy and ovariectomy (Oriel, 2000). Oral testosterone is rarely prescribed in the United States because available preparations are hepatotoxic in the dosages needed for masculinizing therapy (Rhoden & Morgentaler, 2004). Progesterone is occasionally prescribed along with testosterone to help suppress menses (Schlatterer et al., 1996; Gooren, 1999).

Testosterone therapy typically results in deepening of the voice (Meyer et al., 1986), enlargement of the clitoris (Meyer et al., 1986), increased muscle mass and decreased subcutaneous fat (Elbers et al., 1997, 1999), slight reduction in breast size (Meyer et al., 1986), increased facial and body hair (Schlatterer et al., 1996), male pattern scalp hair loss (Giltay et al., 2004), and cessation of menses (Meyer et al., 1986; Schlatterer et al., 1996). Some of these changes are reversible if testosterone is discontinued, but voice deepening, clitoral enlargement, facial and body hair changes, and scalp hair loss must be assumed to be permanent.

Masculinizing hormone therapy has emotional and psychological effects in addition to its physical effects. Van Goozen et al. (1995) observed increases in aggressiveness, anger-proneness, and sexual interest and arousability in testosterone-treated FtM transsexuals. Slabbekoorn et al. (2001) found that masculinizing hormone therapy decreased the intensity of both positive and negative emotions in FtM transsexuals but increased anger-readiness and frequency of sexual feelings and behaviors. Perrone et al. (2003) observed decreased feelings of depression and increased sexual interest and arousability following testosterone therapy in FtM transsexuals. In a large Internet-based survey of self-identified FtM transgender persons, Newfield et al. (in press) found that testosterone use was associated with higher quality-of-life scores in domains related to social functioning and overall mental health.

The HBIGDA *Standards of Care* (Meyer et al., 2001) state that FtM transsexuals should be counseled about reproductive considerations before beginning masculinizing hormone therapy. At present, embryo cryopreservation is the only practical fertility preservation option available to FtM transsexuals, but ovarian tissue banking may become practical in the future (De Sutter, 2001).

2.3.2 *Complications of Masculinizing Hormone Therapy*

Masculinizing hormone therapy has not been shown to be associated with increased mortality (van Kesteren et al., 1997). However, side effects and complications of masculinizing hormone therapy have been reported; they include acne (van Kesteren et al., 1997), weight gain (Elbers et al., 1997), increased red cell mass with possible polycythemia (Futterweit, 1998), liver disease (van Kesteren et al., 1997), insulin resistance (Polderman et al., 1994), fluid retention and edema (van Kesteren et al., 1997; Futterweit, 1998), increases in plasma homocysteine levels (Giltay et al., 1998), decreases in arterial reactivity (McCredie et al., 1998), and shift of lipid profiles toward a more male-typical pattern (Meyer et al., 1986; McCredie et al., 1998; Elbers et al., 2003; Giltay et al., 2004) with the potential for increased cardiovascular risk. Elevated prolactin levels have occasionally been reported in FtM transsexuals and may be attributable to breast binding (Schlatterer et al., 1998b).

Testosterone treatment typically produces changes in ovarian histology similar to those observed in women with polycystic ovarian syndrome (Futterweit & Deligdisch, 1986; Spinder et al., 1989). The significance of this finding is uncertain, especially as untreated FtM transsexuals often have elevated testosterone levels (Futterweit et al., 1986; Bosinski et al., 1997) and polycystic ovaries (Futterweit et al., 1986; Balen et al., 1993; Bosinski et al., 1997). Gooren (1999) observed that polycystic ovaries were more likely to undergo malignant changes and consequently recommended that testosterone-treated FtM transsexuals undergo ovariectomy soon after successful transition to the male gender role.

Bone mineral density in testosterone-treated FtM transsexuals is generally well preserved prior to ovariectomy (van Kesteren et al., 1996a; Goh & Ratnam, 1997) and following ovariectomy if testosterone is taken regularly and in adequate dosage (Lips et al., 1996; Goh & Ratnam, 1997). However, decreases in bone mineral density following ovariectomy have been reported in FtM transsexuals who stop taking testosterone or use testosterone irregularly (Goh & Ratnam, 1997) or in whom testosterone dosage is not high enough to suppress luteinizing hormone (LH), a gonadotropin (van Kesteren et al., 1998). Van Kesteren et al. (1998) proposed that measuring serum LH may be a better indicator of the adequacy of testosterone dosage for preservation of bone mass in FtM transsexuals following ovariectomy than measuring testosterone itself.

Greenman (2004) and Michel et al. (2001) expressed concerns about endometrial hyperplasia, which may be a risk factor for endometrial carcinoma, in testosterone-treated FtM transsexuals. These concerns apparently derive from a report of three instances of mild hyperplasia observed following hysterectomy among 19 testosterone-treated FtM patients (Futterweit & Deligdisch, 1986); no information was provided about estradiol levels in these patients. Chadha et al. (1994) and Miller et al. (1986) detected no instances of endometrial hyperplasia in their respective series of 6 and 32 testosterone-treated FtM patients. Futterweit (1998) asserted that the risks associated with possible endometrial hyperplasia in testosterone-treated FtM patients were such that hysterectomy should be performed "at the earliest possible time" (p. 217) consistent with the patient's psychological and clinical progress, an opinion shared by Michel et al. (2001).

2.4 Hormone Therapy in Transgender Adolescents

It is not unusual for adolescents with GID to seek cross-sex hormone therapy (Cohen-Kettenis & Pfäfflin, 2003). Such requests pose dilemmas for caregivers, parents, and transsexual adolescents themselves. Some adolescents with GID will not sustain the wish to live as members of the opposite sex into adulthood (Meyenburg, 1999), which would argue against the provision of cross-sex hormone therapy, with its relatively irreversible physical effects, to transgender adolescents. On the other hand, the physical changes of puberty can be extremely distressing to adolescents with GID, and prevention of unwanted masculinization or feminization can also make physical presentation in the desired gender role much easier if the adolescent does decide to live full-time as a member of the opposite sex (Cohen-Kettenis & Pfäfflin, 2003).

One option for the treatment of adolescents with GID is to prescribe puberty-blocking hormones, such as GnRH agonists (Gooren & Delemarre-van de Waal, 1996; Cohen-Kettenis & van Goozen, 1998). GnRH agonists suppress the production of endogenous testosterone in male adolescents and the production of estrogen and progesterone in female adolescents, thereby preventing irreversible masculinization or feminization. Puberty-blocking hormones thus give adolescents time to consider their options. If living full-time in the opposite gender role is still desired in adulthood, feminizing or masculinizing hormones can be prescribed; if not, puberty-blocking hormones can be discontinued and normal puberty will occur. Since 1998, the HBIGDA *Standards of Care* have authorized the prescription of puberty-blocking hormones for selected transgender adolescents (Levine et al., 1998; Meyer et al., 2001).

Carefully selected adolescents with GID who are allowed to begin the sex reassignment process during adolescence, including adminis-tration of puberty-blocking hormones in some cases, experience relief of gender dysphoria, high levels of satisfaction, and good psychologi-cal functioning following sex reassignment (Cohen-Kettenis & van Goozen, 1997; Smith et al., 2001). At present it is unclear which ado-lescents with GID are the most appropriate candidates for puberty-blocking hormones. Cohen-Kettenis and Pfäfflin (2003) proposed that their use should be limited to those gender-dysphoric adolescents who had consistently manifested extreme cross-gender behavior since child-hood, who clearly desired to adopt the social role of the opposite sex, whose gender dysphoria had increased significantly with the onset of puberty, who displayed minimal or no comorbid psychopathology, and whose parents consented and were cooperative. Zucker (2001) observed, however, that limiting puberty-blocking hormones to persons without significant coexisting psychopathology was likely to exclude the "vast majority" (p. 2086) of gender-dysphoric adolescents and that the issue was further complicated by the possibility that co-morbid psychopathology can sometimes be a direct consequence of chronic gender dysphoria. He proposed that randomized controlled trials would help clarify whether coexisting psychopathology is an appropriate exclusion criterion for puberty-blocking hormones.

2.5 Use of Nonprescribed and Unsupervised Hormones

Many transgender persons use nonprescribed cross-sex hormones obtained from friends, black market sources, or suppliers in foreign countries. In a survey conducted in Washington, DC, 58% of a combined group of MtF and FtM transgender persons reported having used nonprescribed hormones (Xavier, 2000). In a New York City survey, 39% of MtF transsexuals and 9% of FtM transgender persons reported using nonprescribed hormones (McGowan, 1999); and in a San Francisco survey, the figures were 29% for MtF transgender persons and 3% for FtM transgender persons (Clements-Nolle et al., 2001). Dosages of nonprescribed hormones often exceed those typically prescribed by physicians. Moore et al. (2003) found that 28% of presurgical MtF patients presenting at a gender clinic reported using hormone dosages more than three times greater than what is typically prescribed, although hormone dosages used by FtM patients were in an appropriate range. Despite the apparent widespread use of nonprescribed hormones and the high dosages frequently employed, there is little information available concerning complications of this practice.

Notwithstanding the potential risks, many transgender persons are willing to use nonprescribed hormones to achieve the physical and psychological changes they desire. The benefits of nonprescribed hormones can be genuine. For example, Leavitt et al. (1980) reported that MtF transsexuals who used medically unsupervised hormones displayed better psychological adjustment than transsexuals who were not receiving hormone treatment.

3 Surgical Treatment for Transgender Persons

3.1 Surgical Treatment for Male-to-Female Transsexuals

The desire for feminizing genitoplasty, usually called MtF "sex reassignment surgery" (SRS), is arguably the defining characteristic of MtF transsexuals. SRS been performed in MtF transsexuals for more than 70 years (Karim et al., 1996) and has reached a high state of technical refinement. In expert hands, it yields excellent cosmetic and functional results and highly favorable subjective outcomes (Green & Fleming, 1990; Muirhead-Allwood et al., 1999; Lawrence, 2003). MtF SRS usually involves orchiectomy, penectomy, vaginoplasty, and vulvoplasty. Typically the neovagina is lined with the inverted skin of the penis (penile inversion vaginoplasty); this is widely regarded as the technique of choice for MtF SRS (Karim et al., 1996; Giraldo et al., 2002). Most surgeons construct a sensate clitoris from a portion of the glans penis, a technique that is "recognized today as the best choice for neoclitoroplasty" (Giraldo et al., 2002, p. 1308).

Although all elements of the sex reassignment process contribute to relief of gender dysphoria (Kuiper & Cohen-Kettenis, 1988), MtF SRS appears to provide particular psychological and social benefits. In a randomized, controlled, prospective study of MtF SRS outcomes, Mate-Kole et al. (1990) observed that, in comparison to a wait-list control group, MtF patients who underwent SRS on an expedited basis experienced better psychosocial outcomes, displaying fewer neurotic symptoms and greater engagement in social activities. Satisfaction following MtF SRS is extremely high, and MtF transsexuals rarely express regret after undergoing SRS. In two large SRS follow-up surveys ($n = 140$ and 232, respectively), no respondents reported outright regret, and only

6% expressed even occasional regret, which often was unrelated to SRS per se (Muirhead-Allwood et al., 1999; Lawrence, 2003).

Potential complications of MtF SRS include vaginal stenosis, genital pain, clitoral necrosis, urethral stenosis, and rectovaginal or vesicovaginal fistulas (Krege et al., 2001; Lawrence, in press). Not surprisingly, good surgical results and lack of complications are usually associated with higher levels of subjective satisfaction and better psychosocial outcomes (Ross & Need, 1989; Muirhead-Allwood et al., 1999; Schroder & Carroll, 1999; Lawrence, 2003, in press).

MtF SRS performed in North America typically costs between $15,000 and $20,000 and is usually not covered by health insurance policies in the United States; this makes SRS prohibitively expensive for many patients. Some MtF transsexuals who cannot afford SRS undergo only orchiectomy, a much less expensive procedure that eliminates testosterone production by the testes and allows lower dosages of feminizing hormones to be used (Israel & Tarver, 1997).

Because they often feel that hormone-induced breast development is inadequate, many MtF transsexuals and transgender persons undergo augmentation mammaplasty (breast-enlargement surgery). In the Netherlands, about two thirds of MtF transsexuals who undergo vaginoplasty also undergo augmentation mammaplasty (Kanhai et al., 2001). Approximately 75% of patients express satisfaction after augmentation mammaplasty; the most frequent complaint by dissatisfied patients is that their breasts were not made large enough (Kanhai et al., 2000).

3.2 Surgical Treatment for Female-to-Male Transsexuals

Reduction mammaplasty, often referred to as chest reconstruction, is the surgical procedure most frequently sought by FtM transsexuals and transgender persons. The principal techniques and aesthetic considerations are outlined by Hage and van Kesteren (1995). Even with careful placement and orientation of incisions, scar revisions are frequently required following FtM chest reconstruction. Newfield et al. (in press) found that FtM transgender persons who had undergone chest reconstruction reported higher quality-of-life scores in domains related to general health, social functioning, and mental health.

In contrast to the situation in MtF transsexuals, there are currently no entirely satisfactory masculinizing genitoplasty techniques available to FtM transsexuals, which led Green and Fleming (1990) to conclude that "those [FtMs] with a weak interest in [phalloplasty] have a better prognosis" (p. 172). A variety of FtM genitoplasty techniques are available, but two have achieved the widest acceptance. In *metoidioplasty* (sometimes spelled *metaidoioplasty*), the hypertrophied clitoris is released from its suspensory ligament, creating a microphallus that retains sexual sensation; urethral lengthening can also be performed if desired (Hage, 1996). The small size of the resulting phallus is the principal disadvantage of this technique. In *radial forearm flap phalloplasty* (e.g., Gottlieb et al., 1999; Rohrmann & Jakse, 2003), a free flap of skin from the forearm is used to create a tube-within-a-tube neophallus that permits standing voiding and that often has both protective and sexual sensation. Sometimes a hydraulic penile prosthesis can be inserted to achieve rigidity (Hoebeke et al., 2003). Major disadvantages of the radial forearm flap technique include frequent urethral stenoses and fistulas (Rohrmann & Jakse, 2003), unattractive donor site healing, and formidable expense. De Cuypere et al. (2005) observed the FtM phalloplasty patients who received hydraulic penile prostheses displayed a trend toward greater realization of their sexual expectations than patients who did not, but were also more likely to report pain during intercourse. With both metoidioplasty and phalloplasty, the labia majora are usually brought together to create a neoscrotum in which testicular prostheses are inserted (Sengezer & Sadove, 1993). Because there is significant room for improvement in current techniques, masculinizing genitoplasty procedures will continue to evolve.

4 Screening for Neoplasia in Hormone-Treated Transgender Persons

It is not known whether cross-sex hormone therapy affects the incidence of neoplasia in transgender persons; however, case reports of neoplasia in transgender persons treated with cross-sex hormones are uncommon. Case reports in MtF transsexuals include five breast carcinomas (Symmers, 1968; Pritchard et al., 1988; Ganly & Taylor, 1995; Grabellus et al., 2005), two breast fibroadenomas (Kanhai et al., 1999; Lemmo et al., 2003), four prolactinomas (Gooren et al., 1988; Kovacs et al., 1994; Serri et al., 1996; Futterweit, 1998), four prostatic carcinomas (Markland, 1975; Thurston, 1994; Gooren et al., 1997; van Haarst et al., 1998), one neovaginal carcinoma (Harder et al., 2002), and one case of neovaginal intraepithelial neoplasia (Lawrence, 2001). Case reports in FtM transsexuals include three ovarian carcinomas (Hage et al., 2000; Dizon et al., 2006), one cervical carcinoma (Driak & Samudovsky, 2004), and two cases of breast carcinoma in residual breast tissue following mastectomy (Gooren, 1999; Burcombe et al., 2003). In these cases, there may be a plausible causal link with cross-sex hormone therapy. In addition, van Kesteren et al. (1997) observed seven cancer deaths in MtF transsexuals (three cases of pulmonary carcinoma, one case each of gastric carcinoma, leukemia, glioblastoma, and meningioma) and one cancer death in a FtM transsexual (from colon carcinoma); in these cases a possible causal link with cross-sex hormone therapy is not obvious.

The HBIGDA *Standards of Care* (Meyer et al., 2001) state that transgender patients, "whether on hormones or not, should be screened for pelvic malignancies as are other persons" (p. 23), but there are no data to suggest what screening techniques or intervals might be optimal. The *Standards of Care* recommendations imply that FtM transsexuals who have not undergone hysterectomy should have periodic Pap smears performed (Moore et al., 2003; Tangpricha et al., 2003), although Greenman (2004) suggested that this may not always be necessary. Testosterone treatment is associated with cervical mucosal atrophy in many cases, which can result in a misdiagnosis of cervical dysplasia (Miller et al., 1986). Moore et al. (2003) proposed that testosterone-treated FtM transsexuals should also undergo regular uterine ultrasonography examinations to detect endometrial hyperplasia, a risk factor for endometrial carcinoma.

There is disagreement as to whether MtF transsexuals who have undergone penile inversion vaginoplasty should be screened for neovaginal cancer with Pap smears. Kirk (2001) argued that regular screening Pap smears were indicated for MtF transsexuals following vaginoplasty. Lawrence (2001) observed that if MtF transsexuals were screened for pelvic malignancies according to the recommendations for natal women, then vaginal Pap smears would not be indicated because they are not recommended for natal women who lack a cervix and who have no history of cancer or abnormal cytology (American Academy of Family Physicians, 2004). Vaginal and neovaginal cancers are rare, and vaginal Pap smears lack sensitivity and specificity; consequently, most positive Pap smears from MtF transsexuals would be false positives. Annual pelvic examination without routine Pap smears probably provides optimal screening for most MtF transsexuals who have undergone penile inversion vaginoplasty; exceptions might be patients in whom penile glans tissue was inverted along with penile skin (nowadays an uncommon practice) because of a possible increased potential for malignancy in glans tissue (Lawrence, 2001).

According to the *Standards of Care* (Meyer et al., 2001), hormone-treated MtF transsexuals should be monitored for prostate and breast cancer, but there are no data demonstrating the benefits of such monitoring. The value of prostate-specific antigen (PSA) screening in MtF transsexuals appears to be especially doubtful: PSA testing has not been shown to be beneficial in natal males (Harris & Lohr, 2002), and estrogen strongly suppresses PSA levels in MtF transsexuals (Jin et al., 1996; van Kesteren et al., 1996b).

It is unclear whether monitoring for breast cancer in MtF transsexuals should include mammography, and which if any transsexuals might benefit from it. Feldman and Bockting (2003) recommended annual "mammograms starting at age 40 for patients on hormones who have even modest breast development" (p. 31); Tangpricha et al. (2003) suggested that "mammography may be indicated in high-risk [MtF] patients" (p. 16); and Moore et al. (2003) advised considering mammography for MtF patients over age 50. However, MtF transsexuals are likely to have had many fewer years of estrogen exposure, a known risk factor for breast cancer (Dunn et al., 2005), than natal women of similar age, which might argue against routine mammography for most MtF transsexuals. The potential benefits of mammography must be balanced against the risks of false-positive results and overdiagnosis. Most MtF transsexuals take estrogen indefinitely, and current or recent estrogen use significantly increases the likelihood of false positive mammography (Banks et al., 2004). The problem of overdiagnosis—detection of lesions of low malignant potential that would otherwise not have come to clinical attention during the person's lifetime—is also significant when screening mammography is performed in older persons: Zahl et al. (2004) estimated that in Norway and Sweden one-third of invasive breast cancers detected with screening mammography in persons 50 to 69 years old were overdiagnosed. Moreover, many MtF transsexuals undergo breast augmentation (Kanhai et al., 2001), which lowers the sensitivity of screening mammography in natal women (Miglioretti et al., 2004); mammography in persons who have undergone breast augmentation also carries a small risk of implant rupture (Brown et al., 2004).

The *Standards of Care* state that hormone-treated FtM transsexuals who have "undergone mastectomies and who have a family history of breast cancer should be monitored for this disease" (Meyer et al., 2001, p. 23). Although testosterone is not believed to induce premalignant changes in breast tissue (Burgess & Shousha, 1993), detection of carcinoma in residual breast tissue following mastectomy in two FtM transsexuals (Gooren, 1999; Burcombe et al., 2003) suggests that periodic breast examinations would be prudent in all FtM transgender persons.

5 Liquid Silicone Injection in Transgender Persons

Some MtF transgender persons undergo subcutaneous injection of liquid silicone in an attempt feminize their appearance. The hips and buttocks are the areas most frequently injected (Hage et al., 2001); other reported sites include the face, breasts, and legs. Silicone injection, which may be performed by medical personnel or, more often, by nonmedical practitioners, is seen by some MtF transgender persons as a quick, inexpensive alternative to conventional cosmetic surgical procedures. The total volume injected can be up to 8 liters (Hage et al., 2001), typically over multiple sessions (Wiessing et al., 1999). Occasionally, other viscous fluids, such as mineral oil or olive oil, are injected or are combined with silicone. In some urban areas such as New York City, silicone injection occurs frequently enough to have been called "epidemic" (Fox et al., 2004, p. 452). In a New York City survey of MtF transsexuals, 11% reported receiving silicone injections from professional providers and 18% from "black market" providers (McGowan, 1999). In Rotterdam, Wiessing et al. (1999) found that more than half of transgender street prostitutes surveyed had received silicone injections to the face, breasts, thighs, or buttocks; on average, they had received injections about twice a year.

Liquid silicone injection has been associated with a variety of devastating complications. Embolism of silicone to the lungs can cause acute pneumonitis, leading to severe respiratory distress (e.g., Duong et al., 1998; Kim et al., 2003; Rosioreanu et al., 2004) or death (Ellenbogen & Rubin, 1975; Rodriguez et al., 1989). Pneumonitis typically occurs within hours or a few days of injection but has been observed up to months (Duong et al., 1998) or years after injection, sometimes following trauma (Chastre et al., 1987). Acute silicone pneumonitis has been reported after injection of volumes as small as 10 cc (Kim et al., 2003).

Facial injection of liquid silicone has been associated with the development of granulomatous reactions and cellulitis (Bigatà et al., 2001) and loss of vision (Shin et al., 1988). Silicone-related granulomatous hepatitis has been described (Ellenbogen & Rubin, 1975). Liquid silicone is affected by gravity and can migrate in the body, sometimes resulting in severe disfigurement and disability (Hage et al., 2001). Injection or migration of silicone into the legs can cause chronic ulceration (Rae et al., 1989) and lymphedema (Gaber, 2004), often after a latent period of many years. Multiple cases of *Mycobacterium abscessus* infection have been reported in New York City following liquid silicone injection (Fox et al., 2004). In view of the severity of associated complications, transgender persons should be strongly counseled to avoid liquid silicone injections (Hage et al., 2001).

6 HIV/AIDS and Other Sexually Transmitted Infections in Transgender Persons

Some groups of MtF transgender persons in the United States have disproportionately high HIV seropositivity prevalences and seroconversion rates. Reported HIV seropositivity prevalences from studies conducted with convenience samples of MtF transgender persons include these figures: 25% in New York City (McGowan, 1999); 19% in Philadelphia (Kenagy, 2002); 48%, 35%, and 16% in San Francisco (Nemoto et al., 1999; Clements-Nolle et al., 2001; Kellogg et al., 2001); 32% in Washington, DC (Xavier, 2000); and 22% in Los Angeles (Simon et al., 2000). In comparison, the estimated overall prevalence of HIV infection among U.S. adolescents and adults in 2003 was 0.13% (Centers for Disease Control and Prevention, 2004). Factors associated with HIV seropositivity in MtF transgender persons include lower levels of income and education (Simon et al., 2000), African American ethnicity, nonhormonal injection drug use, and large numbers of lifetime sexual partners (Clements-Nolle et al., 2001). Very high seroconversion rates have also been reported in some samples of MtF transgender persons: 3.4 per 100 person-years in a Los Angeles study (Simon et al., 2000) and 7.8 per 100 person-years in a San Francisco study (Kellogg et al., 2001). In the study by Kellogg et al. (2001), factors associated with higher seroconversion rates included African American ethnicity and engaging in receptive anal sex.

HIV seropositivity is especially high among MtF transgender persons who engage in sex work and in MtF persons of color, especially African Americans. In a study of MtF transgender sex workers in Atlanta (more than 80% of whom were African American), 68% were HIV seropositive (Elifson et al., 1993). In a sample of MtF transgender persons of color in San Francisco, all of whom had a history of exchanging sex for money or drugs, Nemoto et al. (2004) found an overall HIV seropositivity prevalence of 26%, with seropositivity significantly associated with engaging in unprotected receptive anal sex with casual partners. African Americans had the highest HIV seropositivity prevalence, 41%, followed by Latinas, 23%, and Asians/Pacific Islanders, 13% (Nemoto et al., 2004).

Reported HIV seropositivity prevalence figures in FtM transgender persons are much lower than among MtF persons: 0% in Philadelphia and New York City (McGowan, 1999; Kenagy, 2002), 2% in San Francisco (Clements-Nolle et al., 2001), and 5% or less in Washington, DC (Xavier, 2000).

MtF transgender persons also report a high lifetime prevalence of STIs other than HIV/AIDS. Kenagy (2002) found that 41% of a convenience sample of MtF transgender persons reported having been diagnosed with an STI other than HIV / AIDS at some time in their lives; among FtM transgender persons, only 6% reported this. In comparison, in a national probability sample of U.S. adults, about 17% reported having had an STI other than HIV (Laumann et al., 1994). In a survey of MtF transgender persons of color, 14% reported having had an STI other than HIV / AIDS during the past 12 months (Nemoto et al., 2004); among all U.S. adults, the comparable figure was about 1.6% (Laumann et al., 1994).

7 Mental Health Concerns of Transgender Persons

7.1 Transgenderism as a Mental Disorder

Four diagnoses in the DSM-IV-TR (APA, 2000) are specifically applicable to transgender persons; all of these diagnoses require the presence of clinically significant distress or disability, which implies that transgender identity or behavior per se is not sufficient for the diagnosis of a mental disorder under the DSM-IV-TR. The diagnoses of GID in Children and GID in Adolescents or Adults are usually reserved for severely gender-dysphoric persons who are seeking treatment under the HBIGDA *Standards of Care* (Meyer et al., 2001). The diagnosis of Transvestic Fetishism could be applicable to some cross-dressers who experience distress or disability associated with cross-dressing. Gender Identity Disorder Not Otherwise Specified (GIDNOS), the broadest of the four DSM-IV-TR diagnoses, could be applicable to other transgender persons who experience sufficient distress or disability to meet diagnostic criteria.

There is disagreement among transgender persons and their caregivers concerning the value of these DSM diagnostic categories. Some believe that the diagnoses unnecessarily pathologize behavior that may be deviant but that is not pathologic per se, thereby inviting stigmatization of transgender persons (Lev, 2004). Others argue that medical diagnoses such as GID and GIDNOS are needed to justify the provision of medical and surgical services that transsexuals and other transgender persons seek (Meyer et al., 2001). However one may feel about these diagnoses, their presence in the DSM is a reminder that the central mental health concern for many transgender persons, and the issue that underlies many other transgender health concerns, is the suffering associated with gender dysphoria, especially the profoundly distressing sense of "wrong embodiment" (Prosser, 1998, p. 69) that transsexuals experience.

7.2 Other Mental Health Concerns in Transgender Persons

There is conflicting evidence concerning the prevalence of other mental health problems in transgender persons, with some studies reporting elevated levels of psychopathology relative to population norms and others reporting few or no differences. Interpretation of the evidence is complicated by the small sample sizes of many studies and by methodologic problems, such as averaging of pooled scores from the Minnesota Multiphasic Personality Inventory (MMPI) or assigning psychiatric diagnoses without the use of standardized interviews or instruments.

Many investigators have used the MMPI to assess mental health in transgender persons. Results have been inconsistent: Cole et al. (1997) and Hunt et al. (1981) found both MtF and FtM transsexuals to be, for the most part, "notably free of psychopathology" (Cole et al., 1997, p. 13) based on MMPI results; Miach et al. (2000), Michel et al. (2002), and Tsushima and Wedding (1979) reached similar conclusions in studies of MtF transsexuals. However, Beatrice (1985) and Langevin et al. (1977) reported significant psychopathology in some MtF transsexuals based on MMPI studies, as did Fleming et al. (1981) in both MtF and FtM transsexuals; the most common findings included antisocial tendencies, thought disorder, or hypomania. MMPI data suggest, however, that transsexuals tend to experience less psychopathology than transgender persons who meet criteria for the DSM-III-R diagnosis of Gender Identity Disorder of Adolescence and Adulthood, Nontranssexual Type (GIDAANT) (Miach et al., 2000; Michel et al., 2002). MMPI data also suggest that mental health typically improves following gender transition in MtF transsexuals (Langevin et al., 1977) and following SRS in both MtF and FtM transsexuals (Fleming et al., 1981; but see Beatrice, 1985). Beatrice (1985) found no evidence of psychopathology in a small group of male cross-dressers based on MMPI results.

Conclusions about psychopathology based on assessment using the Derogatis Sexual Functioning Inventory (DSFI) have also been inconsistent. Derogatis et al. (1978) reported that, relative to male norms, MtF transsexuals described more severe current psychological symptoms, especially depression and anxiety, on the Brief Symptom Inventory (BSI) scale of the DSFI. FtM transsexuals, however, gave unremarkable responses regarding current symptoms on the BSI (Derogatis et al., 1981). Brown et al. (1996) subsequently used the DFSI to study a large sample of MtF transsexuals, transgenderists, and cross-dressers; for 9 of 10 DFSI subscales, including the BSI, the transgender participants scored within one standard deviation of male norms, and the three transgender groups were not significantly different from each other based on BSI scores.

Studies using other assessment methods likewise have produced conflicting results. Hoenig and Kenna (1974) observed that, based on clinical criteria, about 50% of the MtF and FtM transsexuals they examined displayed significant current psychopathology, including about 12% with either schizophrenia or an affective psychosis. Bodlund and Armelius (1994) diagnosed a current Axis I disorder other than GID in 44% of a small group of MtF and FtM transsexuals, although half of these cases involved only adjustment disorders; in comparison, they found that 82% of patients with a DSM-III-R diagnosis of GIDAANT had another Axis I disorder, with only one third of these being adjustment disorders. De Cuypere et al. (1995) diagnosed a current Axis I disorder other than GID in 23% of their MtF transsexual patients but in none of their FtM transsexual patients. Haraldsen and Dahl (2000) reported that, in a group of MtF and FtM transsexuals undergoing hormone therapy, 33% had a current Axis I disorder. Hepp et al. (2005) diagnosed a current comorbid Axis I disorder in 39% of a small group of patients undergoing treatment for GID; no significant differences between MtF and FtM patient groups were observed. To put these figures in perspective, the 1-year prevalence among U.S. adults for major Axis I mental disorders, excluding adjustment disorders, is about 26% (Kessler et al., 2005b). Verschoor and Poortinga (1988) found that 21% of MtF transsexuals and 33% of FtM transsexuals reported having received treatment for a psychiatric disorder other than GID at some time in their lives; in the study by De Cuypere et al. (1995), these figures were 45% and 38%, respectively. Hepp et al. (2005) observed a lifetime prevalence of comorbid Axis I disorders in 80% among MtF patients and 54% among FtM patients. In comparison, the lifetime prevalence for major Axis I mental disorders among U.S. adults is about 46% (Kessler et al., 2005a).

Abuse of alcohol and other substances appears to be a problem for many transgender persons, although prevalence estimates vary widely. Cole et al. (1997) documented lifetime histories of substance abuse in 29% of MtF transsexuals and 26% of FtM transsexuals studied. De Cuypere et al. (1995) found even higher lifetime prevalences of substance abuse: 50% in MtF transsexuals and 62% in FtM transsexuals. Verschoor and Poortinga (1988), however, observed much lower substance-abuse prevalences: 11% among MtF transsexuals and only 4% among FtM transsexuals. Clements-Nolle et al. (2001) found that 18% of MtF transgender persons surveyed in San Francisco reported injecting street drugs within the last 6 months. In Philadelphia, Kenagy (2002) observed that 20% of MtF transgender persons but only 6% of FtM transgender persons reported having used injected drugs. In Washington, DC, Xavier (2000) found that 34% of transgender persons believed that they had an alcohol problem, and 36% thought they had a drug problem. Weinberg et al. (1999) surveyed MtF transgender sex workers in San Francisco: 35% used marijuana at least once a week, and 25% used hard drugs at least once a week. For comparison purposes, the 1-year prevalence for substance abuse disorders in U.S. adults is about 9% (Grant et al., 2004b).

Personality disorders are frequently observed in transgender persons. Hoenig and Kenna (1974) diagnosed personality disorders in 18% of their transsexual patients; Haraldsen and Dahl (2000) reported a comparable figure, 20%. Hepp et al. (2005) diagnosed a personality disorder in 42% of their GID patients. The prevalence of personality disorders appears to be higher in persons with nontranssexual types of GID: Bodlund and Armelius (1994) diagnosed a personality disorder in 33% of their transsexual patients but in 73% of their patients with GIDAANT. Similarly, Miach et al. (2000) diagnosed personality disorders in 27% of their transsexual patients but in 65% of their patients with GIDAANT. In comparison, the estimated prevalence of personality disorders in U.S. adults is about 15% (Grant et al., 2004a).

8 Suicide and Self-Harm in Transgender Persons

Transgender persons, and MtF persons especially, appear to be at increased risk for completed suicide, suicide attempts, and other forms of self-harm. In The Netherlands, van Kesteren et al. (1997) reported that 13 (1.6%) of 816 MtF hormone-treated MtF transsexuals had died of suicide, a percentage more than nine times that of the general population; none of 293 hormone-treated FtM transsexuals had died of suicide. Many transgender persons report having made suicide attempts: Dixen et al. (1984) observed that about 25% of applicants for MtF sex reassignment and 19% of applicants for FtM reassignment gave a history of suicide attempts. Verschoor and Poortinga (1988) found a history of suicide attempts in about 19% of both MtF and FtM transsexuals. Cole et al. (1997) reported that 12% of MtF transsexuals and 21% of FtM transsexuals had attempted suicide. Clements-Nolle et al. (2001) found a lifetime attempted suicide prevalence of 32% in both MtF and FtM transsexuals. De Cuypere et al. (1995) observed still higher lifetime prevalence figures for attempted suicide: 55% in MtF transsexuals and 46% in FtM transsexuals.

Self-mutilation of genitals and breasts is not rare in transgender persons. Dixen et al. (1984) found such a history in 9.4% of applicants for MtF sex reassignment and 2.4% of applicants for FtM reassignment. Cole et al. (1997) observed similar percentages: 8% among MtF transsexuals and 1% among FtM transsexuals. Lothstein (1992) suggested that attempted genital self-mutilation was an underreported symptom of childhood gender dysphoria in boys. Incarcerated transgender persons who are denied access to cross-sex hormones may be at increased risk for this type of self-harm (Meyer et al., 2001). There are multiple case reports of self-castration in MtF transgender persons who are unable to undergo SRS or who anticipate long waiting times for surgery (Krieger et al., 1982; Rana & Johnson, 1993; McGovern, 1995; Murphy et al., 2001; Baltieri & de Andrade, 2005).

9 Violence as a Health Concern in Transgender Persons

Transgender persons appear to be at increased risk for assault, rape, and sexual assault. In a survey of 402 transgender persons, most of whom were cross-dressers or transsexuals, 16% of respondents reported having been a victim of assault within the past year and 3% having been a victim of rape or attempted rape (Lombardi et al., 2001). Respondents' lifetime prevalence of assault was 47% and their lifetime prevalence of rape or attempted rape was 14% (Lombardi et al., 2001). In comparison, in a telephone survey of U.S. adults, only 1.9% of women and 3.4% of men reported having been a victim of assault during the past year, and only 0.3% of women and 0.1% of men reported having been a victim of rape or attempted rape (Tjaden & Thoennes, 2000). Lifetime prevalence of assault among the U.S. adults surveyed was 52% for women and 66% for men, and lifetime prevalence of rape or attempted rape was 18% for women and 3% for men (Tjaden & Thoennes, 2000). Lombardi et al. (2001) found that transgender persons who were younger, who had lower incomes, who were not employed full time, and who identified as transsexual were more likely to report having been a victim of violence at some time in their lives. The prevalence of assault, rape, and attempted rape appears to be especially high among transgender sex workers. Among a small group of MtF transgender sex workers in Washington, DC, 65% reported having been assaulted since beginning sex work and 35% reported having been raped (Valera et al., 2001).

10 Summary, Conclusions, and Future Perspectives

Some transgender health issues overlap with those of the lesbian, gay, and bisexual (LGB) communities, whereas other transgender health issues are more specialized. The phenomenon that unites the LGB and transgender communities is gender variance. The gender variance of transgender persons is obvious, but LGB persons are also gender-variant in their sexual partner preference and most are gender-variant in other ways as well. Many of the health concerns of LGB communities—especially issues related to mental health, suicide and self-harm, violence, and the sequelae of high-risk sexual behaviors, including HIV infection and other STIs—are plausibly linked to the psychological, social, and economic consequences of living as gender-variant persons in an intolerant society. To the extent that this is true, the health concerns of LGB persons and transgender persons overlap and may find similar solutions. Other transgender health concerns, however, are specific to transgender persons and derive largely from the powerful desire of many transgender persons to change their bodies to more closely reflect their identities. Specific health concerns related to hormone therapy, masculinizing and feminizing surgery, and liquid silicone injection, for example, all reflect transgender persons' often relentless pursuit of bodily transformation.

Cross-sex hormone therapy is highly effective in relieving gender dysphoria and is at least moderately effective in producing physical transformation, especially in FtM transgender persons. Hormone therapy could potentially benefit many more transgender persons than currently receive it, including the many male cross-dressers whose interest in hormones plausibly reflects untreated gender dysphoria. Although potentially the risks of hormone therapy should not be disregarded, reported complications are remarkably infrequent. Postpubertal hormone therapy is, however, limited in the degree of physical transformation it can produce, especially in MtF transgender persons, whose bodies have been irreversibly masculinized by testosterone. The key to increasing the effectiveness of hormone therapy may be earlier intervention, especially increasing the availability of puberty-blocking hormones during the early teenage years. Although earlier hormonal intervention is likely to be controversial in many quarters, initial experience has been encouraging. Transgender health advocates who take issues of prevention seriously should make the initiation of controlled trials of puberty-blocking hormones a high priority.

Transgender persons seek surgery and quasisurgical interventions, such as liquid silicone injections, to try to achieve the physical transformations that hormone therapy alone cannot produce. The quality of transgender surgical procedures is decidedly uneven: MtF SRS is now highly successful, but there are still no really satisfactory FtM SRS techniques and no satisfactory lower-body tissue augmentation techniques for MtF transgender persons. The deficiencies and complications of FtM SRS and the continued use of liquid silicone injections by MtF transgender persons largely reflect the limitations of current surgical techniques: Although surgeons are very good at removing and rearranging tissue, they are still limited in their ability to augment tissue or to create it de novo. It is likely that FtM SRS will improve incrementally, but developing a truly satisfactory FtM SRS procedure and eliminating the tragic consequences of liquid silicone injections in MtF transgender persons may ultimately depend on advances in biotechnology, especially the development of improved tissue augmentation materials and effective techniques for in vitro tissue and organ culture. Given these difficult realities, the specialized health concerns of transgender persons are likely to continue to challenge clinicians and researchers for the foreseeable future.

References

American Academy of Family Physicians. (2004) *Summary of policy recommendations for periodic health examinations.* AAFP, Leawood, KS.

American Psychiatric Association. (1987) *Diagnostic and Statistical Manual of Mental Disorders*, 3rd ed., revised. APA, Washington, DC.

American Psychiatric Association. (2000) *Diagnostic and Statistical Manual of Mental Disorders*, 4th ed., text revision. APA, Washington, DC.

Asscheman, H., and Gooren, L.J.G. (1992) Hormone treatment in transsexuals. *Journal of Psychology and Human Sexuality* 5(4):39–54.

Asscheman, H., Gooren, L.J.G., Assies, J., Smits, J.P.H., and de Slegte, R. (1988) Prolactin levels and pituitary enlargement in hormone-treated male-to-female transsexuals. *Clinical Endocrinology (Oxford)* 28:583–588.

Asscheman, H., Gooren, L.J.G., and Eklund, P.L. (1989) Mortality and morbidity in transsexual patients with cross-gender hormone treatment. *Metabolism* 38:869–873.

Bakker, A., van Kesteren, P.J., Gooren, L.J.G., and Bezemer, P.D. (1993) The prevalence of transsexualism in The Netherlands. *Acta Psychiatrica Scandinavica* 87:237–238.

Balen, A.H., Schachter, M.E., Montgomery, D., Reid, R.W., and Jacobs, H.S. (1993) Polycystic ovaries are a common finding in untreated female to male transsexuals. *Clinical Endocrinology (Oxford)* 38:325–329.

Baltieri, D.A., and de Andrade, A.G. (2005) Transsexual genital self-mutilation. *American Journal of Forensic Medicine and Pathology* 26:268–270.

Banks, E., Reeves, G., Beral, V., Bull, D., Crossley, B., Simmonds, M., Hilton, E., Bailey, S., Barrett, N., Briers, P., English, R., Jackson, A., Kutt, E., Lavelle, J., Rockall, L., Wallis, M.G., Wilson, M., and Patnick, J. (2004) Impact of use of hormone replacement therapy on false positive recall in the NHS breast screening programme: results from the Million Women Study. *BMJ* 328:1291–1292.

Beatrice, J. (1985) A psychological comparison of heterosexuals, transvestites, preoperative transsexuals, and postoperative transsexuals. *Journal of Nervous and Mental Disease* 173:358–365.

Bigatà, X., Ribera, M., Bielsa, I., and Ferrándiz, C. (2001) Adverse granulomatous reaction after cosmetic dermal silicone injection. *Dermatologic Surgery* 27:198–200.

Block, N.L., and Tessler, A.N. (1971) Transsexualism and surgical procedures. *Surgery, Gynecology & Obstetrics* 132:517–525.

Bodlund, O., and Armelius, K. (1994) Self-image and personality traits in gender identity disorders: an empirical study. *Journal of Sex and Marital Therapy* 20:303–317.

Bosinski, H.A.G., Peter, M., Bonatz, G., Arndt, R., Heidenreich, M., Sippell, W.G., and Wille, R. (1997) A higher rate of hyperandrogenic disorders in female-to-male transsexuals. *Psychoneuroendocrinology* 22:361–380.

Brown, G.R., Wise, T.N., Costa, P.T., Jr., Herbst, J.H., Fagan, P.J., and Schmidt, C.W., Jr. (1996) Personality characteristics and sexual functioning of 188 cross-dressing men. *Journal of Nervous and Mental Disease* 184:265–273.

Brown, S.L., Todd, J.F., and Luu, H.M. (2004) Breast implant adverse events during mammography: reports to the Food and Drug Administration. *Journal of Womens Health* 13:371–378.

Burcombe, R.J., Makris, A., Pittam, M., and Finer, N. (2003) Breast cancer after bilateral subcutaneous mastectomy in a female-to-male trans-sexual. *Breast* 12:290–293.

Burgess, H.E., and Shousha, S. (1993) An immunohistochemical study of the long-term effects of androgen administration on female-to-male transsexual breast: a comparison with normal female breast and male breast showing gynaecomastia. *Journal of Pathology* 170:37–43.

Centers for Disease Control and Prevention. (2004) *HIV/AIDS surveillance report*. U.S. Department of Health and Human Services, Centers for Disease Control and Prevention, Atlanta.

Chadha, S., Pache, T.D., Huikeshoven, J.M., Brinkmann, A.O., and van der Kwast, T.H. (1994) Androgen receptor expression in human ovarian and uterine tissue of long-term androgen-treated transsexual women. *Human Pathology* 25:1198–1204.

Chastre, J., Brun, P., Soler, P., Basset, F., Trouillet, J.L., Fagon, J.Y., Gibert, C., and Hance, A.J. (1987) Acute and latent pneumonitis after subcutaneous injections of silicone in transsexual men. *American Review of Respiratory Disease* 135:236–240.

Clements-Nolle, K., Marx, R., Guzman, R., and Katz, M. (2001) HIV prevalence, risk behaviors, health care use, and mental health status of transgender persons: implications for public health intervention. *American Journal of Public Health* 91:915–921.

Cohen-Kettenis, P.T., and Gooren, L.J.G. (1992) The influence of hormone treatment on psychosexual functioning in transsexuals. *Journal of Psychology and Human Sexuality* 5(4):55–67.

Cohen-Kettenis, P.T., and Pfäfflin, F. (2003) *Transgenderism and intersexuality in childhood and adolescence*. Sage, Thousand Oaks, CA.

Cohen-Kettenis, P.T., and van Goozen, S.H. (1997) Sex reassignment of adolescent transsexuals: a follow-up study. *Journal of the American Academy of Child and Adolescent Psychiatry* 36:263–271.

Cohen-Kettenis, P.T., and van Goozen, S.H. (1998) Pubertal delay as an aid in diagnosis and treatment of a transsexual adolescent. *European Child & Adolescent Psychiatry* 7:246–248.

Cole, C.M., O'Boyle, M., Emory, L.E., and Meyer, W.J., III. (1997) Comorbidity of gender dysphoria and other major psychiatric diagnoses. *Archives of Sexual Behavior* 26:13–26.

Coronary Drug Project Research Group. (1970) The Coronary Drug Project: initial findings leading to modifications of its research protocol. *JAMA* 214:1303–1313.

Dahl, M., Feldman, J.L., Goldberg, J., and Jaberi, A. (2006) Endocrine therapy for transgender adults in British Columbia: suggested guidelines. Retrieved

April 10, 2006, from http://www.vch.ca/transhealth/resources/library/tcpdocs/guidelines-endocrine.pdf.

Damewood, M.D., Bellantoni, J.J., Bachorik, P.S., Kimball, A.W., Jr., and Rock, J.A. (1989) Exogenous estrogen effect on lipid/lipoprotein cholesterol in transsexual males. *Journal of Endocrinological Investigation* 12:449–454.

De Cuypere, G., Jannes, C., and Rubens, R. (1995) Psychosocial functioning of transsexuals in Belgium. *Acta Psychiatrica Scandinavica* 91:180–184.

De Cuypere, G., T'Sjoen, G., Beerten, R., Selvaggi, G., De Sutter, P., Hoebeke, P., Monstrey, S., Vansteenwegen, A., and Rubens, R. (2005) Sexual and physical health after sex reassignment surgery. *Archives of Sexual Behavior* 34:679–690.

Derogatis, L.R., Meyer, J.K., and Boland, P. (1981) A psychological profile of the transsexual. II. The female. *Journal of Nervous and Mental Disease* 169:157–168.

Derogatis, L.R., Meyer, J.K., and Vazquez, N. (1978) A psychological profile of the transsexual. I. The male. *Journal of Nervous and Mental Disease* 166:234–254.

De Sutter, P. (2001) Gender reassignment and assisted reproduction: present and future reproductive options for transsexual people. *Human Reproduction* 16:612–614.

De Sutter, P., Kira, K., Verschoor, A., and Hotimsky, A. (2003) The desire to have children and the preservation of fertility in transsexual women: a survey. *International Journal of Transgenderism* 6(3). Retrieved August 18, 2004 from http://www.symposion.com/ijt/ijtvo06no03_02.htm.

Dittrich, R., Binder, H., Cupisti, S., Hoffmann, I., Beckmann, M.W., and Mueller, A. (2005) Endocrine treatment of male-to-female transsexuals using gonadotropin-releasing hormone agonist. *Experimental and Clinical Endocrinology & Diabetes* 113:586–592.

Dixen, J.M., Maddever, H., Van Maasdam, J., and Edwards, P.W. (1984) Psychosocial characteristics of applicants evaluated for surgical gender reassignment. *Archives of Sexual Behavior* 13:269–276.

Dizon, D.S., Tejada-Berges, T., Koelliker, S., Steinhoff, M., and Granai, C.O. (2006) Ovarian cancer associated with testosterone supplementation in a female-to-male transsexual patient. *Gynecologic and Obstetric Investigation* 62:226–228.

Docter, R.F., and Fleming, J.S. (1992) Dimensions of transvestism and transsexualism: the validation and factorial structure of the Cross-Gender Questionnaire. *Journal of Psychology and Human Sexuality* 5(4):15–37.

Docter, R.F., and Fleming, J.S. (2001) Measures of transgender behavior. *Archives of Sexual Behavior* 30:255–271.

Docter, R.F., and Prince, V. (1997) Transvestism: a survey of 1032 cross-dressers. *Archives of Sexual Behavior* 26:589–605.

Driak, D., and Samudovsky, M. (2004) Cervical cancer in a female-to-male trans-sexual [letter to the editor]. *European Journal of Cancer* 40:1795.

Dunn, B.K., Wickerham, D.L., and Ford, L.G. (2005) Prevention of hormone-related cancers: breast cancer. *Journal of Clinical Oncology* 23:357–367.

Duong, T., Schonfeld, A.J., Yungbluth, M., and Slotten, R. (1998) Acute pneumopathy in a nonsurgical transsexual. *Chest* 113:1127–1129.

Elbers, J.M., Asscheman, H., Seidell, J.C., Frolich, M., Meinders, A.E., and Gooren, L.J.G. (1997) Reversal of the sex difference in serum leptin levels upon cross-sex hormone administration in transsexuals. *Journal of Clinical Endocrinology and Metabolism* 82:3267–3270.

Elbers, J.M., Asscheman, H., Seidell, J.C., and Gooren, L.J.G. (1999) Effects of sex steroid hormones on regional fat depots as assessed by magnetic resonance imaging in transsexuals. *American Journal of Physiology* 276(2, Pt. 1): E317–325.

Elbers, J.M., Giltay, E.J., Teerlink, T., Scheffer, P.G., Asscheman, H., Seidell, J.C., and Gooren, L.J.G. (2003) Effects of sex steroids on components of the insulin resistance syndrome in transsexual subjects. *Clinical Endocrinology (Oxford)* 58:562–571.

Elifson, K.W., Boles, J., Posey, E., Sweat, M., Darrow, W., and Elsea, W. (1993) Male transvestite prostitutes and HIV risk. *American Journal of Public Health* 83:260–262.

Ellenbogen, R., and Rubin, L. (1975) Injectable fluid silicone therapy: human morbidity and mortality. *JAMA* 234:308–309.

Feldman, J. (2002) New onset of type 2 diabetes mellitus with feminizing hormone therapy: case series. *International Journal of Transgenderism* 6(2). Retrieved August 18, 2004 from http://www.symposion.com/ijt/ijtvo06no02_01.htm.

Feldman, J., and Bockting, W. (2003) Transgender health. *Minnesota Medicine* 86(7):25–32.

Fleming, M., Cohen, D., Salt, P., Jones, D., and Jenkins, S. (1981) A study of pre- and postsurgical transsexuals: MMPI characteristics. *Archives of Sexual Behavior* 10:161–170.

Fox, L.P., Geyer, A.S., Husain, S., Della-Latta, P., and Grossman, M.E. (2004) Mycobacterium abscessus cellulitis and multifocal abscesses of the breasts in a transsexual from illicit intramammary injections of silicone. *Journal of the American Academy of Dermatology* 50:450–454.

Futterweit, W. (1998) Endocrine therapy of transsexualism and potential complications of long-term treatment. *Archives of Sexual Behavior* 27:209–226.

Futterweit, W., and Deligdisch, L. (1986) Histopathological effects of exogenously administered testosterone in 19 female to male transsexuals. *Journal of Clinical Endocrinology and Metabolism* 62:16–21.

Futterweit, W., Gabrilove, J.L., and Smith, H., Jr. (1984) Testicular steroidogenic response to human chorionic gonadotropin of fifteen male transsexuals on chronic estrogen treatment. *Metabolism* 33:936–942.

Futterweit, W., Weiss, R.A., and Fagerstrom, R.M. (1986) Endocrine evaluation of forty female-to-male transsexuals: increased frequency of polycystic ovarian disease in female transsexualism. *Archives of Sexual Behavior* 15:69–78.

Gaber, Y. (2004) Secondary lymphoedema of the lower leg as an unusual side-effect of a liquid silicone injection in the hips and buttocks. *Dermatology* 208:342–344.

Ganly, I., and Taylor, E.W. (1995) Breast cancer in a trans-sexual man receiving hormone replacement therapy. *British Journal of Surgery* 82:341.

Giltay, E.J., and Gooren, L.J.G. (2000) Effects of sex steroid deprivation/administration on hair growth and skin sebum production in transsexual males and females. *Journal of Clinical Endocrinology and Metabolism* 85:2913–2921.

Giltay, E.J., Hoogeveen, E.K., Elbers, J.M., Gooren, L.J.G., Asscheman, H., and Stehouwer, C.D. (1998) Effects of sex steroids on plasma total homocysteine levels: a study in transsexual males and females. *Journal of Clinical Endocrinology and Metabolism* 83:550–553.

Giltay, E.J., Toorians, A.W., Sarabdjitsingh, A.R., de Vries, N.A., and Gooren, L.J.G. (2004) Established risk factors for coronary heart disease are unrelated to androgen-induced baldness in female-to-male transsexuals. *Journal of Endocrinology* 180:107–112.

Giraldo, F., Mora, M.J., Solano, A., Gonzáles, C., and Smith-Fernández, V. (2002) Male perineogenital anatomy and clinical applications in genital reconstructions and male-to-female sex reassignment surgery. *Plastic and Reconstructive Surgery* 109:1301–1310.

Goh, H.H., and Ratnam, S.S. (1997) Effects of hormone deficiency, androgen therapy and calcium supplementation on bone mineral density in female transsexuals. *Maturitas* 26:45–52.

Gooren, L.J.G. (1999) Hormonal sex reassignment. *International Journal of Transgender* 3(3). Retrieved August 18, 2004 from http://www.symposion.com/ijt/ijt990301.htm.

Gooren, L. (2005) Hormone treatment of the adult transsexual patient. *Hormone Research* 64(Suppl. 2):31–36.

Gooren, L., and Delemarre-van de Waal, H. (1996) The feasibility of endocrine interventions in juvenile transsexuals. *Journal of Psychology and Human Sexuality* 8(4):69–74.

Gooren, L., Asscheman, H., and Newling, D. (1997) Prostate cancer in male-to-female transsexual. Presented at the XV Harry Benjamin International Gender Dysphoria Association Symposium, Vancouver, BC, Canada.

Gooren, L.J.G., Assies, J., Asscheman, H., de Slegte, R., and van Kessel, H. (1988) Estrogen-induced prolactinoma in a man. *Journal of Clinical Endocrinology and Metabolism* 66:444–446.

Gooren, L.J.G., Harmsen-Louman, W., and van Kessel, H. (1985) Follow-up of prolactin levels in long-term oestrogen-treated male-to-female transsexuals with regard to prolactinoma induction. *Clinical Endocrinology (Oxford)* 22:201–207.

Gottlieb, L.J., Levine, L.A., and Zachary, L.S. (1999) Radial forearm free flap for phallic reconstruction. In: Ehrlich, R., and Alter, G. (eds) *Reconstructive and plastic surgery of the external genitalia.* Saunders, Philadelphia, pp. 294–300.

Grabellus, F., Worm, K., Willruth, A., Schmitz, K.J., Otterbach, F., Baba, H.A., Kimmig, R., and Metz, K.A. (2005) ETV6-NTRK3 gene fusion in a secretory carcinoma of the breast of a male-to-female transsexual. *Breast* 14:71–74.

Grant, B.F., Hasin, D.S., Stinson, F.S., Dawson, D.A., Chou, S.P., Ruan, W.J., and Pickering, R.P. (2004a) Prevalence, correlates, and disability of personality disorders in the United States: results from the national epidemiologic survey on alcohol and related conditions. *Journal of Clinical Psychiatry* 65:948–958.

Grant, B.F., Stinson, F.S., Dawson, D.A., Chou, S.P., Dufour, M.C., Compton, W., Pickering, R.P., and Kaplan, K. (2004b) Prevalence and co-occurrence of substance use disorders and independent mood and anxiety disorders: results from the National Epidemiologic Survey on Alcohol and Related Conditions. *Archives of General Psychiatry* 61:807–816.

Green, R., and Fleming, D.T. (1990) Transsexual surgery follow-up: status in the 1990s. *Annual Review of Sex Research* 1:163–174.

Greenman, Y. (2004) The endocrine care of transsexual people [letter to the editor]. *Journal of Clinical Endocrinology and Metabolism* 89:1014.

Hage, J.J. (1996) Metaidoioplasty: an alternative phalloplasty technique in transsexuals. *Plastic and Reconstructive Surgery* 97:161–167.

Hage, J.J., and Karim, R.B. (2000) Ought GIDNOS get nought? Treatment options for nontranssexual gender dysphoria. *Plastic and Reconstructive Surgery* 105:1222–1227.

Hage, J.J., and van Kesteren, P.J. (1995) Chest-wall contouring in female-to-male transsexuals: basic considerations and review of the literature. *Plastic and Reconstructive Surgery* 96:386–391.

Hage, J.J., Dekker, J.J., Karim, R.B., Verheijen, R.H., and Bloemena, E. (2000) Ovarian cancer in female-to-male transsexuals: report of two cases. *Gynecologic Oncology* 76:413–415.

Hage, J.J., Kanhai, R.C., Oen, A.L., van Diest, P.J., and Karim, R.B. (2001) The devastating outcome of massive subcutaneous injection of highly viscous fluids in male-to-female transsexuals. *Plastic and Reconstructive Surgery* 107:734–741.

Haraldsen, I.R., and Dahl, A.A. (2000) Symptom profiles of gender dysphoric patients of transsexual type compared to patients with personality disorders and healthy adults. *Acta Psychiatrica Scandinavica* 102:276–281.

Harder, Y., Erni, D., and Banic, A. (2002) Squamous cell carcinoma of the penile skin in a neovagina 20 years after male-to-female reassignment. *British Journal of Plastic Surgery* 55:449–451.

Harris, R., and Lohr, K.N. (2002) Screening for prostate cancer: an update of the evidence for the U.S. Preventive Services Task Force. *Annals of Internal Medicine* 137:917–929.

Hepp, U., Kraemer, B., Schnyder, U., Miller, N., and Delsignore, A. (2005) Psychiatric comorbidity in gender identity disorder. *Journal of Psychosomatic Research* 58:259–261.

Hoebeke, P., de Cuypere, G., Ceulemans, P., and Monstrey, S. (2003) Obtaining rigidity in total phalloplasty: experience with 35 patients. *Journal of Urology* 169:221–223.

Hoenig, J., and Kenna, J.C. (1974) The nosological position of transsexualism. *Archives of Sexual Behavior* 3:273–287.

Hunt, D.D., Carr, J.E., and Hampson, J.L. (1981) Cognitive correlates of biologic sex and gender identity in transsexualism. *Archives of Sexual Behavior* 10:65–77.

Israel, G.E., and Tarver, D.E., II. (1997) *Transgender care: recommended guidelines, practical information, and personal accounts*. Temple University Press, Philadelphia.

Jequier, A.M., Bullimore, N.J., and Bishop, M.J. (1989) Cyproterone acetate and a small dose of oestrogen in the pre-operative management of male transsexuals: a report of three cases. *Andrologia* 21:456–461.

Jin, B., Turner, L., Walters, W.A., and Handelsman, D.J. (1996) The effects of chronic high dose androgen or estrogen treatment on the human prostate. *Journal of Clinical Endocrinology and Metabolism* 81:4290–4295.

Kanhai, R.C., Hage, J.J., and Karim, R.B. (2001) Augmentation mammaplasty in male-to-female trans-sexuals: facts and figures from Amsterdam. *Scandinavian Journal of Plastic and Reconstructive Surgery and Hand Surgery* 35:203–206.

Kanhai, R.C., Hage, J.J., and Mulder, J.W. (2000a) Long-term outcome of augmentation mammaplasty in male-to-female transsexuals: a questionnaire survey of 107 patients. *British Journal of Plastic Surgery* 53:209–211.

Kanhai, R.C., Hage, J.J., Bloemena, E., van Diest, P.J., and Karim, R.B. (1999) Mammary fibroadenoma in a male-to-female transsexual. *Histopathology* 35:183–185.

Kanhai, R.C., Hage, J.J., van Diest, P.J., Bloemena, E., and Mulder, J.W. (2000b) Short-term and long-term histologic effects of castration and estrogen treatment on breast tissue of 14 male-to-female transsexuals in comparison with two chemically castrated men. *American Journal of Surgical Pathology* 24:74–80.

Karim, R.B., Hage, J.J., and Mulder, J.W. (1996) Neovaginoplasty in male transsexuals: review of surgical techniques and recommendations regarding eligibility. *Annals of Plastic Surgery* 37:669–675.

Kellogg, T.A., Clements-Nolle, K., Dilley, J., Katz, M.H., and McFarland, W. (2001) Incidence of human immunodeficiency virus among male-to-female transgendered persons in San Francisco. *Journal of Acquired Immune Deficiency Syndrome* 28:380–384.

Kenagy, G.P. (2002) HIV among transgendered people. *AIDS Care* 14:127–134.

Kessler, R.C., Berglund, P., Demler, O., Jin, R., Merikangas, K.R., and Walters, E.E. (2005a) Lifetime prevalence and age-of-onset distributions of DSM-IV disorders in the National Comorbidity Survey Replication. *Archives of General Psychiatry* 62:593–602.

Kessler, R.C., Chiu, W.T., Demler, O., Merikangas, K.R., and Walters, E.E. (2005b) Prevalence, severity, and comorbidity of 12-month DSM-IV disorders in the National Comorbidity Survey Replication. *Archives of General Psychiatry* 62:617–627.

Kim, C.H., Chung, D.H., Yoo, C.G., Lee, C.T., Han, S.K., Shim, Y.S., and Kim, Y.W. (2003) A case of acute pneumonitis induced by injection of silicone for colpoplasty. *Respiration* 70:104–106.

Kirk, S. (2001) Human papilloma virus infection: a potential menace in the transsexual community and the importance of gynecologic evaluation for the postoperative male to female transsexual. Presented at the XVII Harry Benjamin International Symposium on Gender Dysphoria, Galveston, TX.

Kovacs, K., Stefaneanu, L., Ezzat, S., and Smyth, H.S. (1994) Prolactin-producing pituitary adenoma in a male-to-female transsexual patient with protracted estrogen administration: a morphologic study. *Archives of Pathology & Laboratory Medicine* 118:562–565.

Krege, S., Bex, A., Lümmen, G., and Rübben, H. (2001) Male-to-female transsexualism: a technique, results, and long-term follow-up in 66 patients. *BJU International* 88:396–402.

Krieger, M.J., McAninch, J.W., and Weimer, S.R. (1982) Self-performed bilateral orchiectomy in transsexuals. *Journal of Clinical Psychiatry* 43:292–293.

Kuiper, B., and Cohen-Kettenis, P.T. (1988) Sex reassignment surgery: a study of 141 Dutch transsexuals. *Archives of Sexual Behavior* 17:439–457.

Kwan, M., Van Maasdam, J., and Davidson, J.M. (1985) Effects of estrogen treatment on sexual behavior in male-to-female transsexuals: experimental and clinical observations. *Archives of Sexual Behavior* 14:29–40.

Langevin, R., Paitich, D., and Steiner, B. (1977) The clinical profile of male transsexuals living as females vs. those living as males. *Archives of Sexual Behavior* 6:143–154.

Langstrom, N., and Zucker, K.J. (2005) Transvestic fetishism in the general population: prevalence and correlates. *Journal of Sex & Marital Therapy* 31:87–95.

Laumann, E.O., Gagnon, J.H., Michael, R.T., and Michaels, S. (1994) *The social organization of sexuality: sexual practices in the United States*. University of Chicago Press, Chicago.

Lawrence, A.A. (2001) Vaginal neoplasia in a male-to-female transsexual: case report, review of the literature, and recommendations for cytological screening. *International Journal of Transgenderism* 5(1). Retrieved August 18, 2004, from http://www.symposion.com/ijt/ijtvo05no01_01.htm.

Lawrence, A.A. (2003) Factors associated with satisfaction or regret following male-to-female sex reassignment surgery. *Archives of Sexual Behavior* 32:299–315.

Lawrence, A.A. (in press) Self-reported complications and functional outcomes of male-to-female sex reassignment surgery. *Archives of Sexual Behavior*.

Lawrence, A.A., Shaffer, J.D., Snow, W.R., Chase, C., and Headlam, B.T. (1996) Health care needs of transgendered patients [letter to the editor]. *JAMA* 276:874.

Leavitt, F., Berger, J.C., Hoeppner, J.-A., and Northrop, G. (1980) Presurgical adjustment in male transsexuals with and without hormonal treatment. *Journal of Nervous and Mental Disease* 168:693–697.

Leinonen, P., Ruokonen, A., Kontturi, M., and Vihko, R. (1981) Effects of estrogen treatment on human testicular unconjugated steroid and steroid sulfate production in vivo. *Journal of Clinical Endocrinology and Metabolism* 53:569–573.

Lemmo, G., Garcea, N., Corsello, S., Tarquini, E., Palladino, T., Ardito, G., and Garcea, R. (2003) Breast fibroadenoma in a male-to-female transsexual patient after hormonal treatment. *European Journal of Surgery Supplement* 588:69–71.

Lev, A.I. (2004) *Transgender emergence: therapeutic guidelines for working with gender-variant people and their families*. Haworth Clinical Practice Press, Binghamton, NY.

Levine, S.B., Brown, G., Coleman, E., Cohen-Kettenis, P., Hage, J.J., Van Maasdam, J., Petersen, M., Pfäfflin, F., and Schaefer, L.C. (1998) *The standards of care for gender identity disorders*, 5th ed. Symposion, Düsseldorf.

Lips, P., van Kesteren, P.J., Asscheman, H., and Gooren, L.J.G. (1996) The effect of androgen treatment on bone metabolism in female-to-male transsexuals. *Journal of Bone and Mineral Research* 11:1769–1773.

Lombardi, E.L., Wilchins, R.A., Priesing, D., and Malouf, D. (2001) Gender violence: transgender experiences with violence and discrimination. *Journal of Homosexuality* 42(1):89–101.

Lothstein, L.M. (1992) Clinical management of gender dysphoria in young boys: genital mutilation and DSM-IV implications. *Journal of Psychology and Human Sexuality* 5(4):87–106.

Lübbert, H., Leo-Rossberg, I., and Hammerstein, J. (1992) Effects of ethinyl estradiol on semen quality and various hormonal parameters in a eugonadal male. *Fertility and Sterility* 58:603–608.

Markland, C. (1975) Transexual surgery. *Obstetrics and Gynecology Annual* 4:309–330.

Mate-Kole, C., Freschi, M., and Robin, A. (1990) A controlled study of psychological and social change after surgical gender reassignment in selected male transsexuals. *British Journal of Psychiatry* 157:261–264.

McCredie, R.J., McCrohon, J.A., Turner, L., Griffiths, K.A., Handelsman, D.J., and Celermajer, D.S. (1998) Vascular reactivity is impaired in genetic females taking high-dose androgens. *Journal of the American College of Cardiology* 32:1331–1335.

McCrohon, J.A., Walters, W.A., Robinson, J.T., McCredie, R.J., Turner, L., Adams, M.R., Handelsman, D.J., and Celermajer, D.S. (1997) Arterial reactivity is enhanced in genetic males taking high dose estrogens. *Journal of the American College of Cardiology* 29:1432–1436.

McGovern, S.J. (1995) Self-castration in a transsexual. *Journal of Accident & Emergency Medicine* 12:57–58.

McGowan, C.K. (1999) *Transgender needs assessment*. HIV Prevention Planning Unit, New York City Department of Health, New York.

Meyenburg, B. (1999) Gender identity disorder in adolescence: outcomes of psychotherapy. *Adolescence* 34:305–313.

Meyer, W., III, Bockting, W.O., Cohen-Kettenis, P., Coleman, E., DiCeglie, D., Devor, H., Gooren, L., Hage, J.J. , Kirk, S., Kuiper, B., Laub, D., Lawrence, A., Menard, Y., Monstrey, S., Patton, J., Schaefer, L., Webb, A., and Wheeler, C.C. (2001) *The standards of care for gender identity disorders*, 6th ed. Symposion, Düsseldorf.

Meyer, W.J., III, Webb, A., Stuart, C.A., Finkelstein, J.W., Lawrence, B., and Walker, P.A. (1986) Physical and hormonal evaluation of transsexual patients: a longitudinal study. *Archives of Sexual Behavior* 15:121–138.

Miach, P.P., Berah, E.F., Butcher, J.N., and Rouse, S. (2000) Utility of the MMPI-2 in assessing gender dysphoric patients. *Journal of Personality Assessment* 75:268–279.

Michel, A., Ansseau, M., Legros, J.J., Pitchot, W., Cornet, J.P., and Mormont, C. (2002) Comparisons of two groups of sex-change applicants based on the MMPI. *Psychological Reports* 91:233–240.

Michel, A., Mormont, C., and Legros, J.J. (2001) A psycho-endocrinological overview of transsexualism. *European Journal of Endocrinology* 145:365–376.

Miglioretti, D.L., Rutter, C.M., Geller, B.M., Cutter, G., Barlow, W.E., Rosenberg, R., Weaver, D.L., Taplin, S.H., Ballard-Barbash, R., Carney, P.A., Yankaskas, B.C., and Kerlikowske, K. (2004) Effect of breast augmentation on the accuracy of mammography and cancer characteristics. *JAMA* 291:442–450.

Miller, N., Bedard, Y.C., Cooter, N.B., and Shaul, D.L. (1986) Histological changes in the genital tract in transsexual women following androgen therapy. *Histopathology* 10:661–669.

Moore, E., Wisniewski, A., and Dobs, A. (2003) Endocrine treatment of transsexual people: a review of treatment regimens, outcomes, and adverse effects. *Journal of Clinical Endocrinology and Metabolism* 88:3467–3473.

Mueller, A., Dittrich, R., Binder, H., Kuehnel, W., Maltaris, T., Hoffmann, I., and Beckmann, M.W. (2005) High dose estrogen treatment increases bone mineral density in male-to-female transsexuals receiving gonadotropin-releasing hormone agonist in the absence of testosterone. *European Journal of Endocrinology* 153:107–113.

Muirhead-Allwood, S.K., Royle, M.G., and Young, R. (1999) *Sexuality and satisfaction with surgical results in male-to-female transsexuals.* Poster presented at the Harry Benjamin International Gender Dysphoria Association XVI Biennial Symposium, London.

Murphy, D., Murphy, M., and Grainger, R. (2001) Self-castration. *Irish Journal of Medical Science* 170:195.

Nemoto, T., Luke, D., Mamo, L., Ching, A., and Patria, J. (1999) HIV risk behaviours among male-to-female transgenders in comparison with homosexual or bisexual males and heterosexual females. *AIDS Care* 11:297–312.

Nemoto, T., Operario, D., Keatley, J., Han, L., and Soma, T. (2004) HIV risk behaviors among male-to-female transgender persons of color in San Francisco. *American Journal of Public Health* 94:1193–1199.

New, G., Timmins, K.L., Duffy, S.J., Tran, B.T., O'Brien, R.C., Harper, R.W., and Meredith, I.T. (1997) Long-term estrogen therapy improves vascular function in male to female transsexuals. *Journal of the American College of Cardiology* 29:1437–1444.

Newfield, E., Hart, S., Dibble, S., and Kohler, L. (in press) Female-to-male transgender quality of life. *Quality of Life Research.*

Orentreich, N., and Durr, N.P. (1974) Mammogenesis in transsexuals. *Journal of Investigative Dermatology* 63:142–146.

Oriel, K.A. (2000) Medical care of transsexual patients. *Journal of the Gay and Lesbian Medical Association* 4:185–194.

Perego, E., Scaini, A., Romano, F., Franciosi, C., and Uggeri, F. (2004) Estrogen-induced severe acute pancreatitis in a male. *JOP* 5:352–356. Retrieved March 3, 2006, from http://www.joplink.net/prev/200409/200409_06.pdf.

Perrone, A.M., Cerpolini, S., D'Emidio, L., Mollo, F., Pelusi, G., and Meriggiola, M.C. (2003) *Effects of long-term testosterone administration on sexual behavior and mood in female to male subjects.* Presented at the XVIII Biennial Symposium of the Harry Benjamin International Gender Dysphoria Association, Ghent, Belgium.

Polderman, K.H., Gooren, L.J.G., Asscheman, H., Bakker, A., and Heine, R.J. (1994) Induction of insulin resistance by androgens and estrogens. *Journal of Clinical Endocrinology and Metabolism* 79:265–271.

Prior, J.C., Vigna, Y.M., and Watson, D. (1989) Spironolactone with physiological female steroids for presurgical therapy of male-to-female transsexualism. *Archives of Sexual Behavior* 18:49–57.

Pritchard, T.J., Pankowsky, D.A., Crowe, J.P., and Abdul-Karim, F.W. (1988) Breast cancer in a male-to-female transsexual: a case report. *JAMA* 259:2278–2280.

Prosser, J. (1998) *Second skins: the body narratives of transsexuality.* Columbia University Press, New York.

Rae, V., Pardo, R.J., Blackwelder, P.L., and Falanga, V. (1989) Leg ulcers following subcutaneous injection of a liquid silicone preparation. *Archives of Dermatology* 125:670–673.

Rana, A., and Johnson, D. (1993) Sequential self-castration and amputation of penis. *British Journal of Urology* 71:750.

Reutrakul, S., Ongphiphadhanakul, B., Piaseu, N., Krittiyawong, S., Chanprasertyothin, S., Bunnag, P., and Rajatanavin, R. (1998) The effects of oestrogen exposure on bone mass in male to female transsexuals. *Clinical Endocrinology (Oxford)* 49:811–814.

Rhoden, E.L., and Morgentaler, A. (2004) Risks of testosterone-replacement therapy and recommendations for monitoring. *New England Journal of Medicine* 350:482–492.

Rodriguez, M.A., Martinez, M.C., Lopez-Artiguez, M., Soria, M.L., Bernier, F., and Repetto, M. (1989) Lung embolism with liquid silicone. *Journal of Forensic Science* 34:504–510.

Rohrmann, D., and Jakse, G. (2003) Urethroplasty in female-to-male transsexuals. *European Urology* 44:611–614.

Rosenmund, A., Köchli, H.P., and König, M.P. (1988) Sex-related differences in hematological values: a study on the erythrocyte and granulocyte count, plasma iron and iron-binding proteins in human transsexuals on contrasexual hormone therapy. *Blut* 56:13–17.

Rosioreanu, A., Brusca-Augello, G.T., Ahmed, Q.A., and Katz, D.S. (2004) CT visualization of silicone-related pneumonitis in a transsexual man. *American Journal of Roentgenology* 183:248–249.

Ross, M.W., and Need, J.A. (1989) Effects of adequacy of gender reassignment surgery on psychological adjustment: a follow-up of fourteen male-to-female patients. *Archives of Sexual Behavior* 18:145–153.

Scarabin, P.Y., Oger, E., and Plu-Bureau, G. (2003) Differential association of oral and transdermal oestrogen-replacement therapy with venous thromboembolism risk. *Lancet* 362:428–432.

Schlatterer, K., Auer, D.P., Yassouridis, A., von Werder, K., and Stalla, G.K. (1998a) Transsexualism and osteoporosis. *Experimental and Clinical Endocrinology & Diabetes* 106:365–368.

Schlatterer, K., von Werder, K., and Stalla, G.K. (1996) Multistep treatment concept of transsexual patients. *Experimental and Clinical Endocrinology & Diabetes* 104:413–419.

Schlatterer, K., Yassouridis, A., von Werder, K., Poland, D., Kemper, J., and Stalla, G.K. (1998b) A follow-up study for estimating the effectiveness of a cross-gender hormone substitution therapy on transsexual patients. *Archives of Sexual Behavior* 27:475–492.

Schroder, M., and Carroll, R. (1999) New women: sexological outcomes of male-to-female gender reassignment surgery. *Journal of Sex Education and Therapy* 24:137–146.

Schulze, C. (1988) Response of the human testis to long-term estrogen treatment: morphology of Sertoli cells, Leydig cells and spermatogonial stem cells. *Cell and Tissue Research* 251:31–43.

Sengezer, M., and Sadove, R.C. (1993) Scrotal construction by expansion of labia majora in biological female transsexuals. *Annals of Plastic Surgery* 31:372–376.

Serri, O., Noiseux, D., Robert, F., and Hardy, J. (1996) Lactotroph hyperplasia in an estrogen treated male-to-female transsexual patient. *Journal of Clinical Endocrinology and Metabolism* 81:3177–3179.

Shin, H., Lemke, B.N., Stevens, T.S., and Lim, M.J. (1998) Posterior ciliary-artery occlusion after subcutaneous silicone-oil injection. *Annals of Ophthalmology* 20:342–344.

Simon, P.A., Reback, C.J., and Bemis, C.C. (2000) HIV prevalence and incidence among male-to-female transsexuals receiving HIV prevention services in Los Angeles County. *AIDS* 14:2953–2955.

Slabbekoorn, D., van Goozen, S., Gooren, L., and Cohen-Kettenis, P. (2001) Effects of cross-sex hormone treatment on emotionality in transsexuals. *International Journal of Transgenderism* 5(3). Retrieved August 18, 2004, from http://www.symposion.com/ijt/ijtvo05no03_02.htm.

Smith, Y.L., van Goozen, S.H., and Cohen-Kettenis, P.T. (2001) Adolescents with gender identity disorder who were accepted or rejected for sex reassignment surgery: a prospective follow-up study. *Journal of the American Academy of Child and Adolescent Psychiatry* 40:472–481.

Sosa, M., Jódar, E., Arbelo, E., Domínguez, C., Saavedra, P., Torres, A., Salido, E., de Tejada, M.J., and Hernández, D. (2003) Bone mass, bone turnover, vitamin D, and estrogen receptor gene polymorphisms in male to female transsexuals: effects of estrogenic treatment on bone metabolism of the male. *Journal of Clinical Densitometry* 6:297–304.

Sosa, M., Jódar, E., Arbelo, E., Domínguez, C., Saavedra, P., Torres, A., Salido, E., Limiñana, J.M., Gómez de Tejada, M.J., and Hernández, D. (2004) Serum lipids and estrogen receptor gene polymorphisms in male-to-female transsexuals: effects of estrogen treatment. *European Journal of Internal Medicine* 15:231–237.

Spinder, T., Spijkstra, J.J., van den Tweel, J.G., Burger, C.W., van Kessel, H., Hompes, P.G., and Gooren, L.J.G. (1989) The effects of long term testosterone administration on pulsatile luteinizing hormone secretion and on ovarian histology in eugonadal female to male transsexual subjects. *Journal of Clinical Endocrinology and Metabolism* 69:151–157.

Symmers, W.S. (1968) Carcinoma of breast in trans-sexual individuals after surgical and hormonal interference with the primary and secondary sex characteristics. *British Medical Journal* 2:82–85.

Tangpricha, V., Afdhal, N.H., and Chipkin, S.R. (2001) Case report: auto-immune hepatitis in a male-to-female transsexual treated with conjugated estrogens. *International Journal of Transgenderism* 5(3). Retrieved August 18, 2004, from http://www.symposion.com/ijt/ijtvo05no03_03.htm.

Tangpricha, V., Ducharme, S.H., Barber, T.W., and Chipkin, S.R. (2003) Endocrinologic treatment of gender identity disorders. *Endocrine Practice* 9:12–21.

Thurston, A.V. (1994) Carcinoma of the prostate in a transsexual. *British Journal of Urology* 73:217.

Tjaden, P., and Thoennes, N. (2000) Full report of the prevalence, incidence, and consequences of violence against women: findings of the National Violence Against Women Survey. Publication no. NCJ 183781. U.S. Department of Justice, National Institute of Justice, Rockville, MD.

Tom Waddell Health Center Transgender Teamerican (2001) *Protocols for hormonal reassignment of gender*. Retrieved August 18, 2004, from http://www.dph.sf.ca.us/chn/HlthCtrs/HlthCtrDocs/TransGendprotocols.pdf.

Toorians, A.W., Thomassen, M.C., Zweegman, S., Magdeleyns, E.J., Tans, G., Gooren, L.J., and Rosing, J. (2003) Venous thrombosis and changes of hemostatic variables during cross-sex hormone treatment in transsexual people. *Journal of Clinical Endocrinology and Metabolism* 88:5723–5729.

T'Sjoen, G., Rubens, R., De Sutter, P., and Gooren, L. (2004) The endocrine care of transsexual people [letter to the editor]. *Journal of Clinical Endocrinology and Metabolism* 89:1014–1015.

Tsushima, W.T., and Wedding, D. (1979) MMPI results of male candidates for transsexual surgery. *Journal of Personality Assessment* 43:385–387.

Valera, R.J., Sawyer, R.G., and Schiraldi, G.R. (2001) Violence and posttraumatic stress disorder in a sample of inner city street prostitutes. *American Journal of Health Studies* 16:149–155.

Van Goozen, S.H., Cohen-Kettenis, P.T., Gooren, L.J.G., Frijda, N.H., and Van de Poll, N.E. (1995) Gender differences in behaviour: activating effects of cross-sex hormones. *Psychoneuroendocrinology* 20:343–363.

Van Haarst, E.P., Newling, D.W., Gooren, L.J.G., Asscheman, H., and Prenger, D.M. (1998) Metastatic prostatic carcinoma in a male-to-female transsexual. *British Journal of Urology* 81:776.

Van Kemenade, J.F.L.M., Cohen-Kettenis, P.T., Cohen, L., and Gooren, L.J.G. (1989) Effects of the pure antiandrogen RU 23.903 (anandron) on sexuality, aggression, and mood in male-to-female transsexuals. *Archives of Sexual Behavior* 18:217–228.

Van Kesteren, P.J., Asscheman, H., Megens, J.A., and Gooren, L.J. (1997) Mortality and morbidity in transsexual subjects treated with cross-sex hormones. *Clinical Endocrinology (Oxford)* 47:337–342.

Van Kesteren, P., Lips, P., Deville, W., Popp-Snijders, C., Asscheman, H., Megens, J., and Gooren, L.J.G. (1996a) The effect of one-year cross-sex hormonal treatment on bone metabolism and serum insulin-like growth factor-1 in transsexuals. *Journal of Clinical Endocrinology and Metabolism* 81:2227–2232.

Van Kesteren, P., Lips, P., Gooren, L.J.G., Asscheman, H., and Megens, J. (1998) Long-term follow-up of bone mineral density and bone metabolism in transsexuals treated with cross-sex hormones. *Clinical Endocrinology (Oxford)* 48:347–354.

Van Kesteren, P., Meinhardt, W., van der Valk, P., Geldof, A., Megens, J., and Gooren, L. (1996b) Effects of estrogens only on the prostates of aging men. *Journal of Urology* 156:1349–1353.

Verschoor, A.M., and Poortinga, J. (1988) Psychosocial differences between Dutch male and female transsexuals. *Archives of Sexual Behavior* 17:173–178.

Weinberg, M.S., Shaver, F.M., and Williams, C.J. (1999) Gendered sex work in the San Francisco tenderloin. *Archives of Sexual Behavior* 28:503–521.

Wiessing, L.G., van Roosmalen, M.S., Koedijk, P., Bieleman, B., and Houweling, H. (1999) Silicones, hormones and HIV in transgender street prostitutes [letter to the editor]. *AIDS* 13:2315–2316.

Women's Health Initiative Steering Committee. (2004) Effects of conjugated equine estrogen in postmenopausal women with hysterectomy: the Women's Health Initiative randomized controlled trial. *JAMA* 291:1701–1712.

Writing Group for the Women's Health Initiative Investigators. (2002) Risks and benefits of estrogen plus progestin in healthy postmenopausal women: principal results from the Women's Health Initiative randomized controlled trial. *JAMA* 288:321–333.

Xavier, J. (2000) *Final report of the Washington Transgender Needs Assessment Survey*. Administration for HIV and AIDS, Government of the District of Columbia, Washington, DC.

Zahl, P.H., Strand, B.H., and Maehlen, J. (2004) Incidence of breast cancer in Norway and Sweden during introduction of nationwide screening: prospective cohort study. *BMJ* 328:921–924.

Zucker, K.J. (2001) Gender identity disorder in children and adolescents. In: Gabbard, G.O. (ed) *Treatment of psychiatric disorders*, 3rd ed. American Psychiatric Publishing, Washington, DC, pp. 2069–2094.

Zwirska-Korczala, K., Ostrowska, Z., and Fryczkowski, M. (1996) Effect of long-term androgen treatment on the function of hypothalamo-hypophysial and -adrenal axes in transsexual agonadal women. *Endocrine Regulations* 30:163–172.

20

Health Care of Lesbians and Bisexual Women

Katherine A. O'Hanlan and Christy M. Isler

1 Introduction

Historically, survey data reveal that lesbians have experienced ostracism, rough treatment, and derogatory comments by their medical practitioners (Stevens & Hall, 1988; Kass et al., 1992). As a result, many lesbians have decided not to tell their physicians about their orientation (Hughes, 2004). Some patients have perceived the negative attitudes some of their caregivers have toward them, causing them to hesitate about returning or obtaining routine health maintenance visits. Surveys of physicians (Mathews et al., 1986) and nursing professionals (Eliason, 1998) confirm that about 30% of caregivers have discomfort providing care to lesbian patients and have received little training about issues of orientation (Albarran & Salmon, 2000; Risdon et al., 2000) Additionally, some lesbians are limited in their access to health care because they cannot participate in their partners' employment benefit package, as a married spouse is entitled to do (O'Hanlan, 1999).

Gay and lesbian medical students describe hearing frequent, overtly hostile comments about lesbians and gays by attending physicians during clinical teaching rounds (Tinmouth & Hamwi, 1994; Risdon et al., 2000). One-fourth of second-year medical students in an Illinois survey reported that they believed that homosexuality is immoral and dangerous to the family, expressing an aversion to socializing with homosexuals (Klamen et al., 1999). Nine percent believed homosexuality to be a mental disorder. Negative attitudes of health care providers, if left unchallenged, will preclude a healthy doctor-patient relationship and may cause a decrease in patients' willingness to disclose sensitive issues or even return for routine care.

Recently, health care providers have begun to focus on many minority populations in an effort to maximize utilization of standard screening techniques and prevent common ailments and premature death. The lesbian population has been studied during the last decade, and these is evidence that this population may have a specific health demographic profile (O'Hanlan, 1996). In response to requests from the Gay and Lesbian Medical Association and lay lesbian health organizations made from 1993 until 1997, the Institute of Medicine (IOM) convened a committee to study whether lesbians in the United States comprised a special population that deserved research focus and funding from the National Institutes of Health (Solarz, 1999). The Committee recommended government funding for the following:

- Population-based studies to determine the incidence of cancer, heart disease, infectious diseases, and mental illness and their attendant risk factors in the lesbian population
- Investigation of effective methods of encouraging health promotion, breast and cervical cancer screening, utilization of mental and medical health care facilities and smoking cessation plans
- Study of possible mechanisms to reduce human immunodeficiency virus (HIV) transmission among bisexual women
- Examining what constitutes a healthy "coming out," including factors that help/hinder development of healthy self-esteem, relationships, childbearing and motherhood patterns, family relations
- Studies of the impact of prejudice and discrimination and the necessary coping and resilience patterns

In March 2000, the National Institutes of Health (NIH) convened health experts to recommend methods for implementing the IOM study. These scientists requested that ongoing NIH-funded projects stratify their demographic data by sexual orientation, especially those focusing on cancer, cardiovascular disease, infectious disease, life-span development, and mental health (Haynes, 2000). It was also recommended that ongoing public health surveys include the question of sexual orientation, and that medical specialty associations and training programs disseminate information on lesbian health to health care providers, researchers, and the public. When clinicians demonstrate cultural competence and are more familiar with health issues related to sexual orientation and gender, lesbian and bisexual patients are more likely to adhere to standards of routine care (Yali & Revenson, 2004). Such expertise in lesbian health concerns is especially important to clinicians treating young women who are first discovering and seeking to understand their sexuality and gender expression as they access health care for the first time.

2 Medical Definition and Prevalence

There are three generally recognized components of sexual orientation used in medical research: behavior, attraction, and identity (Laumann, et al., 1999). Between 4.4% and 13.4% of women report a same-gender attraction, 4.5% to 11.0% report having had same-gender sexual activity since puberty, and 1.3% identify as lesbian (Laumann et al., 1999; Mosher et al., 2005). In the longitudinal, observational Nurses Health Study II (NHS-II) initiated in 1995, among 116,671 nurses ages 31 to 49 years 0.8% identified as lesbian and 0.3% as bisexual; 0.9% refused to categorize themselves (Case et al., 2004). The Women's Health

Initiative (WHI) had enrolled 96,007 women ages 50 to 70 in this longitudinal study by February 1997, reporting that 2.8% preferred not to answer an orientation identification question, 0.6% identified as lesbian, and 0.8% identified as bisexual (Valanis et al., 2000). In the Women Physicians Health Study of American physicians, 3% of respondents identified as lesbian (Brogan, et al., 2001). Using capture-recapture statistical analyses of the 1990 United States census revealed estimates that 1.87% of women were lesbians (Aaron et al., 2003). Analyses of the U.S. census 2000 data suggest that there may be about 10 million homosexuals, with about half being female (Smith & Gates, 2001).

3 Adolescent Lesbian, Bisexual, or Questioning Girls

Children as young as 10 years old can recognize their sexual orientation by their attraction to a particular gender (Smith et al., 2005). By high school, about 10% of Minnesota girls responding to a statewide health questionnaire say they are unsure about their orientation, with 4.5% reporting lesbian attraction and 1.0% having had lesbian behavior (Remafedi et al., 1992). The Committee on Adolescence of the American Academy of Pediatrics stated that while homosexual youth are attempting to reconcile their feelings with negative societal attitudes, they must then confront a "lack of accurate knowledge, [a] scarcity of positive role models, and an absence of opportunity for open discussion. Youth who self-identify as lesbian or gay during high school report higher rates of unintended pregnancy, victimization, sexual risk behaviors, substance use and all at an earlier age than are their peers (Garofalo et al., 1998) Rejection by family and peers based on popular misconceptions about homosexuality may lead to isolation, domestic violence, depression, school or job failure, run-away behavior, homelessness, and suicide" (American Academy of Pediatrics, Committee on Adolescence, 1993) On a Centers for Disease Control and Prevention (CDC) health questionnaire administered in Massachusetts to all students in grades 7 to 12, among the 1.3% of females identified as lesbian or not sure, the risk of suicide behavior was twice that of the controls during the past 12 months, especially if they had experienced severe harassment from peers or family (Garofalo et al., 1999).

Among 3816 Minnesota high school girls surveyed in 1997, the 1% who identified as lesbian, bisexual, or unsure of their sexual orientation had a significantly higher prevalence of pregnancy (12%) and physical or sexual abuse than heterosexual or unsure adolescents (Saewyc et al., 1999). Multiple other reports suggest that lesbians may have experienced more physical and sexual abuse as children (Saewyc et al., 1999; Tjaden et al., 1999; Welch et al., 2000) and physical abuse from males as adults (Tjaden & Theonnes, 2000). Such abuse, when present, was found to be a strong risk factor for suicide among adolescent homosexuals (Remafedi et al., 1991). The Institute of Medicine has suggested that further research be focused on the prevention of abuse and the impact of such mistreatment (Solarz, 1999). Whether adult males are more likely to beat a woman with androgynous features or whom they suspect or know to be a lesbian or whether these young girls are more likely to later identify as lesbian deserves further study.

Among the youth who were aware of their homosexual orientation, three-fourths in one study had told one of their parents, usually their mother, with the remainder anticipating parental disapproval (D'Augelli et al., 1998). Parental lack of information about homosexuality is still widespread, with many parents trying to alter their children's gender expression or extinguish their gender-atypical or prehomosexual behavior at "camps."

The American Psychological Association, the American Psychiatric Association, the National Education Association, the American Academy of Pediatrics, and many other mental health, child health, and education groups have reviewed the literature with regard to sexual orientation and youth and report the "unanimity of the health and mental health professions on the normality of homosexuality" (American Psychological Association, 2000). These same mental health associations condemn "reparative therapy" and the "transformational ministries" for stigmatizing gender-variant children, imposing their unsubstantiated views of gender-normative behavior and attempting to coerce heterosexuality. Because social stigma per se is the primary factor motivating some to seek change of orientation, youth and parents should be educated about the normal spectrum of human sexual attraction and behavior. Such educational initiatives should be in schools, public libraries, and clinicians' offices (Fikar & Keith, 2004). Also, when parents, teachers, and faith-leaders recognize a gender-atypical or homosexual youth, they should facilitate the youth's in creating and maintaining self-confidence and honest relationships with family and friends. Age-appropriate education about family diversity (e.g., two-female, grandparent) in grade schools, high school education about homosexuality, after-school clubs such as gay-straight alliances, and counseling may help lesbian youth navigate their teens without smoking, drug abuse, sexual risk-taking, unintended pregnancy, or social alienation. Social relaxation of social pressures on girls to conform to rigid gender roles can also reduce alienation and the risk of suicidal symptoms, and it can improve peer acceptance and support (Fitzpatrick et al., 2005). Participation of other lesbian and bisexual youth in the community can lead to more satisfaction with peer friendships, higher levels of confidant and appraisal support, less hopelessness, higher self-esteem, and lower levels of depression (Vincke & van Heeringen, 2004). We can conclude that gender atypia or homosexuality per se does not lead to social pathology, drug abuse, suicide, prostitution, or HIV infection. Rather, it is the pervasive misconceptions and negative social attitudes that alienate and marginalize these youth and cause them preventable injury.

4 Sexual Activity, Contraception, STDs, and HIV

Most of the surveys of lesbian health confirm that 70% to 90% of lesbians are or have been sexual with men, especially at younger ages while they were questioning and exploring their orientation. In one survey of young lesbians, 25% had been pregnant, 16% had an abortion, and more than half had used oral contraceptives for more than 3 years (Marrazzo & Stine, 2004). Providers of reproductive health care and family planning services should not assume that pregnant teenagers are heterosexual or that adolescents who say they are bisexual, lesbian, or unsure of their sexual orientation are not in need of contraceptive counseling and prevention of sexually transmitted diseases.

Although the overall incidence of vaginitis and sexually transmitted diseases (STDs) appears quite low in the lesbian population, all types of STDs have been diagnosed and should remain in the differential for pelvic pain and vaginal discharge (Patel et al., 2000). Exclusive lesbian sexual activity is associated with the lowest rates of all types of infection, although it must be noted that lesbians have contracted bacterial vaginosis, *Trichomonas*, yeast, herpes, and gonorrhea, all of which correlate with extent of their heterosexual activity (Johnson et al., 1987). As many as one-third of lesbians have had bacterial vaginosis, and one-fifth have had yeast infections (Bailey et al., 2004). Fewer than 2% have had genital warts, genital herpes, or trichomoniasis; and fewer than 1% have had *Chlamydia* infection or gonorrhea, which have occured mostly in women who had histories of sex with men (Bailey et al., 2004). However, there is lesbian sexual transmission of herpes type 2, human papilloma virus (HPV), HIV, syphilis, and *Trichomonas* (Troncoso et al., 1995; Kellock & O'Mahony, 1996; O'Hanlan & Crum, 1996; Campos-Outcalt & Hurwitz, 2002; Marrazzo et al., 2003). Routine screening for *Chlamydia*, herpes, *Trichomonas*, gonorrhea, and syphilis does not seem indicated for asymptomatic lesbians who are not having sex with men, but testing for STDs in symptomatic lesbians should incorporate all the same standards as those currently used for heterosexual women.

There are many literature reports of cases of suspected lesbian sexual transmission of HIV (Marmor et al., 1986; Chu, et al., 1990; Einhorn & Polgar, 1994; Lemp et al., 1995). The Institute of Medicine has reviewed the issue and concludes that the risk of transmitting HIV between women is unclear, noting that bisexual women have the highest rates of seropositivity in comparison with both lesbians and heterosexual women (Solarz, 1999). In a convenience sample survey of HIV risk behavior among 1086 inner-city lesbians and bisexual women, 16% reported having sex with a bisexual man, 2.5% reported injecting drugs, 4% had sex with an injection drug-using man, and 8% had sex with an injection drug using woman; also, 21% engaged in risky behavior: 75% failed to use safer-sex techniques, and only 9% used safer-sex techniques during their subsequent homosexual activity (Einhorn & Polgar, 1994).

Prevention of STDs should start with social inclusion and diverse education in schools (Nelson, 1997). Lesbian and bisexual youth with gay-sensitive health instruction in their schools reported fewer sexual partners, less recent sex, and less substance use during sexual activity than did lesbian youth in other schools (Blake et al., 2001). To reduce risk of HIV transmission, some lesbian health groups have advocated use of various latex barriers such as dental dams, gloves, and even plastic kitchen wrap. Many lesbians do not know what safer-sexual practices entail (Fishman & Anderson, 2003). However, there are no prospective studies on which to base recommendations about safer sex for lesbians. Studies on drug use and sexual activity have been urged by the Scientific Workshop on Lesbian Health to investigate transmission of HIV among lesbians (Haynes, 2000).

5 Lesbian Family, Insemination, and Parenting

According to Maslow's hierarchy of needs, once the basic physical survival needs are met an individual naturally seeks to fulfill higher needs such as community, intimacy, and family (Maslow, 1970). More than 60% of lesbians in one survey were in long-term relationships (Bradford et al., 1994), similar to the 2000 US census statistic of 62% of heterosexual women who are married (Usdansky, 1993). A 1991 convenience survey of gay and lesbian couples revealed that 75% of lesbian couples shared their income, 88% had held a wedding ceremony or ritual celebrating their union, 91% were monogamous, 7% broke their agreement, and 92% were committed to their partners for life.

Lesbians who did not hide their homosexuality had better psychological health (Morrow, 1996; LaSala, 2000) and satisfaction with their relationships (Berger, 1990); however, relationship instability in lesbian couples can occur because of the same common relational conflicts observed in all couples. It can be compounded, however, by the effects of cultural homophobia: dealing with the disdain, coming out issues, maintaining a self-concept in a hostile dominant culture (Igartua, 1998; Ridge & Feeney, 1998).

The definition of "family" for lesbian couples often involves creation of a network of close and accepting friends as a family-of-choice, especially if their family-of-origin has rejected them (Kurdek, 1988). The most frequent sources of support for lesbians who had recently developed breast cancer were partners, friends, prior partners, family, and coworkers (Fobair et al., 2001). Without contracts for mutual medical conservatorship, a domestic partner may be unable to make decisions for her domestic partner. A comprehensive review of published studies of children raised in gay and lesbian households concluded that the children developed normally regarding gender identity, sex-role behavior, sexual orientation, self-concept, locus of control, moral judgment, and intelligence (American Psychological Association Working Group on Same-Sex Families and Relationships, 2004). Although 5% of children are taunted by their peers because of their parents' orientation, children still fare better when informed early, when their mothers are psychologically healthy, and when their biologic fathers, if known and present, are not homophobic.

Until recent years, societal heterosexism has resulted in many lesbians coming to accept their orientation after leading heterosexual lives for many years. They may have married and borne children. Younger lesbians are increasingly choosing to become parents through donor insemination, adoption, and foster care (Solarz, 1999). Among women seeking insemination services, the clinical pregnancy rate and complications have been confirmed to be among lesbians and heterosexual women (Ferrara et al., 2000).

A growing body of scientific literature demonstrates that children who grow up with one or two gay and/or lesbian parents fare as well in emotional, cognitive, social, and sexual functioning as do children whose parents are heterosexual. Children's optimal development seems to be influenced more by the nature of the relationships and interactions within the family unit than by the particular structural form it takes. [American Academy of Pediatrics Committee on Psychosocial Aspects of Child and Family Health, 2002]

In a study comparing heterosexual couples with lesbian couples seeking insemination services, there were no observed differences in individual's self-esteem, psychiatric symptoms or relationship adjustment, except that lesbians reported greater dyadic cohesion than heterosexual couples (Jacob et al., 1999). Lesbian and heterosexual mothers in another study self-reported similar scores on stress, adjustment, competence, and the quality of their relationships with their families (McNeill et al., 1998).

Lesbians desiring insemination should be advised to employ the services of an established sperm bank to reduce infectious diseases and genetic abnormalities and to establish custody. In the absence of access to civil marriage contracts, it may be valuable to refer lesbians planning to have children to a lawyer who can help them establish parental authority for both the biologic mother and the lesbian co-parent. Four states currently prohibit lesbians from adopting children. In a survey of members of the Society of Assisted Reproduction Technology, it was reported that only 55% accept lesbians as eligible recipients (Kingsberg et al., 2000). Based on all available evidence, there is no ethical justification for obstetrician-gynecologists to refuse insemination to lesbian couples or individuals.

The NHS-II respondents were between 31 and 49 years of age, and the WHI respondents were between 50 and 79 years (Valanis et al., 2000; Case et al., 2004). Both studies demonstrate significantly lower parity among lesbians and bisexuals, with nulligravidity rates of 51% to 76% for lesbians and 19% to 49% for bisexuals, compared with 8% to 22% for heterosexuals (Valanis et al., 2000; Case et al., 2004). Younger lesbians appear to be conceiving at higher rates than the NHS-II and WHI populations and have been described as creating a "gayby boom." Fertility should be similar in lesbians and heterosexual women. Serum hormone levels of testosterone, androstenedione, estradiol, and progesterone of lifelong lesbians, lesbians who realized their orientation at a later age, and heterosexual women were measured at the same points in the menstrual cycle and revealed no differences (Dancey, 1990; Agrawal et al., 2004). Conception rates have been reported to be similar as well.

6 Obstetric Issues

Many physicians who provide care for lesbian patients do not view them as potentially fertile women who may desire to inseminate and create a family. They may similarly miss the opportunity to perform preconception counseling. Furthermore, ignoring or excluding the patient's partner in counseling sessions, prenatal appointments, and peripartum care is a major source of anxiety and frustration to lesbian patients (Wilton & Kaufmann, 2001). Preconception counseling also includes testing for sexually transmittable infections prior to pregnancy or at the initial prenatal visit. Additionally, repeat screening for STDs later in pregnancy should be considered if sperm from a source other than an established sperm bank is used to achieve pregnancy. Lack of previous exposure to the donor's sperm increases the risk of preeclampsia in the gravida (Trupin, et al., 1996).

Several health risks are more prevalent in lesbians than in heterosexual women (Valanis et al., 2000) and, if present, pose risks to pregnancy. Tobacco and alcohol use should be firmly discouraged. Achieving a normal body mass index (BMI) and improving nutritional intake should be addressed before conception. Finally, depression and anxiety (Bailey, 1999) should be specifically discussed during both antepartum and postpartum care and aggressively managed. A strong family-of-choice support system for the couple should be established, particularly if the families-of-origin are not supportive of the pregnancy.

7 Domestic Violence

In a population-based survey of 8000 women by the U.S. Department of Justice in 1999, about 11% of lesbians reported being raped, physically assaulted, and/or stalked by a female cohabitant, and 30% reported being raped, physically assaulted, and/or stalked by a prior male cohabitant or husband. Just over 20% of heterosexual women reported violence by the husband or male cohabitant (Tjaden & Theonnes, 2000). In comparison, in a convenience sampling of lesbians and gays matched with their heterosexual siblings in 2005, lesbian participants reported more partner psychological and physical victimization and more sexual assault experiences during adulthood (Balsam et al., 2005). As with heterosexual couples, battering is correlated with abuse of alcohol and drugs (Schilit et al., 1990). Current studies also reveal many similarities between opposite-gender and same-gender domestic violence regarding the types of abuse and various violent dynamics (McClennen, 2005); however, in areas such as help-seeking behaviors and correlates, lesbians have fewer resources and require unique assessment and intervention strategies. Clinicians should be alert to the signs and symptoms of battery in all relationships. Shelters for battered women are needed to provide services to lesbian clients.

8 Suicide and Substance Abuse Among Lesbians

After stratifying data from the 1996 National Household Survey of Drug Abuse, it was found that lesbians were more likely to be classified with alcohol and drug dependence syndromes (Cochran & Mays, 2000). Gay and lesbian study respondents in two large southern metropolitan areas had significantly higher prevalence rates for use of marijuana, inhalants, and alcohol during the past year (Skinner & Otis, 1996). Whereas lesbian and gay people reported drinking alcohol more frequently during the month than the predominantly heterosexual respondents of the National Household Survey on Drug Abuse, few differences were observed between the two samples for heavy alcohol consumption (Skinner & Otis, 1996). However, the Nurses' Health Study and the Women's Health Initiative reported that the women who identify as lesbian or who have sex with women have higher rates of alcohol use and self-reported abuse, and they are more likely to smoke cigarettes (Koh, 2000; Valanis et al., 2000; Case et al., 2004).

Both the NHS-II and the WHI have reported that the women who identify as lesbian or who have sex with women are more likely to admit to having depression (Valanis et al., 2000; Case et al., 2004) and to be taking antidepressants (Case et al., 2004). When questioned about causes of depressive stress in their lives, most lesbians report stress due to isolation and social ascription of inferior status (Savin-Williams, 1994; Safren & Heimberg, 1999) as well as the lack of support from families and friends (Oetjen & Rothblum, 2000). In some studies, as many as 70% to 80% of lesbians report having sought counseling services (Bradford et al., 1994; Cochran, 2001).

The Institute of Medicine recognizes that lesbians "experience stress related to the difficulties of living in a homophobic society. Stress may result from the burden of keeping one's lesbian identity secret from family or coworkers, of being excluded by physicians from making health care decisions for a gravely ill lesbian partner, or, among many other factors, being the target of violence or other hate crimes. Hostility and isolation are potent forms of stress that contribute to the allostatic load by leading to elevated levels of the stress hormones "[which] may be greatest for lesbians who are subject to multiple forms of discriminations, for example, lesbians who are members of racial and ethnic minority groups" (Solarz, 1999). It is recognized that there are many factors protecting individuals from negative outcomes from this stress, such as close relations with one or both parents, participation in supportive educational systems and religious groups, and involvement in the larger lesbian community (Solarz, 1999; Meyer, 2003).

9 Healthy Aging

9.1 Cardiovascular Disease and Obesity

Lesbian women appear to weigh more, eat slightly fewer fruits and vegetables, exercise similarly, have a similar rate of hypertension but a higher rate of reported heart attacks, and smoke more than heterosexual women (Valanis et al., 2000; Case et al., 2004). Obesity and smoking are also reported to be more common among African American women and have similarly been shown to correlate with stress in their lives (Baltrus et al., 2005). Although lesbians do not subscribe to strict rules of body shape and rules for dress, they do have rates of body dissatisfaction similar to those of heterosexual women (Beren et al., 1996). Lesbians with a high BMI were more likely to be older, have a lower socioeconomic status, and got less exercise. They had accurate perceptions of their being overweight and often reported a health condition that limited their exercise (Yancey et al., 2003). Given that heart disease kills many women, it would be prudent to investigate culturally competent, effective prevention strategies for heart disease in the lesbian community because this community carries a rich concentration of cardiac and cancer risk factors (Cochran et al., 2001).

9.2 Gynecologic Cancers

Lower parity and less use of oral contraceptives, (Valanis et al., 2000) combined with higher rates of obesity and endometriosis than among heterosexual women may give rise to a higher rate of ovarian carcinoma in the lesbian population (O'Hanlan, 1995). The opportunity for prevention of ovarian cancer occurs during the routine gynecologic examination, which should include inquiry about dysmenorrhea/endometriosis, consideration of oral contraceptives for prevention of pain and regulation of menses, advice about lowering the BMI, and consideration of familial breast and ovarian cancer screening. In a recent survey of Boston area women, annual routine examinations were obtained at a higher rate than in prior years' studies, but the rates were still lower than those of heterosexual women (Roberts, et al., 2004).

The risk factors for endometrial cancer include obesity, a high fat diet, and low parity. Endometrial cancer remains the most curable gynecologic malignancy because women recognize and report their spotting early, resulting in early diagnosis and surgery. Although hysterectomy rates appear similar between lesbians and heterosexual women in the Women's Health Initiative (Valanis et al., 2000), lesbians remain at higher risk of more advanced disease and lower cure probability if they do not obtain routine care and access to their gynecologist (O'Hanlan, 1995).

Many physicians incorrectly think that lesbian patients do not require a yearly Pap smear because they also assume that lesbians have not had sex with men and cannot transmit HPV by their sexual activity. However, most lesbians have had sex with men (Saewyc et al., 1999), and HPV can be transmitted by exclusive lesbian sexual contact (O'Hanlan & Crum, 1996). Lesbians and bisexuals also appear to have higher rates of cigarette abuse (Valanis et al., 2000; Case et al., 2004), another risk factor for cervical dysplasia. Bisexual women were significantly less compliant with Pap smear screening recommendations than either lesbian or heterosexual women in the WHI (Valanis et al., 2000). It is prudent to recommend yearly Pap tests to all women with any of the known risk factors for cervical cancer and to offer triennial Pap tests to women with none of the cervical cancer risk factors and a history of normal Pap tests over the prior 3 years (O'Hanlan & Crum, 1996; Marrazzo et al., 2000).

9.3 Other Cancer Risks: Breast, Colon, and Lung

Among the WHI population, lesbians and bisexual women had more breast cancer than heterosexual women despite similar mammography screening rates as study protocol participants (Valanis et al., 2000). Lesbians appear to have more risk factors for breast cancer, including nulliparity, alcohol and cigarette abuse, menopausal hormone replacement therapy, and obesity (Valanis et al., 2000; Case et al., 2004) and they may undergo mammography less frequently than in the general population (Koh, 2000).

Most studies have confirmed that lesbian adults have high rates of smoking (Rankow & Tessaro, 1998; Valanis et al., 2000; Case et al., 2004), placing them at higher risk of lung cancer than heterosexuals. Estimated rates of adolescent lesbians and bisexuals smoking are 38% to 50% (Ryan et al., 2001). More than 50% of African American and Hispanic American lesbians smoked in one survey, which also reported that Hispanic lesbians were less likely to have tried to quit than Black lesbians (Sanchez et al., 2005). Culturally sensitive interventions are needed to prevent smoking and to help all lesbian and bisexual women move from the precontemplative to action stage of quitting. Prevention programs must address the psychosocial stresses and cultural underpinnings of tobacco use by encouraging healthy psychosocial development (Remafedi & Carol, 2005).

Smoking, obesity, and high alcohol intake have been shown to increase rates of colon polyp formation as well as colon and gastric cancer. From the WHI and the NHS-II data, lesbians on these protocol studies were shown to have obtained fecal occult blood tests and to have developed colon cancer at rates similar to those of heterosexuals and bisexuals (Valanis et al., 2000; Case et al., 2004), but in studies of the general population, there may be less screening and more smoking and drinking, posing a higher risk for colon cancer (Giovannucci et al., 1993, 1994).

9.4 Aging Lesbians

Age, poverty, and health issues can render the older lesbian invisible (Fullmer et al., 1999). For aging lesbians, acceptance of the aging process and high levels of life satisfaction are associated with connection to and activity in the lesbian community (Quam & Whitford, 1992; Slusher et al., 1996). Currently, many lesbian seniors find they must give up their gay identity as they progress into senior age and retirement communities in a generation that is still predominantly homophobic (Brogan, 1996). Toward this end there have been a few retirement communities created and advertised in the lesbian and gay communities that specifically enable residents to maintain their identities as they age.

In a 2001 survey about attitudes on end-of-life care, lesbian and gay respondents' were more likely to have completed advance directives (Stein & Bonuck, 2001) and to support legalization of physician-assisted suicide, preferring a palliative approach to end-of-life care. Denial of legal marriage to lesbian couples prevents them from receiving social security benefits as a senior couple. As with heterosexual couples, often one spouse earns less than the other spouse in order to manage the home and enable the other spouse to earn their mutual support. Treating the two as legal strangers prohibits the lesbian couple from receiving the retirement support and disability and death benefits that are essential to the health of aging heterosexual couples. Finally, when one lesbian dies, her surviving spouse is taxed on the "inherited half" of the estate she enabled her partner to create, unlike in civil marriage, where no tax is levied on a surviving marriage partner.

10 Future Directions

Although lesbians and bisexual women have not been well studied and reported in the medical literature, more research has been funded and is forthcoming. With more accurate information and more familiarity with lesbians, clinicians' offices will be more welcoming, and lesbians will access routine care more easily. When America has greater familiarity with lesbians and bisexual women, it is likely that legislators will feel more comfortable voting to afford lesbians and gays equal civil rights. With equal civil rights, it is likely that the homophobia and heterosexism that marginalizes lesbians and gays will be reduced. When homophobia and heterosexism are reduced, the health disparities can be ameliorated and demographic disparities lost in favor of better American public health.

References

Aaron, D.J., Chang, Y.F., Markovic, N., and LaPorte, R.E. (2003) Estimating the lesbian population: a capture-recapture approach. *Journal of Epidemiology and Community Health* 57:207–209.

Agrawal, R., Sharma, S., Bekir, J., Conway, G., Bailey, J., Balen, A.H., et al. (2004) Prevalence of polycystic ovaries and polycystic ovary syndrome in lesbian women compared with heterosexual women. *Fertility and Sterility*, 82: 1352–1357.

Albarran, J.W., and Salmon, D. (2000) Lesbian, gay and bisexual experiences within critical care nursing, 1988–1998: a survey of the literature. *International Journal of Nursing Studies*, 37:445–455.

American Academy of Pediatrics, Committee on Adolescence. (1993) Homosexuality and adolescence. *Pediatrics* 92:631–634.

American Academy of Pediatrics Committee on Psychosocial Aspects of Child and Family Health. (2002) Coparent or second-parent adoption by same-sex parents; homosexuality and adolescence, sexuality education for children and adolescents. *Pediatrics* 92, 108, 109(2), 341–344.

American Psychological Association. (2000) *Just the facts about sexual orientation and youth: a primer for principals, educators and school personnel.* American Academy of Pediatrics, American Counseling Association, American

Association of School Administrators, American Federation of Teachers, American Psychological Association, American School Health Association, Interfaith Alliance Foundation, National Association of School Psychologists, National Association of Social Workers, National Education Association, Washington, DC.

American Psychological Association Working Group on Same-Sex Families and Relationships. (2004) *APA briefing sheet on same-sex families and relationships.* APA, Washington, DC.

Bailey, J.M. (1999) Homosexuality and mental illness. *Archives of General Psychiatry* 56:883–884.

Bailey, J.V., Farquhar, C., Owen, C., and Mangtani, P. (2004) Sexually transmitted infections in women who have sex with women. *Sexually Transmitted Infections* 80:244–246.

Balsam, K.F., Rothblum, E.D., and Beauchaine, T.P. (2005) Victimization over the life span: a comparison of lesbian, gay, bisexual, and heterosexual siblings. *Journal of Consulting and Clinical Psychology* 73:477–487.

Baltrus, P.T., Lynch, J.W., Everson-Rose, S., Raghunathan, T.E., and Kaplan, G.A. (2005) Race/ethnicity, life-course socioeconomic position, and body weight trajectories over 34 years: the Alameda County Study. *American Journal Public Health* 95:1595–1601.

Beren, S.E., Hayden, H.A., Wilfley, D.E., and Grilo, C.M. (1996) The influence of sexual orientation on body dissatisfaction in adult men and women. *International Journal of Eating Disordors* 20:135–141.

Berger, R.M. (1990) Passing: impact on the quality of same-sex couple relationships. *Social Work* 35:328–332.

Blake, S.M., Ledsky, R., Lehman, T., Goodenow, C., Sawyer, R., and Hack, T. (2001) Preventing sexual risk behaviors among gay, lesbian, and bisexual adolescents: the benefits of gay-sensitive HIV instruction in schools. *American Journal Public Health* 91:940–946.

Bradford, J., Ryan, C., and Rothblum, E.D. (1994) National Lesbian Health Care Survey: implications for mental health care. *Journal of Consulting and Clinical Psychology* 62:228–242.

Brogan, D.J., Frank, E., and O'Hanlan, K.A. (2001) Characteristics of lesbian vs. heterosexual women physicians. *In preparation.*

Brogan, M. (1996) The sexual needs of elderly people: addressing the issue. *Nursing Standard* 10(24):42–45.

Campos-Outcalt, D., and Hurwitz, S. (2002) Female-to-female transmission of syphilis: a case report. *Sexually Transmitted Diseases* 29:119–120.

Case, P., Austin, S.B., Hunter, D.J., Manson, J.E., Malspeis, S., Willett, W.C., et al. (2004) Sexual orientation, health risk factors, and physical functioning in the Nurses' Health Study II. *Journal of Womens Health (Larchmont)* 13:1033–1047.

Chu, S.Y., Buehler, J.W., Fleming, P.L., and Berkelman, R.L. (1990) Epidemiology of reported cases of AIDS in lesbians, United States 1980–89. *American Journal of Public Health* 80:1380–1381.

Cochran, S.D. (2001) Emerging issues in research on lesbians' and gay men's mental health: does sexual orientation really matter? *The American Psychologist* 56:931–947.

Cochran, S.D., and Mays, V.M. (2000) Relation between psychiatric syndromes and behaviorally defined sexual orientation in a sample of the US population. *American Journal of Epidemiology*, 151:516–523.

Cochran, S.D., Mays, V.M., Bowen, D., Gage, S., Bybee, D., Roberts, S.J., et al. (2001) Cancer-related risk indicators and preventive screening behaviors among lesbians and bisexual women. *American Journal of Public Health* 91:591–597.

Dancey, C. (1990) Sexual orientation in women: an investigation of hormonal and personality variables. *Biology and Psychology* 30:251–264.

D'Augelli, A.R., Hershberger, S.L., and Pilkington, N.W. (1998) Lesbian, gay, and bisexual youth and their families: disclosure of sexual orientation and its consequences. *American Journal of Orthopsychiatry* 68:361–371.

Einhorn, L., and Polgar, M. (1994) HIV-risk bahavior among lesbians and bisexual women. *AIDS Education and Prevention* 6:514–523.

Eliason, M.J. (1998) Correlates of prejudice in nursing students. *Journal of Nursing Education* 37(1):27–29.

Ferrara, I., Balet, R., and Grudzinskas, J.G. (2000) Intrauterine donor insemination in single women and lesbian couples: a comparative study of pregnancy rates. *Human Reproduction* 15:621–625.

Fikar, C.R., and Keith, L. (2004) Information needs of gay, lesbian, bisexual, and transgendered health care professionals: results of an Internet survey. *Journal of the Medical Library Association* 92(1):56–65.

Fishman, S.J., and Anderson, E.H. (2003) Perception of HIV and safer sexual behaviors among lesbians. *Journal of the Association of Nurses AIDS Care* 14(6):48–55.

Fitzpatrick, K.K., Euton, S.J., Jones, J.N., and Schmidt, N.B. (2005) Gender role, sexual orientation and suicide risk. *Journal of Affective Disordors* 87(1), 35–42.

Fobair, P., O'Hanlan, K., Koopman, C., Classen, C., Dimiceli, S., Drooker, N., et al. (2001) Comparison of lesbian and heterosexual women's response to newly diagnosed breast cancer. *Psychooncology* 10(1):40–51.

Fullmer, E.M., Shenk, D., and Eastland, L.J. (1999) Negating identity: a feminist analysis of the social invisibility of older lesbians. *Journal of Women and Aging* 11:131–148.

Garofalo, R., Wolf, R.C., Kessel, S., Palfrey, S.J., and DuRant, R.H. (1998) The association between health risk behaviors and sexual orientation among a school-based sample of adolescents. *Pediatrics* 101:895–902.

Garofalo, R., Wolf, R.C., Wissow, L.S., Woods, E.R., and Goodman, E. (1999) Sexual orientation and risk of suicide attempts among a representative sample of youth. *Archives of Pediatric and Adolescent Medicine* 153:487–493.

Giovannucci, E., Rimm, E.B., Stampfer, M.J., Colditz, G.A., Ascherio, A., Kearney, J., et al. (1994) A prospective study of cigarette smoking and risk of colorectal adenoma and colorectal cancer in U.S. men. *Journal of the National Cancer Institute* 86:183–191.

Giovannucci, E., Stampfer, M.J., Colditz, G.A., Rimm, E.B., Trichopoulos, D., Rosner, B.A., et al. (1993) Folate, methionine, and alcohol intake and risk of colorectal adenoma. *Journal of the National Cancer Institute* 85:875–884.

Haynes, S.G. (2000) *Scientific workshop on lesbian health 2000: steps for implementing the IOM report*. Department of Health and Human Services, Washington, DC.

Hughes, D. (2004) Disclosure of sexual preferences and lesbian, gay, and bisexual practitioners. *British Medical Journal* 328:1211–1212.

Igartua, K.J. (1998) Therapy with lesbian couples: the issues and the interventions. *Canadian Journal of Psychiatry* 43:391–396.

Jacob, M.C., Klock, S.C., and Maier, D. (1999) Lesbian couples as therapeutic donor insemination recipients: do they differ from other patients? *Journal of Psychosomatic Obstetrics and Gynaecology* 20:203–215.

Johnson, S.R., Smith, E.M., and Guenther, S.M. (1987) Comparison of gynecologic health care problems between lesbians and bisexual women: a survey of 2345 women. *Journal of Reproductive Medicine* 32:805–811.

Kass, N.E., Faden, R.R., Fox, R., and Dudley, J. (1992) Homosexual and bisexual men's perceptions of discrimination in health services. *American Journal of Public Health* 82:1277–1279.

Kellock, D., and O'Mahony, C.P. (1996) Sexually acquired metronidazole-resistant trichomoniasis in a lesbian couple. *Genitourinary Medicine* 72(1): 60–61.

Kingsberg, S.A., Applegarth, L.D., and Janata, J.W. (2000) Embryo donation programs and policies in North America: survey results and implications for health and mental health professionals. *Fertility and Sterility* 73:215–220.

Klamen, D.L., Grossman, L.S., and Kopacz, D.R. (1999) Medical student homophobia. *Journal of Homosexuality* 37(1):53–63.

Koh, A.S. (2000) Use of preventive health behaviors by lesbian, bisexual, and heterosexual women: questionnaire survey. *Western Journal of Medicine* 172:379–384.

Kurdek, L.A. (1988) Perceived social support in gays and lesbians in cohabitating relationships. *Journal of Personality and Social Psychology* 54:504–509.

LaSala, M.C. (2000) Lesbians, gay men, and their parents: family therapy for the coming-out crisis. *Family Process* 39(1):67–81.

Laumann, E.O., Paik, A., and Rosen, R.C. (1999) Sexual dysfunction in the United States: prevalence and predictors. *Journal of the American Medical Association* 281:537–544.

Lemp, G.F., Jones, M., Kellogg, T.A., Nieri, G.N., Anderson, L., Withum, D., et al. (1995) HIV seroprevalence and risk behaviors among lesbians and bisexual women in San Francisco and Berkeley, California. *American Journal of Public Health* 85:1549–1552.

Marmor, M., Weiss, L.R., Lyden, M., Weiss, S.H., Saxinger, W.C., Spira, T.J., et al. (1986) Possible female-to-female transmission of human immunodeficiency virus [letter]. *Annals of Internal Medicine* 105:969.

Marrazzo, J.M., and Stine, K. (2004) Reproductive health history of lesbians: implications for care. *American Journal of Obstetrics and Gynecology* 190:1298–1304.

Marrazzo, J.M., Stine, K., and Koutsky, L.A. (2000) Genital human papillomavirus infection in women who have sex with women: a review. *American Journal of Obstetrics and Gynecology* 183:770–774.

Marrazzo, J.M., Stine, K., and Wald, A. (2003) Prevalence and risk factors for infection with herpes simplex virus type-1 and -2 among lesbians. *Sexually Transmittal Diseases* 30:890–895.

Maslow, A.L. (1970) *Motivation and personality*. Harper and Row, New York.

Mathews, W.C., Booth, M.W., Turner, J.D., and Kessler, L. (1986) Physicians' attitudes toward homosexuality—survey of a California County Medical Society. *Western Journal of Medicine* 144:106–110.

McClennen, J.C. (2005) Domestic violence between same-gender partners: recent findings and future research. *Journal of Interpersonal Violence* 20:149–154.

McNeill, K.F., Rienzi, B.M., and Kposowa, A. (1998) Families and parenting: a comparison of lesbian and heterosexual mothers. *Psychology Reports* 82(1):59–62.

Meyer, I.H. (2003) Prejudice, social stress, and mental health in lesbian, gay, and bisexual populations: conceptual issues and research evidence. *Psychological Bulletin* 129:674–697.

Morrow, D.F. (1996) Coming-out issues for adult lesbians: a group intervention. *Social Work* 41:647–656.

Mosher, W.D., Chandra, A., and Jones, J. (eds). (2005) *Sexual behavior and selected health measures: men and women 15–44 years of age, United States* 2002, vol. 362. U.S. Dpartment of Health and Human Services, Centers for Disease Control and Prevention, National Center for Health Statistics, Atlanta.

Nelson, J.A. (1997) Gay, lesbian, and bisexual adolescents: providing esteem-enhancing care to a battered population. *Nurse Practitioner* 22(2), 94, 99, 103 passim.

Oetjen, H., and Rothblum, E.D. (2000) When lesbians aren't gay: factors affecting depression among lesbians. *Journal of Homosexuality* 39(1):49–73.

O'Hanlan, K.A. (1995) Lesbian health and homophobia: perspectives for the treating obstetrician/gynecologist. *Current Problems in Obstetrics and Gynecology and Fertility* 18(4):94–133.

O'Hanlan, K.A. (1996) Do we really mean preventive medicine for all? *American Journal of Preventive Medicine* 12:411–414.

O'Hanlan, K.A. (1999) Domestic partnership benefits at medical universities. *Journal of the American Medical Association* 282:1289, 1292.

O'Hanlan, K.A., and Crum, C.P. (1996) Human papillomavirus-associated cervical intraepithelial neoplasia following lesbian sex. *Obstetrics and Gynecology* 88(4 Pt 2):702–703.

Patel, A., DeLong, G., Voigl, B., and Medina, C. (2000) Pelvic inflammatory disease in the lesbian population-lesbian health issues: asking the right questions. *Obstetrics and Gynecology* 95(Supplement 1):S29-S30.

Quam, J.K., and Whitford, G.S. (1992) Adaptation and age-related expectations of older gay and lesbian adults. *Gerontologist* 32:367–374.

Rankow, E.J., and Tessaro, I. (1998) Cervical cancer risk and Papanicolaou screening in a sample of lesbian and bisexual women. *Journal of Family Practice* 47:139–143.

Remafedi, G., and Carol, H. (2005) Preventing tobacco use among lesbian, gay, bisexual, and transgender youths. *Nicotine & Tobacco Research* 7:249–256.

Remafedi, G., Farrow, J.A., and Deisher, R.W. (1991) Risk factors for attempted suicide in gay and bisexual youth. *Pediatrics* 87:869–875.

Remafedi, G., Resnick, M., Blum, R., and Harris, L. (1992) Demography of sexual orientation in adolescents. *Pediatrics* 89:714–721.

Ridge, S.R., and Feeney, J.A. (1998) Relationship history and relationship attitudes in gay males and lesbians: attachment style and gender differences. *Australian and New Zealand Journal of Psychiatry* 32:848–859.

Risdon, C., Cook, D., and Willms, D. (2000) Gay and lesbian physicians in training: a qualitative study. *Canadian Medical Association Journal* 162:331–334.

Roberts, S.J., Patsdaughter, C.A., Grindel, C.G., and Tarmina, M.S. (2004) Health related behaviors and cancer screening of lesbians: results of the Boston Lesbian Health Project II. *Women and Health* 39(4):41–55.

Ryan, H., Wortley, P.M., Easton, A., Pederson, L., and Greenwood, G. (2001) Smoking among lesbians, gays, and bisexuals: a review of the literature. *American Journal of Preventive Medicine* 21(2):142–149.

Saewyc, E.M., Bearinger, L.H., Blum, R.W., and Resnick, M.D. (1999) Sexual intercourse, abuse and pregnancy among adolescent women: does sexual orientation make a difference? *Family Planning Perspective* 31:127–131.

Safren, S.A., and Heimberg, R.G. (1999) Depression, hopelessness, suicidality, and related factors in sexual minority and heterosexual adolescents. *Journal of Consulting and Clinical Psychology* 67:859–866.

Sanchez, J.P., Meacher, P., and Beil, R. (2005) Cigarette smoking and lesbian and bisexual women in the Bronx. *Journal of Community Health* 30:23–37.

Savin-Williams, R.C. (1994) Verbal and physical abuse as stressors in the lives of lesbian, gay male, and bisexual youths: associations with school problems, running away, substance abuse, prostitution, and suicide. *Journal of Consulting and Clinical Psychology* 62:261–269.

Schilit, R., Lie, G.Y., and Montagne, M. (1990) Substance use as a correlate of violence in intimate lesbian relationships. *Journal of Homosexuality* 19(3):51–65.

Skinner, W.F., and Otis, M.D. (1996) Drug and alcohol use among lesbian and gay people in a southern U.S. sample: epidemiological, comparative, and methodological findings from the Trilogy Project. *Journal of Homosexuality* 30(3) 59–92.

Slusher, M.P., Mayer, C.J., and Dunkle, R.E. (1996) Gays and Lesbians Older and Wiser (GLOW): a support group for older gay people. *Gerontologist* 36:118–123.

Smith, D.H., and Gates, G.J. (2001) Gay and lesbian families in the United States: same-sex unmarried partner households. In: *A preliminary analysis of 2000 United States census data*, 12.

Smith, S.D., Dermer, S.B., and Astramovich, R.L. (2005) Working with non-heterosexual youth to understand sexual identity development, at-risk behaviors, and implications for health care professionals. *Psychological Reports* 96(3 Pt 1):651–654.

Solarz, A. (1999) *Lesbian health: current assessment and directions for the future.* Institute of Medicine, National Institutes of Health, United States Department of Health and Human Services. National Academy Press, Washington, DC.

Stein, G.L., and Bonuck, K.A. (2001) Attitudes on end-of-life care and advance care planning in the lesbian and gay community. *Journal of Palliative Medicine* 4:173–190.

Stevens, P.E., and Hall, J.M. (1988) Stigma, health beliefs and experiences with health care in lesbian women. *Image Journal of Nursing School* 20(2):69–73.

Tinmouth, J., and Hamwi, G. (1994) The experience of gay and lesbian students in medical school. *Journal of the American Medical Association* 271:714–715.

Tjaden, P., and Theonnes, N. (2000) *Extent, nature, and consequences of intimate partner violence: findings from the National Violence Against Women Survey.* National Institutes of Justice and National Insititutes of Health, Washington, DC.

Tjaden, P., Thoennes, N., and Allison, C.J. (1999) Comparing violence over the life span in samples of same-sex and opposite-sex cohabitants. *Violence and Victims* 14:413–425.

Troncoso, A.R., Romani, A., Carranza, C.M., Macias, J.R., and Masini, R. (1995) [Probable HIV transmission by female homosexual contact.] *Medicina (Buenos Aires)* 55:334–336.

Trupin, L.S., Simon, L.P., and Eskenazi, B. (1996) Change in paternity: a risk factor for preeclampsia in multiparas. *Epidemiology* 7:240–244.

Usdansky, M. (1993) Gay couples, by the numbers, data suggest they're fewer than believed, but affluent. *USA Today*, p. 1a.

Valanis, B.G., Bowen, D.J., Bassford, T., Whitlock, E., Charney, P., and Carter, R.A. (2000) Sexual orientation and health: comparisons in the Women's Health Initiative sample. *Archives of Family Medicine* 9:843–853.

Vincke, J., and van Heeringen, K. (2004) Summer holiday camps for gay and lesbian young adults: an evaluation of their impact on social support and mental well-being. *Journal of Homosexuality* 47(2):33–46.

Welch, S., Collings, S.C., and Howden-Chapman, P. (2000) Lesbians in New Zealand: their mental health and satisfaction with mental health services. *Australian and New Zealand Journal of Psychiatry* 34:256–263.

Wilton, T., and Kaufmann, T. (2001) Lesbian mothers' experiences of maternity care in the UK. *Midwifery* 17:203–211.

Yali, A.M., and Revenson, T.A. (2004) How changes in population demographics will impact health psychology: incorporating a broader notion of cultural competence into the field. *Health and Psychology* 23:147–155.

Yancey, A.K., Cochran, S.D., Corliss, H.L., and Mays, V.M. (2003) Correlates of overweight and obesity among lesbian and bisexual women. *Preventive Medicine* 36:676–683.

Cancer and Sexual Minority Women

Deborah J. Bowen, Ulrike Boehmer, and Marla Russo

1 Introduction

1.1 Issues and Trends

Cancer is the leading cause of death in the United States, outpacing deaths due to heart disease. During the year 2005, an estimated 1,372,910 persons in the United States were expected to be diagnosed with cancer, and 570,280 persons were expected to die from it—more than 1500 people per day (American Cancer Society, 2005). These estimates do not include noninvasive (in situ) cancers and most skin cancers; new cases of skin cancer are estimated to exceed 1 million per year (American Cancer Society, 2005). About three-fourths of all cancers occur in people age 55 and older (American Cancer Society, 2005).

After adjusted for normal life expectancy (accounting for factors such as dying of heart disease, injuries, and other diseases of old age), a relative 5-year survival rate of 64% is seen for all cancers (American Cancer Society, 2005). This rate means that the chance of a person recently diagnosed with cancer being alive in 5 years is 64% of the chance of someone not diagnosed with cancer. Five-year relative survival rates commonly are used to monitor progress in the early detection and treatment of cancer and include persons who are living 5 years after diagnosis, whether in remission, disease-free, or under treatment. Currently almost 10 million people in the United States are cancer survivors (American Cancer Society, 2005) and more than half of the cancer survivors are women (National Cancer Institute, 2003). Therefore, the number of sexual minority women who are cancer survivors is likely to be considerable. In addition to the human toll of cancer, the financial costs of cancer are substantial (Brown et al., 1996; American Cancer Society, 2005). These costs include the financial cost of cancer treatment and/or survival (essentially, costs for health care provision and for long-term care due to disability) and the financial costs of cancer due to economic loss of individuals who work less or leave the workforce due to cancer (Yabroff et al., 2004).

These data allow us to make two points. First, cancer is a relatively frequent disease that takes a toll on the population's health. Therefore, it is likely that cancer takes a toll on the health of sexual minority women as well. Whether it affects sexual minority women disproportionally is the topic of much discussion, but a definitive answer is still unknown. Second, there are opportunities for both improving the quality of cancer treatment and survivorship for the general population and for identifying opportunities for testing and disseminating methods to prevent cancer from occurring and for detecting it early. It is likely that sexual minority women could benefit from these opportunities as well as the general population.

1.2 Disparities in the General Population

The cancer burden is unequally distributed in the population in that different demographic and socioeconomic characteristics are linked to cancer-related disparities. The American Cancer Society links the following characteristics to disparities: "income, race/ethnicity, culture, geography (urban/rural), age, sex, sexual orientation, literacy" (American Cancer Society, 2004, (p. 21)). For instance, death rates vary by gender (Wingo et al., 1999) in that lung cancer death rates in men have declined since 1990 yet have increased among women for several decades until recently when they reached a plateau (American Cancer Society, 2005).

Racial and ethnic minority groups have lower survival rates than Whites for most cancers (Jemal et al., 2005). All racial and ethnic groups, except Asian/Pacific Islander women, are more likely to die from all cancers combined within 5 years of diagnosis compared with Whites (Ward et al., 2004; Jemal et al., 2005). African American women are about 20% more likely to die of cancer in general than are Whites, yet they are twice as likely to die of stomach or cervical cancer than Whites (Jemal et al., 2005). African American women are more likely to die of breast and colon cancers than are women of any other racial and ethnic group (Ward et al., 2004). The incidence also differs among ethnic groups in that Asian Americans/Pacific Islanders have the highest incidence of stomach, liver, and intrahepatic bile duct cancer, Hispanic women the highest incidence of cancer of the cervix, and African American women the highest incidence of colon, rectum, and stomach cancer (Ward et al., 2004). Across all racial or ethnic groups, persons who live in more affluent areas have higher survival rates than do those in poorer areas (American Cancer Society, 2004; Ward et al., 2004).

These disparities in cancer incidence, survival, and mortality rates represent a challenge to understand the reasons that cause them. Healthy People 2010 calls for the elimination of these disparities to improve the nation's health (U.S. Department of Health and Human Services, 2000). We know that complex interactions of social, cultural, and economic factors cause cancer disparities, yet disparities as they relate to sexual minority women have yet to be identified in population-based data, and the factors that cause them must be carefully examined. The challenge of detecting factors of cancer disparities related to sexual minority women is further compounded by the fact that sexual minority women are also of different race/ethnicity, age, socioeconomic status, religion, and education, providing additional complexities in understanding subgroups of sexual minority women.

1.3 Definition of Sexual Minority Women

Different labels for sexual minority women are used in the literature cited in this chapter because of the diversity of labels, identities, and sexual behaviors investigated in the research. The issue of measuring sexual orientation status has received attention in the theoretical and empirical literature (Laumann et al., 1994; Young & Meyer, 2005). For this review we use the term "sexual minority women" (SMW) to refer generally to lesbian, gay, and bisexual women. When possible we use the term SMW to describe the general group of women.

Typically, this definition also includes transgender individuals; however, existing research on cancer does not generally focus on this population. As a result, in this discussion we do not include transgender individuals under the general description of SMW and, instead, refer to them separately in the text. Research studies on SMW sometimes group lesbians and bisexual women together because of their overlapping sexual practices whereas at other times separate them when sexual behaviors differ (Johnson et al., 1987). As a result, lesbian and bisexual are terms we use in addition to SMW when a study's focus dictates this distinction. We define *lesbians* as "women whose emotional, social, and sexual relationships are primarily with women" (p. 315) (Phillips-Angeles et al., 2004). The lesbian identity, like other sexual orientations, encompasses different dimensions, including sexual identity or how one self-identifies, the sexual desire or attraction a person feels for another, and sexual behavior (Bonvicini & Perlin, 2003). *Bisexual women*, as described by Tucker and Colleagues (1995), have the potential for attraction to both men and women and are attracted to the individual rather than a person of a particular biologic sex or gender (Tucker et al., 1995).

2 What is Known About Cancer Incidence and Risks in Sexual Minority Women?

2.1 Cancer Rates Among Sexual Minority Women

Little is known about potential cancer incidence disparities in SMW owing primarily to the lack of collection of appropriate data in national registries and databases. MEDLINE searches crossing the cancer site by homosexuality, female, and lesbian (October 26, 2005) provided no comparative population-based incidence data. Possible disparities regarding the health status of lesbians and possible barriers to access to health services by lesbians have been identified by the Institute of Medicine (IOM) as a research priority (Solarz, 1999). The January 2001 newsletter of the Mary-Helen Mautner Project for Lesbians with Cancer points out that "each year 23,000 women are diagnosed with ovarian cancer, and 14,000 die from the disease, making it the deadliest of the gynecologic cancers and the fifth leading cause of cancer death among women" (Boyd, 2001). Several investigators have hypothesized that SMW have a higher breast cancer incidence than heterosexual women. A small-scale study found higher rates of breast cancer among SMW; but because the cohort was small and the research methodology was not population-based, the reliability of these findings has been questioned (Dibble et al., 1997). One study found a higher risk of breast cancer among lesbians using a reasonable sample (Kavanaugh-Lynch et al., 2002). None of the existing studies has been truly population-based, as are the cancer incidence publications for the United States (Greenlee et al., 2000).

A Danish group found similar rates of cancer between SMW and heterosexual women using a registry approach, where same-sex marriage-like relationships are registered as well as heterosexual marriages (Frisch et al., 2003). However, the median age of the female registry participants at the time of registry was 37, leaving a relatively small sample at the older years, when cancer is more prevalent. SMW receive less frequent gynecologic care than heterosexual women (Robertson & Schachter, 1981) and therefore might be at greater risk for mortality and morbidity from a range of gynecologic cancers. Both of these risks are likely compounded by the difficulties many SMW experience in communicating with or receiving standard clinical care from physicians and health care systems.

Each year more women die from lung cancer than breast cancer (American Cancer Society, 2004). Lung cancer rates are likely to be higher in SMW owing to smoking differences (summarized below), although data on incidence and prevalence are lacking. The three most common cancers in women—breast, lung, colon—were expected to claim the lives of more than 140,000 women during 2005 (Jemal et al., 2005). Little is known about the prevalence and incidence of other cancers among SMW, and more research is thus needed. Even less is known about cancer in transsexual persons, and research is thus needed to determine rates, risk factors, and screening needs (Balen et al., 1993; Lawrence, 2005).

2.2 Risk Factors for Common Cancers Among Sexual Minority Women

Risk factor levels or risk factors themselves may differ between SMW and heterosexual women. However, published population-based data on these risk factors are sparse. The hypothesis that SMW have higher rates of breast cancer came about because of the potential higher rates of risk factors such as obesity, alcohol consumption, and null parity (Denenberg, 1995; Haynes, 1995) in addition to lower screening rates. Although definitive studies in this area have yet to be completed, data on the prevalence of each of the risk factors confirm the plausibility of this hypothesis (Dibble et al., 1997; Valanis et al., 2000; Cochran et al.,

2001; Case et al., 2004). There are risk factors for ovarian cancer that are common among all women (e.g., personal or family history of ovarian, breast, and colon cancer; increasing age), but there is discussion that SMW may be at increased risk for ovarian cancer as well (Boyd, 2001). Among the risk factors responsible for this possible increased risk are lower frequency of childbearing, lack of oral contraceptive use, lack of access of health care, lower utilization of the health care system, and possibly the use of fertility drugs (Boyd, 2001).

The single exception to the striking lack of data on risk factors for cancer among SMW is in the area of smoking. Smoking is the most important risk factor for lung cancer and many other chronic diseases; SMW are more likely than heterosexual women to use tobacco products, as documented in reviews and population-based studies (Diamant et al., 2000; Valanis et al., 2000; Cochran et al., 2001; Gruskin et al., 2001; Ryan et al., 2001; Case et al., 2004; Tang et al., 2004). Data collected using strong methodology have documented approximately double the rates of smoking for SMW compared to heterosexual women in California (Tang et al., 2004; Burgard et al., 2005). This single risk factor difference could account for up to one-third of disparity-related deaths, given national estimates on the impact of smoking on health. No intervention studies are published, but one such study is ongoing at the University of California, San Francisco (2005); and the American Legacy Foundation (2005) is supporting community inter-vention for LGBT adults in several major cities in the United States. These activities are encouraging starts at reducing the behavioral disparity of smoking use by SMW.

3 Primary and Secondary Prevention Opportunities

3.1 Primary Prevention in Sexual Minority Women

Evidence suggests that several types of cancer can be prevented and that the prospects for surviving cancer continue to improve. The ability to reduce cancer death rates depends, in part, on the existence and application of various resources, in particular the means to provide cul-turally and linguistically appropriate information to the public and to health care providers on primary prevention actions, such as changing or reducing behaviors known to increase the likelihood of developing cancer. It is estimated that 50% or more of cancers can be prevented through smoking cessation and improved dietary habits, such as reduc-ing fat consumption and increasing fruit and vegetable consumption (U.S. Department of Health and Human Services, 1990; Willet, 1996). Physical activity and weight control can also contribute to cancer pre-vention (Greenwald et al., 1995; U.S. Department of Health and Human Services, 1996). These are all relevant to SMW owing to differences in the behavioral characteristics of this group.

As previously discussed, tobacco use is clearly higher among SMW than among heterosexual women. Given the importance of tobacco use in causing most major diseases and premature deaths, this is a critical disparity that needs research attention. Unfortunately, little has been published on methods to reduce this disparity in SMW.

Considerable literature has linked healthy dietary behaviors, physical activity, and more recently obesity to rates of several cancers. One review concluded that obesity levels were higher in SMW than in heterosexual controls (Bowen & Balsam, 2005). The small literature comparing dietary behaviors and physical activity between SMW and heterosexual women indicates poorer dietary quality and lower rates of overall physical activity. The literature in these areas is sporadic and poorly sampled, and therefore it is difficult to draw reliable conclusions from the available articles.

3.2 Secondary Prevention and Sexual Minority Women

Data suggest that mammography, the best proven breast cancer screening method to date, is used less frequently by SMW. There are few population-based studies, but regional and local surveys of SMW and reasonable comparison samples indicate 10% differences in mammography rates between these two groups (Valanis et al., 2000; Bowen et al., 2004; Case et al., 2004). Although there are no national data on rates of mammography among SMW and transgender populations, the existing data indicate that a possible disparity by sexual minority status may exist. Access barriers may inhibit appropriate mammography screening, and specific interventions should be designed for both providers and patients to increase access to mammography screening. Breast and cervical health programs funded by the Centers for Disease Control and Prevention (CDC) may serve as a potential model for replication in sexual minority communities, but no evaluation data on these programs have been published. After such a program was implemented, a reduction in breast cancer deaths could be expected to occur after a delay of roughly 7 years (Fletcher et al., 1993).

Evidence shows that a reduction in colorectal cancer deaths can be achieved through detection and removal of precancerous polyps and treatment in the earliest stages of the disease. The findings from randomized, controlled trials indicate that biennial screening with fecal occult blood tests can reduce deaths from colorectal cancer (Mandel et al., 1993, 1999; Hardcastle et al., 1996; Kronborg et al., 1996; Winawer et al., 1997). The U.S. preventive services task force recommends annual tests, with follow-up endoscopy for those with positive screens. We have no data on rates of colon cancer screening among SMW.

To reduce the number of cervical cancer deaths, a high percentage of women in the United States aged 18 years and older must comply with screening recommendations. Evidence from randomized preventive trials is unavailable, but expert opinion suggests that a beneficial impact on cervical cancer death rates would be expected to occur after a delay of a few years. There are no national data on Pap test rates among women of sexual minority orientation or nonconformative gender identity. Recent survey data suggest lower Pap test rates among lesbians (Diamant et al., 2000). This lack of established medical care could lead to higher rates of cervical cancer, and research is needed to identify methods for reducing this disparity. Issues regarding access to appropriate care could be one explanation (Cochran et al., 2001) and should form the basis of interventions to improve provision of care. Little or no population-based data on lesbians, bisexual women, or male-to-female (MtF) transgender people are obtained through national-level surveys or studies.

Cancer has been related to human papilloma virus (HPV) infection. Data indicate that sexual behaviors between women can result in HPV transmission (Marrazzo, 1996; O'Hanlan & Crum, 1996), and there is some indication that SMW and their providers may not perceive women who have sex with women as an at-risk group, contributing to a lack of Pap tests among SMW (Marrazzo, 2004). Similarly, gay men, who are at higher risk for anal cancer, often do not receive preventive care, including Pap tests. Therefore, it is likely that SMW do not receive adequate care as well.

For MtF transgender individuals, the belief among many providers that they are still biologically male may interfere with preventive gyne-cologic care. Also, tissue remaining after sex reassignment may still produce cancer cells. Female-to-male (FtM) transgender people who have a cervix remain at risk for cervical cancer and require regular Pap tests. However, there are no existing data on actual risk. Specific guide-lines for recommended prevention efforts have not been developed, but the Harry Benjamin International Gender Dysphoria Association (HBIGDA) recommends that transgender persons be screened for malignancies "as are all other persons" (Association, 1998). MtF trans-sexuals who have undergone vaginoplasty also may not be perceived as being at risk. However, persons who have undergone penile-inversion vaginoplasty with the penile gland retained as a neocervix should be offered neocervical Pap tests because of the risk of penile cancer in this group (Lawrence, 2005).

4 What of the Future? Research on Cancer in Sexual Minority Women

The above discussion illustrates the dearth of data to guide policy and practice in the area of cancer prevention and control in SMW. Here we list areas of immediate need for research into this area.

4.1 Call for Research into Cancer Risks and Risk Factors for Sexual Minority Women

More research using innovative methodologies and standard registries is needed to determine differences in cancer risk and risk factors for SMW. For example, a cohort design using studies of records in New York and California cancer registries and the National Death Index found gay and bisexual men to be at excess risk for anal cancer, non-Hodgkin's lymphoma, and Hodgkin's disease. These data accounted for an increased risk for all cancers in this population. The authors found no difference in the incidence of cancers at any other site, includ-ing lip, oral cavity, and pharynx; digestive system and peritoneum;

respiratory system; bone and connective tissues; skin; genital and urinary organs; bone marrow (multiple myeloma); blood and tissues (leukemia); or other and unspecified sites (Koblin et al., 1996). This type of design could be implemented with SMW to identify increased risk of all types of cancer.

Population-based national data sets, such as Surveillance Epidemiology and End Results (SEER), could include sexual orientation in specific circumstances and could encourage the publication of data using sexual orientation as a subgrouping variable. Current examples of national public health surveys that do include sexual orientation are the National Health and Nutrition Examination Survey, the National Survey of Family Growth, and others that are tracked at http://www.gaydata.org. Individual states are now including sexual orientation on selected Behavioral Risk Factor Surveillance System surveys, but this does not provide us with a national picture. Once this simple, easily collected variable is in place in multiple surveys, risks and risk factors for a variety of diseases could be identified for SMW.

4.2 Call for Research into Prevention in Sexual Minority Women

Mechanisms or systems must exist for providing SMW with access to state-of-the-art risk assessment, preventive services, and treatment. Where suitable, application for participation in clinical trials should be encouraged. A mechanism for maintaining continued research programs and for fostering new research is essential. New information on genetic markers or environmental linkages that can be used to improve disease prevention strategies and healthy behavior counseling is emerging for many cancers and may provide the foundation for improved effectiveness in clinical care and preventive counseling services.

There is a continuing and vital need to foster new partnerships for innovative research on both the causes of cancer (including genetic and environmental causes) and on methods to translate biologic and epidemiologic findings into effective prevention and control programs through publicly funded programs and community organizations (Lasker et al., 2001), and research with SMW is no exception (Durfy et al., 1999). This research can provide new opportunities for cancer prevention and control in the future and further reduce many burdens associated with cancer. This need can be met, in part, with the network of cancer control resources now in place, as it has the organizational and personnel capacity for various cancer interventions. Despite the extent of these resources, they alone are insufficient to reduce deaths from cancer. Gaps exist in information dissemination, information on optimal practice patterns and clinical guidelines, research capabilities, and research underway in other countries. These gaps must be recognized and filled to meet cancer prevention and control needs.

Rigorous evaluation of interventions that target SMW for screening and health behavioral change interventions comprise the most critical gap in the literature. For example, a pilot study evaluating the feasibility of a didactic session to encourage cancer screening among lesbians (Dibble & Roberts, 2003) ended with a call for a carefully evaluated study in this area. Few other research on interventions to improve the health of SMW have been published (Bowen et al., 2006) but much more is needed to provide evidence-based ideas for public health and clinical practice changes. Intervention research involves first identifying the changeable risk factors, developing methods to support change in these risk factors, and conducting rigorous research to identify the ability of these interventions to change the targeted behaviors. Previously mentioned intervention research and public health practice to reduce smoking among lesbian, gay, bisexual, transgender (LGBT) communities is a cutting edge example of intervention opportunity. As disparities are identified, we must move more quickly to intervention research to reduce or eliminate them.

4.3 Research Needs Regarding Treatment and Survivorship of Sexual Minority Women

For all cancers, treatments proven to increase survival are needed along with improved access to state-of-the-art screening and postdetection care. In addition to measurements of survival, indices of quality of life for both the short term and long term are important considerations. Appropriate treatment relies on full access to care, which is likely lacking in SMW. Therefore, this could form another area of need for both research and practice improvement. Although we have no good data on the cancer treatment SMW receive (Dibble & Roberts, 2002), it is possible that differences in cancer treatments may exist that influence SMW's survival. Studies of the general population with cancer indicated that differences in treatment exist; for example, patients who are older are less likely to receive aggressive therapy (Goodwin et al., 1993, 1996; Ballard-Barbash et al., 1996; Silliman et al., 1997), as do patients who are uninsured (Ayanian & Guadagnoli, 1996; Roetzheim et al., 2000; Bradley et al., 2002; Voti et al., 2005). We do not know if potential treatment disparities for SMW is due to aspects of the provider–SMW patient relationship that interfere with treatment adherence or to provider prescription itself. Furthermore, lesbians are likely to express interest in complementary and alternative therapies (Bowen et al., 2002; Matthews et al., 2005), and how this affects SMW's choices and preferences for standard treatment and adjuvant therapy should form the basis of research in the future.

Coping with and responses to cancer, including cancer survivors' perceptions of well-being, have been widely researched, and interventions to improve cancer survivors' psychosocial outcomes have been developed. Similar studies of the social context and the psychosocial outcomes of SMW with cancer are mostly lacking (Fobair et al., 2001, 2002; McGregor et al., 2001; Boehmer et al., 2005b). Although there are sparse data on long-term follow-up of SMW cancer survivors and their social context, it is reasonable to suggest that several factors may affect survivorship. Social support through partners and friends rather than family, a lack of community support, health care access barriers, and barriers in provider–patient communication may jeopardize the adjustment of SMW diagnosed with cancer and their long-term survival. One study determined that lesbians were less frequently partnered, yet were more likely to obtain social support from their partners and friends than heterosexuals (Fobair et al., 2001). Another study found that almost one-fourth of SMW with breast cancer did not have a significant support person to rely on and suggested that relationship status may be of importance for the availability of such a person (Boehmer et al., 2005a). The single intervention study with SMW breast cancer survivors indicated that emotional distress can be reduced and the coping of SMW can be altered; yet SMW reported also a decline in the level of their social support after the intervention (Fobair et al., 2001). Additional research is needed to verify that these are barriers and to design appropriate solutions to improve SMW's well-being and to increase their survival.

4.4 General Research Needs in This Area

Difficulty assessing sexual orientation in the general population may lead to bias in any existing studies on LGBT participants and their risk for various cancers. Available studies typically use study respondents who live in urban areas and are perhaps more open about their sexual orientation, usually of midlife age. It is not known to what extent the results are applicable to the less "out," older, or younger SMW populations.

There has been little research concerning cancer among transgender persons. One population-based study from The Netherlands suggests that overall cancer morbidity and mortality rates among transsexuals are comparable to those of the general population (van Kesteren et al., 1997). Nevertheless, transsexuals' exposure to hormone therapy over an extended period of time might be expected to increase the risk of certain hormone-related cancers. For example, estrogen is a risk factor for cancer of the breast, and there have been four case reports of breast cancer in MtF transsexuals treated with estrogens (Symmers, 1968; Pritchard et al., 1988; Ganly & Taylor, 1995). There have also been two case reports of ovarian cancer in FtM transsexuals, and it has been suggested that testosterone therapy may be a risk factor for such cancers in FtM transsexuals (Hage et al., 2000). These case reports might welcome follow-up research attention.

There are no national data on the degree to which physicians and dentists recommend preventive measures or deliver clinical preventive screens for cancer among LGBT patients. However, there is a significant amount of data, cited in other chapters, to suggest that SMW are less likely to have health insurance and have limited access to appropriate care, including culturally appropriate health education materials, cancer screening, and prevention counseling. There is also evidence that health care providers from a variety of disciplines are uncomfortable providing care to SMW and therefore may not address their specific needs or even general prevention strategies.

The negative impact of homophobia and heterosexism cause much more than a lack of population-based data on LGBT persons and SMW's cancer-related disparities, respectively. They also cause a lack of recognition of LGBT persons as a population subgroup with a shared culture consisting of "customs, beliefs, values, knowledge, and skills that guide a people's behavior along shared paths" (p. 14) (Gay and Lesbian Medical Association & LGBT Health Experts, 2001). Although we need population-based data to measure the magnitude of the cancer burden in SMW, we also need research that seeks to examine SMW's culture to understand how to reach this population appropriately and effectively for cancer-related messages and provide cancer-related care. Many of the disparities outlined in this document could be linked to cultural differences between SMW and heterosexual women. For example, there is some consideration of body image and perceptions that could prevent SMW from feeling comfortable with providers who do not understand issues of sexuality and gender roles prevalent in SMW (Boehmer et al., in press). These cultural issues deserve more research attention and could form the basis of a research program that could benefit SMW and contribute to the larger field of gender studies.

There are currently a wide variety of demonstration projects that provide services to SMW in large urban areas living with cancer. These cancer projects provide services for survivors of cancer and other chronic diseases. There is no available research on the efficacy of these projects, but their continued wide use and availability speaks to the role they fill in communities.

5 Summary

Cancer is a serious health issue for many people, including LGBT persons. Research suggests that some risk factors for cancer are more prevalent in sexual minority women than heterosexual women, and sexual minority women may be disproportionately affected by some cancers, including breast cancer, lung cancer, and cancers caused by HPV. Data are needed on rates of risk factors and cancers in sexual minority women, with participants identified by sexual orientation in population-based research efforts and data surveillance systems. Heterosexism and homophobia in the health care system may make LGBT persons less likely to receive needed prevention information and treatment, putting them at risk of higher cancer-related morbidity and mortality. Finally, public health programs to improve health behaviors to prevent cancer are lacking for sexual minority women. Therefore, research is needed to determine culturally appropriate methods of prevention- and treatment-oriented interventions for sexual minority women, so targeted health education, care services, and planning policies can be implemented.

References

American Cancer Society. (2004) *Cancer facts and figures 2004* (web version). American Cancer Society, Atlanta.
American Cancer Society. (2005) Cancer facts and figures 2005. ACS, Washington, DC.

American Legacy Foundation. (2005) From http://www.americanlegacy.org/americanlegacy/skins/alf/home.aspx.

Association: Harry Benjamin International Gender Dysphoria Association. (1998) *The standards of care for gender identity disorders.* HBIGD, Dusseldorf.

Ayanian, J.Z., and Guadagnoli, E. (1996) Variations in breast cancer treatment by patient and provider characteristics. *Breast Cancer Research and Treatment* 40(1):65–74.

Balen, A.H., Schachter, M.E., Montgomery, D., Reid, R.W., and Jacobs, H.S. (1993) Polycystic ovaries are a common finding in untreated female to male transsexuals. *Clinical Endocrinology* 38:325–329.

Ballard-Barbash, R., Potosky, A.L., Harlan, L.C., Nayfield, S.G., and Kessler, L.G. (1996) Factors associated with surgical and radiation therapy for early stage breast cancer in older women. *Journal of the National Cancer Institute* 88:716–726.

Boehmer, U., Freund, K.M., and Linde, R. (2005a) Support providers of sexual minority women with breast cancer who they are and how they impact the breast cancer experience. *Journal of Psychosomotion Research* 59:307–314.

Boehmer, U., Linde, R., and Freund, K.M. (In Press) Breast reconstruction following mastectomy for breast cancer: the decisions of sexual minority women. *Plastic and Reconstructive Surgery*

Boehmer, U., Linde, R., and Freund, K.M. (2005b). Sexual minority women's coping and psychological adjustment after a diagnosis of breast cancer. *Journal of Women's Health* 14:214–224.

Bonvicini, K.A., and Perlin, M.J. (2003) The same but different: clinician-patient communication with gay and lesbian patients. *Patient Education and Counseling* 51:115–122.

Bowen, D.J., and Balsam, K. (2005). A review of obesity issues in sexual minority women.

Bowen, D.J., Anderson, J., White, J., Powers, D., and Greenlee, H. (2002) Preferences for alternative and traditional health care: relationship to health behaviors, health information sources, and trust of providers. *Journal of Gay and Lesbian Medical Association*, 6(1):3–7.

Bowen, D.J., Powers, D., Bradford, J., McMorrow, P., Linde, R., Murphy, B.C., et al. (2004) Comparing women of differing sexual orientations using population-based sampling. *Women & Health* 40(3):19–34.

Bowen, D.J., Powers, D., and Greenlee, H. (2006) Effects of breast cancer risk counseling for sexual minority women. *Health Care for Women International* 27:59–74.

Boyd, N.C. (2001) *Lesbians and ovarian cancer: ending the epidemic of silence.* Mary-Helen Mautner Project for Lesbians with Cancer, Washington, DC.

Bradley, C.J., Given, C.W., and Roberts, C. (2002) Race, socioeconomic status, and breast cancer treatment and survival. *Journal of the National Cancer Institute* 94:490–496.

Brown, M.L., Hodgson, T.A., and Rice, D.P. (1996) Economic impact of cancer in the united states. In: Schottenfeld, D., Fraumeni, J., and Joseph, F. (eds) *Cancer epidemiology and prevention*, 2nd ed. Oxford University Press, New York.

Burgard, S.A., Cochran, S.D., and Mays, V.M. (2005) Alcohol and tobacco use patterns among heterosexually and homosexually experienced California women. *Drug and Alcohol Dependence* 77(1):61–70.

Case, P., Austin, S.B., Hunter, D.J., Manson, J.E., Malspeis, S., Willett, W.C., et al. (2004) Sexual orientation, health risk factors, and physical functioning in the nurses' health study ii. *Journal of Women's Health (Larchmont)* 13:1033–1047.

Cochran, S.D., Mays, V.M., Bowen, D.J., Gage, S., Bybee, D., Roberts, S.J., et al. (2001) Cancer-related risk indicators and preventive screening behaviors among lesbians and bisexual women. *American Journal of Public Health* 91:591–597.

Denenberg, R. (1995) Report on lesbian health. *Women's Health Issues* 5(2): 51–91.

Diamant, A.L., Wold, C., Spritzer, K., and Gelberg, L. (2000) Health behaviors, health status, and access to and use of health care: a population-based study of lesbian, bisexual, and heterosexual women. *Archives of Family Medicine* 9:1043–1051.

Dibble, S.L., and Roberts, S.A. (2002) A comparison of breast cancer diagnosis and treatment between lesbian and heterosexual women. *Journal of the Gay and Lesbian Medical Association* 6(1):9–17.

Dibble, S.L., and Roberts, S.A. (2003) Improving cancer screening among lesbians over 50: results of a pilot study. *Oncology Nursing Forum* 30(4):E71–E79.

Dibble, S.L., Vanoni, J.M., and Miaskowski, C. (1997) Women's attitudes toward breast cancer screening procedures: differences by ethnicity. *Women's Health Issues* 7(1):47–54.

Durfy, S.J., Bowen, D.J., McTiernan, A., Sporleder, J., and Burke, W. (1999) Attitudes and interest in genetic testing for breast and ovarian cancer susceptibility in diverse groups of women in western Washington. *Cancer Epidemiology, Biomarkers & Prevention* 8(4 Pt 2):369–375.

Fletcher, S.W., Black, W., Harris, R., Rimer, B.K., and Shapiro, S. (1993) Report of the international workshop on screening for breast cancer. *Journal of the National Cancer Institute* 85:1644–1656.

Fobair, P., Koopman, C., Dimiceli, S., O'Hanlan, K., Butler, L., Classen, C., et al. (2002) Psychosocial intervention for lesbians with primary breast cancer. *Psycho-oncology* 11:427–438.

Fobair, P., O'Hanlan, K., Koopman, C., Classen, C., Dimiceli, S., Drooker, N., et al. (2001) Comparison of lesbian and heterosexual women's response to newly diagnosed breast cancer. *Psycho-oncology* 10(1):40–51.

Frisch, M., Smith, E., Grulich, A., and Johansen, C. (2003) Cancer in a population-based cohort of men and women in registered homosexual partnerships. *American Journal of Epidemiology* 157:966–972.

Ganly, I., and Taylor, E.W. (1995) Breast cancer in a trans-sexual man receiving hormone replacement therapy. *British Journal of Surgery* 82:341.

Gay and Lesbian Medical Association and LGBT health experts. (2001) Healthy people 2010 companion document for lesbian, gay, bisexual and transgender (LGBT) health. http://wwwglmaorg/policy/hp2010/.

Goodwin, J.S., Hunt, W.C., and Samet, J.M. (1993) Determinants of cancer therapy in elderly patients. *Cancer* 72:594–601.

Goodwin, J.S., Samet, J.M., and Hunt, W.C. (1996) Determinants of survival in older cancer patients. *Journal of the National Cancer Institute* 88:1031–1038.

Greenlee, R.T., Murray, T., Bolden, S., and Wingo, P.A. (2000) Cancer statistics, 2000. *CA: A Cancer Journal for Clinicians* 50:7–33.

Greenwald, P., Kramer, B., and Weed, D.L. (1995) *Cancer prevention and control.* Marcel Dekker, New York.

Gruskin, E.P., Hart, S., Gordon, N., and Ackerson, L. (2001) Patterns of cigarette smoking and alcohol use among lesbians and bisexual women enrolled in a large health maintenance organization. *American Journal of Public Health* 91:976–979.

Hage, J.J., Dekker, J.J., Karim, R.B., Verheijen, R.H., and Bloemena, E. (2000) Ovarian cancer in female-to-male transsexuals: report of two cases. *Gynecologic Oncology* 76:413–415.

Hardcastle, J.D., Chamberlain, J.O., Robinson, M.H.E., Moss, S.M., Amar, S.S., Balfour, T.W., et al. (1996) Randomized controlled trial of faecal-occult-blood screening for colorectal cancer. *Lancet* 348:1472–1477.

Haynes, S. (1995) Breast cancer risk: comparisons of lesbians and heterosexual women. In: Bowen, D.J. (ed) *Cancer and cancer risks among lesbians*. Fred Hutchinson Cancer Research Center Liasion Program, Seattle.

Jemal, A., Murray, T., Ward, E., Samuels, A., Tiwari, R.C., Ghafoor, A., et al. (2005) Cancer statistics, 2005. *CA Cancer J Clin* 55:10–30.

Johnson, S.R., Smith, E.M., and Guenther, S.M. (1987) Comparison of gynecologic healthcare problems between lesbians and bisexual women: a survey of 2,345 women. *Journal of Reproductive Medicine* 32:805–811.

Kavanaugh-Lynch, M., White, E., Daling, J., and Bowen, D.J. (2002) Correlates of lesbian sexual orientation and the risk of breast cancer. *Journal of the Gay and Lesbian Medical Association* 6:91–96.

Koblin, B.A., Hessol, N.A., Zauber, A.G., Taylor, P.E., Buchbinder, S.P., Katz, M.H., et al. (1996) Increased incidence of cancer among homosexual men, New York City and San Francisco, 1978–1990. *American Journal of Epidemiology* 144:916–923.

Kronborg, O., Fenger, C., Oslen, J., Jorgensen, O.D., and Sondergaard, O. (1996) Randomized study of screening for colorectal cancer with faecal-occult-blood-test. *Lancet* 348:1467–1471.

Lasker, R.D., Weiss, E.S., and Miller, R. (2001) Partnership synergy: a practical framework for studying and strengthening the collaborative advantage. *Milbank Quarterly* 79:179–205, III–IV.

Laumann, E.O., Gagnon, J.H., Michael, R.T., and Michael, S. (1994) *The social organization of sexuality: sexual practices in the United States.* University of Chicago Press, Chicago.

Lawrence, A.A. (2001). Vaginal neoplasia in a male-to-female transsexual: case report, review of the literature, and recommendations for cytological screening. *The International Journal of Transgenderism* 5:1, http://www.symposion.com/ijt/ijtvo05no01_01.htm.

Mandel, J.S., Bond, J.H., Church, T.R., and Snover, D.C. (1993) Reducing mortality from colorectal cancer by screening for fecal occult blood. *The New England Journal of Medicine* 328:1365–1371.

Mandel, J.S., Church, T.R., Ederer, F., and Bond, J.H. (1999) Colorectal cancer mortality: effectiveness of biennial screening for fecal occult blood. *Journal of the National Cancer Institute* 91:434–437.

Marrazzo, J. (1996). *STDs and cervical neoplasia amoung lesbians: research review and update.* Presented at the 19th Annual National Lesbian and Gay Health Association Conference, Seattle, WA.

Marrazzo, J.M. (2004) Barriers to infections disease care among lesbians. *Emerging Infections Diseases* 10:1974–1978.

Matthews, A.K., Hughes, T.L., Osterman, G.P., and Kodl, M.M. (2005) Complementary medicine practices in a community-based sample of lesbian and heterosexual women. *Health Care for Women International* 26:430–447.

McGregor, B.A., Carver, C.S., Antoni, M.H., Weiss, S., Yount, S.E., and Ironson, G. (2001) Distress and internalized homophobia among lesbian women treated for early stage breast cancer. *Psychology of Women Quarterly* 25(1):1–9.

National Cancer Institute. (2003) Women's health report, fiscal years 2001–2002. NCI, Bethesda, MD.

O'Hanlan, K.A., and Crum, C.P. (1996) Human papvillomavirus-associated cervical intraepithelial neoplasia following lesbian sex. *Obstetrics and Gynecology* 88:702–703.

Phillips-Angeles, E., Wolfe, P., Myers, R., Dawson, P., Marrazzo, J., Soltner, S., et al. (2004) Lesbian health matters: Pap test education campaign nearly thwarted by discrimination. *Health Promotion Practice* 5:314–325.

Pritchard, T.J., Pankowsky, D.A., Crowe, J.P., and Abdul-Karim, F.W. (1988) Breast cancer in a male-to-female transsexual: a case report. *Journal of the American Medical Association* 259:2278–2280.

Robertson, P., and Schachter, J. (1981) Failure to identify venereal disease in a lesbian population. *Sexually Transmitted Diseases* 8(20):75–76.

Roetzheim, R.G., Gonzalez, E.C., Ferrante, J.M., Pal, N., Van Durme, D.J., and Krischer, J.P. (2000) Effects of health insurance and race on breast carcinoma treatments and outcomes. *Cancer* 89:2202–2213.

Ryan, H., Wortley, P.M., Easton, A., Pederson, L., and Greenwood, G. (2001) Smoking among lesbians, gays, and bisexuals: a review of the literature. *American Journal of Preventive Medicine* 21:142–149.

Silliman, R.A., Troyan, S.L., Guadagnoli, E., Kaplan, S.H., and Greenfield, S. (1997) The impact of age, marital status, and physician-patient interactions on the care of older women with breast carcinoma. *Cancer* 80:1326–1334.

Solarz, A.L. (1999) *Lesbian health: current assessment and direction for the future.* National Academy Press, Washington, DC.

Symmers, W.S. (1968) Carcinoma of breast in trans-sexual individuals after surgical and hormonal interference with the primary and secondary sex characteristics. *British Medical Journal* 2:82–85.

Tang, H., Greenwood, G.L., Cowling, D.W., Lloyd, J.C., Roeseler, A.G., and Bal, D.G. (2004) Cigarette smoking among lesbians, gays, and bisexuals: how serious a problem? (United States). *Cancer Causes Control* 15:797–803.

Tucker, N., Highleyman, L., and Kaplan, R. (1995) *Bisexual politics: theories, queries, and visions.* Haworth Press, Binghamton, NY.

University of California, San Francisco. (2005) From http://www.ucsf.edu/.

U.S. Department of Health and Human Services (DHHS). (1990) *The health benefits of smoking cessation.* DHHS Publ. No. CDC 90-8416. CDC, Atlanta.

U.S. Department of Health and Human Services. (1996) *Physical activity and health: a report of the Surgeon General.* DHHS, Bethesda, MD.

U.S. Department of Health and Human Services. (2000) *Healthy people 2010: understanding and improving health* (conference edition). Electronic version: http://www.health.gov/healthypeople/default.htm.

Valanis, B.G., Bowen, D.J., Bassford, T., Whitlock, E., Charney, P., and Carter, R.A. (2000) Sexual orientation and health: comparisons in the Women's Health Initiative sample. *Archives of Family Medicine* 9:843–853.

Van Kesteren, P.J., Asscheman, H., Megans, J.A.J., and Gooren, L.J.G. (1997) Mortality and morbidity in transsexual subjects treated with cross-sex hormones. *Clinical Endocrinology* (Oxford) 47:337–342.

Voti, L., Richardson, L.C., Reis, I., Fleming, L.E., Mackinnon, J., and Coebergh, J.W. (2005) The effect of race/ethnicity and insurance in the administration of standard therapy for local breast cancer in florida. *Breast Cancer Research and Treatment* 1–7.

Ward, E., Jemal, A., Cokkinides, V., Singh, G.K., Cardinez, C., Ghafoor, A., et al. (2004) Cancer disparities by race/ethnicity and socioeconomic status. *CA: a Cancer Journal for Clinicians* 54:78–93.

Willet, W. (1996) Diet and nutrition. In: Schottenfeld, D., and Fraumeni, J.F. (eds) *Cancer epidemiology and prevention,* 2nd ed. Oxford University Press, New York, pp. 438–461.

Winawer, S.J., Fletcher, R.H., Miller, L., Godlee, F., Stolar, M.H., Mulrow, C.D., et al. (1997) Colorectal cancer screening: clinical guidelines and rationale. *Gastroenterology* 112:594–642.

Wingo, P.A., Ries, L.A.G., Giovino, G.A., Miller, D.S., Rosenberg, H.M., Shopland, D.R., et al. (1999) Annual report to the nation on the status of cancer, 1973–1999, with a special section on lung cancer and tobacco smoking. *Journal of the National Cancer Institute* 91:675–690.

Yabroff, K.R., Lawrence, W.F., Clauser, S., Davis, W.W., and Brown, M.L. (2004) Burden of illness in cancer survivors: findings from a population-based national sample. *Journal of the National Cancer Institute* 96:1322–1330.

Young, R.M., and Meyer, I.H. (2005) The trouble with "MSM" and "WSW": erasure of the sexual-minority person in public health discourse. *American Journal of Public Health* 95:1144–1149.

22

HIV/AIDS Prevention Research Among Black Men Who Have Sex with Men: Current Progress and Future Directions

Gregorio A. Millett, David Malebranche, and John L. Peterson

1 Introduction

The social demography of the human immunodeficiency virus (HIV) epidemic among Black men in the United States has changed over the last two decades. Black men who have sex with men (MSM) now account for the largest proportion (30%) of all Black men diagnosed with HIV (CDC, 2004a). Moreover, Black men constitute a sizable proportion (27%) of all MSM diagnosed with HIV (CDC, 2004a,b). Similarly, most studies of MSM have reported that rates of HIV infection are higher among Black MSM than all other racial or ethnic MSM groups (Easterbrook et al., 1993; Lemp et al., 1994; Valleroy et al., 2000; CDC, 2001; Mansergh et al., 2002; Harawa et al., 2004).

Given the toll of the HIV epidemic on Black MSM, there is a pressing need to provide effective interventions that prevent HIV transmission and progression to the acquired immunodeficiency syndrome (AIDS). These interventions depend on the availability of sufficient research that describes and explains the factors that influence HIV transmission. Studies in public health and in the social or behavioral sciences provide evidence of potential factors that prevent HIV infection or an AIDS diagnosis among Black MSM. In primary prevention research, studies focus on factors associated with HIV serostatus, HIV risk behaviors, and protective behaviors associated with the initial infection with HIV. Secondary prevention research focuses on the factors that affect disease progression among HIV-infected individuals. Both research areas may involve intervention research to determine the types of intervention approaches to prevent HIV transmission or disease progression.

This chapter reviews the evidence relevant to HIV prevention among Black MSM in the United States from peer-reviewed literature indexed in online databases. Three topic sections address the main areas of research in the field: (1) factors associated with HIV-positive status,

HIV risk behaviors (e.g., unprotected anal sex, multiple sex partners, drug use), and HIV protective behaviors (e.g., HIV testing, condom use, help seeking) among Black MSM; (2) prevention of disease progression among HIV-positive Black MSM; and (3) HIV intervention research among Black MSM. In the first section, we discuss the descriptive studies that identify the demographic, behavioral, psychological, sociocultural, structural, and genetic or biologic factors associated with HIV-positive status, risk, and protective behaviors. These studies examine the specific individual, interpersonal, and contextual factors that affect HIV infection, HIV risk, or protective behaviors. In the second section, we discuss the effect of controlled HIV interventions to modify HIV risk behaviors among Black MSM and the components of effective interventions. Finally, we discuss patterns of health care access, mental health status, and sexual behaviors among HIV-positive Black MSM.

2 HIV-Positive Status, HIV Risk, and HIV-Protective Behavior Factors Among Black MSM

Most HIV research among MSM involves comparative studies that examine racial or ethnic differences in HIV prevalence or HIV risk behaviors. Typically, however, these comparative studies only report predictors of HIV status or risk behavior separately by race or ethnicity when the results confirm significant interactions with race. Relatively few MSM studies examine predictors of HIV status, HIV-related risk, or HIV-protective mechanisms exclusively among Black MSM. Factors significantly associated with HIV-positive status, HIV-related risk behavior, or an HIV-protective effect in Black MSM samples are listed in Table 1 and discussed below.

2.1 Demographic Factors

We defined variables that described characteristics of a research participant (e.g., education level, socioeconomic level, age) as demographic factors. Demographic factors of HIV-positive status, HIV-protective behavior, and sexual risk behavior among Black MSM are summarized below.

Only one demographic factor was associated with an outcome variable in more than one study. Both Peterson et al. (1992) and Myers et al. (2003) found that Black MSM from lower socioeconomic levels engaged in greater sexual risk behavior than black MSM from higher income levels.

Among all of the studies, only age was significantly associated with each of the outcome variables in samples of Black MSM. Being 22 to 25 years of age was only associated with HIV infection among Black men in a sample of young MSM (ages 17 to 29) (Ruiz et al., 1998). Older Black MSM were significantly more likely than younger Black MSM to be tested for HIV in one study (Mashburn et al., 2004), but another study found no association between age and condom use in a sample

Table 1. Predictors[a] of HIV Seropositivity, HIV Risk Behavior, and HIV-Protective Behavior Among Black MSM in Studies Published Between 1987 and 2005

Category	Factor
Outcome 1: HIV seropositivity factors	
Biologic and genetic	Previous gonorrhea infection[b]
Behavioral	Sexuality disclosure
Interpersonal	Age of sex partner
	Knowing a person who died of AIDS
Outcome 2a: HIV risk—Factors associated with sexual risk-taking	
Behavioral	Injection drug use
	Sexuality disclosure[c]
Demographic	Older age
Interpersonal	Low income[b]
	Gay identity
	HIV-negative status
	Being in a relationship
Psychological	Low condom peer norms
	Not carrying a condom
	High life satisfaction
	High psychological distress[b]
Sociocultural	Social support[c]
Outcome 2b: HIV risk—Factors associated with drug use	
Demographic	HIV-negative status
Outcome 3a: HIV-protective behavior—Factors associated with HIV testing	
Behavioral	Sexuality disclosure[b]
	Help-seeking for HIV risk behavior
Demographic	Older age
Interpersonal	Main and casual partners during past year
Psychological	HAART knowledge
Sociocultural	High social support
Structural	Comfortable HIV testing venue
Outcome 3b: HIV-protective behavior—Factors associated with condom use	
Psychological	High condom use expectations
	High condom use self-efficacy
	High safer-sex peer norms
Outcome 3c: HIV-protective behavior—Factors associated with professional counseling	
Demographic	HIV-positive status

HIV, human immunodeficiency virus; AIDS, acquired immunodeficiency syndrome; HAART, highly active antiretroviral therapy; MSM, men who have sex with men.
[a]Some of the listed correlates may have been significant in one study and not another.
[b]Correlate is significantly associated with the specified dependent variable in more than one study, and the direction of the relation is similar across studies.
[c]Correlate is significantly associated with the specified dependent variable in more than one study, but the direction of the relation varies.

of black MSM (Peterson et al., 1992). Similar conflicting results were reported for associations between age and HIV risk behavior. Myers et al. (2003) found that older Black MSM engaged in more sexual risks than younger Black MSM, but two other studies found no association between age and HIV risk behavior among Black MSM (Peterson et al.,

1992; Hart & Peterson, 2004). There was also conflicting evidence for the relation between HIV status and HIV risk behavior. Being HIV-negative compared to being HIV-positive was associated with greater risk behavior in one study (Myers et al., 2003), but HIV status was unrelated to unprotected anal intercourse or condom use among black MSM in a second study (Peterson et al., 1992).

Several demographic correlates were unrelated to any of the dependent variables. Although sexual identity was associated with HIV risk in one study and not associated in another study, the only study that examined sexual identity and HIV status among Black MSM found no association (CDC, 2004b). Neither education level nor employment status were associated with sexual risk taking (Hart & Peterson, 2004); and education level, employment status, and sexual identity were unrelated to HIV testing (Mashburn et al., 2004).

2.1.1 Summary of Demographic Predictors and Gaps

Of all the demographic factors reviewed, only one factor was associated with any of the dependent variables in more than one Black MSM study. Two studies found that low-income Black MSM were significantly more likely than high-income Black MSM to report sexual risk behaviors (Peterson et al., 1992; Myers et al., 2003).

There were notable gaps in the demographic variables tested in the available studies. None of the studies examined associations between HIV-positive status and education, income, or employment among Black MSM. Future studies should evaluate the few associations found between demographic variables and dependent variables and examine other demographic variables that have been previously neglected.

2.2 Interpersonal Factors

Sex partner characteristics and relationship status were broadly categorized as interpersonal factors. Only four interpersonal factors were significantly correlated with any of the outcome variables. Knowing someone who had died of AIDS was associated with HIV infection among young Black MSM (Ruiz et al., 1998). Age of sex partners was also associated with HIV infection in one study of young black MSM (Bingham et al., 2003) but was unrelated to HIV infection in another sample of young Black MSM (CDC, 2004b).

Relationship status was associated with HIV risk-taking and HIV-protective behavior in two studies of black MSM. Black MSM who reported a main male sexual partner were more likely than Black MSM with a casual male sex partner to engage in insertive and receptive anal sex (Hart & Peterson, 2004). Similarly, Black MSM who had main and casual male sex partners during the past year were more likely to report having had a past HIV test than Black MSM who had only casual male sex partners (Mashburn et al., 2004).

Many interpersonal factors were unrelated to any of the dependent variables. Having a sex partner with AIDS, having sex with a person from a high HIV prevalence city (Easterbrook et al., 1993), or having a recent female sex partner (CDC, 2004b) were each unrelated to HIV infection among Black MSM. Furthermore, the HIV-positive status of sex partners was unrelated to unprotected anal intercourse among Black MSM, and having an HIV-positive sex partner was unrelated to condom use among Black MSM (Peterson et al., 1992). A separate study of young Black MSM found that a sex partner's race was not associated with HIV infection (CDC, 2004b).

2.2.1 Summary of Interpersonal Predictors and Gaps

None of the interpersonal factors were tested across more than one study for a specific outcome. Only four interpersonal factors were associated with any of the outcomes. Given the disproportionately high HIV prevalence among black MSM, it is surprising that few studies have examined the characteristics of sex partners of homosexually active black men.

2.3 Behavioral Factors

We defined sexual behavior, drug use, carrying a condom, and other actions as behavioral factors. A few behavioral variables were correlated with HIV-positive status in Black MSM samples. Valleroy et al. (2000) found that having 5 to 19 male sex partners or more than 20 male sex partners was associated with HIV infection among black MSM. Wohl et al. (2002) reported that HIV-positive Black MSM who were aware of their serostatus were significantly less likely than HIV-negative Black MSM to report alcohol or drug use during sex. In addition, Peterson et al. (1995) found that self-identified HIV-positive Black MSM were more likely than self-identified HIV-negative Black MSM to seek help for risky sexual behavior. Last, one study found no relationship between sexuality disclosure and HIV status in a small sample of Black MSM (CDC, 2004b), whereas another investigation found that Black MSM who disclosed their sexuality were more likely than Black MSM nondisclosers to be HIV-positive (CDC, 2003).

Sexuality disclosure was also associated with sexual risk behavior, but the studies show mixed results. One study reported that Black MSM who did not disclose their sexuality to others engaged in fewer sexual risks than Black MSM who disclosed their sexuality (Crawford et al., 2002). Another study found that, compared with disclosing Black MSM, Black MSM nondisclosers reported more lifetime female partners, more female casual or sex trade partners, and more unprotected vaginal sex with female partners; but nondisclosing Black MSM also reported fewer lifetime male sex partners or acts of unprotected anal intercourse with men than disclosing Black MSM (CDC, 2003). A third study found that Black MSM who did not disclose their sexuality engaged in more risky sexual activities with male sex partners than did Black MSM who disclosed their sexuality (Peterson et al., 1992).

Other behavioral correlates, in addition to sexuality disclosure, were associated with HIV risk behaviors among Black MSM. Unprotected anal intercourse was associated with injection drug use in a sample of Black MSM (Peterson et al., 1992), and Black MSM who reported a recent episode of unprotected receptive anal intercourse were less likely than Black MSM who reported a recent episode of protected anal intercourse to carry a condom (Hart & Peterson, et al., 2004).

HIV protective behavior was significantly correlated with only a few behavioral variables. Both help seeking and sexuality disclosure were associated with HIV testing in samples of Black MSM. Peterson et al. (1995) reported that Black MSM who had previously taken an HIV test were more likely than Black MSM who had never been tested for HIV to seek help for high risk behaviors; and two studies found that Black MSM who disclosed their sexuality to others were more likely than Black MSM nondisclosers to be tested for HIV (Cochran & Mays, 1992; CDC, 2003).

A few behavioral variables were not associated with any of the dependent variables in samples of Black MSM. HIV-positive status was not correlated with a history of HIV testing (CDC, 2004b), recreational drug use, injection drug use, receptive anal sex, anorectal douching, oral sex, digital-anal contact, or dildo usage among Black MSM (Easterbrook et al., 1993). Number of sex partners (Easterbrook et al., 1993; CDC, 2004b), receptive anal sex (Easterbrook et al., 1993), and unprotected receptive anal sex (CDC, 2004b) were also not associated with HIV seropositivity in Black MSM samples. Furthermore, unprotected insertive anal sex was unrelated to condom carrying (Hart & Peterson, et al., 2004); HIV testing was unrelated to unprotected sex with men or women during the past 3 months (Mashburn et al., 2004), and sexuality disclosure was unrelated to condom use (Peterson et al., 1992).

2.3.1 Summary of Behavioral Predictors and Gaps

One behavioral correlate was associated with HIV-protective behavior in more than one study. Black MSM who disclosed their sexuality to others were more likely than Black MSM nondisclosers to be tested for HIV (Cochran & Mays, 1992; CDC, 2003). No behavioral variables were uniformly associated with HIV-positive status or HIV risk behavior across studies. The lack of behavioral correlates associated with HIV seropositivity among Black MSM is not a finding unique to this review. Even though HIV seroprevalence rates among Black MSM are higher than those of other MSM (Easterbrook et al., 1993; Lemp et al., 1994; Valleroy et al., 2000; Peterson et al., 2001; Mansergh et al., 2002; Harawa et al., 2004), several studies have found that known HIV-related risk behaviors (i.e., unprotected sex, number of partners, drug use) do not sufficiently explain the disproportionately high HIV seroprevalence rates among Black MSM (Samuel & Winkelstein, 1987; Easterbrook et al., 1993; Harawa et al., 2004). Future studies should explore which additional behavioral factors may contribute to the high HIV seroprevalence rates among Black MSM (Malebranche et al., 2003; Harawa et al., 2004; Millett et al., 2006).

2.4 Psychological Factors

We defined variables that measured knowledge, attitudes, beliefs, perceptions or mood as psychological factors. None of the psychological factors in the available studies that recruited Black MSM were significantly associated with HIV-positive status. Depressive mood (Peterson et al., 1996b), perceived risk for HIV infection (Easterbrook et al., 1993; CDC, 2004b), and perceived helpfulness of various resources

(Peterson et al., 1995) each did not significantly differ between HIV-positive and HIV-negative Black MSM.

Although no psychological variables were associated with HIV status, several psychological variables were associated with sexual risk behavior. High psychological distress was correlated with sexual risk behavior among Black MSM in two studies (Crawford et al., 2002; Myers et al., 2003). Sexual risk behavior was also associated with low perceived condom-use peer norms (Hart & Peterson, 2004) and high life satisfaction among Black MSM (Crawford et al., 2002).

Psychological correlates of HIV-protective behaviors were also reported in studies of Black MSM. Condom use was associated with high condom self-efficacy (Peterson et al., 1992), high condom outcome expectations (Peterson et al., 1992), and high safer-sex peer norms (Peterson et al., 1995). In addition, knowledge of highly active anti-retroviral therapy (HAART) and a comfortable place to be tested were each associated with HIV testing in a multisite sample of Black MSM (Mashburn et al., 2004).

Some psychological variables included in studies of Black MSM were unrelated to any dependent variable. Sexual risk-taking among Black MSM was unrelated to prevention self-efficacy, low self-esteem, or male gender role stress in a Chicago sample of Black MSM (Crawford et al., 2002). AIDS knowledge and cultural beliefs about HIV transmission were not associated with unprotected anal intercourse in a study of Black MSM in the San Francisco Bay area (Peterson et al., 1992). Psychiatric history, psychological hardiness, internal locus of control, and role strain were unrelated to HIV risk behavior among Black MSM in a Los Angeles sample (Myers et al., 2003). Condom-use peer norms were not associated with HIV testing in a three-city sample of Black MSM (Mashburn et al., 2004); and there was no correlation between condom use and cultural beliefs, AIDS knowledge, or perceived risk among Black MSM in northern California (Peterson et al., 1992).

2.4.1 Summary of Psychological Predictors and Gaps
Psychological distress was the only psychological variable consistently associated with sexual risk behavior across the available studies of Black MSM. No psychological variables in Black MSM samples were associated with HIV-positive status.

Psychological correlates of HIV-protective behaviors were either not included across studies or if included did not always yield significant associations. Few Black MSM studies examined associations between any of the dependent variables and HIV knowledge, mental health status, cultural beliefs, or self-esteem. None of the studies examined whether HIV-related risk behavior among Black MSM was associated with HIV treatment optimism. Moreover, associations between HIV-positive status and normative safer-sex beliefs or condom-use expectations were not explored in any of the studies.

2.5 Sociocultural Factors

Interpersonal interactions and societal forces were broadly categorized as sociocultural variables. Few Black MSM studies tested for associations between sociocultural variables and HIV risk or HIV-protective behavior, and no Black MSM studies tested for associations between sociocultural variables and HIV-positive status.

Of all the sociocultural variables, social support was most often examined in the available studies. Social support was also the only sociocultural variable that produced statistically significant results. Black MSM who reported higher levels of social support were significantly more likely than Black MSM with lower levels of social support to be tested for HIV (Mashburn et al., 2004). Likewise, Black MSM who reported higher levels of social support were less likely than Black MSM who reported lower levels of social support to engage in unprotected anal intercourse during the past 6 months (Peterson et al., 1992). Social support was also correlated with HIV risk behavior among Black MSM who were HIV-positive, but the association was inversely related. HIV-positive Black MSM who reported low social support engaged in fewer unprotected sexual risk activities than HIV-positive Black MSM who reported higher levels of social support (Ostrow et al., 1991). The same study found that low social support was associated with sexual risk-taking among HIV-positive White MSM in the study. Ostrow and his colleagues (1991) suggested that the counterintuitive results among HIV-positive Black MSM either were due to culturally inappropriate measures of social support or reflected genuine racial differences in the nature of social support systems between Black and White HIV-positive MSM.

Two additional sociocultural variables, racial discrimination and homophobia, were examined in a separate study (Crawford et al., 2002). Neither variable was significantly associated with sexual risk-taking among Black MSM.

2.5.1 Summary of Sociocultural Predictors and Gaps
Only three sociocultural variables in studies of Black MSM have been examined for associations with the HIV outcome variables. Although social support was the only sociocultural variable significantly associated with any dependent variable, none of the significant associations was observed more than once for the same dependent variable.

Several issues must be addressed in future studies of Black MSM that examine sociocultural factors of HIV outcome variables. First, none of the studies reviewed examined the association between sociocultural variables and HIV seropositivity in Black MSM. Second, few studies have examined the association of racism or homophobia with HIV risk behavior among Black MSM. Third, future research should examine the influence of other sociocultural variables (i.e., religiosity, gay community acculturation, Black community acculturation) that may provide further context for behaviors that place Black MSM at risk of contracting or transmitting HIV.

2.6 Structural-Level Factors

Ecologic or contextual aspects of the environment—both physical (e.g., buildings, public spaces) and nonphysical (e.g., policies, laws)—were categorized as structural factors. Few studies tested associations between structural-level factors and HIV-dependent variables. In fact, structural-level variables were examined for their association with HIV-positive status in only three studies that included Black MSM. A small case-control study of an HIV outbreak among young Black MSM in North Carolina found that the locations in which Black MSM met male sex partners (e.g., bars, Internet, school, telephone chat lines) were not associated with HIV-positive status (CDC, 2004b). Likewise, a second Black MSM study found that HIV status was not significantly associated with incarceration in a Los Angeles sample (Wohl et al., 2000). However, a third study found that HIV infection was associated with Black MSM in only one of three participating southern California counties (Ruiz et al., 1998).

2.6.1 Summary of Structural-Level Predictors and Gaps

Few studies of Black MSM have included structural-level variables in their analyses. Neither of the two studies reviewed found significant associations between the selected structural-level variables and HIV-positive status or HIV risk behavior. In addition, none of the studies in the review tested associations between structural-level variables and HIV-protective behavior. Additional work in this area of research is needed, especially studies that examine the association between structural-level variables that regulate behavior (i.e., laws, policies) and the HIV outcome variables among Black MSM.

2.7 Genetic or Biologic Factors

We defined hereditary or cellular-level mechanisms associated with HIV infection as genetic or biologic factors. The most commonly discussed genetic factor of HIV infection is the CCR5 base 32 deletion. CCR5 receptors facilitate the capacity of HIV to infect cells. Worldwide, Caucasian populations are more likely than other racial or ethnic groups to express the CCR5 genetic variant (Fowke et al., 1998; Martinson et al., 2000; Williamson et al., 2000). A few studies have examined the distribution of the variant among MSM (Paxton et al., 1998; Marmor et al., 2001; Stephenson, 2001). Although it is likely that CCR5 is equally distributed among Black populations, irrespective of sexual orientation, no studies have examined the impact of the genetic variant on HIV infection among Black MSM.

Biologic factors may also influence HIV susceptibility. Chief among these factors are circumcision and sexually transmitted diseases (STDs). Both factors have a behavioral component with biologic consequences: Circumcision is a practice grounded in cultural beliefs, and STDs are a consequence of unprotected sexual activity. Studies reveal that circumcised men are less likely than uncircumcised men to become infected with HIV (Laumann et al., 1997; Quinn et al., 2000). However, most of the studies that have found associations between circumcision and HIV status have been conducted with heterosexual men or in international settings. Only three studies have tested associations between circumcision and HIV infection among racially diverse samples of MSM, and none were stratified by the Black race (Kreiss & Hopkins,

1993; Grulich et al., 2001; Buchbinder et al., 2005). Despite the lack of data on circumcision rates among Black MSM, the available data show that circumcision rates in the United States are significantly lower among Black men than white men (Smith et al., 1987; Cook, et al., 1993; Laumann 1997). Given the greater likelihood of circumcision among white men than Black men in the United States, it is plausible that the higher HIV prevalence and incidence among Black MSM may be partially due to a lower prevalence of circumcision.

Prior research has demonstrated that STDs facilitate acquisition and transmission of HIV (Rothenberg 1998; Fleming & Wasserheit, 1999). STD infection has also been associated with HIV-positive status among Black MSM (Celentano et al., 2005; Torian et al., 2002). A recent case-control study reported that HIV-positive Black MSM were more likely than HIV-negative Black MSM to report a prior history of gonorrhea (CDC, 2004b). Previous history of gonorrhea infection was also significantly related to HIV-positive status in a separate sample of Black MSM (Easterbrook et al., 1993).

Bacterial and viral infections that were not associated with HIV-positive status among Black MSM included a history of *Chlamydia* infection (CDC, 2004b), cytomegalovirus infection (Easterbrook et al., 1993), hepatitis-positive serology (Easterbrook et al, 1993), or a lifetime history of syphilis (Easterbook et al., 1993; CDC, 2004b).

2.7.1 *Summary of Genetic or Biologic Predictors and Gaps*

The only biologic factor in the literature that is associated with HIV-positive status among Black MSM is a history of gonorrhea infection. Although Black populations are less likely than white populations to express the CCR5 delta 32 variant and African American men are less likely to be circumcised than European American men, neither the CCR5 delta 32 deletion nor the circumcision studies that exclusively recruited MSM were stratified by the Black race in their analyses. The lack of data specific to Black MSM for these two known and important contributors to HIV seropositivity is a significant research gap.

2.8 Section Summary of Factors

Although the available literature on Black MSM identifies many factors that are associated with one of the three dependent variables, few of the factors were (1) tested for associations with the same dependent variable across studies or (2) showed the same relationship with a specific dependent variable across studies.

There are limitations to our approach of summarizing predictors of HIV-positive status, HIV risk, and HIV-protective behavior. First, counting the number of studies that included specific factors for the specified outcomes is imperfect. Presenting results from one study that assessed a factor is not equivalent, in terms of importance, as results from several studies that assessed the same factor. Second, contradictory results across studies for a given factor may be due to differences in methodology or measurement and may not indicate whether a given factor is genuinely associated or not associated with a specific outcome. Third, there were too few studies to conduct a meta-analysis to determine definitively which predictors were related to which outcome. Nevertheless, there is important information that can be gleaned from the available data.

Only four correlates showed similar relationships across studies for any specific dependent variable: (1) Black MSM who reported a history of gonorrhea were more likely than Black MSM who did not report previous infection with gonorrhea to be HIV-positive; (2) Black MSM who reported low incomes were more likely than Black MSM who reported comparatively higher incomes to engage in greater sexual risk behaviors; (3) Black MSM who reported high psychological distress were more likely than Black MSM with lower psychological distress to engage in sexual risk behavior; and (4) Black MSM who disclosed their sexual behavior to others were more likely than Black MSM nondisclosers to have been tested for HIV.

This dearth of information is, in large part, due to the scarcity of studies that recruited exclusively Black MSM samples or conducted separate regression analyses by racial group. The lack of identifiable predictors also stems from the fact that fewer potential factors were tested for associations with the same dependent variable in more than one study. Only 14 factors in the literature were tested across multiple studies. Additional research must be undertaken to determine the degree to which identified factors are associated with specific dependent variables across studies. Future research must also evaluate the degree to which any of these factors can be generalized to all communities of Black MSM. Last, future research must test with samples of Black MSM additional factors that have been associated with the outcome variables in other at-risk populations. For instance, childhood sexual abuse, which has been significantly associated with HIV risk behavior (Lemp et al., 1994; O'Leary et al., 2003; Newman et al., 2004), and HIV-positive status (Bartholow et al., 1994; Jinich et al., 1996; Diaz et al., 1999) in other populations of MSM have not been tested with any of the dependent variables in Black MSM studies.

3 HIV Primary Prevention Interventions for Black MSM

3.1 HIV Prevention Intervention Research

Intervention research remains an essential aspect of the public health response to HIV prevention among MSM in the United States. Such research provides the extensive information needed to adequately develop and rigorously test the efficacy of behavioral and social interventions (Wolitski et al., 2003). Outcome and impact evaluation studies that employ experimental and quasi-experimental research designs provide the best evidence of effective intervention programs. Meta-analyses and literature reviews have documented that behavioral interventions can produce significant reductions in unsafe sexual behavior that transmit HIV (Choi & Coates, 1994; Oakley et al., 1995; Kalichman et al., 1996; Kegeles & Hart, 1998; Semaan et al., 2002). The documented success of HIV intervention research over the past two decades offers strong evidence that prevention works and science-based prevention programs have been widely disseminated (Wolitski et al., 2003). Effective interventions, based on sound science, have been adopted and tailored by health departments and community organizations to offer prevention services that reflect local needs and good public health practice. This section of the chapter explores the components of effective HIV prevention interventions, the effectiveness of culturally tailored interventions, previous effective interventions with Black MSM, and recommendations for future intervention studies targeting Black MSM.

3.2 Components of Effective HIV Prevention Interventions

Typically, HIV prevention interventions emphasize previously identified and successful intervention approaches (Des Jarlais & Semaan, 2002). These approaches include strong cognitive information on HIV/AIDS (e.g., knowledge, attitudes), persistent efforts to enhance sexual negotiation skills, and attempts to change normative influences on risk behavior, which vary between behavioral and social interventions. Intervention activities may emphasize changes in individuals and small groups or in entire communities and subgroups within communities (Wolitski et al., 2003). Efforts are made at the individual or small group level to influence directly the knowledge, attitudes and behavior of people who participate in the intervention activities. The delivery of the intervention may involve professionals, peers, and the media (e.g., brochures, radio, Internet). Inherent in an individual-level approach is face-to-face interactions intended to assist individuals to make and maintain risk reduction in sexual behavior through the promotion of positive attitudes and intentions toward safer sex; behavioral skills to enact risk reduction behavior changes; risk reduction, problem-solving, and self-management skills; and positive appraisals of self-identity, self-esteem, and relationship goals (Ross & Kelley, 2000).

At the community level, intervention efforts directly and indirectly attempt to influence the knowledge, attitudes, and behavior of the entire community or subgroup within the community through emphasis on changes in social norms (Wolitski et al., 2003). Delivery of the intervention may involve professionals, peers, and/or the media; and it may include multiple intervention components. These social interventions can theoretically affect risk behaviors of large numbers of people at the city, state, or national level through changes in structures, laws, or public policies that influence HIV transmission or availability of prevention resources (Wolitski et al., 2003).

A recently published meta-analysis of 20 interventions to reduce sexual risk behavior among MSM found four characteristics that were associated with statistically significant reductions in sexual risk (Herbst et al., 2005). These characteristics included (1) interventions with a theoretical underpinning, particularly diffusion of innovations theory and the model of relapse prevention; (2) interventions that included interpersonal skills training to communicate about and negotiate safer sex; (3) interventions that offered multiple methods (e.g., counseling, group discussions, role play, lecture, live demonstrations) of imparting relevant information; and (4) interventions that offered more than one session, lasted 4 hours or more, and applied over 3 or more weeks.

3.3 What Has Culture Got to Do with It?

Evidence suggests that efforts made to consider cultural influences in the design of the intervention are beneficial for achieving success (Darbes et al., 2002). Wilson and Miller (2003) reviewed HIV risk reduction intervention studies published between 1985 and 2001 that included culturally tailored components (e.g., by racial/ethnicity, gender, sexual orientation) in the intervention design. In their review, Wilson and Miller identified the populations studied, the methodologies used, and the strategies used to make the selected interventions culturally specific. Only 17 among more than 1700 articles the authors reviewed satisfied inclusion criteria of interventions that explicitly made culture a central component in the program design.

Two primary strategies that investigators used to integrate culture into intervention research across the reviewed studies were presentation strategies and content strategies. Presentation strategies frequently used to make the intervention program culturally appropriate included use of facilitators, models, and video actors of the same race and ethnicity as study participants; use of scripts with cultural terminology; and the use of appropriate forms and styles of expression by facilitators or video actors. Additionally, several studies, considered multiple aspects of the intervention's aesthetics (e.g., images of Black men and the use of culturally specific language). Most of the studies Wilson and Miller selected for review attempted to match the appearance and sound of the intervention to the target population. Fewer studies used strategies to ensure that the content of the intervention program was culturally grounded in the experiences, values, and norms of the study population. Wilson and Miller concluded that future research is needed that more adequately defines and describes strategies that incorporate cultural aspects of targeted communities to enhance intervention studies.

3.4 Prior HIV Intervention Research with Black MSM

There is a striking scarcity of intervention research with MSM, particularly racial and ethnic minority MSM. Several reviews of effective behavioral interventions have each found few interventions that target Black MSM.

One systematic review of controlled trials for MSM reported that only nine MSM intervention studies qualified for inclusion in the comprehensive synthesis of rigorous HIV/AIDS prevention research (Johnson et al., 2002). Six of the MSM studies examined small group interventions, and three examined community-level approaches. Overall, the selected interventions reported a moderate (26%) reduction in the prevalence of unprotected anal intercourse in the intervention group compared with the control group. The most favorable effects were obtained by interventions that promoted interpersonal skills for practicing safer sex. However, none of the selected intervention studies

552   G.A. Millett et al.

targeted Black MSM (Semaan et al., 2002). Similarly, in an updated systematic review and meta-analysis of 54 MSM interventions, Johnson et al. (2005) identified only one intervention that targeted Black MSM.

In a second review, the HIV/AIDS Prevention Program Archive (HAPPA), a collection of promising prevention programs, was compiled and reviewed by an independent panel of scientists (Card et al., 2001). Of 23 promising HIV prevention programs, only two interventions targeted MSM of color. One of the two MSM of color interventions targeted Black MSM (Peterson et al., 1996a).

A third review of HIV behavioral prevention research found that 52 of 129 intervention studies that included African Americans satisfied several rigorous methodologic criteria (Darbes et al., 2002). Studies that met the inclusion criteria included behavioral, social, and policy interventions, and each study was rated good, fair, or limited. Results indicated that the most successful intervention studies that were derived from theory included skills training, addressed cultural sensitivity of Blacks, and were conducted over multiple sessions for relatively long periods of time. However, few interventions that recruited African American participants included Black MSM. Of the effective behavioral interventions targeting Black participants, eight targeted homosexually active men, and only one provided separate analyses for Black MSM.

The lack of outcome studies that evaluate HIV prevention interventions among Black and other ethnic minority MSM severely limits the ability to determine the effectiveness of existing risk reduction approaches in these populations. Two of the three systematic reviews found only one published methodologically rigorous and effective HIV prevention intervention targeting Black MSM. The Brother to Brother intervention is a small group randomized trial that emphasizes sexual negotiation skills based on the cultural influences in the lives of Black MSM (Peterson et al., 1996a). The study enrolled a sample of 318 African American gay and bisexual men recruited from community venues in San Francisco, Berkeley, and Oakland who were randomly assigned to single-session workshop groups, triple-session workshop groups, or waiting-list control groups, with a 6-, 12-, and 18-month follow-up. Workshop activities included risk education, sexual assertiveness and negotiation skill exercises, activities to strengthen behavioral change commitment, and conversations to foster positive self-identity and support as African American gay and bisexual men. Results revealed that control group participants showed little change in unprotected anal intercourse, single workshop participants showed modest change in unprotected anal intercourse, and multiple-session participants showed considerable reduction in risk behavior: from 45% at baseline to 20% at 18 months' follow-up.

3.5 Directions for Future Research Interventions with Black MSM

Several considerations emerge as future issues in HIV intervention research among Black MSM. In particular, an expansion of intervention trials is necessary to identify effective prevention strategies for Black

MSM. The few rigorously evaluated interventions are inadequate given the disproportionate rate of HIV infection in this population. Substantial efforts should also be expended to consider structural and environmental factors that impede HIV risk reduction in this population. Structural interventions are needed to examine factors that influence HIV risk at the community level that result from differential access to social, educational, economic, and medical resources and that are affected by cultural prejudice and discrimination (e.g., racism, sexism, homophobia, HIV stigma) (Sumartojo et al., 2000). In addition, Internet and social network approaches offer innovative opportunities to reach Black MSM who may be more difficult to locate and access through individual-level interventions (Peterson & Carballo-Dieguez, 2000; Wolitski et al., 2001). These community-level efforts provide a greater opportunity to reach larger segments of the MSM population and examine the influence of social networks and norms in HIV transmission (Myrick, 1999; Hart & Peterson, 2004; Mays et al., 2004). Community-level interventions may improve the ability to address concurrently other health problems that increase the likelihood of HIV exposure (e.g., substance abuse, sexual abuse, depression, internalized homophobia). For example, the pervasive influence of stigma and discrimination require much greater attention in intervention research to determine their consequences for HIV risk reduction. Such intervention efforts might especially consider the influence of homophobia in HIV risk reduction (Stokes & Peterson, 1998; Huebner et al., 2002) and how to reduce the detrimental effects of stigma and discrimination (e.g., racial and sexual prejudice) on HIV risk behavior.

4 HIV-Positive Black MSM and Secondary Prevention

Secondary HIV prevention refers to the prevention or alleviation of adverse conditions among persons who already have HIV infection (Kelly & Kalichman, 2002). This may involve, but is not limited to, the social and emotional adjustment of people living with HIV/AIDS, treatment access and utilization, treatment adherence, and prevention of morbidity and mortality from opportunistic infections (OIs). Additionally, HIV secondary prevention includes efforts to reduce sexual behaviors that facilitate HIV transmission. However, despite current medical advances in HIV treatment and OI prevention, translation of these breakthroughs into improved morbidity and mortality rates for HIV-positive Black MSM has lagged behind that of MSM of other ethnicities (Blair et al., 2002). To understand why mortality rates remain highest among HIV-positive Black MSM compared with all other racial groups of MSM, it is necessary to examine the HIV testing practices, health care access and utilization, treatment adherence, mental health, and sexual behaviors of HIV-positive Black MSM.

4.1 HIV Testing Practices

HIV testing and counseling may facilitate access to HIV/AIDS services and referrals for seropositive persons; but HIV-positive individuals who are unaware of their infection may be less likely to receive treatment early after their diagnosis. These issues have been underscored by recent studies of Black MSM. A cross-sectional survey of young MSM found that most (64%) of 920 Black MSM reported having had a previous HIV test, but the median number of lifetime tests was one test (CDC, 2002b; Bingham et al., 2003). Furthermore, of the 536 Black MSM in the study who reported testing negative during their last test, 16% were HIV-positive and nearly all were unaware of their seropositive status. Likewise, high rates of unrecognized HIV infection among Black MSM were reported in a separate multisite cross-sectional study of MSM (CDC, 2005). Studies have also found that a significantly larger proportion of HIV-positive Black MSM test late in their HIV infection (within 2 months to a year of an AIDS diagnosis) compared to their white peers (Wortley et al., 1995). However, other studies report comparable or higher HIV testing rates among Black MSM relative to other MSM (McKirnan et al., 1995; Heckman et al., 1999; Torian et al., 2002).

4.2 Healthcare Access and Utilization

An important component of secondary prevention involves access to and utilization of health care facilities. Studies have found that the racial disparity in AIDS morbidity and mortality among African Americans in general is partially attributable to differential access to care, lower outpatient utilization practices, and possible racial bias among medical providers of medical treatment (Siegel et al., 2000; Asch et al., 2001; Bird & Bogart, 2001; Bogart et al., 2001).

Although not as extensive as the literature on health care access among the general African American population, there are studies that have examined health care access and utilization among HIV-positive MSM. The available research show that HIV-positive Black MSM are as equally likely as HIV-positive white MSM to report having health insurance (Kass et al., 1999; Halikitis et al., 2003), including private health insurance (Kass et al., 1999). In addition, no racial or ethnic differences among HIV-positive MSM are found in emergency department visits (Kass et al., 1999), inpatient visits (Kass et al., 1999), or recent hospitalizations (Zucconi et al., 1994). However, a few notable differences exist between HIV-positive Black MSM and other racial or ethnic groups of HIV-positive MSM. Compared with other groups of HIV-positive MSM, Black MSM are less likely to have access to private clinics (Halikitis et al., 2003) or to express HIV-related health concerns to their medical providers (Mason et al., 1997). Moreover, although one study found no racial or ethnic differences among HIV-positive MSM in outpatient visits (Zucconi et al., 1994), another study found that Black MSM with high CD4 counts (>500 cells/mm^3) were significantly less likely than white MSM with similar CD4 counts to utilize outpatient health services. Additionally, Black MSM in that study were significantly less likely than white MSM to have visited the dentist within the past 6 months.

Qualitative investigations have also evaluated health care access and utilization of HIV-positive Black MSM. Among 81 Black MSM (50%

HIV-positive) recruited for focus groups in New York and Atlanta, Malebranche et al. (2004) found that participants reported frustration with medical personnel in outpatient settings and discriminatory practices of medical staff; and they distrusted the quality and competence of outpatient medical services. Likewise, Siegel and Raveis (1997) reported that among HIV-positive men of color Black MSM expressed more critical and distrustful attitudes toward physicians than Latino MSM. The authors also reported that HIV-positive Black MSM and Latino MSM felt that their race and socioeconomic status negatively influenced the information, health care, or advocacy they received from AIDS service organizations (Siegel & Raveis, 1997).

4.3 HIV Treatment Access and Adherence

A limited number of studies have explored HIV treatment access and patterns among HIV-positive Black MSM. Stall and colleagues (2001) found that a comparison group of minority (Black and Latino) MSM were less likely than white MSM to receive recommended levels of antiretroviral care. Jacobson et al. (2001) also reported that HIV-positive Black MSM were less likely than men of other races or ethnicities to be on HAART. Similarly, a study involving 322 HIV-positive MSM found that Black MSM were more likely than MSM of other ethnicities to report low perceived access to medications (Halikitis et al., 2003). In contrast, race was not significantly related to being on highly active antiretroviral therapy (HAART) in other multiracial samples of HIV-positive MSM (Kass et al., 1999).

Studies of HAART adherence among MSM are mixed. In a sample of 539 MSM, Kleeberger et al. (2001) reported that Black race was a significant predictor of lower HAART adherence at baseline (Kleeberger et al., 2001) and at the 2-year follow-up (Kleeberger et al., 2004). In contrast, Halikitis et al. (2003) found no racial differences in HAART adherence among 322 HIV-positive MSM.

4.4 Mental Health and Social Support

Several studies have explored the association between HIV-positive status and psychological distress among Black MSM. Richardson et al. (1999) found high rates of depression or dysthymia (11.5%) in a sample of 243 Black gay and bisexual men but noted no significant relation between HIV status and depression or dysphoric mood. Likewise, another study of 234 Black MSM found that HIV-positive status, regardless of disease stage, was not associated with increased risk for anxiety or depressive disorders (Myers & Durvasula, 1999). In contrast, Peterson et al. (1996b) found a direct relation between depressed mood and physical health symptoms in a sample of Black men of mixed HIV serostatus and sexual orientation ($n = 139$). However, there were no differences in reports of physical health symptoms among the men in the study by either HIV status or sexual orientation (Peterson et al., 1996b).

A few studies of HIV-positive Black MSM have examined the association between social support and HIV risk behavior or social support and mental health. A pilot study of 40 HIV-positive MSM (50% Black) found that, in contrast to white MSM, social support was inversely correlated with mental health among Black MSM (Ostrow et al., 1991). These findings were mirrored by a small comparative study of 16 White and 17 Black MSM in Detroit, which found a borderline significant inverse relation between material social support from friends or family and adverse mental health outcomes among Black MSM (Gant & Ostrow, 1995).

4.5 Sexual Risks

Understanding the sexual behavior patterns of HIV-positive Black MSM is important for both primary and secondary prevention of HIV. Studies that examine sexual risk behaviors of HIV-positive Black MSM comprise two general categories: (1) comparative studies that stratify samples of MSM by race and (2) comparative studies that stratify Black men by sexual behavior.

Among racially diverse samples of HIV-positive MSM, there is evidence of racial differences in sexual risk behaviors. Bingman et al. (2001) provided data from a small subsample ($n = 71$) of HIV-positive men who reported recent sex with HIV-negative partners or partners whose HIV status was unknown. The prevalence of unprotected anal intercourse (UAI) was significantly higher among HIV-positive Black MSM (50%) than HIV-positive Latino (37%) or White (11%) MSM. Likewise, Gomez and Halikitis (1998) found ethnic differences in HIV risk behaviors among another small sample of 71 HIV-positive MSM. Significantly more Black MSM (29%) than White MSM (0%) reported that they had engaged in unprotected insertive anal intercourse with seronegative men during the past 3 months (Gomez & Halikitis, 1998). However, the authors did not find any racial or ethnic differences among MSM who had unprotected insertive anal sex with partners of unknown HIV serostatus during the past 3 months. In another study, Siegel et al. (2004) surveyed a sample of 59 HIV-positive White and Black men 50 years of age and older. The authors found that, compared with white MSM, Black MSM were more likely to report unprotected anal or vaginal sex during the past 6 months.

Two other studies with substantially larger racially diverse samples of HIV-positive MSM found few racial differences in sexual risk behaviors other than UAI. There were no racial or ethnic differences in the number of male or female partners of bisexually active HIV-positive MSM in a multisite study ($n = 5156$) (Montgomery et al., 2003). Likewise, Parsons et al. (1998) found no racial or ethnic differences among HIV-positive MSM ($n = 300$) who sought sex in public venues (i.e., parks or public restrooms). However, the authors found that HIV-positive Black MSM were significantly less likely than white MSM to report looking for sex in commercial venues (i.e., bathhouses and sex clubs).

Sexual risk behaviors among HIV-positive Black MSM have also been documented in studies that recruited only Black men. A recent Los Angeles study that recruited 185 self-reported HIV-positive Black men and 308 self-reported HIV-negative Black men found that HIV-positive Black MSM engaged in fewer sexual risks than their HIV-negative counterparts (Myers et al., 2003). Another study reported that 100% of self-identified HIV-positive Black MSM and 33% of self-identified HIV-negative Black MSM used condoms consistently during anal sex with another man (Wohl et al., 2002). Another article from the same study found that 59% of the HIV-positive Black men had previously been incarcerated, and 23% reported anal sex with men while in custody (Wohl et al., 2000). The authors also found that history of incarceration was not related to HIV status. However, HIV-positive Black MSM were significantly less likely than HIV-negative Black MSM to use condoms during anal sex while incarcerated; and HIV-positive Black MSM reported more sexual partners and more episodes of coercive sex in prison than HIV-negative Black MSM with a history of incarceration.

4.6 Future Directions for HIV Secondary Prevention for Black MSM

The available data suggest future secondary prevention research initiatives for Black MSM with HIV. First, proportionally more HIV-positive Black MSM test infrequently or later in their disease progression than other HIV-positive MSM. Interventions that include strong social support, information about HIV testing and treatment, and comfortable or neutral spaces for testing might persuade more Black MSM to learn their serostatus and engage in honest communication with sexual partners. Second, the health care access and utilization literature suggests that HIV-positive Black MSM are less likely to seek outpatient services than are HIV-positive White MSM. Additional work to improve cultural competence programs for medical staff, empowerment initiatives for patients, and provider–patient communication strategies may increase utilization of outpatient services. Third, HIV-positive Black MSM are less likely than HIV-positive MSM of other races and ethnicities to have access to HAART. Improving treatment access and adherence practices of HIV-positive Black MSM may require tailored patient counseling and education efforts that emphasize current HIV treatment options, official recommendations for initiating or delaying HAART, potential side effects of medications, and consequences of missed doses (viral resistance, progression of disease, opportunistic infections). Fourth, small studies have found that HIV-positive Black MSM engage in greater sexual risks than HIV-positive MSM of other races or ethnicities. Larger probability samples of HIV-positive MSM are needed to explore the generalizability of these racial differences.

5 Summary

This chapter highlights several crucial points related to HIV/AIDS among Black MSM. First, although correlates of HIV-positive status, HIV risk, or HIV-protective behavior among Black MSM have been identified, most of the correlates have not been tested across studies.

Second, there is a dearth of effective HIV prevention interventions targeting HIV-negative Black MSM and no identified effective risk reduction interventions for HIV-positive Black MSM. Finally, HIV-positive Black MSM are less likely than other HIV-positive MSM to access care from private clinics, report access or adherence to HAART medications, or engage in safer-sex behaviors.

There are several research implications for future investigations of predictors of HIV status or HIV-related (promoting or preventive) behaviors among Black MSM. Studies of resiliency factors—variables associated with keeping Black MSM from becoming infected or engaging in HIV-related risks—are largely absent from the available literature. Future research studies should emphasize identifying which resiliency factors are associated with HIV-protective behaviors among Black MSM. Moreover, in the available literature the correlates tested for associations with HIV status, HIV risk, or HIV-protective behaviors are primarily demographic, behavioral, or psychological. Few studies that recruited Black MSM tested sociocultural or structural-level correlates for associations with the dependent variables. The degree to which religion, discrimination, identity (both sexual and racial), or incarceration predict HIV infection or risk behavior among Black MSM should be explored in future scientific investigations (Brooks et al., 2003; Beatty et al., 2004).

The lack of proven effective HIV prevention interventions is particularly glaring given the disproportionate HIV disease burden among Black MSM compared with MSM of other races or ethnicities. Most notable is the absence of risk reduction efforts focused on HIV-positive Black MSM. Although individual-level skills-building interventions are important, they do not address the multiple structural and community factors that may influence HIV seroconversion and progression of disease among Black MSM. The mechanisms that drive HIV-related risk among Black MSM are multifactorial and necessitate intervening on multiple levels. Future HIV intervention research targeting Black MSM should emphasize an ecologic approach and address the dynamics of social and sexual networks that facilitate transmission of the virus between members of this population.

Future qualitative and quantitative investigations of HIV-positive Black MSM must explore several topic areas, including (1) the factors that influence health care utilization and HIV treatment adherence among Black MSM; (2) whether racial or sexual discrimination or distrust of medical research or medical professionals affect health care utilization and treatment adherence among HIV-positive Black MSM; (3) the degree to which treatment knowledge and optimism influences the sexual risks of HIV-positive Black MSM; (4) whether nondisclosure of HIV status to sex partners is associated with greater sexual risk-taking; (5) the extent to which knowing a sex partner's status influences sexual risk taking among HIV-positive Black MSM; and (6) the prevalence of bisexual behavior among HIV-positive Black MSM and unprotected sexual activity with female sex partners.

The preponderance of data from racial comparative MSM studies clearly indicates that Black MSM are at greater risk for HIV seroconversion and suffer greater AIDS morbidity and mortality rates than other MSM. To move the Black MSM HIV research and prevention agenda forward, it is important to focus future research efforts on the three major areas highlighted in this chapter: (1) defining and exploring existing correlates of HIV status, risk, and protective behavior; (2) developing and evaluating culturally specific interventions for both HIV-negative and HIV-positive Black MSM; and (3) emphasizing secondary prevention among HIV-positive Black MSM. The first step in accomplishing this involves oversampling Black MSM in racial comparative studies to ensure sufficient sample sizes to determine race-specific effects, as well as recruiting exclusively Black MSM samples. Only when the demographics of HIV research and prevention initiatives adequately reflect the current racial disparity of the epidemic will we begin to understand, and subsequently slow down, the transmission of HIV among Black MSM.

References

Asch, S.M., Gifford, A.L., Bozzette, S.A., Turner, B., Matthews, C.W., Kuromiya, K., Cunningham, W., Anderson, R., Shapiro, M., Rastegar, A., and McCutchan, J.A. (2001) Underuse of primary Mycobacterium avium complex and Pneumocystis carinii prophylaxis in the United States. *Journal of Acquired Immune Deficiency Syndrome* 28:340–344.

Bartholow, B.N., Doll, L.S., Joy, D., Douglas J.M. Jr., Bolan, G., Harrison, J.S., Moss, P.M., and McKirnan, D. (1994) Emotional, behavioral, and HIV risks associated with sexual abuse among adult homosexual and bisexual men. *Child Abuse & Neglect* 18:747–761.

Beatty, L.A., Wheeler, D., and Gaiter, J. (2004) HIV prevention research for African Americans: current and future directions. *Journal of Black Psychology* 30(1):40–58.

Bingham, T.A., Harawa, N.T., Johnson, D.F., Secura, G.M., MacKellar, D.A., and Valleroy, L.A. (2003) The effect of partner characteristics on HIV infection among African American men who have sex with men in the Young Men's Survey, Los Angeles, 1999–2000. *AIDS Education and Prevention* 15:39–52.

Bingman, C.R., Marks, G., and Crepaz, N. (2001) Attributions about one's HIV infection and unsafe sex in seropositive men who have sex with men. *AIDS Behavior* 5:283–289.

Bird, S.T., and Bogart, L.M. (2001) Perceived race-based and socioeconomic status-based discrimination in interactions with health care providers. *Ethnicity & Disease* 11:554–563.

Blair, J.M., Fleming, P.L., and Karon, J.M. (2002) Trends in AIDS incidence and survival among racial/ethnic minority men who have sex with men, United States, 1990–1999. *Journal of Acquired Immune Deficiency Syndrome* 31:339–347.

Bogart, L.M., Catz, S.L., Kelly, J.A., and Benotsch, E.G. (2001) Factors influencing physicians' judgments of adherence and treatment decisions for patients with HIV disease. *Medical Decision Making* 21(1):28–36.

Brooks, R., Rotheram-Borus, M., Bing, E.G., Ayala, G., and Henry, C.L. (2003) HIV and AIDS among men of color who have sex with men and men of color who have sex with men and women: an epidemiological profile. *AIDS Education and Prevention* 15(Supplement A):1–6.

Buchbinder, S.P., Vittinghoff, E., Heagerty, P.J., et al. (2005) Sexual risk, nitrite inhalant use, and lack of circumcision associated with HIV seroconversion in men who have sex with men in the United States. *Journal of Acquired Immune Deficiency Syndrome* 39:82–89.

Card, J.J., Benner, T., Shields, J.P., and Feinstein, N. (2001) The HIV/AIDS Prevention Program Archive (HAPPA): a collection of promising prevention programs in a box. *AIDS Education and Prevention* 13(1):1–28.

Celentano, D.D., Sifakis, F., Hylton, J., Torian, L.V., Guilin, V., and Koblin, B.A. (2005) Race/ethnic differences in HIV prevalence and risks among adolescent and young adult men who have sex with men. *Journal of Urban Health* 82(4):610–621.

Centers for Disease Control and Prevention (CDC) (2001) HIV incidence among young men who have sex with men—seven U.S. cities, 1994–2000. *MMWR Morbidity and Mortality Weekly Report* 50:440–444.

Centers for Disease Control and Prevention. (2002a) STDs among men who have sex with men. Division of STD Prevention STD Surveillance 2001: Special Focus Profiles.

Centers for Disease Control and Prevention. (2002b) Unrecognized HIV infection, risk behaviors, and perceptions of risk among young Black men who have sex with men—six US cities, 1994–1998. *MMWR Morbidity and Mortality Weekly Report* 51:733–736.

Centers for Disease Control and Prevention. (2003) HIV/STD risks in young men who have sex with men who do not disclose their sexual orientation, six U.S. cities, 1994–2000. *MMWR Morbidity and Mortality Weekly Report* 52:81–85.

Centers for Disease Control and Prevention. (2004a) AIDS cases, deaths, and persons living with AIDS by year, 1985–2002—United States.

Centers for Disease Control and Prevention. (2004b) HIV transmission among Black college student and non-student men who have sex with men—North Carolina, 2003. *MMWR Morbidity and Mortality Weekly Report* 53(32):731–734.

Centers for Disease Control and Prevention. (2005) HIV prevalence, unrecognized infection, and HIV testing among men who have sex with men—five U.S. cities, June 2004–April 2005. *MMWR Morbidity and Mortality Weekly Report* 54:597–601.

Choi, K.H., and Coates, T.J. (1994) Prevention of HIV infection. *AIDS* 8:1371–1389.

Cochran, S.D., and Mays, V.M. (1992) Disclosure rates of potential HIV transmission risks to physicians and dentists by U.S. Black gay and bisexual men. In: *Proceeding of the International Conference on AIDS 1992*. Abstract Puc. 8039.

Cook, L.S., Koutsky, L.A., and Holmes, K. (1993) Clinical presentation of genital warts among circumcised and uncircumcised heterosexual men attending an urban STD clinic. *Genitourinary Medicine* 69:262–264.

Crawford, I., Allison, K.W., Zamboni, B.D., and Soto, T. (2002) The influence of dual-identity development on the psychosocial functioning of African-American gay and bisexual men. *Journal of Sexual Research* 39:179–189.

Darbes, L.A., Kennedy, G.E., Peersman, G., Zohbrabyan, L., and Rutherford, G.W. (2002) Systematic review of HIV behavioral prevention research in African Americans. From http://hivinsite.ucsf.edu/InSite.jsp.

Des Jarlais, D.C., and Semaan, S. (2002) HIV prevention research: cumulative knowledge or accumulating studies. *Journal of Acquired Immune Deficiency Syndrome* 30(Supplement 1):S1–S7.

Diaz, R.D., Ayala, G., and Bein, E. (1999) Social oppression, resiliency and sexual risk: findings from the national Latino gay men's study. In: *Proceedings of the National HIV Prevention Conference 1999* Abstract 287.

Easterbrook, P.J., Chmiel, J.S., Hoover, D.R., Saah, A.J., Kaslow, R.A., Kingsley, L.A., and Detels, R. (1993) Racial and ethnic differences in human immunodeficiency virus type 1 (HIV-1) seroprevalence among homosexual and bisexual men. *American Journal of Epidemiology* 138:415–429.

Fleming, D.T., and Wasserheit, J.N. (1999) From epidemiological synergy to public health policy: the contribution of other sexually transmitted diseases to sexual transmission of HIV infection. *Sexually Transmitted Infections* 75:3–17.

Fowke, K.R., Dong, T., Rowland-Jones, S.L., Oyugi, J., Rutherford, W.J., Kimani, J., Krausa, P., Bwayo, J., Simonsen, J.N., Shearer, G.M., and Plummer, F.A. (1998) HIV type 1 resistance in Kenyan sex workers is not associated with altered cellular susceptibility to HIV type 1 infection or enhanced beta-chemokine production. *AIDS Research and Human Retroviruses* 17:1521–1530.

Gant, L.M., and Ostrow, D.G. (1995) Perceptions of social support and psychological adaptation to sexually acquired HIV among White and African American men. *Social Work* 40:215–224.

Gomez, C.A., and Halkitis, P. (1998) Culture counts: understanding the context of unprotected sex for HIV positive men in a multi-ethnic urban sample in the U.S. Presented at the International Conference on AIDS, San Francisco.

Grulich, A.E., Hendry, O., Clark, E., Kippax, S., and Kaldor, J.M. (2001) Circumcision and male-to-male sexual transmission of HIV. *AIDS* 15:1188–1189.

Halkitis, P.N., Parsons, J.T., Wolitski, R.J., and Remien, R.H. (2003) Characteristics of HIV antiretroviral treatments, access and adherence in an ethnically diverse sample of men who have sex with men. *AIDS Care* 15:89–102.

Harawa, N.T., Greenland, S., Bingham, T.A., Johnson, D.F., Cochran, S.D., Cunningham, W.E., Celentano, D.D., Koblin, B.A., LaLota, M., MacKellar, D.A., McFarland, W., Shehan, D., Stoyanoff, S., Thiede, H., Torian, L., and Valleroy, L. (2004) Associations of race/ethnicity with HIV prevalence and HIV-related behaviors among young men who have sex with men in 7 urban centers in the United States. *Journal of Acquired Immune Deficiency Syndrome* 35:526–536.

Hart, T., and Peterson, J. (2004) Predictors of risky sexual behavior among young African American men who have sex with men. *American Journal of Public Health* 94:1122–1123.

Heckman, T.G., Kelly, J.A., Bogart, L.M., Kalichman, S.C., and Rompa, D.J. (1999) HIV risk differences between African-American and White men who have sex with men. *Journal of the National Medical Association* 91:92–100.

Herbst, J.H., Sherba, R.T., Crepaz, N., DeLuca, J.B., Zohrabyan, L., Stall, R.D., Lyles, C.M., and the HIV/AIDS Prevention Research Synthesis Team (2005) A metaanalytic review of HIV behavioral interventions for reducing sexual risk behavior of men who have sex with men. *Journal of Acquired Immune Deficiency Syndrome* 39:228–241.

Heubner, D.M., Davis, M.C., Nemeroff, C.J., and Aiken, L.S. (2002) The impact of internalized homophobia on HIV preventive interventions. *American Journal of Community Psychology* 30:327–348.

Jacobson, J.L., Gore, M.E., Strathdee, S.A., Phair, J.P., Riddler, S., and Detels, R. (2001) Therapy naivete in the era of potent antiretroviral therapy. *Journal of Clinical Epidemiology* 54:149–156.

Jinich, S., Stall, R., Acree, M., Paul, J., Kegeles, S., Hoff, C., and Coates T.J. (1996) Childhood sexual abuse predicts HIV risk sexual behavior in adult gay and bisexual men. In: *Proceeding of the International Conference on AIDS* 11:177 (abstract Mo.D.1718).

Johnson, W.D., Holtgrave, D.R., McClellan, W.M., Flanders, W.D., Hill, A.N., and Goodman, M. (2005) HIV intervention research for men who have sex with men: a 7-year update. *AIDS Education and Prevention* 17(6):568–589.

Johnson, W.D., Semaan, S., Hedges, L.V., Ramirez, G., Mullen, P.D., and Sogolow, E. (2002) A protocol for the analytical aspects of a systematic review of HIV prevention research. *Journal of Acquired Immune Deficiency Syndrome* 30(Supplement 1):S62–S72.

Kalichman, S.C., Carey, M.P., and Johnson, B.T. (1996) Prevention of sexually transmitted HIV infection: a met-analytic review of the behavioral outcome literature. *Annals of Behavioral Medicine* 18:6–15.

Kass, N., Flynn, C., Jacobson, L, Chmiel, J.S., and Bing, E. (1999) Effect of race on insurance coverage and health service use for HIV-infected gay men. *Epidemiology* 20:85–92.

Kegeles, S.M., and Hart, G.J. (1998) Recent HIV-prevention interventions for gay men: individual, small group and community-based studies. *AIDS* 12(Supplement A):S209–S215.

Kelly, J.A., and Kalichman, S.C. (2002) Behavioral research in HIV/AIDS primary and secondary prevention: recent advances and future directions. *Journal of Consulting and Clinical Psychology* 70:626–639.

Kleeberger, C.A., Buechner, J., Palella, F., Detels, R., Riddler, S., Godfrey, R., and Jacobson, L.P. (2004) Changes in adherence to highly active antiretroviral therapy medications in the Multicenter AIDS Cohort Study. *AIDS* 18:683–688.

Kleeberger, C.A., Phair, J., Strathdee, S.A., Detels, R., Kingsley, L., and Jacobson, L.P. (2001) Determinants of heterogeneous adherence to HIV-antiretroviral therapies in the Multicenter AIDS Cohort Study. *Journal of Acquired Immune Deficiency Syndrome* 26:82–92.

Kreiss, J.K., and Hopkins, S.G. (1993) The association between circumcision status and human immunodeficiency virus infection among homosexual men. *Journal of Infections Diseases* 168:1404–1408.

Laumann, E.O., Masi, C.M., and Zuckerman, E.W. (1997) Circumcision in the United States: prevalence, prophylactic effects, and sexual practice. *Journal of the American Medical Association* 277:1052–1057.

Lemp, G.F., Hirozawa, A.M., Givertz, D., Nieri, G.N., Anderson, L., Lindegren, M.L., Janssen, R.S., and Katz, M. (1994) Seroprevalence of HIV and risk behaviors among young homosexual and bisexual men: the San Francisco/Berkeley Young Men's Survey. *Journal of the American Medical Association* 272:449–454.

Malebranche, D. (2003) Black men who have sex with men and the HIV epidemic: next steps for public health. *American Journal of Public Health* 93:862–865.

Malebranche, D.J., Peterson, J.L., Fullilove, R.E., and Stackhouse, R.W. (2004) Race and sexual identity: perceptions about medical culture and healthcare among men who have sex with men. *Journal of the National Medical Association* 96:97–107.

Mansergh, G., Marks, G., Colfax, G.N., Guzman, R., Rader, M., and Buchbinder, S. (2002) "Barebacking" in a diverse sample of men who have sex with men. *AIDS* 14:653–659.

Marmor, M., Haynes, S.W., Donnell, D., et al. (2001) Homozygous and heterozygous CCR5-Δ32 genotypes are associated with resistance to HIV infection. *Journal of Acquired Immune Deficiency Syndrome* 27:472–481.

Martinson, J.J., Hong, L., Karanicolas, R., Moore, J.P., and Kostrikis, L.G. (2000) Global distribution of the CCR2-64I/CCR5-59653T HIV-1 disease-protective haplotype. *AIDS* 14:483–489.

Mashburn, A.J., Peterson, J.L., Bakeman, R., Miller, R.L., Clark, L.F., and the Community Intervention Trials for Youth Study Team. (2004) Influences on HIV testing among young African-American men who have sex with men and the moderating effect of geographic setting. *Journal of Community Psychology* 32:45–60.

Mason, H.R.C., Simoni, J.M., Marks, G., Johnson, C.J., and Richardson, J.L. (1997) Missed opportunities? Disclosure of HIV Infection and support seeking among HIV+ African-American and European-American men. *AIDS Behavior* 1:155–162.

Mays, V.M., Cochran, S.D., and Zamudio, A. (2004) HIV prevention research: are we meeting the needs of African American men who have sex with men? *Journal of Bleek Psychology* 30:78–105.

McKirnan, D., Stokes, J., Doll, L., and Burzette, R. (1995) Bisexually active men: social characteristics and sexual behavior. *Journal of Sex Research* 32:65–76.

Millett, G.A., Peterson, J.L., Wolitski, R.J., and Stall, R. (2006) Greater risk for HIV infection of black men who have sex with men: a critical literature review. *American Journal of Public Health* 96:1007–1019.

Montgomery, J.P., Mokotoff, E.D., Gentry, A.C., and Blair, J.M. (2003) The extent of bisexual behaviour in HIV-infected men and implications for transmission to their female sex partners. *AIDS Care* 15:829–837.

Myers, H.F., and Durvasula, R.S. (1999) Psychiatric disorders in African American men and women living with HIV/AIDS. *Cultural Diversity & Ethnic Minority Psychology* 5:249–262.

Myers, H.F., Javanbakht, M., Martinez, M., and Obediah, S. (2003) Psychosocial predictors of risky sexual behaviors in African American men: implications for prevention. *AIDS Education and Prevention* 15(Supplement A):66–79.

Myrick, R. (1999) In the life: culture-specific HIV communication programs designed for African American men who have sex with men. *Journal of Sex Research* 36:159–170.

Newman, P.A., Rhodes, F., and Weiss, R.E. (2004) Correlates of sex trading among drug-using men who have sex with men. *American Journal of Public Health* 94:1998–2003.

Oakley, A., Fullerton, D., and Holland, J. (1995) Behavioral interventions for HIV/AIDS prevention. *AIDS* 9:479–486.

O'Leary, A., Purcell, D., Remien, R.H., and Gomez, C. (2003) Childhood sexual abuse and sexual transmission risk behavior among HIV-positive men who have sex with men. *AIDS Care* 15(1):17–26.

Ostrow, D.G., Whitaker, R.E., Frasier, K., Cohen, C., Wan, J., Frank, C., and Fisher, E. (1991) Racial differences in social support and mental health in men with HIV infection: a pilot study. *AIDS Care* 3(1):55–63.

Parsons, J., Halkitis, P.N., Stirratt, M.J., and O'Leary, A. (1998) Sexual behavior among HIV seropositive men-who-have-sex-with-men who frequent public and commercial sex environments. In: *Proceedings of the International Conference on AIDS* 12:423 (abstract 23405).

Paxton, W.A., Kang, S., and Koup, R.A. (1998) The HIV type 1 coreceptor CCR5 and its role in viral transmission and disease progression. *AIDS Research and Human Retroviruses* 14:S89–S92.

Peterson, J.L., and Carballo-Diéguez, A. (2000) HIV prevention among African-American and Latino men who have sex with men. In: Peterson, J.L., and DiClemente, R.J. (eds) *Handbook of HIV Prevention*. Kluwer Academic/Plenum, New York, pp. 217–224.

Peterson, J.L., Bakeman, R., Stokes, J., and Community Intervention Trial for Youth Study Team. (2001) Racial ethnic patterns of HIV sexual risk behaviors among young men who have sex with men. *Journal of the Gay and Lesbian Medical Association* 5:155–162.

Peterson, J.L., Coates, T., Catania, J., Hauck, W.W., Acree, M., Daigle, D., Hilliard, B., Middleton, L., and Hearst, N. (1996a) Evaluation of an HIV risk reduction intervention among African-American gay and bisexual men. *AIDS* 10:319–325.

Peterson, J.L., Coates, T.J., Catania, J.A., Hilliard, B., Middleton, L., and Hearst, N. (1995) Help-seeking for AIDS high-risk sexual behavior among gay and bisexual African-American men. *AIDS Education and Prevention* 7(1):1–9.

Peterson, J.L., Coates, T.J., Catania, J.A., Middleton, L., Hilliard, B., and Hearst, N. (1992) High-risk sexual behavior and condom use among gay and bisexual African-American men. *American Journal of Public Health* 82:1490–1494.

Peterson, J.L., Folkman, S., and Bakeman, R. (1996b) Stress, coping, HIV status, psychosocial resources and depressive mood in African American gay, bisexual and heterosexual men. *American Journal of Community Psychology* 24:461–487.

Quinn, T.C., Wawer, M.J., Sewankambo, N., Serwadda, D., Li, C., Wabwire-Mangen, F., Meehan, M.O., Lutalo, T., and Gray, R.H. (2000) Viral load and heterosexual transmission of human immunodeficiency virus type 1; Rakai Project Study Group. *New England Journal of Medicine* 342:921–929.

Richardson, M.A., Satz, P., Meyers, H.F., Miller, E.N., Bing, E.G., Fawzy, F.I., and Maj, M. (1999) Effects of the depressed mood versus clinical depression on neuropsychological performance among African American men impacted by HIV/AIDS. *Journal of Clinical and Experimental Neuropsychology* 21:769–783.

Ross, M.S., and Kelly, J.A. (2000) Interventions to reduce HIV transmission among homosexual men. In: Peterson, J.L., and DiClemente, R.J. (eds) *Handbook of HIV Prevention*. Kluwer Academic/Plenum, New York, pp. 201–216.

Rothenberg, R., Wasserheit, J., and St. Louis, M. (1998) Estimating the effect of treating sexually transmitted diseases (STDs) on HIV transmission; National HIV/STD Interaction Study Group. Presented at the International Conference on AIDS.

Ruiz, J., Facer, M., and Sun, R.K. (1998) Risk factors for human immunodeficiency virus infection and unprotected anal intercourse among young men who have sex with men. *Sexually Transmitted Diseases* 25:100–107.

Samuel, M., and Winkelstein, W., Jr. (1987) Prevalence of human immunodeficiency virus infection in ethnic minority homosexual/bisexual men. *Journal of the American Medical Association* 257:1901–1902.

Semaan, S., Kay, L., Strouse, D., Sogolow, E., Mullen, P.D., Neumann, M.S., Flores, S.A., Peersman, G., Johnson, W.D., Lipman, P.D., Eke, A., and Des Jarlais, D.C. (2002) A profile of U.S.-based trials of behavioral and social interventions for HIV risk reduction. *Journal of Acquired Immune Deficiency Syndrome* 30(Supplement 1):S3–S50.

Siegel, K., and Raveis, V. (1997) Perceptions of access to HIV-related information, care and services among minority men. *Qualitative Health Research* 7(1):9–31.

Siegel, K., Karus, D., and Schrimshaw, E.W. (2000) Racial difference in attitudes toward protease inhibitors among older HIV-infected men. *AIDS Care* 12:423–434.

Siegel, K., Schrimshaw, M.A., and Karus, D. (2004) Racial disparities in sexual risk behaviors and drug use among older gay/bisexual and heterosexual men living with HIV/AIDS. *Journal of the National Medical Association* 96:215–223.

Smith, G.L., Greenup, R., and Takafuji, E. (1987) Circumcision as a risk factor for urethritis in racial groups. *American Journal of Public Health* 77:452–452.

Stall, R., Pollack, L., Mills, T.C., et al. (2001) Use of antiretroviral therapies among HIV-infected men who have sex with men: a household-based sample of 4 major American cities. *American Journal of Public Health* 91:767–773.

Stephenson, J. (2001) Gene mutation link with HIV resistance. *Journal of the American Medical Association* 286:1441–1442.

Stokes, J.P., and Peterson, J.L. (1998) Homophobia, self-esteem and risk for HIV among African American men who have sex with men. *AIDS Education and Prevention* 10:278–292.

Sumartojo, E., Doll, L., Holtgrave, D., Gayle, H., and Merson, M. (2000) Enriching the mix: incorporating structural factors into HIV prevention. *AIDS* 14(Supplement 1):S1–S2.

Torian, L.V., Makki, H.A., Menzies, I.B., Murrill, C.S., and Weisfuse, I.B. (2002) HIV infection in men who have sex with men, New York City Department of Health sexually transmitted disease clinics, 1990–1999: a decade of sero-surveillance finds that racial disparities and associations between HIV and gonorrhea persist. *Sexually Transmitted Diseases* 29:73–78.

Valleroy, L.A., MacKellar, D.A., Karon, J.M., Rosen, D.H., McFarland, W., Shehan, D.A., Stoyanoff, S.R., LaLota, M., Celentano, D.D., Koblin, B.A., Thiede, H., Katz, M.H., Torian, L.V., and Janssen, R.S. (2000) HIV prevalence and associated risks in young men who have sex with men. *Journal of the American Medical Association* 284:198–204.

Williamson, C., Loubser, S.A., Brice, B., Joubert, G., Smit, T., Thomas, R., Visagie, M., Cooper, M., and van der Ryst, E. (2000) Allelic frequencies of host genetic variants influencing susceptibility to HIV-1 infection and disease in South African populations. *AIDS* 14:449–451.

Wilson, B.D.M., and Miller, R.L. (2003) Examining strategies for culturally grounded HIV prevention. *AIDS Education and Prevention* 15:184–202.

Wohl, A.R., Johnson, D., Jordan, W., Lu, S., Beall, G., Currier, J., and Kerndt, P.R. (2000) High-risk behaviors during incarceration in African American men treated for HIV at three Los Angeles public medical centers. *Journal of Acquired Immune Deficiency Syndrome* 24:386–392.

Wohl, A.R., Johnson, D.F., Lu, S., Jordan, W., Beall, G., Currier, J., and Simon, P.A. (2002) HIV risk behaviors among African American men in Los Angeles County who self-identify as heterosexual. *Journal of Acquired Immune Deficiency Syndrome* 31:354–360.

Wolitski, R.J., Janssen, R.S., Holtgrave, D.R., and Peterson, J.L. (2003) The public health response to the HIV epidemic in the United States. In: Wormser, G.R. (ed) *AIDS and other manifestations of HIV infection*, 4th ed. Elsevier Science, Philadelphia, pp. 983–999.

Wolitski, R.J., Valdiserri, R.O., Denning, P.H., and Levine, W.C. (2001) Are we headed for a resurgence in HIV infections among men who have sex with men? *American Journal of Public Health* 91:883–888.

Wortley, P.M., Chu, S.Y., Diaz, T., Ward, J.W., Doyle, B., Davidson, A.J., Checko, P.J., Herr, M., Conti, L., Fann, S.A., Sorvillo, F., Mokotoff, E., Levy, A., Hermann, P., and Norris-Walczak, E. (1995) HIV testing patterns: where, why, and when were persons with AIDS tested for HIV? *AIDS* 9:487–492.

Zucconi, S.L., Jacobson, L.P., Schrager, L.K., et al. (1994) Impact of immuno-suppression on health care use by men in the Multicenter AIDS Cohort Study (MACS). *Journal of Acquired Immune Deficiency Syndrome* 7:607–616.

23

LGBT Tobacco and Alcohol Disparities

Gregory L. Greenwood and Elisabeth P. Gruskin

1 Introduction

The literature is replete with a discussion of the health disparities facing the lesbian, gay, bisexual, transgender (LGBT) population in the United States. Against the backdrop of effective, comprehensive tobacco and alcohol control programs at the state and local levels during the past decade (Fichtenberg, 2000; Scott, 2003) are the high rates of smoking (Stall et al., 1999; Gruskin et al., 2001; Ryan et al., 2001; Greenwood, 2005; Tang, 2004) and drinking (Cochran & Mays, 2000a,b; Greenwood et al., 2001; Gruskin et al., 2001; Stall et al., 2001) reported for the LGBT population. It makes sense that there are tobacco and alcohol health disparities for LGBTs given the evidence of well known risk factors facing this community that other priority populations such as ethnic/racial minorities and lower socioeconomic communities have confronted.

LGBT people face high levels of daily stress due to stigma, homophobia, and discrimination as well as sexism, racism, and transphobia for LBT women, LGBT people of color, and transgenders, respectively (Meyer, 1995; Friedman, 1999; Dean et al., 2000; Clements-Nolle et al., 2001; Mays & Cochran, 2001; Meyer 2003a,b). Smoking and drinking among LGBTs is also supported by the centrality of bars (Kelly et al., 1997; Warwick et al., 2003)—which provide safe spaces to congregate, socialize, find acceptance and support, and meet prospective friends and partners—where tobacco and alcohol use is common. Co-morbid conditions that seem to be more prevalent among LGBT individuals than their heterosexual counterparts, such as depression (Cochran & Mays 2000a,b; Mays & Cochran, 2001; Mills et al., 2004), substance abuse (Cochran & Mays 2000a,b; Stall et al., 2001), victimization (Greenwood et al., 2002), and childhood trauma (Paul et al., 2001), likely contribute to higher rates of use and misuse. Finally, usage rates are further encouraged by tobacco and alcohol industry support of the LGBT population through direct advertisement, sponsorship, and promotional events (Lippman, 1992; Goebel, 1994; Elliot, 1997; Washington, 2002; Smith & Malone, 2003; Stevens et al., 2004).

This chapter is limited to drinking and smoking in the adult LGBT population. First, we review key behavioral outcome measures from published studies of tobacco and alcohol use and misuse, respectively (i.e., prevalence of current tobacco and alcohol use and misuse). It is important to note that precise estimates of disparities in smoking and drinking for LGBTs have been difficult to gauge for three primary reasons: (1) enumerating the LGBT population living in the United States is extraordinarily difficult; (2) obtaining data on LGBT consumption patterns from population-based surveillance studies has not been possible because sexual orientation, same-sex behavior, and transgender identity are not often indexed; and (3) obtaining data from large samples of LGBTs has been difficult.

Second, we summarize the varied health and social consequences of using tobacco or alcohol for LGBTs. Third, we present a conceptual model of tobacco and alcohol disparities by identifying the major risk factors for each level of influence: individual, peer/family, social, environmental. Finally, we discuss key considerations for advancing tobacco and alcohol control programs for the LGBT population to reduce consumption patterns and use-related disease burden and to increase treatment efficacy.

2 LGBT Tobacco Consumption Patterns

2.1 Studies

Skinner and Otis (1996) were among the first to publish smoking prevalence rates drawn from self-report measures collected during the late 1980s from lesbian/gay respondents recruited via mailing lists of LGBT organizations, from research referrals, and from outreach during a gay pride event in the Midwest. Current smoking was reported by 42.7% of lesbians and 34.9% of gay men.

Stall et al. (1999) found high rates of current smoking among men who have sex with men (MSM) (i.e., self-identified as gay or bisexual, or reported same-sex behavior within the past 5 years). Telephone surveys were completed in 1992 using random-digit-dial (RDD) household-based sampling of MSM ($n = 696$), and self-administered questionnaires (SAQs) were collected during the same year from a convenience sample of bar patrons ($n = 1897$). Altogether, 41.5% of the household-based subgroup and 50.1% of the convenience subgroup were current smokers. Even when controlling for key sociodemographics such as age, education, and race/ethnicity, the gay/bisexual men smoked at higher rates than a general sample of men.

Diamant (2000a) collected via mail SAQs from a convenience sample ($n = 6935$) of self-identified lesbians from national LGB magazines. They found that 27.0% of lesbians were current smokers compared to 22.6% of a general sample of women.

Valanis et al. (2000) measured smoking using convenience samples of postmenopausal women (50 to 79 years) participating in 40 Women's Health Initiative Centers during 1993 to 1996. Of these participants, 264 were *lifetime* lesbians (sex only with women during lifetime), 309 were *adult* lesbians (sex only with women since age 45), and 740 were bisexual women (sex with both women and men). Current smoking prevalence rates were 10.0% for *lifetime* lesbians, 14.4% for *adult* lesbians, and 12.0% for bisexual women. When comparing these smoking rates to those from a general sample of women, the researchers found that lesbian and bisexual women were more likely to report being current smokers [odds ratio (OR) = 2.58] than were women in general.

Gruskin et al. (2001) examined smoking among women (120 lesbians and bisexuals and 7993 heterosexuals) by measuring current smoking status from completed SAQs by members of a larger Health Maintenance Organization (HMO). Altogether, 25.4% of lesbians were current smokers, which was significantly different from the rate for women in general (12.6%). When controlling for sociodemographic characteristics, the youngest (20–34 years) and the middle age group (35–49 years) of lesbian and bisexual women were more likely to be smokers than were the youngest and middle age groups of heterosexual women (OR 3.2 and 3.4, respectively). However, the differences in the oldest age group (50+ years) were not statistically significant.

Cochran et al. (2001) measured current smoking by combining self-report data gathered from 11,876 lesbians participating in health research studies from 1987 to 1996. They also found that lesbian and bisexual women were more likely to report current smoking than women in a national sample (21.2% vs. 16.1%).

Aaron et al. (2001), in a study of 1010 self-identified lesbians, also found higher rates of current smoking than in a general sample of women (35.5% vs. 20.5%).

Greenwood et al. (2005) is the first published study that we know of to use state-of-science sampling and data collection methods to compare measures of smoking more rigorously. This cross-sectional study [Gay Men's Tobacco Study (GMTS), January 1999 to December 1999] was conducted with a previously recruited household-based RDD sample of adult MSM in four U.S. cities [Urban Men's Health Study (UMHS), November 1996 to February 1998] who were eligible for follow-up (1780/2402, 74%). They found that MSM had higher rates of current smoking than the general population: 31.4% vs. 24.7% ($p < 001$).

Tang et al. (2004) is the first published study we know of to report prevalence rates of current smoking among a *statewide, household-based sample* of lesbians, gay men, and bisexual women and men. The 2000 California Health Interview Survey asked (for the first time) respondents to report their sexual orientation. Of 44,606 completed telephone interviews, 343 were lesbians, 593 were gay men, and 793 were bisexual (511 women, 282 men). The results confirmed earlier findings that LGBs smoke at significantly higher rates than the general population. More than one-fourth of the lesbians smoked [25.3%; 95% confidence interval (CI): 19.5%, 31.0%]. The rate is about 70% higher than that of heterosexual women, who had a smoking prevalence of 14.9% (95% CI: 14.3%, 15.5%). Gay men had a smoking prevalence of 33.2% (95% CI: 27.8%, 38.7%), which is 55.9% higher than that of heterosexual men. Bisexual women and lesbians had similar smoking prevalence, and the rate for bisexual men was close to that of heterosexual men (21.3%; 95% CI: 20.5%, 22.1%). These differences were still evident after controlling for key demographic characteristics (i.e., age, race/ethnicity, education, household income, and urban/rural status.

2.2 Summary

The studies above found that the rates of smoking were higher for the LGB population than for the general population. The report by Greenwood et al. (2005) was the first probability sample to measure and support high rates of smoking among MSM in particular; and the findings by Tang et al. (2004) was the first population-based survey to ask about sexual orientation and support high prevalence rates among LGBs in general. It is important to note that the costs of constructing the probability sample of urban MSM in the study by Greenwood et al. (2005) were high, whereas the benefits of simply adding a couple of questions to a population-based survey clearly outweigh the costs, as demonstrated by Tang et al. (2004). This study is an example of how one small step (i.e., adding two questions to a statewide general household interview survey) can substantially advance the state of the science of LGB tobacco use and cessation research. It is the first large statewide probability sample of adult lesbians, gay men, and bisexuals of which we know. As such, it allowed comparisons between a sample of the LGB population and a sample of men and women in general. The use of a standard measurement of smoking not only allows comparisons as reported herein, it enables future investigators to conduct longitudinal comparisons or meta-analyses, which are both commonly performed in tobacco research, particularly with priority populations.

Taken together, the findings from these studies advance the argument that LGBTs should be identified as a priority population for intensive, targeted tobacco control efforts. Tobacco prevention and treatment research has not adequately dealt with the LGBT population even though they are targeted by tobacco companies and disproportionately affected by smoking. This is particularly worrisome given the negative synergy between smoking and HIV/AIDS (Craib et al., 1992; Conley et al., 1996; Page-Shafer et al., 1996; Begtrup et al., 1997; Galai et al., 1997; Cole, 2004) and other co-morbid conditions such as perceived stress, depression, and substance abuse that appear to be high for LGBTs (Cochran & Mays 2000a,b; Dean et al., 2000; Greenwood et al., 2001; Gruskin et al., 2001; Mays & Cochran, 2001; Stall et al., 2001, 2003; Mills et al., 2004). Basic surveillance data necessary to monitor and track the effects of current tobacco control efforts are missing, for example. Beyond simply measuring the prevalence of tobacco use (i.e., current smoking), we have few or no data on average consumption patterns, lifetime use patterns, use of other tobacco products, the effects of antitobacco advertising, tobacco attitudes, exposure to smoking bans at home or work, the rates of cessation, the mean number of quit attempts, the methods used to quit, or the characteristics and correlates of quitting. At minimum, collecting basic data would be an essential first step in addressing these issues.

3 LGBT Alcohol Consumption Patterns

3.1 Studies

Stall and Wiley (1988) measured alcohol use and alcohol-related problems using telephone survey data collected in the first household-based sample of gay and bisexual men. They found that gay and bisexual men did not differ from their heterosexual neighbors in reported alcohol-related problems, yet they were more likely to be frequent/heavy drinkers (19% vs. 11%).

McKirnan and Peterson (1989) collected SAQs from a convenience sample of 3400 lesbians and gay men from a community sample. Gay/bisexual men compared to men in general reported higher rates of frequent/heavy drinking (17% vs. 8%), and alcohol problems (23% vs. 16%, respectively). Similarly, lesbians compared to women in general reported higher rates of alcohol problems (23% vs. 8%).

Greenwood et al. (2001) measured alcohol use among young (18–29 years) gay and bisexual men (n = 428) who completed telephone surveys during 1992 and 1993 during a multistage RDD sample of men living in San Francisco. A total of 13.6% of gay/bisexual men reported frequent/heavy alcohol use compared to 10.4% of a general sample of similarly aged men.

Diamant (2000a) found higher levels of alcohol use and of frequent/heavy drinking in a large sample (n = 6935) of self-identified lesbians recruited from national LGB magazines.

Valanis et al. (2000) compared alcohol consumption patterns between lesbian- and heterosexual-identified women ages 50 to 79 participating in 40 Women's Health Initiative centers during 1993 to 1996. Researchers found that lesbian and bisexual women were more likely than heterosexuals to drink alcohol and to drink in larger quantities than their heterosexual counterparts.

Nawyn et al. (2000) surveyed a college sample of 40 lesbian and 1254 heterosexual employees at a large American university. They found that lesbians were more likely to report drinking to intoxication, heavy episodic drinking, and consumption of greater quantities than heterosexual women.

Gruskin et al. (2001) examined smoking and drinking among women (120 lesbians/bisexuals and 7993 heterosexuals) by measuring prevalence rates from completed SAQs by members of a large HMO. Higher rates of heavy drinking were found for lesbians ages 20 to 49.

Cochran and Mays (2000b) found that among respondents to the 1996 National Household Survey of Drug Abuse, the 96 homosexual women were more likely than the 5792 heterosexual women to be classified with alcohol or drug dependence when controlling for age, ethnicity/race, education, and income (OR 1.6). However, there were no differences in normative alcohol consumption.

Aaron et al. (2001) surveyed 1158 self-identified lesbians and compared the results to a national sample. Researchers found that lesbians were more likely to report current alcohol use and heavy drinking.

Dibble et al. (2002), in a study of 324 lesbians and their heterosexual sisters, found that although there were no differences in drinking rates lesbians were more likely than their sisters to report ever having had a drinking problem.

Stall et al. (2001) measured alcohol use and alcohol-related problems among MSM in four major U.S. cities (UMHS). Alcohol use was especially common, with 85% of the overall sample reporting at least some drinking during the past 6 months. Comparable rates of heavy/frequent drinking were found between this probability sample of MSM and men in general (8.0% vs. 9.1%). Altogether, 12.4% (95% CI: 10.8–14.3) of MSM also reported three or more alcohol-related problems.

3.2 Summary

Although many of the studies above found higher consumption patterns and alcohol-related problems for the LGB population than for women and men in general, others did not. Alcohol use and misuse among the transgender population has been underinvestigated. Similar to findings on tobacco use for LGBT, there is a general lack of basic surveillance data on relevant outcomes such as average per-capita consumption, intoxication, binge drinking, alcohol attitudes, quit rates, and more. Such basic information is needed to gauge more clearly the level of alcohol use and misuse and to establish priorities that advance alcohol control programs to reduce its use (and alcohol-related diseases) among the LGBT population and to increase abstinence.

4 Health and Social Consequences

Diseases and other adverse health effects for which smoking is identified as a cause in the 2004 Surgeon's General Report (U.S. Department of Health and Human Services, 2004) include cancer (bladder, cervical, esophageal, kidney, and laryngeal cancer; leukemia; lung, oral, pancreatic, and stomach cancer); cardiovascular disease, cerebrovascular disease, coronary heart disease, respiratory disease, reproductive effects (fertility, low birth weight); other effects such as cataracts, diminished health status/morbidity, hip factures, low bone density, and peptic ulcer disease. Adverse medical consequences for which alcohol is identified as a cause include gastrointestinal, cardiovascular, endocrine, hematologic, and neurologic diseases (Gambert & Katsoyannis, 1995; National Institute on Alcohol Abuse and Alcoholism, 2000). It is important to clarify that health consequences of tobacco use occur at any level of use, in contrast to alcohol use, the consequences of which generally occur at excessive levels of use.

4.1 Benefits of Cessation

Because smoking and alcohol abuse have both long-term and short-term health consequences, stopping or reducing use decreases morbidity and mortality. For example, quitting smoking decreases cancers affecting the lung, mouth, nasal cavities, larynx, pharynx, esophagus, stomach, liver, pancreas, kidney, bladder, and uterine cervix as well as myeloid leukemia (Gambert & Katsoyannis, 1995; National Institute on Alcohol Abuse and Alcoholism, 2000; U.S. Department of Health and Human Services, 2004). In addition, research has consistently indicated that people who quit smoking live longer than people who continue to smoke.

4.2 LGBT Special Considerations

LGBTs (general) may experience psychosocial consequences of tobacco or alcohol use and misuse that are commonly encountered in the general population. For example, smoking/drinking and treatment failure may be associated overall with higher levels of negative moods and perceived stress (Hall et al., 1993, 1994, 1996, 1998). High levels of alcohol use and misuse have been associated with unsafe sexual encounters, poor treatment adherence, and poor treatment outcomes for LGBTs in general (Stall et al., 2000). Even though the direction of causality is not clear, the negative synergy of elevated levels of substance abuse and the central role of bars and clubs in LGBT culture may exacerbate smoking or drinking as well as hinder cessation or abstinence (Stall et al., 2000).

Lesbian/bisexual women who smoke or drink face may face challenges related to changes in their menstrual cycle. Smoking can cause changes to a women's menstrual cycle, such as increased risk of painful menstruation, absence of menstruation, and menstrual irregularity (O'Hara et al., 1989). Quitting smoking at the beginning of the menstrual cycle could result in more severe withdrawal symptoms and smoking-related cravings (O'Hara et al., 1989). Like women in general, it is reasonable to expect that lesbian and bisexual women who take estrogen (as a form of birth control or treatment of menopausal symptoms) are at greater risk of heart disease and cancer. Lesbian and bisexual women may be less likely to undergo screening for risk factors related to smoking and drinking because studies show they seek health services less frequently than other women (Diamant et al., 2000b).

Gay/bisexual men who smoke may face (like men in general) increased risks of impotence and prostate cancer (Opalinska et al., 2003). Weight concerns may be more pronounced for gay men given the value placed on physical appearance in some parts of the gay community (Kassel & Franko, 2000). Some gay men may be reluctant to quit smoking for fear that doing so will cause them to gain weight.

Transgender persons, particularly male-to-female (MtF), who take hormones may experience an increased risk of blood clots. The risk increases in women who smoke (Anonymous, 1995), particularly after the age of 40. For transgender female-to-male (FtM), smoking may increase the risk of coronary heart disease. This happens to men using testosterone and can lead to an increased risk of heart attack and stroke (Phillips et al., 2004). Studies have shown that it takes longer for wounds to heal in people who smoke. The same delays could occur following surgery, including plastic or reconstructive surgery.

Human immunodeficiency virus (*HIV*)-*positive LGBTs*. High rates of smoking have been reported in numerous HIV-positive cohorts (Craib et al., 1992). Some research has indicated that smoking is related to the development of *Pneumocystis carinii* pneumonia (PCP), predicts a shorter time of progression to diagnosis with AIDS, and is associated with a higher risk of death (Page-Shafer et al., 1996), but these findings are not consistent (Craib et al., 1992; Conley et al., 1996; Begtrup et al., 1997). This is a particular concern among smokers, as researchers have consistently found an association between smoking and oral candidiasis (Galai et al., 1997) and hairy leukoplakia (Conley et al., 1996). Recently, researchers found that HIV-positive gay/bisexual men who have not received highly active antiretroviral therapy (HAART) are at increased risk for both ischemic stroke and intracerebral hemorrhage, reinforcing theories that HIV induces a prothrombotic state or induces vasculopathy (Cole, 2004). High rates of drinking among the HIV-positive population has been shown to affect negatively treatment adherence and medication effects, to increase HIV sexual risk transmission, and to predict a shorter time of disease progression and impaired immune system functioning.

5 Conceptual Model of LGBT Tobacco and Alcohol Use

The theoretical and empirical literature suggests that there is a complex combination of factors at the level of the individual, peer/family, social, and environment directly and indirectly associated with of tobacco and alcohol disparities in the LGBT population. We need a conceptual framework that at once identifies known or hypothesized associations and their interactions and one that also allows exploration into uncharted territory.

Such a framework built from the social science and public health literature (Peterson and DiClemente, 2000; Dolcini et al., 2004) is depicted in Figure 23.1. We present this model as a heuristic to advance LGBT tobacco and alcohol control programs. However, our conceptual framework cannot and should be empirically tested as a single, definitive model that provides a full account of all the possible dynamically interconnected array of factors. Instead, it can be used to enhance our understanding and guide future explorations. It is of importance to examine LGBT subgroup differences in tobacco and alcohol use disparities. That is, whether (and how) the major risk and protective factors of use and misuse vary by key sociodemographic factors, such as sexual identity, gender, age, and ethnicity/race.

5.1 Individual-Level Factors

The importance of genetic and biologic factors is well established in the tobacco and alcohol literature. Other individual-level factors that influence tobacco and alcohol use include developmental (e.g., sexual identity development and acceptance, disclosure versus concealment),

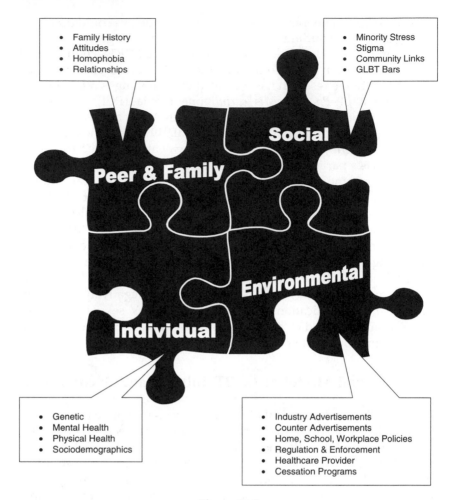

Figure 23.1

sociodemographic (e.g., age, gender, ethnicity/race, education, socioeconomic status, marital or intimate partner status), mental health (e.g., depression, anxiety, substance abuse), internalized homophobia, expectancies, attitudes, attributions, and behavior (e.g., coping behavior and sexual practices).

5.2 Peer/Family-Level Factors

The literature of tobacco and alcohol use has identified a number of peer/family factors: parental and family history of lifetime and current use and consumption patterns; tobacco and alcohol use patterns of peers; and attitudes of peer/family toward tobacco and alcohol use. Other factors may affect tobacco and alcohol use as well: adverse family events such as domestic violence, victimization, and childhood sexual abuse; peer/family use attitudes and expectations; parental/family acceptance or rejection of LGBT status; and parental/family homophobia.

5.3 Social Factors

Standard social factors such as social support, perceived stress, stressful life events, poverty, stigma, discrimination, tobacco and alcohol use of the social network, and network characteristics have been related to tobacco or alcohol use. Potentially strong LGBT-related social determinants of tobacco or alcohol use include minority stress, homophobia, LGBT bar attendance, and LGBT community involvement.

5.4 Environmental Factors

A number of environmental factors have been found or hypothesized to affect tobacco or alcohol use: unequal access among some LGBT people to quality health care; exposure to tobacco and alcohol advertising; exposure to tobacco and alcohol promotional items; exposure to antismoking messages; access to and regulation of tobacco and alcohol products; and smoking or drinking policies in the workplace and home.

6 LGBT Tobacco and Alcohol Control Programs

The LGBT population can benefit from comprehensive tobacco and alcohol control programs to the degree that we are able to (1) share a common vision of LGBT wellness goals; (2) develop theoretically and empirically derived strategies to achieve this vision; (3) identify benchmarks and individual performance indicators; (4) anticipate key barriers and manage risks; and (5) track our progress on short-term and longer-term population outcomes. The need for the LGBT population to be identified as a priority population by national, state, and local tobacco and alcohol control programs is fundamental to take full advantage of existing best practice guidelines and interventions (MacDonald et al., 2001) and, where necessary, to begin to tailor control efforts to meet the needs of LGBTs. It makes sense not only to begin to implement best-practice treatment interventions (Centers for Disease Control and Prevention, 1999) but to begin simultaneously to develop, implement, and evaluate whether (and how) LGBT-tailored cessation services result in higher utilization, satisfaction, and ultimately quit rates.

In the meantime, the current best practice model of tobacco control programs (MacDonald et al., 2001; Centers for Disease Control and Prevention, 2003) provides a useful framework for developing LGBT-targeted programs to reduce smoking and drinking in this population. To illustrate, we focus on the best practice model of tobacco control. This model includes multilevel efforts (e.g., prevention, treatment, media advocacy, and economic, legislative, and public policy) aimed at reducing use and misuse, decreasing disease-related morbidity and mortality, increasing treatment access, utilization, and success, and reducing environmentally related hazards (e.g., second-hand smoke, drunk driving arrests). For example, the CDC recommended a best practice control model (MacDonald et al., 2001; Centers for Disease

Control and Prevention, 2003) for tobacco use and prevention that includes the following interconnected inputs, activities, outputs, and outcomes:

- *Inputs* include (1) federal programs, litigation, and other inputs; (2) state tobacco control programs; and (3) community and national partners and organizations.
- *Activities* sponsored by state (or local) tobacco control programs generally include four primary activities: (1) counter-marketing advertising; (2) community prevention and treatment; (3) policy and regulatory action; and (4) efforts targeted to disparate populations.
- *Outputs* include (1) exposure to no-smoking and pro-health messages; (2) increased use of services; and (3) creation of no-smoking regulations and policies (e.g., clean indoor air regulation and smoking bans in the home).
- *Short-term outcomes*
  - Changes in knowledge and attitudes
  - Adherence to and enforcement of bans, regulations, and policies
- *Intermediate outcomes*
  - Reduced smoking initiation among young people
  - Increased smoking cessation among all
  - Increased number of non-smoking environments
- *Long-term outcomes*
  - Decreased smoking
  - Reduced exposure to second-hand smoke
  - Reduced tobacco-related morbidity and mortality
  - Decreased tobacco-related health disparities

6.1 LGBT-Targeted Cessation and Treatment Programs

6.1.1 Tobacco

The only study we know that examined LGBT-targeted smoking cessastion is a pilot community-level intervention conducted by Harding et al. (2005). Using a noncomparison, pre- and post-test study design, the authors examined the efficacy of a 7-week group cessation program that combined nicotine replacement therapy and peer support with a convenience sample of 98 gay men. At 7 weeks, 44 (76%) participants were confirmed to have quit using a standard measurement of abstinence. The only significant independent baseline predictor of quitting was prior number of quit attempts (OR 1.48, $p = 0.04$). This targeted community-level intervention is the first one we know of to conduct a process evaluation and outcome monitoring of smoking cessation designed for the LGBT population.

6.1.2 Alcohol

We do not know of any peer-reviewed published treatment research that has examined the efficacy of LGBT-targeted alcohol interventions. Irwin and Morgenstern (2005) found that treatment-seeking MSM with an alcohol or drug diagnosis had high rates of comorbid disorders, which would need to be addressed by any treatment program designed for this population.

7 Summary and Future Directions

A basic foundation for state-based chronic disease surveillance programs is data collection, which allows monitoring and tracking of key indicators to establish a basic understanding of the problem, identify high risk groups, inform policies, programs, and legislation, and justify and direct research and surveillance (Giovino, 2003). Although the general population and some key priority populations have benefited from such comprehensive targeting and monitoring, the LGBT population has been largely ignored. There are limited data on its size, geographic distribution, demographic composition, and other characteristics. A key priority, therefore, is research and surveillance. We need population-based data that (1) more precisely and accurately measure prevalence rates; and (2) examine in greater depth the patterns of use and misuse, the attempts to quit or abstain, and the outcomes of a host of other tobacco- and alcohol-related factors needed to close the gap in science and to help inform and guide future tobacco and alcohol control efforts.

7.1 Research and Surveillance

A fundamental start is for local, state, and national surveillance systems to include measures of sexual orientation (same-sex behavior) and transgender identification to begin to monitor and track basic short-, intermediate-, and long-term outcomes related to tobacco and alcohol use and misuse in the LGBT population. Furthermore, surveillance research is necessary to identify which subsegments in the LGBT population shoulder a disproportionate burden of tobacco or alcohol use. For example, assuming that trends observed in the general population hold true for LGBT, we might find that LGBT persons of color or lower socioeconomic status smoke and drink at higher rates, shoulder a heavier burden of morbidity and mortality, have less access to health care services or prevention and treatment initiatives, and benefit less from environmental efforts aimed at regulating or minimizing the effects of tobacco or alcohol. Finally, research studies should use quantitative and qualitative methodologies to uncover *how* identity (gender, sexual, ethnic), socioeconomic status, geography (urban, suburban, rural), and related issues contribute to smoking and drinking by LGBTs; how LGBTs successfully quit or cut down; and how LGBTs remain smoke- and/or alcohol-free.

7.2 Treatment

Given the high rates of tobacco and alcohol use and misuse, the prevalence of co-morbid conditions and factors that exacerbate the health and social consequences of use, and the exposure to targeted industry marketing, it is critical that LGBTs are able to take full advantage of existing best practice treatments. For example, equal access and utilization of available health services and treatment resources need to be in place for risk screening procedures and systems to identify the LGBT smoker or drinker, particularly the heavy or problematic user. Technical assistance, training, and education should be provided to ensure that the LGBT receives culturally competent treatment and, at the very least, stands to benefit from evidence-based cessation or treatment approaches. There is yet to be research evaluating the outcomes of best practice treatments aimed at the LGBT smoker or drinker. As with other priority populations (Anonymous, 2004), it is necessary to design, implement, and evaluate culturally appropriate programs specifically for LGBT smokers. The need for evidenced-based LGBT-tailored interventions has been directly addressed in Healthy People 2010 (http://www.glma.org/home.html), and the Program Announcement on LGBT Health released by the National Institutes of Health (http://grants.nih.gov/grants/guide/pa-files/PA-01-096.html).

As a start, substance abuse providers caring for LGBT smokers or drinkers should be aware of the following issues:

- Where the individual is in his or her life cycle. The LGBT individual has different needs depending on age and maturity. Substance abuse plays a varying role throughout their lives. For example, whereas most LGBT individuals frequent bars at some point early in their lives, as they age they tend to spend more of their social life outside bars and may therefore be less likely to rely on alcohol as a social lubricant.
- The stage they are in at the time of their coming out process. LGBT individuals go through various stages during which they become more accepting of their sexual orientation. They may use substances for different reasons throughout this process. For example, in the early stages, when they first start identifying as an LGBT they may seek out role models—friends and sexual partners at the LGBT bars—and use alcohol as a coping mechanism to deal with their insecurities. Whereas later, when their sexual orientation is more established, alcohol as a social lubricant may be less important, and they may drink to cope with other difficulties that individuals experience as they age.
- The degree and impact of internalized homophobia. LGBTs develop in a world that is not accepting of their behavior in perhaps one of the most important areas, their love life. Most LGBTs internalize these negative attitudes at some point in their lives and may use alcohol as a coping mechanism.
- Their social support networks. It is important for a substance abuse treatment provider to know the people in the client's support system as they are often incorporated in the treatment.
- Their relationships with their family of origin. Often the family-of-origin has an impact on the substance abuse of LGBT individuals whether it is to avoid the alcoholism they experienced in their families or as they model substance abusing behavior. It is also important to know who in their family-of-origin is a potential support and which family members create stress for the LGBT individual.

- Their relationship history. LGBTs' drinking often reflects the drinking of their partners. It is often important for the substance abuse treatment provider to understand the role of partners in their clients' lives.
- Their sexual behavior with an emphasis on how their drinking and using behavior has in the past and currently affects their sex life. Many LGBTs use substances to enhance their sex lives or to deal with sexuality with which they are uncomfortable. Substances also affect the practice of safer sex. Understanding the relation between substance abuse and sex can help the substance abuse treatment provider work with clients to practice safer sex and limit the need for substances to enhance their sex lives.
- Their experiences with alcohol, smoking, and drugs. It is always important for treatment providers to understand the role that alcohol, smoking, and drugs have in their LGBT patients' lives and explore ways to help them minimize their use.
- Their participation in complementary treatments such as counseling, 12-step programs, and other support groups. Providers may be in a good position to evaluate the potential help that 12-step programs and other support groups can play in the LGBT substance abusers' lives. Knowing of LGBT-specific programs may help them find the support they need outside of the bars.
- Their participation in the bar scene. The bar scene plays a role for most LGBTs at some point in their lives. Understanding this role can help find alternatives to bars in the LGBT individuals' lives.

7.3 Collaborative Partnerships and Capacity

LGBT medical and public health professionals, researchers, service agency providers, and community activists/advocates should take part in mainstream tobacco and alcohol control movements. Similarly, members of local and state control programs need to assist and take part in LGBT-targeted efforts. In fact, it would be ideal for key LGBT leaders and researchers to participate with mainstream control groups when identifying "requests for proposals" and when reviewing grant proposals. Finally, future LGBT tobacco and alcohol researchers, providers, and advocates should be supported and mentored, particularly those from historically disenfranchised communities of the LGBT population.

References

Aaron, D., Markovic, N., Danielson, M., Honnold, J., Janosky, J., and Schmidt, N. (2001) Behavioral risk factors for disease and preventive health practices among lesbians. *American Journal of Public Health* 91:972–975.
Anonymous (1995) The truth about oral contraceptives, heart attack, stroke and blood clots. *Contraceptive Report* 6:1–2.
Anonymous (2004) *Making cancer health disparities history: Trans-HSS Cancer Health Disparities Progress Review Group.* U.S. Department of Health and Human Services, Washington, DC.

Begtrup, K., Melbye, M., et al. (1997) Progression to acquired immunodeficiency syndrome is influenced by CD4 T-lymphocyte count and time since seroconversion. *American Journal of Epidemiology* 145:629–635.

Centers for Disease Control and Prevention. (1999) *Best practices for comprehensive tobacco control programs—1999.* U.S. Department of Health and Human Services, Centers for Disease Control and Prevention, National Center for Chronic Disease Prevention and Health Promotion, Office on Smoking and Health. CDC, Atlanta.

Centers for Disease Control and Prevention. (2003) *Promising practices in chronic disease prevention and control.* U.S. Department of Health and Human Services, Centers for Disease Control and Prevention. CDC, Atlanta.

Clements-Nolle, K., Marx, R., et al. (2001) HIV prevalence, risk behaviors, health care use, and mental health status of transgender persons: implications for public health intervention. *American Journal of Public Health* 91:915–921.

Cochran, S.D., and Mays, V.M. (2000a) Lifetime prevalence of suicide symptoms and affective disorders among men reporting same-sex sexual partners: results from NHANES III. *American Journal of Public Health* 90:573–578.

Cochran, S.D., and Mays, V.M. (2000b) Relation between psychiatric syndromes and behaviorally defined sexual orientation in a sample of the US population. *American Journal of Epidemiology* 151:516–523.

Cochran, S.D., Mays, V.M., Bowen, D., Gage, S., Bybee, D., Roberts, S., Goldstein, R., Robison, A., Rankow, E., and White, J. (2001) Cancer-related risk indicators and preventive screening behaviors among lesbian and bisexual women. *American Journal of Public Health* 91:591–597.

Cole, E.A. (2004) HIV infection and stroke. *Stroke* 35:51–56.

Conley, L.J., Bush, T.J., et al. (1996) The association between cigarette smoking and selected HIV-related medical conditions. *AIDS* 10:1121–1126.

Craib, K.J., Schechter, M.T., et al. (1992) The effect of cigarette smoking on lymphocyte subsets and progression to AIDS in a cohort of homosexual men. *Clinical and Investigative Medicine. Medecine Clinique et Experimentale* 15:301–308.

Dean, L., Meyer, I., Sell, R., Sember, R., Silenzio, V., Bowen, D., et al. (2000) Lesbian, gay, bisexual and transgender health: findings and concerns. *Journal of the Gay and Lesbian Medical Association* 4:101–151.

Diamant, A.L., Schuster, M.A., et al. (2000a) Receipt of preventive health care services by lesbians. *American Journal of Preventive Medicine* 19:141–148.

Diamant, A.L., Wold, C., et al. (2000b) Health behaviors, health status, and access to and use of health care: a population-based study of lesbian, bisexual, and heterosexual women. *Archives of Family Medicine* 9:1043–1051.

Dibble, S.L., Roberts, S.A., Robertson, P.A., and Paul, S.M. (2002) Risk factors for ovarian cancer: lesbian and heterosexual women. *Oncology Nursing Forum* 29:E1–E7.

Dolcini, M.M., Canin, L., Gandelman, A., and Skolnik, H. (2004) Theoretical domains: a heuristic for teaching behavioral theory in HIV/STD prevention courses. *Health Promotion Practice* 5:404–417.

Elliot, S. (1997) A campaign urges gay men and lesbians to resist tobacco ads. *New York Times.*

Fichtenberg, C.M., and Glantz, S.A. (2000) Association of the California Tobacco Control Program with declines in cigarette consumption and mortality from heart disease. *New England Journal of Medicine* 343:1772–1777.

Friedman, R.C. (1999) Homosexuality, psychopathology, and suicidality. *Archives of General Psychiatry* 56:887–888.

Galai, N., Park, L.P., et al. (1997) Effect of smoking on the clinical progression of HIV-1 infection. *Journal of Acquired Immune Deficiency Syndromes and Human Retrovirology* 14:451–458.

Gambert, S.R., and Katsoyannis, K.K. (1995) Alcohol-related medical disorders of older heavy drinkers. In: Beresford, T.P., and Gomberg, E.S. (eds) *Alcohol and Aging*. Oxford University Press, New York, pp. 70–81.

Giovino, G.A. (2003) Tobacco surveillance in the U.S. Presented at the National Conference on Tobacco or Health, Boston.

Goebel, K. (1994) Lesbians and gays face tobacco targeting. *Tobacco Control* 3:65–67.

Greenwood, G.L., Paul, J., Pollack, L., Binson, D., Chang, J., Catania, J., Humfleet, G., and Stall, R. (2005) Tobacco use and cessation among a household-based sample of urban men who have sex with men (MSM) in the U.S. *American Journal of Public Health* 95:145–151.

Greenwood, G.L., Relf, M., et al. (2002) Battering victimization among a probability-based sample of men who have sex with men (MSM). *American Journal of Public Health* 92:1964–1969.

Greenwood, G.L., White, E.W., et al. (2001) Correlates of heavy substance use among young gay and bisexual men: the San Francisco Young Men's Health Study. *Drug & Alcohol Dependence* 61:105–112.

Gruskin, E.P., Hart, S., et al. (2001) Patterns of cigarette smoking and alcohol use among lesbians and bisexual women enrolled in a large health maintenance organization. *American Journal of Public Health* 91:976–979.

Hall, S., et al. (1993) Nicotine, negative affect, and depression. *Journal of Consulting and Clinical Psychology* 61:761–767.

Hall, S., Munoz, R., and Reus, V. (1994) Cognitive-behavioral intervention increase abstinence rates for depressive-history smokers. *Journal of Consulting and Clinical Psychology* 62:141–146.

Hall, S., et al. (1996) Mood management and nicotine gum in smoking treatment: a therapeutic contact and placebo controlled study. *Journal of Consulting and Clinical Psychology* 64:1003–1009.

Hall, S., et al. (1998) Nortriptyline and cognitive behavioral therapy in the treatment of cigarette smoking. *Archives of General Psychiatry* 55:681–693.

Harding, R., Bensley, J., and Corrigan, N. (2004) Targeting smoking cessation to high prevalence communities: outcomes from a pilot intervention for gay men. *BMC Public Health* 4:43.

Irwin, T.W., and Morgenstern, J. (2005) Drug-use patterns among men who have sex with men presenting for alcohol treatment: differences in ethnic and sexual identity. *Journal of Urban Health* 82(Supplement 1):i127–i133.

Kassel, P., and Franko, D.L. (2000) Body image disturbance and psychodynamic psychotherapy with gay men. *Harvard Review of Psychiatry* 8:307–317.

Kelly, J.A., Murphy, D.A., et al. (1997) Randomised, controlled, community-level HIV-prevention intervention for sexual-risk behaviour among homosexual men in US cities: Community HIV Prevention Research Collaborative. *Lancet* 350:1500–1505.

Lippman, J. (1992) Philip Morris to push brand in gay media. *Wall Street Journal* p. 13.

MacDonald, G., Starr, G., Schooley, M., Yee, S., Klimowski, K., and Turner, K. (2001) Introduction to program evaluation for comprehensive tobacco control programs. Centers for Disease Control and Prevention, Atlanta.

Mays, V., and Cochran, S. (2001) Mental health correlates of perceived discrimination among lesbian, gay, and bisexual adults in the U.S. *American Journal of Public Health* 91:1869–1876.

McKirnan, D.J., and Peterson, P.L. (1989) Alcohol and drug use among homosexual men and women: epidemiology and population characteristics. *Addictive Behaviors* 14:545–553.

Meyer, I.H. (1995) Minority stress and mental health in gay men. *Journal of Health and Social Behavior* 36:38–56.

Meyer, I.H. (2003a) Prejudice as stress: conceptual and measurement problems. *American Journal of Public Health* 93:262–265.

Meyer, I.H. (2003b) Prejudice, social stress, and mental health in lesbian, gay, and bisexual populations: conceptual issues and research evidence. *Psychological Bulletin* 129:674–697.

Mills, T., Paul, J., Stall, R., Pollack, L., Canchola, J., Chang, J., Moskowitz, J., and Catania, J.A. (2004) Distress and depression in men who have sex with men: the Urban Men's Health Study. *American Journal of Psychiatry* 16:278–285.

National Institute on Alcohol Abuse and Alcoholism. (2000) *10th Special report to the U.S. Congress on alcohol and health*. Department of Health and Human Services, Washington, DC.

Nawyn, S.J., Richman, J.A., et al. (2000) Sexual identity and alcohol-related outcomes: contributions of workplace harassment. *Journal of Substance Abuse* 11:289–304.

O'Hara, P., Portser, S.A., and Anderson, B.P. (1989) The influence of menstrual cycle changes on the tobacco withdrawal syndrome in women. *Addictive Behaviors* 14:595–600.

Opalinska, E., Michalak, A., Stoma, F., Latalski, M., and Goniewicz, M. (2003) Increasing level of prostate-specific antigen and prostate cancer risk factors among 193 men examined in screening procedure. *Annals of the University Mariae Curie Sklodowska* 58:57–63.

Page-Shafer, K., Delorenze, G.N., et al. (1996) Comorbidity and survival in HIV-infected men in the San Francisco Men's Health Survey. *Annals of Epidemiology* 6:420–430.

Paul, J., Catania, J., et al. (2001) Understanding childhood sexual abuse as a predictor of sexual risk-taking among men who have sex with men: the Urban Men's Health Study. *Child Abuse and Neglect* 25:557–584.

Peterson, J.L., and DiClemente, R.J. (2000) *Handbook of HIV prevention*. Kluwer/Plenum, New York.

Phillips, G.B., Pinkernell, B.H., and Jing, T.Y. (2004) Are major risk factors for myocardial infarction the major predictors of degree of coronary artery disease in men? *Metabolism* 53:324–329.

Ryan, H., Wortley, P.M., et al. (2001) Smoking among lesbians, gays and bisexuals: a review of the literature. *American Journal of Preventive Medicine* 21:142–149.

Scott, L.C., Cowling, D.A., Schumacher, J.R., Kwong, S.L., and Heogh, H.J. (2003) Tobacco and cancer in California: 1988–1999. California Department of Health Services, Cancer Surveillance Section, Sacramento, CA.

Skinner, W.F., and Otis, M.D. (1996) Drug and alcohol use among lesbian and gay people in a southern U.S. sample: epidemiological, comparative and methodological findings from the Trilogy Project. *Journal of Homosexuality* 30:59–62.

Smith, E.A., and Malone, R.E. (2003) The outing of Philip Morris: advertising tobacco to gay men. *American Journal of Public Health* 93:988–993.

Stall, R., and Wiley, J. (1988) A comparison of alcohol and drug use patterns of homosexual and heterosexual men: the San Francisco Men's Health Study. *Drug and Alcohol Dependence* 22:63–73.

Stall, R.D., Greenwood, G.L., et al. (1999) Cigarette smoking among gay and bisexual men. *American Journal of Public Health* 89:1875–1878.

Stall, R.D., Hays, R.B., et al. (2000) The gay '90s: a review of research in the 1990s on sexual behavior and HIV risk among men who have sex with men. *AIDS* 14(Supplement 3):S101–S114.

Stall, R., Mills, T., Williamson, J., Hart, T., Greenwood, G., Paul, J., Pollack, L., Binson, D., Osmond, D., and Catania, J. (2003) Association of co-occurring psychosocial health problems and increased vulnerability to HIV/AIDS among urban men who have sex with men (MSM). *American Journal of Public Health* 93:939–942.

Stall, R., Paul, J., et al. (2001) Alcohol use, drug use and alcohol-related problems among men who have sex with men: the Urban Men's Health Study. *Addiction* 96:1589–1601.

Stevens, P., Carlson, L., and Hinman, J. (2004) An analysis of tobacco industry marketing to lesbian, gay, bisexual and transgender (LGBT) populations: Strategies for mainstream tobacco control and prevention. *Health Promotion Practice* 5:129S–134S.

Tang, H., Greenwood, G.L., Cowling, D., Lloyd, J., Roeseler, A., and Bal, D. (2004) Cigarette smoking among lesbians, gays, and bisexuals: how serious a problem? *Cancer Causes and Control* 15:797–803.

U.S. Department of Health and Human Services (DHHS). (2004) *The health consequences of smoking: a report from the Surgeon General.* U.S. Department of Health and Human Services, Centers for Disease Control and Prevention, National Center for Chronic Disease Prevention and Health Promotion, Office on Smoking and Health, Atlanta.

Valanis, B., Bowen, D., Bassford, T., Whitlock, E., Charney, P., and Carter R. (2000) Sexual orientation and health: comparisons in the women's health initiative sample. *Archives of Family Medicine* 9:843–853.

Warwick, L., Douglas, N., Aggleton, P., and Boyce, P. (2003) Context matters: the educational potential of gay bars revisited. *AIDS Education & Prevention* 15:320–333.

Washington, H.A. (2002) Burning love: big tobacco takes aim at LGBT youths. *American Journal of Public Health* 92:1086–1095.

24

Methamphetamine Use and Its Relation to HIV Risk: Data from Latino Gay Men in San Francisco

Rafael M. Díaz

1 Introduction

Latino gay men constitute one of the most vulnerable groups in the nation for the transmission of the human immunodeficiency virus (HIV), showing some of the highest rates of seroprevalence, seroconversion, and unprotected anal intercourse (Lemp et al., 1994; CDC, 2002). In the largest study of young men who have sex with men (MSM) in the United States, Centers for Disease Control and Prevention (CDC) researchers reported an HIV prevalence of 14% among Latinos ages 23 to 29, double the HIV prevalence (7%) of their White same-age counterparts (Valleroy et al., 2000). This finding mirrors a much larger national health disparity where gay men of color—particularly African American and Latinos—show disproportionate rates of HIV infection, acquired immunodeficiency syndrome (AIDS) diagnoses, and both morbidity and mortality related to HIV/AIDS (Blair et al., 2002; CDC, 2004). Public health officials in the United States have called for a national effort to understand, address, and eliminate health disparities in the United States; however, at present it is unclear why gay men of color are disproportionately affected by the HIV/AIDS epidemic (Malebranche, 2003).

In Latino MSM, high risk sexual practices occur in the presence of substantial knowledge about HIV/AIDS and in the presence of relatively strong personal intentions and skills to practice safer sex (Díaz, 1998). A major focus of my research during the last 12 years has been to understand this seemingly paradoxical disconnection between knowledge, intentions, and behavior within the domain of sexuality and the consequent spread of HIV. The findings have been clear and consistent: HIV risk behavior occurs within particular contexts and situations—such as sexual activity aimed to alleviate exhaustion and depression, sexual activity in relationships of unequal power, sexual activity under the influence of drugs and/or alcohol—where it is subjectively difficult to act according to personal intentions for health and sexual safety. Men who are knowledgeable, capable of, and skillful at safer sex practices confess certain helplessness and inability to be safe is those situations we have labeled "risky." Furthermore, participation in those difficult, risky situations are strongly predicted by individual and group histories of social discrimination and financial hardship as well as by the negative impact of such discrimination and hardships on men's social connectedness and sense of self-worth (Diaz & Ayala, 2001; Diaz et al., 2001, 2004a). Because the same individual can act safely in some situations and unsafe in others, my studies have led me to conceptualize "risk" as a property of contexts and situations, rather than as an intraindividual characteristic.

The purpose of this chapter is to take a closer look at the situation of sexual risk that emerges in the context of sex under the influence of stimulants, particularly methamphetamine, in order to understand recent increases in both risky sexual behavior and related increases in HIV and syphilis infections in this population. I also describe other negative health consequences of methamphetamine use beyond the increased risk for HIV infection.

A major concern among researchers and public health officials is the finding of a strong link between new HIV infections and the use of stimulants, particularly methamphetamine (MA), also known as "speed" or "crystal meth." The link is also evident in my data from Latino gay men, where those who use MA report the highest rate (72%) of risky sexual behavior of any Latino subgroup studied to date (Diaz et al., 2004b). However, little is known about patterns and contexts of stimulant use among Latino gay men in the United States and its relation to HIV risk. To address this serious gap in the literature, I recently completed a study funded by the National Institute of Drug Abuse (NIDA) designed to provide a rich description (qualitative and quantitative) of drug use among Latino gay men in the San Francisco Bay Area, with a particular focus on stimulant (MA, cocaine, and crack) use and its relation to HIV risk behavior.

In this chapter, I report some of the basic qualitative and quantitative findings of the 4-year study, particularly the perceived effects of the stimulant—sexual and nonsexual—while under the influence, the consequences or life impact of stimulant use in their lives, and the relation of stimulant use to HIV risk. The focus is mostly on MA use, but I report the data on cocaine use as a point of comparison to underscore, when appropriate, the unique features of MA. The chapter ends with a discussion of opportunities for intervention that our data reveal and that we are currently attempting to develop.

2 The Intertwining MA/HIV Epidemics Among Gay Men

In recent years, we have witnessed a troubling increase in the use of MA within the gay community, and there is ample evidence of its relation to recent waves of new HIV and syphilis infections. A comprehensive review of the literature on drug use among gay/bisexual men

(Halkitis et al., 2001) cites increased rates of MA use among gay men, with prevalence rates ranging from 5% to 25% in various samples and increases in both MA-related emergency room admissions and the number of gay men seeking psychological and medical help for MA-related problems. One of the highest rates of MA use—30% during 1994—was reported in the San Francisco Young Men's Health Study (Gorman, 1994 (May)).

The concern with MA is not only about its increased use among gay/bisexual men reaching epidemic proportions, particularly in the West, but also about its reported impact on potentially risky sexual activity and the consequent transmission of HIV. A 2001 review cites 21 studies that show a significant relation between drug use and sexual risk behavior; 11 of those studies reported more specifically a significant relation between MA use and both sexual risk behavior and/or HIV seroconversion. In the three-city study (Morgan, 1993; Morgan et al., 1994), for example, gay/bisexual men reported MA as the first drug of choice for sex, with heightened and prolonged sexual activity as a major rationale. Many stated that MA increased their desire for anal sex and attributed the prevalence of "fisting" and other aggressive, potentially high-risk sex practices to the effects of MA. MA has been described as the "quintessential gay drug" because of its ability to enhance and prolong states of sexual arousal, increasing the capacity for multiple encounters with multiple partners in a relatively short period of time. Because of its paradoxical effects on penile erection ("crystal dick") and lower sexual inhibition, MA use is associated with the practice of receptive anal intercourse with multiple partners, the riskiest sexual practice for HIV transmission in this population. The fact that MA use is on the rise and that it appears as a powerful predictor of unprotected sexual practices and HIV seroconversion have led experts in the field refer to MA use as the "second" epidemic, and as "intertwining" epidemics when referring to MA use and HIV (Stall & Purcell, 2000; Halkitis et al., 2001).

One of the most detailed profiles of MA users can be found in the study by Reback and Grella (1999) of 908 drug-using gay and bisexual men recruited through street outreach in Los Angeles, 37% of whom reported MA use in the previous 30 days. In comparison to their non-MA drug-using peers, MA users were more likely to be White polydrug users who engage in sex work and more frequently inject drugs. MA users were also less likely to use condoms when engaging in high-risk sexual encounters. It is important to note that MA users in Reback and Grella's study reported multiple adaptive benefits of their MA use, such as the ability to stay awake through the night in potentially dangerous street environments and the ability to engage in a greater number of sexual encounters. Reback and Grella's (1999) study shows that MA use is deeply embedded in a gay street culture, where MA-induced enhanced energy and sexual effects are both functional and adaptive to the demands of street life and sex work.

In contrast to Reback and Grella's street sample in Los Angeles, Halkitis et al. (2003) studied personal characteristics and contexts of use among 49 gay and bisexual MA users who socialize in bars, dance clubs, sex clubs, and bathhouses in New York City. Similar to the L.A. street sample, men in New York were polydrug users, 61% of whom used MA during most or all of their sexual encounters. In contrast to the L.A. street sample, men in New York seldom injected drugs and were more likely to use MA in a friend's or lover's place. Interestingly, the frequency of MA use was related to situations of unpleasant emotions, physical discomfort, and conflict with others, suggesting the functional uses of MA to alleviate physical and emotional discomfort in social and sexual contexts. In Halkitis et al.'s (2003) study, similar rates and frequency of use were found between HIV+ and HIV– men and between White and ethnic minority gay men; group differences were found mostly in the drug combinations used. However, ethnic minority men reported increased use in situations of "social pressure."

Taken together, the studies in Los Angeles and New York City suggest that MA use is well entrenched in the gay community, among both college-educated men who participate in mainstream social and sexual venues and gay men of low socioeconomic status (SES) who participate in a street sex work culture. For all, middle class and poor men alike, MA use is strongly linked subjectively and behaviorally to enhanced and prolonged sexual activity with multiple partners. Both types of men experience MA as an energizing facilitator to navigate and participate in the (both exhilarating and challenging) contexts of multiple anonymous and casual sexual encounters with other men. For both types of men, MA use was related to coping with and adaptation to social and sexual contexts perceived as difficult. The finding that gay men of color report more pressure to use MA in those same social and sexual contexts is intriguing and merits further exploration.

3 A Study of Stimulant Use Among Latino Gay Men

Although recent studies of drug use among (mostly non-Hispanic, White) gay men show a strong link between MA use and HIV infection, no study has directly focused on MA use among Latino gay men and its relation to HIV risk in this particular population. As of this writing, only two published studies, one qualitative and one quantitative, have focused on substance use or sex under the influence of drugs among Latino gay men in the United States. In the qualitative study comparing protected and unprotected sexual episodes among Latino, African American, and non-Latino White gay/bisexual men, unprotected anal intercourse was more likely to occur while under the influence of drugs, particularly MA; this finding was true for all three ethnic groups studied (Díaz, 1999). In the second study, conducted in New York City with a sample of Colombian, Dominican, Mexican, and Puerto Rican MSM, Dolezal et al. (2000) found strong correlations between drug use and unprotected anal sex among three of the four ethnic subgroups studied. Drug use was predictive of unprotected sex particularly with casual sexual partners. However, among men who engaged in both protected and unprotected anal sex episodes, substance use was *not* more common during their unprotected episodes.

The two published studies to date underscore the need to understand more clearly how drug use, and in particular MA use, may create a context that is considered difficult or risky for the practice of safer sex among Latino gay men.

In a recently completed study funded by NIDA, we aimed to provide a rich description (qualitative and quantitative) of drug use among Latino gay men in the San Francisco Bay Area, with a focus on stimulant (MA, cocaine, crack) use and its relation to HIV risk behavior. The "rich" description of drug use included the drugs used, frequency and amount of use, modes of administration, contexts where used, reasons for use, perceived effects while intoxicated, the relation to sexual activity, and the impact of drug use on social relations, work, finances, and physical and mental health. The inclusion of multiple stimulants allowed us to examine the unique features of MA use in comparison to other powerful, frequently used stimulants. The study was designed also to answer a question of theoretical and applied significance: Under what conditions—demographic, psychological, interpersonal, and situational—does the use of MA increase the risk for HIV transmission?

The study was conducted in three phases: First, 70 drug-using Latino gay men (50 of them MA users) who reported at least one instance of unprotected anal intercourse during the last 6 months were interviewed in a 2-hour qualitative semistructured interview. Beyond a detailed qualitative description of both drug use and sexual activity (including behavior, social contexts, and subjective meanings), the interview elicited narratives on specific episodes of drug use with and without sexual activity and narratives on episodes of sex under the influence of drugs with and without condom use. During the second phase, and based on the qualitative findings, we created and pilot-tested a survey instrument to describe quantitatively the various dimensions of stimulant use (with specifics about MA, cocaine, and crack) and assess the relevant constructs to test a model on the relation between stimulant use and HIV risk. For the third and final phase, a random sample of stimulant users was drawn from among men entering or participating in gay-identified venues including bars, sex clubs, public sex environments, internet chat rooms, and sex phone lines. Inclusion criteria were male, Latino, nonheterosexual self-identification, and any stimulant use during the past 6 months. One third of the final sample was snowballed from participants' drug-using networks. Men were interviewed individually and face-to-face using a 2-hour, close-ended survey. For the survey, a total of 2442 Latino MSM were screened, of whom 517 (21%) qualified for stimulant use. A total of 300 men were interviewed.

Although most of the sample were polydrug users, 51% reported MA, 44% reported cocaine, and 5% reported crack as their "most frequently used stimulant" (MFS). Questions on frequency, reasons, effects, and consequences were asked about their particular MFS. When asked about frequency, 6% reported daily, 28% weekly, 40% monthly, and 26% less than monthly use of their MFS. The rich database is currently under analysis and, to date, only one study has been published reporting the participants' stated reasons for stimulant use (Díaz et al.,

2005). In the present chapter, I report on perceived drug effects, negative life consequences, and the relation to HIV risk among MA and cocaine users. Because only 14 men reported crack as their MFS, they were excluded from the present analysis.

4 Perceived Effects of MA Use

During the qualitative interviews, we asked men to tell us about their experiences—physical, psychological, social, sexual—while under the influence of MA, particularly the experiences they attributed specifically to the substance's effects. We refer to those experiences as "perceived effects" of MA use. Participants described a wide variety of effects, ranging from a boost of energy that allowed them to participate in social and sexual activities after an exhausting work week to increased feelings of social connection and prolonged states of sexual arousal. Most of the effects were described as both powerful and enjoyable (at times referred to as "fabulous"), giving men a sense of power, invincibility, beauty, youth, and sexual prowess.

I feel like invincible, you have so much energy, you can do anything you want . . . you can have a hard-on that goes for 6 hours. . . .

Most of the effects reported in the qualitative interviews could be categorized under five headings: (1) Increases in energy level and feelings of well-being, accompanied by a sense of power and invincibility; (2) sexual enhancement, including prolonged periods of sexual arousal and increased capacity for sexual activity with multiple partners in a relatively short period of time; (3) sexual disinhibition, with decreased feelings of shame or guilt, specifically about anal sex and sexual acts that are perceived as daring or "hard core"; (4) social enhancement, including decreased shyness, increased sociability, and talkativeness; and (5) increased desire and ability to do household chores, more focused work, and general productivity. In what follows, I quote and briefly discuss some specific examples from the interviews.

Study participants spoke about the effects of MA in the context of coping with economic hardships and related work demands. Some spoke about the need to work more than one job to keep up with exorbitant housing prices and the general high cost of living in the San Francisco Bay Area coupled with situations of underemployment, public assistance, or the extremely low incomes typical of immigrant groups. Some current MA users spoke of cocaine as the first stimulant they used to cope with pressures related to work and financial worries.

I needed to work many hours, sometimes 20 hours a day or more, sometimes I wouldn't sleep. So I would use cocaine to get by and get through work. I would finish one job and go to another one, perhaps I had errands to run so I couldn't sleep and would resort to the cocaine. I would go back to work and maybe not sleep for 2 or 3 days, but that wasn't for the fun of it, it was for work.

Increased energy and stamina appeared quite frequently as a powerful effect of MA use, particularly for men who felt exhausted by work responsibilities and needed an extra boost of energy to meet the demands of social life:

We each did a line of crystal because I was feeling sleepy. I was yawning. It wasn't that I didn't want to go out, I think I was physically just exhausted from the week. It was just long, and so that kind of gave me a boost of energy.

I started doing it because I was working hard and when the weekend came around I was too tired and I said, 'I don't want to party. I don't want to even hang out.' I was too tired. So, I thought, I need something that will keep me awake and kind of alive to, to, to enjoy the evening. And that was initially my motivation to do it. . . .

For many men, as the last quote suggests, work and financial worries take away both the energy and the desire to go out and participate during the weekend in the gay nightlife San Francisco offers. MA allowed men to participate in both social and sexual activities when they were simply too tired (and in their minds too stressed out) to even go out and play.

It gives me the energy, it gives me the stamina to finish all these projects, it also gives me a feeling of being able to stay up with my friends and partying.

It is important to note that the use of drugs during sexual activity is commonly referred to as "party and play," where "play" refers to sex and "party" refers to drug use. The interviews made clear that for many men sex is indeed the only affordable and accessible way to play (as opposed to "work"), in a way that offers joy and relaxation—a badly needed break between busy work weeks and as a relief from general life worries. When by then end of the week they were too tired—too tired to go out, to socialize, to dance, to find sexual partners—the drug made play possible.

In addition, the energizing effects of MA facilitated the completion of all those weekend domestic chores that are so tedious after a hard week of work.

I would be cleaning my home, I'd be doing my laundry, I'd be doing dinner, [things] I usually don't do because I don't have the energy for it. . . .

The energizing effects were particularly welcome by HIV-positive individuals who perceived the drug as erasing the debilitating effects of HIV infection and the related rigorous medication regimens:

When you have AIDS, you feel like you're slowing down and you're losing all your senses, ok? And speed brings them all back and it makes me feel like I'm 16, 17. . . . When you're 16 or 17 years old you feel like you are invincible.

For most participants, MA was also seen as an enhancer of sexual desire and sexual activity. Men reported prolonged arousal, better sex, more focused sex, more daring sex, and sex with more partners, as described below:

I felt like it rushed to my brain, I felt my skin get hot and I felt the desire to have sex with whomever was around. . . .

Sex is better, much better. . . . I go for like 9 hours. It's more passionate . . . the intensity, it makes me feel incredibly well.

Under the influence of MA, men were more able to focus on their bodies and the present sexual situation, with no other things in mind, when nothing else seems to matter:

When you are high there is nothing on your mind but the contact. There's nothing in your mind but reaching like, like another sensation, like bringing it closer to you, bringing it inside of you, you know, like engulfing it, pretty much you know bringing it all in. And so it's, everything else is totally just ignored.

. . . the focusing on the sex, the focusing means unity in all that time when you are having sex. When I'm having sex under those circumstances there's nothing else to think about. . . .

Men also felt more connected to their bodies and more daring when exploring new sexual behaviors:

I become even more hardcore. Sexual risks and inhibitions are totally gone. I become empowered in feeling, like I can take on the world or anyone that fucked with me. It can be an euphoric rush. You can feel it in your ass, in your balls, where it heats them up all of a sudden. It did help me explore my ass at one point when I refused to even think I had an ass.

This last quote reflects the powerful role of MA to help men explore and feel their bodies, particular those parts of their bodies and activities that have been experienced as dirty or shameful in their socialization within a homophobic society. Anal sex can be difficult for some Latino men, particularly for the receptive partners, given masculinity scripts and messages that receptive homosexuality is equivalent to taking a woman's role and a violation of the honor of manhood (Díaz, 1998). It is thus no surprise that Latino gay men tend to experience an exhilarating sense of sexual liberation when under the influence of MA.

Beyond energy and sexual enhancement, men described many other positive effects of MA, including the lessening of physical and emotional pain, as well as a sense of physical attractiveness, mostly because of MA's perceived positive impact on body weight.

That particular drug [crystal] seems to attach itself to a certain side of the brain that kind of like stimulates endorphin production, or somehow negates emotional, mental, and physical pain.

[With crystal] I find that I am no longer pudgy and plump. I feel that I'm a little bit more physically attractive because I'm not overweight.

In the subsequent quantitative study, we assessed perceived effects under the influence of the most frequently used stimulant (MFS) in a

Table 1. Perceived Positive Effects of Most Frequently Used Stimulant

Factors affected positively	All (n = 300) (%)	Crystal meth (n = 151) (%)	Cocaine (n = 129) (%)	p
Energy	42	48	39	NS
Sexual effects	35	46	19	0.00001
Nonspecified altered state	27	23	30	NS
Interpersonal connection	23	15	35	0.0001
Self-esteem	12	15	8	0.10
Feel good/well-being	14	14	15	NS
Escape/relief/forget problems/ relieve boredom	13	11	15	NS
Focus/attention/get things done	11	10	12	NS

The data are coded from open-ended responses.

open ended way, asking men to describe briefly their experiences, as follows: "The following questions are about what we call the effects of [MFS], that is, what you experience while you are under the influence of this drug. In a few words, please describe the three most satisfying/pleasant effects you experience while under the influence of [MFS]." We then coded the responses into mutually exclusive categories. The coded responses from the quantitative survey mirrored quite accurately the qualitative analysis done with the in-depth interviews. Table 1 shows the percentage of men in the sample, as well as the percentage of men within groups of MA and cocaine users who reported the particular coded effect. Table 1 also shows the results of the statistical significance of the comparison between the two groups determined by chi-squared analysis.

The most highly reported effect while under the influence of MA was "energy" (48%) followed by "sexual enhancement" (46%). Whereas cocaine users also reported energy as their most frequently perceived effect (39%), in contrast to MA users only a small proportion of cocaine users (19%) reported sexual enhancement effects. Interestingly, cocaine users reported effects of increased sociability more often than MA users (35% vs. 15%, $p < 0.0001$). These findings suggest that although both stimulants (MA and cocaine) produce important and highly valued energizing effects, MA is the stimulant most associated with increased and prolonged sexual arousal and behavior.

5 Negative Life Impact of Stimulant Use

Study participants who described powerful pleasant and satisfying effects of MA also described a wide range of negative consequences of MA use in their lives, including mental confusion and paranoia, social isolation, physical depletion, and sexual dysfunction, among others. Unlike "perceived effects," defined as experiences while under the influence of the drug, "consequences" refer to the general impact of drug use in a participants' life. Negative consequences are thus a reflection of the "costs" that participants associate with their drug use. The following quotes illustrate material from the qualitative interviews that was coded under different themes within the category "negative consequences."

5.1 Paranoia

That also makes me want to stop because I have been feeling this horror of someone who is following me, uh . . . who wants to kill me or that is hiding but is following me.

5.2 Social Isolation

I enjoyed doing them but at same time I was in another world . . . living in a world where at times you lose all shame, you lose friends, family, you lose . . . everything. Sometimes I wouldn't even make a phone call, all I cared about was getting high and that was it.

5.3 Physical Depletion

I feel so gross that I can't wash it off anymore. It's like you feel like this inside dirty, like because there's no food in your stomach for the past days, you've been just like running on empty and like you're really gaunt now because you've been in a constant workout.

5.4 Sexual Dissatisfaction and Dysfunction

I couldn't get nobody, and I couldn't get an erection any more. I was so sore that, I kept playing with myself at home, and I rubbed it so sore, it became raw, that's how bad it was. It didn't feel good afterward.

5.5 Discussion

Based on the consequences reported in the qualitative in-depth interviews, we created a set of 14 items to measure the impact of the most frequently used stimulant (MA, cocaine, crack) on the life of participants during the last year. The question was read to participants, as follows: "I would like to know how your use of [MFS] has impacted your life in the last year. Please tell me whether this drug has had a positive or negative influence, or no influence at all in the following aspects of your life, during the last year. How has your use of [MFS] impacted or influenced . . . your physical health?" Participants responded with a four-point categorical scale: not at all; positively; negatively; or both positively and negatively. In addition to inquiring about the impact of drug use on participants' physical health, the other 13 items inquired about the impact of the particular stimulant on mental health, relationships with family, relationships with friends, relationships with lovers or primary partners, sex life, work life, stress level, sense of social connection, finances, self-esteem, ability to think clearly, motivation to improve one's life, and spiritual or religious life. Table 2 reports the percentage of men in the sample who indicated any

Table 2. Perceived Negative Impact in the Last Year of the Most Frequently Used Stimulant

Factors affected negatively	All ($n = 300$) (%)	Crystal meth ($n = 153$) (%)	Cocaine ($n = 133$) (%)	p
Ability to think clearly	58	67	47	0.001
Mental health	55	63	44	0.001
Stress level	54	61	46	0.01
Self-esteem	53	59	44	0.01
Physical health	50	58	39	0.01
Sense of social connection	49	54	39	0.05
Relationships with friends	48	57	37	0.001
Finances	48	53	40	0.05
Relationships with lovers or primary partners	39	47	26	0.001
Motivation to improve your life	39	41	34	NS
Work life	38	48	26	0.001
Sex life	34	41	25	0.01
Relationships with family	32	39	24	0.01
Spiritual or religious life	24	24	23	NS

negative impact of their MFS during the last year. Table 2 also reports the percentage of men who reported negative consequences within groups of MA and cocaine users separately, as well as significance tests (using Chi square analysis) of the differences observed between the two stimulant-using groups.

Table 2 shows the perceived negative effects, from the most frequently experienced to the least, suggesting that stimulant use was related to cognitive and emotional problems for most of the participants. The stimulants were also perceived to affect negatively the participants' self-esteem, their social and romantic relationships, their finances, work life, and personal motivation to improve one's life. Negative sexual effects were reported by one-third of participants. One of the most telling aspects of the findings is that more MA users reported negative effects than did the cocaine users. More than 50% of MA users reported negative consequences on 8 of the 14 domains that were assessed, whereas no single domain of negative consequences was reported by more than 47% of the cocaine users. Paradoxically, MA users who elsewhere reported the most positive sexual enhancement benefits reported negative consequences in their sex lives more often than cocaine users (39% vs. 24%, $p < 0.01$).

6 Relation to HIV Risk

Shortly after we began our qualitative in-depth interviews of Latino drug-using men, it became clear that most of the interview material reporting sexual risk behavior (i.e., unprotected anal intercourse with casual partners of discordant or unknown HIV status) appeared in the context of stimulant use, particularly MA. We thus began to focus the rest of the qualitative study and the entire subsequent quantitative study on the use of the three stimulants (MA, cocaine, crack) that more often appeared in the context of unprotected sex episodes.

In the qualitative interviews, participants were very open about what they perceived to be a strong relation between MA use and sexual risk-taking. In fact, it was truly amazing to witness how clearly and candidly men spoke about the negative impact of stimulants and in particular of MA in their lives. With respect to HIV risk, many men admitted that the drug-induced sexual effects overpowered their concerns for safety, allowing them to take sexual risks they would not normally take when sober. For others, the drug helped them focus away from HIV-related concerns or allowed them to conceptualize the situation in such a way as to minimize the risks involved.

It definitely puts you in a mindset where you feel safe enough to go somewhere where you shouldn't normally go . . . kind of the mindset you fall into when you're doing speed. That, 'oh, it's okay because he's probably positive' and 'I'm probably positive,' and some people think that and probably don't even know if they are. So, it's just kind of a cop-out to make it okay.

For some participants, the drug made them feel sexually insatiable, and at times some felt "out of control," with negative consequences for safer sex.

With drugs you start degenerating and you no longer are satisfied with one person . . . you want another and you want more and you want them all at the same time. So I do see a relationship, drugs do lead to becoming infected with diseases.

I got real high and I got really horny, so horny that it was out of control. It was very out of control. It's like I could have fucked forever. . . .

Regardless of the specific reasoning, most men in the qualitative interviews admitted that MA use was closely related to their episodes of unprotected sex. It is important to note, however, that many HIV-positive men who engaged in unprotected anal sex while under the influence of MA assumed or actually knew that their partners were also positive. HIV-positive men more often than not, disclose their HIV status in their Internet or phone line personal profiles; these profiles are typically read or heard prior to sexual encounters. The assumption of HIV seroconcordance is thus often based on actual information available through the Internet or phone line profiles prior to the sexual encounters.

In the subsequent quantitative study, we were able to obtain five measures of sexual risk behavior during the last 6 months prior to the survey interview: (1) any unprotected anal intercourse (UAI); (2) UAI with more than one partner; (3) UAI with casual partners in their most frequent sexual setting; (4) UAI under the influence of any drug; and (5) UAI under the influence of their MFS. In addition, we asked study participants about their own perceptions regarding their risk of HIV

Table 3. Sexual Risk During the Last 6 Months, by Most Frequently Used Stimulant

	All (n = 300) (%)	Crystal Meth (n = 153) (%)	Cocaine (n = 133) (%)	p
Risk behavior				
Any UAI	68	72	64	NS
UAI with more than one partner	39	45	35	0.10
UAI with casual partner in most frequentsexual setting	37	44	29	0.05
UAI under the influence of any drug	69	73	65	NS
UAI under the influence of most frequently used stimulant	43	53	32	0.001
Risk perception				
Perceived risk of HIV transmission under most frequently used stimulant	47	55	36	0.01
Perceived risk of HIV transmission under most frequently used nonstimulant	28	26	30	NS

UAI, unprotected anal intercourse.

transmission under the influence of their MFS, as well as when they were under the influence of their most frequently used nonstimulant, such as marijuana, hallucinogens, or tranquilizers. For HIV-negative men, we asked about their perception of risk for *acquiring* HIV, whereas for HIV-positive men we asked about their perception of risk for *transmitting* HIV. All these measurements of risk were derived from questions distributed throughout different sections of the survey questionnaire. For the purpose of briefly describing the findings, all five measures of behavioral sexual risk were dichotomized as happening "ever" versus "never" within the last 6 months prior to the interview; perceptions of risk were dichotomized as "yes" versus "no." Table 3 reports the percentage of participants who engaged at least once in the measured sexual risk behavior or who said yes in response to the risk perception questions; percentages are also given separately for groups of MA and cocaine users, together with *p* values for the statistical comparison of the two groups on each of the reported variables of risk.

As can be seen on Table 3, more than two-thirds (68%) of stimulant users reported at least one instance of UAI during the last 6 months. Altogether, 72% of MA users reported at least one instance of UAI during the last 6 months, which constitutes (to my knowledge) the highest HIV risk rate ever reported for any Latino MSM subgroup studied to date. Table 3 also shows that, for both MA and cocaine users, their respective UAI rates are exactly the same as their UAI rates under the influence of *any* drug. This finding suggests that for this group of stimulant-using men most if not all of their unprotected UAI occurs under the influence of drugs. Rates of UAI under their specific MFS are also high, particularly for MA users in contrast to cocaine users (53% vs. 32%, $p < 0.01$), confirming the stronger connection between MA use and perceived sexual effects. Overall, MA users reported higher rates of risky behavior than their cocaine-using counterparts, but the differences were not always statistically significant.

The data on perceptions of risk confirm the fact that men are well aware that MA use is closely connected to their risk for acquiring or transmitting HIV; more MA users report this risk perception in comparison to cocaine users (55% versus 36%, $p < 0.01$). The percentages of men who report UAI under the influence of their MFS and their perceived risk under the influence of their MFS are virtually the same (53% and 55%, respectively, for MA users; 32% and 36%, respectively, for cocaine users). This finding suggests that both groups of stimulant users are well aware that the practice of UAI under the influence of stimulants (MA as well as cocaine) poses the risk of HIV transmission. Interestingly, sex under the influence of nonstimulant drugs is much lower for MA users (55% vs. 26%) but only slightly lower for cocaine users (36% vs. 30%).

7 Frequency of Stimulant Use and Its Relation to Social Isolation, Negative Consequences, and HIV Risk

Our data also revealed a potentially dangerous trajectory for men whose frequency of MA use escalates to weekly or daily use, particularly when the increased use involved a type of binge, called "a run," of several days' duration. While motivated initially by the drug's energizing effects, many users continue to increase the frequency of their MA use mostly because of its powerful sexual effects. As a result of their MA use, men not only have energy to go out and socialize with friends, they also are able to sustain while on "the run" an enormous sexual appetite that allows them to have multiple and long sexual encounters with multiple partners on a daily basis, a shared and valued goal in many circles of gay popular culture. Sex phone lines and Internet chat rooms, where men are able to connect with other men in similar situations—and with similar sexual appetites—are major conduits and facilitators for MA-related patterns of sexual encounters. Internet- and phone line-mediated connections typically lead to sexual encounters in small groups, organized as small orgies in private homes where MA is snorted, smoked, or injected while sexual activity is taking place. Sexual encounters may begin with a pair of men who then bring in other partners to create small sex parties that can last, on average, 9 to 12 hours, sometimes until men's penises literally become raw.

The trajectory of increased use, although leading to sexual encounters with more and more partners, paradoxically seems to create a greater sense of social isolation for the participants. The encounters initiated through phone lines or Internet chat rooms bring together men who are basically strangers and whose sole connection is through these mostly anonymous sexual encounters. During these encounters, the experience of social connection is short-lived, and men need to learn quickly not to become too attached to one another. In several interviews, stories of these sexual encounters were accompanied with expressions of sadness when, for example, a partner whom a participant was romantically interested in decided that he wanted to call someone else to join the sexual event, indicating some degree of boredom with the present company. Many times the sexual encounter was described in ways that seemed interpersonally disconnected, with great emphasis on the particular characteristic of the sexual acts or with reference to environmental characteristics (e.g., videos, dark corners, toys, mirrors) that were made available to increase the erotic charge of the situation.

Above all, men often felt that the men in these encounters were not true friends or people who cared for them for reasons other than their drugs or the pleasure offered by their bodies. The "paranoia" described by the following user reflects some of the social characteristics of the sexual encounters among MA-using men.

I think I'm becoming paranoid. I'm finding that I'm even less trusting of people. It has to do with the people that I'm associating with now, that come with it. There's a lot of people out there, a lot of guys that are on that phone line looking for crystal. They're looking for drugs and they're basically what we call crack whores. They are out there and they are attractive and they're willing to have sex and they'll meet your sexual needs but they'll show up with no money and no drugs. I think that it also brings in . . . it's just bringing in drug addicts, people that I don't know, strangers off the street. And I'm finding that I'm changing my locks on my doors, I'm hiding things when I have strangers over, I'm becoming paranoid and it's with good reason because a lot of these guys don't give a damn about me or my property.

This quote contains a sample of deprecatory labels that participants often used to describe men with whom they connected for sexual encounters: "crack whores," "drug addicts," "strangers off the street." However, these labels were describing individuals who were acting just like themselves in similar situations. It is not surprising that, for men who progressed to increased frequency of use and Internet/phone-line mediated encounters, there was a sense of increased social isolation, particularly isolation from non-drug-using individuals, as well as from other friends and family.

In the subsequent survey, we were able to measure quantitatively participants' gradual isolation from family and friends during the last year with two-stage questions such as: How many people could you call if you need to talk about a problem? And compared to 1 year ago, do you have (1) more people to talk to? (2) fewer people to talk to? (3) about the same? Using a similar format, we asked questions about the number of people who could come and help participants when they were sick and needed help, the number of people from whom they could borrow money in case they needed to, and the number of people with whom they could call to go out if they wanted to go out for fun. For all these questions, we asked participants to make comparisons with the number of people they had a year ago. Based on participants' responses to these two-stage items of social support, we created a "progressive isolation" score based on responses that indicated a lessening of social connections and support during the last year.

For both types of users—MA and cocaine users—increased frequency of use of their MFS was strongly correlated with progressive isolation, with more negative consequences and with increases in HIV risky sexual behavior. For example, the percentage of stimulant users who reported UAI under the influence of their MFS increased from 23% (for less-than-monthly users) to 46% (for monthly users) to 56% (for weekly/daily users); these differences were significant at the $p < 0.0001$ level. We tested the effects of drug type and frequency of use on created scales of Sexual Risk (8-item scale, $\alpha = 0.78$), Progressive Isolation (3-item scale, $\alpha = 0.71$), and Negative Consequences (14-item scale, $\alpha = 0.90$), in three separate 2×2 ANOVAs with factors Drug Type (MA vs. cocaine) and Frequency of Use (weekly vs. monthly vs. less than monthly). The first ANOVA indicated that MA users and more frequent users were more likely to be at risk for transmitting or acquiring HIV [Drug Type: $F(1, 247) = 3.84$, $p < 0.05$; Frequency: $F(2, 247) = 3.43$, $p < 0.05$]. The second ANOVA indicated that more frequent users of both drugs had become more isolated during the last year [Frequency: $F(2, 276) = 4.05$, $p < 0.05$]. The third ANOVA indicated that MA users and more frequent users more often reported negative consequences on account of their stimulant use [Drug Type: $F(1, 272) = 10.11$, $p < 0.01$; Frequency: $F(2, 272) = 9.85$, $p < 0.001$]. None of the interactions between drug type and frequency of use reached the prespecified level of statistical significance.

8 Awareness and Intraventions

Whereas the preceding pages painfully witness the negative impact of MA use on the health, well-being, and HIV risk of Latino gay men, the data from our study also revealed several reasons for hope. First, our study revealed a deep and quite refined level of awareness among participants about the high cost of their MA use. Most men acknowledged negative consequences in their lives as a result of their stimulant use, including their increased risk for HIV transmission. They confessed an ambivalent relationship to the drug.

That's what I was going to say—it's a love/hate relationship.
I love the rush but I hate the effects.

The awareness and frank recognition of negative consequences, together with expressed ambivalence about the cost/benefits of their drug use, signal a certain readiness for interventions that address negative consequences while acknowledging the multiple and powerful functions of stimulant use in their personal, social, and sexual lives.

That whole thing made me reevaluate and I asked myself, "What am I doing with my life?" This is not a road that will take me to success or a good life . . . there comes a time when your body gets tired and you just want to find solace and love in another person.

Second, our study revealed not only awareness of negative effects but also multiple examples of mutual warnings and encouragements to abstain among MA users themselves. Some of these interactions between MA-using friends suggested the presence of what Friedman and colleagues call "intraventions," that is, "prevention activities that are conducted by and sustained through ongoing actions of members of communities at risk" (Friedman et al., 2004, p 250). Intraventions typically occurred in the form of warnings and reminders of negative effects.

I'd heard it before from someone who used it and also had incredible sex, he told me it was incredible, that . . . but he said, "But I don't recommend that you use it."

They were telling me about their experiences. They told me that it wasn't good to take it, to take that drug very often, that maybe if I used it recreation-ally . . . then maybe I could, um, be, have a good time with it. But that I should-n't get hooked on it, that I shouldn't get hooked on that drug, That it wasn't, wasn't very good, it could lead to a lot of things. By the way, I will never forget the saying that they told me that day. They said, "Crystal robs you of every-thing, even your soul." And there was a time when I did feel that way.

Finally, our data also revealed that some men were able to regain their ability to have satisfactory sexual experiences without the use of the drug. Some, in fact, thought that their sexual lives got better after stopping their MA use.

I used to think that I felt the sensation of having sex better with drugs, but I've learned to feel it even better without drugs. And I don't mean to say—I enjoy it both ways—but I prefer it not with drugs, because again your mind gets clouded. And I don't want to go back to the same old behavior with drugs and what it can do—I'm tired of that kind of madness.

9 Summary

The data reported in this chapter suggest that Latino gay men in the San Francisco Bay Area use stimulants, in particular MA, to achieve important and adaptive functions in their work, social, and sexual lives. The data suggest that for many men stimulant use may start as an attempt to cope with work schedules and other life stressors that make them too tired to play or participate in gay social and sexual life. Although most of the stimulant users listed energy-related effects as their main reason for stimulant use, MA use was strongly related to sex-enhancing effects, whereas cocaine was more often related to increased sociability. The energy and sexual effects of MA were described quite strongly with terms such as power and invincibility.

The perceived effects while under the influence, particularly in the sexual domain, were often described as "fabulous." However, the same individuals who described fabulous effects also reported "disastrous" consequences of their MA use, including the increased risk for acquiring or transmitting HIV. Negative life consequences, including HIV transmission, were more frequently reported by MA users than by cocaine users.

Increased use of MA is closely related to its sexual effects, mostly because it allows men to remain sexually aroused for long periods of time and it facilitates multiple sexual encounters with multiple casual partners at late hours of the night. It is important to realize that this pattern of sexual prowess and activity is congruent with values shared by many members of the gay community and is facilitated by technologies (sex phone lines and Internet chat rooms) that mediate social and sexual encounters in our culture. However, this drug-enhanced and technology-mediated sexual activity often leads to social isolation as well as sexual dissatisfaction, and it poses enormous threats to physical and mental health. Increased frequency of MA use to weekly or daily use is also related to increased and progressive social isolation from friends, suggesting that the breakdown of social support networks may be related to the loss of more regulated patterns of stimulant use and vice versa.

The devastating effects of MA use are a cause of major concern for those of us interested in the health of LGBT communities, particularly those of us working toward ending the HIV pandemic. Encouragingly, the data revealed both community readiness and multiple opportunities for pubic health interventions. Many MA users are not only accurately aware of negative consequences and the increased risk of HIV transmission, they also seem to communicate about this with one another in attempts to minimize their friends' MA-related losses. Interventions that encourage, support, and sustain those within-community "intraventions" might be our most efficient tools for addressing the new challenges posed by the intertwining epidemics of MA abuse and HIV.

References

Blair, J.M., Flemming, P.L., and Karon, J.M. (2002) Trends in AIDS incidence and survival among racial/ethnic minority men who have sex with men, United States, 1990–1999. *Journal of Acquired Immune Deficiency Syndromes* 31:339–347.

Centers for Disease Control and Prevention (CDC) (2002) *HIV/AIDS Surveillance Report* 14(1).

Centers for Disease Control and Prevention (CDC) (2004) Health disparities experienced by racial/ethnic minority populations. *MMWR Morbidity and Mortality Weekly Report* 53(33):755.

Díaz, R.M. (1998) *Latino gay men and HIV: culture, sexuality and risk behavior.* Routledge, New York.

Díaz, R.M. (1999) Trips to fantasy island: contexts of risky sex for San Francisco gay men. *Sexualities* 2(1):89–112.

Diaz, R.M., and Ayala, G. (2001) *Social discrimination and health: the case of Latino gay men and HIV risk.* The Policy Institute of the National Gay and Lesbian Task Force, New York.

Díaz, R.M., Ayala, G., and Bein, E. (2004a) Sexual risk as an outcome of social oppression: data from a probability sample of Latino gay men in three US cities. *Cultural Diversity and Ethnic Minority Psychology* 10:255–267.

Diaz, R.M., Ayala, G., Bein, E., Henne, J., and Marin, B.V. (2001) The impact of homophobia, poverty, and racism on the mental health of gay and bisexual men: findings from 3 US cities. *American Journal of Public Health* 91:927–932.

Díaz, R.M., Heckert, A.H., and Sanchez, J. (2004b) Fabulous effects, disastrous consequences: stimulant use among gay men in San Francisco. Invited presentation at the workshop New Dynamics of HIV Risk Among Drug-Using Men Who Have Sex with Men, National Institute on Drug Abuse, Bethesda, MD.

Díaz, R.M., Heckert, A.H., and Sanchez, J. (2005) Reasons for stimulant use among Latino gay men in San Francisco: a comparison between methamphetamine and cocaine users. *Journal of Urban Health* 82 (Supplement 1):71–78.

Dolezal, C., Carballo-Diéguez, A., Nieves-Rosa, L., and Díaz, F. (2000) Substance use and sexual risk behavior: understanding their association among four ethnic groups of Latino men who have sex with men. *Journal of Substance Abuse* 11:323–336.

Friedman, S.R., Maslow, C., Bolyard, M., Sandoval, M., Mateu-Gelabert, P., and Neaigus, A. (2004) Urging others to be healthy: "intravention" by injection drug users as a community prevention goal. *AIDS Education and Prevention* 16:250–263.

Gorman, M. (1994) Substance abuse issues in men who have sex with other men: the particular case with speed. Presented at the Conference on Reinventing HIV Prevention for Men Who Have Sex with Other Men, Seattle, WA (May).

Halkitis, P.N., Parsons, J.T., and Stirratt, M.J. (2001) A double epidemic: crystal methamphetamine drug use in relation to HIV transmission among gay men. *Journal of Homosexuality* 41(2):17–35.

Halkitis, P.N., Parsons, J.T., and Wilton, L. (2003) An exploratory study of contextual and situational factors related to methamphetamine use among gay and bisexual men in New York City. *Journal of Drug Issues* 33:413–432.

Lemp, G.F., Hirozawa, A.M., Givertz, D., Nieri, G.N., Anderson, L., Lindergren, M., Janssen, R.S., and Katz, M. (1994) Seroprevalence of HIV and risk behaviors among homosexual and bisexual men: the San Francisco/Berkeley young men's survey. *Journal of the American Medical Association* 272:449–454.

Malebranche, D.J. (2003) Black men who have sex with men and the HIV epidemic: next steps for public health. *American Journal of Public Health* 93:862–865.

Morgan, P. (1993) Researching hidden communities: a qualitative comparative study of methamphetamine users in three sites. In: *Proceedings of the Community Epidemiology Work Group Public Health Service.* National Institute on Drug Abuse, Bethesda, MD.

Morgan, P., Beck, J., Joe, K., McDonnell, D., and Gutierrez, R. (1994) *Ice and other methamphetamine use: an exploratory study.* Final report of project activities. National Institute on Drug Abuse, Bethesda, MD (grant RO-1DA6853).

Reback, C.J., and Grella, C.E. (1999) HIV risk behaviors of gay and bisexual male methamphetamine users contacted through street outreach. *Journal of Drug Issues* 29:155–166.

Stall, R., and Purcell, D.W. (2000) Interwining epidemics: a review of research on substance use among me who have sex with men and its connection to the AIDS epidemic. *AIDS and Behavior* 4:181–192.

Valleroy, L.A., MacKellar, D.A., Karon, J.M., Rosen, D.H., McFarland, W., Shehan, D.A., Stoyanoff, S.R., Lalota, M., Celentano, D.D., Koblin, B.A., Thiede, H., Katz, M.H., Torian, L.V., and Janssen, R.S. (2000) HIV prevalence and associated risks in young men who have sex with men. *Journal of the American Medical Association* 284:198–204.

Part VI

Healthcare Systems and Services

Improving Access to Health Care Among African-American, Asian and Pacific Islander, and Latino Lesbian, Gay, and Bisexual Populations

Patrick A. Wilson and Hirokazu Yoshikawa

1 Introduction

In the United States, lesbian, gay, and bisexual persons (LGBPs) of color may experience great difficulty obtaining high quality health care and/or health-related interventions. Issues surrounding access to health care may explain the disproportionate numbers of LGB ethnic minorities experiencing poor health outcomes relative to nonminority and non-LGB persons. This chapter presents research that may help to explain why African American, Asian and Pacific Islander (API), and Latino LGBPs have a lack of access to quality health care and a higher prevalence of poor health outcomes than other populations. The chapter also explores the ways in which access to health care can be improved for minority LGBPs and presents suggestions for institutional-, community-, and policy-level interventions.

2 Importance of Understanding Health Disparities Among Ethnic Minority LGB Persons

Ethnic minority LGBPs are at risk for a variety of poor physical health outcomes. Perhaps the most studied of these outcomes are sexuality transmitted infections (STIs), such as human immunodeficiency virus (HIV) infection. HIV has had a tremendous impact on the LGB community, as gay men constituted most of the HIV and acquired immunodeficiency syndrome (AIDS) cases during the 1980s and early 1990s. However, as the epidemic has grown and changed, ethnic minority men who have sex with men (MSM), notably those who are African

American and Latino, represent the highest proportion of new AIDS cases in the United States (CDC, 2002). MSM also show high rates of other STIs, including hepatitis B, gonorrhea, *Chlamydia*, and other bacterial infections (Council on Scientific Affairs, 1996). Inclusive of HIV, ethnic minority MSM have higher rates of most STIs than White MSM (CDC, 2003). Lesbians who are ethnic minorities also face great health challenges relative to other groups. Although lesbian women have a lower incidence of STIs than heterosexual women, some research suggests that these women are at heightened risk for certain cancers including breast, ovarian, and endometrial malignancies (Council of Scientific Affairs, 1996). This greater risk may stem from lesbians' higher likelihood of nulliparity (i.e., to have never given birth to a child) than heterosexual women. Ethnic minority lesbians have a greater chance of experiencing these poor health outcomes and not receiving treatment for them because of their greater likelihood of not having health insurance and not receiving preventive care (Dean et al., 2000; Mays et al., 2003).

Mental health problems also occur with frequency among LGB ethnic minorities. LGBPs are more likely than heterosexuals to experience major depression and anxiety disorders (Gilman et al., 2001; Cochran et al., 2003). Ethnic minority LGBPs may be more likely to experience mental health problems than other populations. For example, when studying depressive distress among gay and lesbian African Americans, Cochran and Mays (1994) found higher rates of depression (as measured by the CES-D) among African-Americans, relative to White gay men and non-LGB African Americans. Similarly, levels of depressive symptoms have been observed in samples of API gay men (Yoshikawa et al., 2004) and Latino gay men (Díaz et al., 2004) that are higher than those obtained in comparable general-population studies of these ethnic groups. Studies specifically examining depression and mental health among lesbians of color are scarce and much needed for this population. Related research suggests that these women may be more likely to experience mental health issues, as many experience stigma based on their ethnicity, sexuality, and gender (Phillip, 1993; Greene, 1997).

Many ethnic minority LGBPs also contend with substance use and addiction and the health problems that may result from substance-using behaviors. Studies indicate that gays and lesbians are more likely to abuse drugs and alcohol than heterosexuals (Council of Scientific Affairs, 1996; Cochran, 2003). Medical professionals report that the prevalence of substance use among LGBP ranges between 28% and 35%, compared to 10% to 12% for heterosexual persons (Cabaj, 1992). Though studies are scant, ethnic minority LGBPs may be more likely to engage in substance use and/or abuse in an effort to reduce stress stemming from stigma and to alleviate the psychological discomfort of engaging in same-sex sexual behavior (Icard & Traunstein, 1987; Semple et al., 2002; Wilson, 2005).

Data collected over the past several years have consistently demonstrated significant health disparities between minority and nonminority groups in the United States. As a result, research aiming to explain disparities in health and access to health care has been called for in both community-based organizations and government organizations. Notably, in 2000 Congress passed the Minority Health and Health Disparities Research and Education Act[1] in response to President Clinton's Healthy People 2010 initiative, which aimed to eliminate health disparities among Americans by 2010. The National Center on Minority Health and Health Disparities was created through the Act, and hundreds of millions of dollars were earmarked for research and intervention aimed at reducing health disparities. The Health Disparities Act, one of the most notable pieces of health legislation over the past decade, gave visibility and much needed funding to interventions created to tackle the health disparities problem in the United States. However, the Act and the five Titles that comprise it focus on health disparities between persons of different racial/ethnic groups and neglect to place attention on the special health needs of LGBPs. In an effort to shed light on the healthcare needs and issues of LGBT people, the Gay and Lesbian Medical Association (GLMA) published an exhaustive report on the state of LGBT health in the United States shortly after passage of the Health Disparities Act (GLMA, 2001). The document served to fill in the gaps in federal initiatives on health disparities and was a supplement to the President's original Healthy People 2010 mandate. Although this work has been useful to highlight the importance of understanding and eliminating health disparities across more than simply race categories in the United States, little work has focused specifically on the health care needs of ethnic minority LGBPs. Most attention to health disparities has been placed either on the needs of ethnic minorities or LGBPs, but not the needs of persons who belong to both groups. Nonetheless, ethnic minority LGBPs may experience a compounded effect of their ethnic and sexual minority statuses with regard to their health, and these effects may result in poorer health outcomes when compared to those of White LGB populations or the U.S. population as a whole.

3 Intersection of Ethnicity, Sexual Orientation, and Immigration Experiences: Their Impact on Health and Healthcare Access

Why are ethnic minority LGBPs at heightened risk for poor health outcomes compared to other populations? Why are ethnic minority LGBPs less likely than White LGBPs to receive high quality health care? These questions must be answered to effectively design and implement interventions that promote health and access to health care among LGB ethnic minorities. The relevant research suggests three major factors that may play a role: (1) the negative impact of discrimination on health and risk behavior; (2) racism and homophobia in health care and

---

[1]The Minority Health and Health Disparities Research and Education Act of 2000, S. 1880, 106th Congress, 2nd Session.

health-related research settings, and (3) immigration experiences and their effects on health care.

3.1 Negative Impact of Discrimination on Health and Risk Behavior

Logically, membership in socially constructed demographic groups defined by race/ethnicity and sexual orientation should not cause poor health. Thus, the relation between demographic characteristics and poor health outcomes must be mediated by factors associated with being a person who belongs to an ethnic and/or sexual minority. One such mediating factor important to consider is discrimination. Discrimination, in all of its forms (i.e., structural, institutional, interpersonal), has an adverse impact on the health of those who experience it (Clark et al., 1999; Krieger, 1999). Several researchers have noted that the psychological and physiologic stress that stems from the experience of discrimination is related to acute and chronic health problems among those who are discriminated against. For example, Williams et al. (1999) found that African Americans who reported recurring experiences of racism were more likely to have chronic health problems (e.g., cardiovascular disease, hypertension) than those who did not have such experiences. Similarly, research has suggested that the strain associated with persistent racism the ethnic minorities experience may be linked to stress-related diseases such as high blood pressure (Krieger & Sidney, 1996) and heart disease (Jiang et al.), as well as psychological disorders such as depression (Rumbaut, 1994), psychological distress (Williams, 2000), and low self-esteem (Broman, 1997).

Discrimination also plays a role in the adverse health outcomes of LGBP, regardless of their ethnicity. Notably, studies have suggested that the chronic experience of stigma linked to sexual orientation and the stress that ensues from such stigmatization is linked to greater risk behavior and poor mental health in LGBP. For example, Meyer (1995) found that gay men were more likely to report psychological distress (including distress linked to demoralization, guilt, suicide, and AIDS traumatic stress response) when they reported experiencing antigay violence and/or discrimination. In a related study, Meyer and Dean (1995) found that gay men who engaged in high levels of sexual risk behavior were more likely to have high levels of internalized homophobia, which the authors posited may result from antigay attitudes and being stigmatized by heterosexuals.

The combined effects of being stigmatized as both a sexual minority and an ethnic minority may have especially adverse health consequences. Studies of ethnic minority gay men have demonstrated a link between discrimination and negative health outcomes, including risky sexual behavior and poor mental health. In one study, Díaz and Ayala (2001) found that experiences of social discrimination (rooted in racism and/or homophobia) were strong predictors of both psychological distress and sexual risk behavior in their study of Latino gay men. Similarly, a study examining the impact of discrimination on HIV risk among API gay men found that experiences of racism were linked to depression, and experiences of antiimmigrant discrimination were related to higher rates of unprotected sex with casual partners (Yoshikawa et al., 2004). The experience of being in a minority within an already disenfranchised group (as is the case with ethnic minority LGBPs) may create difficulty engaging in healthy behaviors and responding to discrimination, notably that which stems from other minority group members. For example, Wilson and Yoshikawa (2004) found that API gay men who experienced discrimination based in stereotypes about Asian gay men as passive, exotic, and/or feminine were more likely to engage in sexual risk behavior than those without such experiences. Participants noted that this form of discrimination was rooted within the White gay community and emphasized the dual minority status of API gay men. Research examining the impact of discrimination on the health of LGBPs is still in its formative stage, and there is a paucity of studies on other ethnic and sexual minority groups, notably ethnic minority lesbians or bisexuals. Nonetheless, the available research suggests that ethnic minority LGBPs' experiences of discrimination are consistently associated with poorer health and health-related behaviors and that they likely contribute to disparities in health.

3.2 Racism and Homophobia in Health Care and Health-Related Research Settings

Discrimination affects not only the health of ethnic minority LGBPs but also their health care experiences. Indeed, U.S. health care and research settings have a long history of discriminatory practices with regard to ethnic and sexual minorities. These practices have created a legacy of distrust and nonutilization of the health care system among ethnic minorities as well as LGBPs. The Tuskegee syphilis experiments may represent the most atrocious form of health- and research-based racism in the United States, with the most lasting effects on African Americans and members of other ethnic groups. During the experiments, which lasted 40 years, hundreds of African American men with syphilis went untreated by medical professionals, who were interested in studying the progression of the disease. Men were deceived by the physicians in the study, who told them they were being treated for "bad blood" and offered several incentives for study participation (for a complete description on the experiments and their impacts, see Jones, 1993). While current medical research is conducted with relatively stringent standards for the protection of human subjects, discriminatory practices in health-related research have affected the way ethnic minorities view and use the healthcare system. Notably, researchers have posited that the deception involved in the Tuskegee experiments may be linked to the belief (predominantly held by ethnic minorities) that HIV/AIDS is a government-made form of genocide (Thomas & Quinn, 1991; Gamble, 1993).

Though such conspiracy theories were much more popular during the 1980s and early 1990s, the core belief that the U.S. healthcare system cannot be trusted persists among many ethnic minorities and is linked to their higher rates of poor health outcomes. For example, Dalton (1989) noted that the African-American community's mistrust of early HIV/AIDS prevention initiatives led to the resistance in accepting AIDS as a significant health issue within the community and delayed the enactment of prevention efforts. Indeed, research suggests that ethnic minority LGBPs are distrustful of medical and mental health professionals and perceive the health care system to be disinterested in minority health needs (Dowd, 1994; Klonoff & Landrine, 1997; Siegel & Raveis, 1997). Distrust of healthcare professionals and the healthcare system is rooted in a legacy of racism in the healthcare system: Ethnic minorities frequently report personal experiences of neglect, misunderstanding, and a lack of cultural competence when accessing health care. For example, Blanchard and Lurie (2004) found that 14% of African Americans, 19% of Latinos, and 20% of APIs reported being looked down upon or treated with disrespect during their interactions with health providers, compared to 9% of Whites. Participants who reported being treated in a disrespectful manner were more likely to report not following their doctor's advice and putting off necessary medical care. Correspondingly, a study of satisfaction with mental health services among people with major mental illness revealed that LGBPs were more likely to report dissatisfaction with their mental health care than non-LGBPs (Avery et al., 2001). However, African American and Latino LGBPs reported dissatisfaction with mental health services more frequently than nonminority LGB participants. Such experiences among LGBP of color lead to nonutilization of the healthcare system among this population: They are likely to believe that healthcare professionals will be insensitive to their mental and physical health needs as both ethnic and sexual minorities (Parés-Avila & Montano-López, 1994; Greene, 1997). A participant's quote in Malebranche and colleagues' (2004) study of perceptions of health care among African American MSM highlights the difficulty of achieving quality care as an LGBP of color.

As being a young black male, if [I] would come and say something's wrong with me, they [medical providers] would say, 'oh, look at this, you know, they probably just hip-hoppin' and screwin' down, and you know, smokin' the blunts, and then he gonna come in here talkin' about he sick.' So it's like I'm stereotyped already. And now, if you say you're gay, everybody can get the picture of the feminine, gay brother. So I guess it can come to sexuality because they [medical professionals] feel, 'oh, he must have been [sexually promiscuous] already'. [pp. 101–102]

As this quote suggests, homophobia is a major barrier to accessing quality health care among ethnic minority LGBPs. Homophobia in health care settings is tied to a lack of training of health professionals and a lack of understanding of the health needs of people who are lesbian, gay, or bisexual. In a literature review of studies examining the utilization of healthcare programs among gay men and lesbians, Maccio and Douceck (2002) observed that LGBPs frequently reported negative attitudes among healthcare workers and a lack of preparedness in handling health issues related to sexual orientation. The researchers examined health care programs in mental health counseling, addiction treatment, pediatric care, and gynecologic care. A survey conducted of gay and lesbian physicians in the United States revealed that whereas 98% of those surveyed believed it was important for patients to disclose their sexual orientation to healthcare providers, 64% also believed that by disclosing homosexual behavior patients risked receiving substandard care (Shatz & O'Hanlan, 1994). Research has shown that physicians frequently assume that all their LGB patients are heterosexual, which contributes to anxiety surrounding the disclosure of sexual orientation and perceptions that disclosure would have negative consequences on their health care (Barbara et al., 2001; Eliason & Schope, 2001). The available research appears to confirm negative health care experiences among LGB persons. Stevens (1998), when detailing the health care experiences of lesbians, found that of the 332 health care interactions reported by the women, less than one-fourth were evaluated positively. For example, one of the study participants stated:

White male doctors make it their job to see to it that Black women do not have anymore babies . . . Whenever I went in [to a doctor's office] they would never let up when I said no, I don't need birth control. So sometimes I would come out as a lesbian, just to get them to move on to other things. The doctors would fumble around and say something like, "Oh . . . I'm sorry." It was so awkward . . . I always felt harassed because I am Black and because I am a lesbian. [p. 84]

Most of the women in Stevens' sample reported negative experiences due to prejudice linked to sexual orientation, race, and socioeconomic status, and almost half of the women stopped seeing their healthcare providers as a result of negative experiences.

Stigma associated with HIV/AIDS in health care settings may also play a role in the discrimination experienced by LGBPs. Many health care professionals, notably those with limited experience working with LGB individuals, associate AIDS is homosexuality. The idea that HIV/AIDS is a gay disease—it was labeled gay-related immune deficiency (GRID) before being identified as HIV—has persisted over time (Caldwell, 1994). Although today most health professionals acknowledge HIV/AIDS as a disease affecting people from all backgrounds, many continue to stigmatize certain at-risk subgroups. Some LGBPs, notably gay men, assume that once they divulge their sexual orientation health care professionals automatically suspect that they have HIV/AIDS or will at some point contract the virus (Malebranche et al., 2004). It is also important to note the lack of discussions about HIV and its prevention and treatment that occur between patients and their primary care physicians (Gerbert et al., 1991; Council on Scientific Affairs, 1996). A lack of discussion about HIV may affect LGBPs of color more than White LGBPs, given that LGBPs of color are less likely to come out to their physician or disclose certain sexual behaviors.

As noted, patients' nondisclosure of their sexual orientation to their healthcare provider may be linked to their poor health. This has serious implications for ethnic minority LGBPs, who may experience more difficulty letting others know their sexual orientation than LGBPs who are not ethnic minorities. Research has shown that a variety of social and cultural factors are linked to discomfort about disclosing sexual orientation among ethnic minorities. These factors include cultural norms of sexual silence (Dowd, 1994; Gomez & Marín, 1996; Díaz, 1998; Chng et al., 2003), prominent religious beliefs (Woodyard et al., 2000), and familial obligations regarding marriage and procreation (Morales, 1990). Actual and expected experiences of homophobia and/or AIDS-related stigma in healthcare settings further promote nondisclosure of sexual orientation and internalized homophobia. Indeed, research has shown that LGBPs who have disclosed their sexual orientation to their health care providers are more likely to be White than African American or Latino (Klitzman & Greenberg, 2002). Research has suggested that LGBPs of color who are not open about their sexual identity may be more likely to engage in sexual risk behaviors (Chng & Geliga-Vargas, 2000). Thus, ethnic minority LGBPs who internalize stigma linked to their sexual orientation may be more likely to engage in sexual risk behavior and less likely to talk openly about their sexual behavior with health care providers. The link between disclosure of sexual orientation, risk behavior, and healthcare provider attitudes around sexuality suggests that the removal of homophobic attitudes from health care settings is pertinent to promote health among LGB ethnic minorities.

3.3 Immigration Experiences and Their Effects on Health Care

Ethnic minority LGBPs who are immigrants to the United States may face unique issues that affect their access to and utilization of the American healthcare system. Findings from the National Survey of America's Families suggest that Black, Latino, and API immigrants are much more likely to be uninsured than their citizen counterparts (Ku & Waidmann, 2003). Research suggests that noncitizen immigrants are more likely to be employed in low-income jobs that do not offer health insurance benefits and are more likely to be concerned that enrolling in public health care programs would jeopardize their residency status compared to immigrants who are citizens and nonimmigrant citizens (Ku & Waidmann, 2003; Yoshikawa & Lugo-Gil, 2004). As is discussed in a later section of this chapter, changes in U.S. immigrant policies may also explain the disproportionate number of immigrants who are uninsured.

Research also suggests that immigrants are less likely to utilize the healthcare system for reasons related to how they assess poor health and their healthcare experiences in their country of origin. For example, Chin et al. (2000) suggest that because of the way many Asian American immigrants define poor or ailing health (i.e., as an extreme dysfunction), they may be less likely to utilize the healthcare system until their health and functioning is so impaired they can no longer fulfill their work and social roles. The same may be true for other immigrant groups. For instance, in a focus group study of Dominican, Mexican, and Central American immigrants in New York City, Shedlin and Shulman (2004) observed that many immigrants reported not receiving treatment for health conditions until they were seriously ill. Participants' neglect of their health problems was based not only on cultural values about what health problems warranted health-based interventions but also a lack of experience in receiving preventive care. For example, participants noted, "We are not even accustomed to having milk for our children . . . we have to be [so] sick to seek services [that] we cannot go backwards or ahead" (p. 439). Indeed, many participants reported not seeking care until they were "falling down."

Language can represent another barrier to receiving high-quality health care that ethnic minority LGB immigrants may experience. Many communities, notably those with large immigrant populations, advertise health care programs in other languages (predominantly Spanish) and have bilingual or multilingual healthcare providers. Nonetheless, data suggest that non-English-speaking immigrants access health care programs less frequently than English-speaking immigrants and citizens (Ku & Waidmann, 2003). A great deal of research on access to HIV prevention services has focused on the language barriers faced by newly immigrated API and Latino gay men who do not speak English as their primary language. Chng and Collins (2000) noted that the numerous languages and dialects spoken by API immigrants in the United States make HIV prevention interventions, notably those that are mass-marketed, ineffective for many people in this population. Furthermore, the translation of HIV prevention and other health-based information from English to other languages may result in a loss of information and/or inaccurate phrasing of messages, as well as removal of the context in which the message should be understood and interpreted. Language issues may also prevent awareness of available healthcare programs among ethnic minority LGB immigrants (Morales, 1990). Public health programs such as free HIV testing, diabetes screening, and testing and treatment for other health problems are often advertised only in English and are not promoted to noncitizen immigrants, much less non-English-speaking immigrants. Thus, to promote health among ethnic minority LGBPs who are immigrants and to reduce disparities in health care accessibility, it is important to consider the difficulties immigrants have in achieving high-quality health care.

4 Intervening at Different Levels of the Healthcare System: Institutional, Community, and Policy

To improve access to health care among African-American, API, and Latino LGBPs, interventions are needed to remove the barriers that stand in the way between these groups and their receipt of high quality health care. Many of the previously described barriers to health care that LGB ethnic minorities experience can be eliminated through interventions occurring at different levels of the healthcare system: institutional, community, and policy levels. It should be noted that because of the nature of the problem we examine here (i.e., health disparities and healthcare access among ethnic minority LGB persons) we are interested in interventions that go beyond the individual and group levels. Although these interventions are undoubtedly valuable in promoting healthy behaviors in individuals, to achieve improved health and healthcare access across an entire population we must implement interventions that can reach entire communities.

4.1 Institutional Responses

We begin by examining intervention strategies at the institutional levels. These interventions are our starting point because institutional responses may need to occur before some community interventions can be effectively implemented. There are three major institutional responses necessary to promote healthcare access among ethnic minority LGBPs: (1) reduce the isolation of healthcare programs who are from ethnic minority LGBPs; (2) train the healthcare professionals who are delivering services and interventions; and (3) conduct research in healthcare settings.

4.1.1 Reducing the Isolation of Healthcare Programs from Ethnic Minority LGBPs

Reducing the isolation of healthcare programs from ethnic minority LGBPs is of critical importance in our efforts to promote accessibility to health care. Ethnic minority LGBPs live and work in diverse settings. Some are in ethnic enclaves, others may live in low-income neighborhoods, and still others may live in rural areas. However, many of the health-related services targeting LGBPs, particularly those that are resource-rich, are located in affluent, predominantly White communities. Notably, these services tend to be in "gay ghettos," or neighborhoods with a large population of LGBPs and/or a preponderance of gay or lesbian bars, stores, and social organizations (e.g., the Castro in San Francisco; Chelsea in New York City). In their four-city study comparing men living in gay ghettos and those living in other neighborhoods, Mills and colleagues (2001) found that MSM living in neighborhoods with a high concentration of same-sex households were more likely to be White, identify as gay, and have a higher income than MSM not living in neighborhoods with a large gay population. The authors also observed that MSM living in gay ghettos were more likely to have been tested for HIV, and posited that these MSM likely had greater access to HIV prevention services. Similar findings have been obtained in studies of ethnic minority LGBPs (Yoshikawa et al., 2002). Thus, by not living in the neighborhoods in which services are located and marketed, LGBPs of color may have limited access to health care targeted to gays and lesbians. For this reason it is important that health care programs for LGBPs be advertised in neighborhoods that do not have the characteristics of a gay ghetto (i.e., a large number gay-identified persons, gay businesses, and so on) but have high proportions of ethnic minority and/or immigrant populations. At a minimum, organizations located in gay ghettos that have programs focused on the health needs of LGBPs should make an effort to locate satellite offices in neighborhoods that house predominantly ethnic minority populations and/or persons of lower income status. It is also important that HIV prevention and other interventions linked to LGB health provide services to suburban, small city, and rural areas, which have been historically overlooked in most HIV prevention interventions (Mancoske, 1997), though many of these areas are experiencing rapid growth in ethnic minority and immigrant populations (Capps et al., 2003).

It is also important that existing healthcare-providing organizations (i.e., hospitals, community health clinics) in neighborhoods with large ethnic populations develop, implement, and market healthcare programs targeted toward LGBPs in the area. This requires eliminating stigma and/or institutional discrimination toward gays and lesbians in health organizations and increasing the resources available to these organizations to develop health programs for LGBPs. Cultural sensitivity trainings for medical professional and antidiscrimination policies in health care organizations are important institutional interventions that need to be implemented, as discussed later. Hospitals and clinics can submit applications to obtain federal, state, and private sector grants to aid in the development and implementation of health promotion and prevention programs for ethnic minority LGBPs. Also, it is important for healthcare organizations currently serving LGBPs of color to make efforts to increase their accessibility to the target population and broaden the services available. Research has shown that ethnic minority LGBPs often believe that minority-focused health organizations are not effective at achieving their goals of promoting health and reducing risk among ethnic minority LGBPs largely due to a lack of resources (Siegel & Raveis, 1997). A deficit of available resources may translate into an organization's limited hours of operation, lack of comprehensive services, and/or inadequate staff to carry out interventions. With the difficulties involved in obtaining funding to support or broaden community-based programs, it is of increasing importance that healthcare organizations strengthen their grassroots organizing efforts and volunteer programs, while developing their ability to apply for and receive external grants.

Healthcare organizations also need to reach out to the ethnic minority LGBPs in the communities they serve by developing ties to existing social groups and organizations in the community. Healthcare providers should make an effort to be aware of the LGBP social groups to the communities they serve so they can collaborate with these groups to promote awareness of available healthcare programs available to LGBPs. Collaboration with community organizations is of dire importance for hospitals and clinics serving largely minority populations, who may have an underground, but nonetheless active, gay and lesbian social scene (Hawkeswood, 1996). For example, ethnic minority LGBPs have a strong presence in faith-based organizations, though they may not be open about their sexuality (Woodyard et al., 2000). Thus, it is important for healthcare organizations to collaborate with churches and faith-based organizations in their efforts to treat ethnic minority LGBPs and inform them about health care programs tailored to their needs. Offering HIV testing, cancer screening, and other diagnostic and preventive medical practices in churches, temples, and synagogues are prime examples of how to achieve a collaborative effort that links health and faith-based organizations. Also, it is important for the staff delivering healthcare interventions to respect and support patients' use of religion and spirituality in coping with and treating illness while providing formal health care and treatment.

LGB healthcare programs also need to be advertised in communities with predominantly ethnic minority and/or immigrant populations, which are frequently overlooked in HIV prevention and other LGB-related health campaigns. Peterson and Carballo-Dieguez (2000) recommended that innovative marketing campaigns deliver HIV prevention messages directed toward both minority MSM and minority heterosexual men in attempts to reach African American and Latino MSM. This could help reduce the negative impact of what could be perceived a "gay ad" by community members and make the message more applicable to ethnic minority MSM who do not identify as gay or bisexual. Similar social marketing and advertising campaigns are needed in immigrant communities and rural areas. Healthcare organizations should advertise programs for LGBPs and conduct outreach programs in venues that may not be commonly understood as places were LGBPs congregate. For example, Yoshikawa and colleagues (2002) noted that HIV prevention interventions targeting Chinese immigrants in New York City were successful when the outreaching was done at ethnic grocery stores and Chinatown pharmacies—social settings with high degrees of interaction and community trust. Thus, successful healthcare interventions are those that make a strong effort to advertise programs in ethnic communities and develop healthcare programs in these communities to promote access to health care among ethnic minority LGBPs.

4.1.2 Training Healthcare Professionals Delivering Services and Interventions

As noted previously, it is important that healthcare providers are trained to be sensitive to ethnic minorities and LGBPs. Government-sponsored training on human subject protection, antidiscrimination policies in clinical trials and health-related research projects, and other similar training is not enough for health care professionals who deliver services and interventions to ethnic minority LGBPs. Health care professionals must be well versed with regard to the LGBP population living, working, and socializing in the communities in which they work. Do predominantly lesbians live in one area of the neighborhood? Are there locations in the community where ethnic minority MSM congregate and/or have sexual encounters? Are LGBPs likely to be stigmatized in the community and unlikely to disclose their sexual orientation? These are all questions that need to be asked and answered by healthcare providers. Healthcare professionals need to understand why ethnic minority LGBP may be uncomfortable in healthcare settings and address their own prejudices and issues surrounding homosexuality and ethnic diversity (Dowd, 1994; Parés-Avila &

Montano-López, 1994). Healthcare organizations must ensure that the staff delivering services and interventions can effectively work with people of all sexual orientations, ethnicities, and socioeconomic status. It is also important that organizations ensure that the health care providers are aware of the diversity extant in the gay community and work to reduce the preconceptions and stereotypes many providers have about LGBPs (Greene, 1997; Brotman et al., 2002). Several interventions have shown to be effective for increasing the cultural competence of healthcare professionals, though none have specifically addressed cultural sensitivity when working with ethnic minority LGB populations. However, these interventions contain features that can be employed by healthcare organizations when training staff to work with LGBPs of color. For example, Holland and Courtney (1998) observed three major strategies that can effectively increase cultural competence among healthcare professionals: increasing educational awareness; employing workers who are members of diverse ethnic and cultural groups; and creating a cultural immersion experience for the workers. Cultural immersion experiences may be the most important way to promote openness and respect for diversity among staff delivering health care to LGBPs of color. Effective interventions of this type have included inviting ethnic minority LGB community members to share experiences and engage in discussions with staff (Neville et al., 1996; Doutrich & Storey, 2004) and have taken the form of even more creative approaches such as going into ethnic minority and/or LGB neighborhoods for "scavenger hunts" that allow staff to be exposed to prominent persons and places in the community (Holland & Courtney, 1998).

Healthcare providers must be trained not only to respect the diversity of ethnic minority LGBPs but to meet clients "where they are." As previously noted, ethnic minority LGBPs are less likely than white LGBPs to disclose their sexual orientation to health care providers (Klitzman & Greenberg, 2002; Chng et al., 2003). Thus, healthcare providers need to be aware that not all of their patients, particularly those who are in ethnic minorities, will be forthcoming with regard to their sexual behaviors. Similarly, providers need to learn sexual history-taking techniques and be taught to screen for HIV and STIs on the basis of risk behaviors, not the risk group (Wheeler, 2003). For example, Malebranche and colleagues (2004) stated, "screen[ing] for HIV risk by targeting risk groups like 'BMSM [Black MSM];' straight, or gay, in essence, tells a patient they are at risk because of who they are and may make them fearful to engage medical facilities for diagnosis just based on their demographic profile" (p. 104). The authors noted that screening for risk groups may perpetuate fear-based miscommunication of risky sexual practices to healthcare providers. The American Medical Association reported that only about one-third of primary care physicians report routinely taking a sexual history from a new adult patient (Council on Scientific Affairs, 1996). Physicians who do not determine their patients' sexual orientation and sexual behaviors deter patients from confiding in them and overlook possibly important health risk factors. Thus, it is of paramount importance that healthcare professionals talk with their clients about sexual health while maintaining a nonjudgmental attitude and ensuring confidentiality.

Last, healthcare professionals should be aware of and adhere to the 14 Community Standards of Practice for the Provision of Quality Health Care Services for LGBT Clients (derived from the LGBT Health Access Project, an intervention aimed at reducing health disparities in LGBP living in Massachusetts) (Table 1). The Standards were reported

Table 1. Community Standards of Practice for the Provision of Quality Healthcare Services for LGBT Clients

Standard 1:	The agency shall establish, promote and effectively communicate an inclusive, nondiscriminatory work place environment for LGBT employees.
Standard 2:	The agency shall support and encourage visibility of LGBT employees.
Standard 3:	The agency shall work toward ensuring that LGBT employees of all ages are subject to the same terms of employment as all other employees.
Standard 4:	The agency shall assure that comprehensive policies are implemented to prohibit discrimination in the delivery of services to LGBT clients and their families. The agency shall ensure that all staff use, and all written forms and policies employ, culturally appropriate language when dealing with LGBT clients and their families. For the purpose of these standards the terms "family" and "families" shall be broadly construed and shall include but not be limited to relatives by blood, adoption, marriage, or declaration of domestic partnership.
Standard 5:	The agency shall ensure that it has comprehensive and easily accessible procedures in place for clients to file and resolve complaints alleging violations of these policies.
Standard 6:	The agency shall develop and implement or revise existing intake and assessment procedures to ensure that they meet the needs of LGBT clients of all ages and their families.
Standard 7:	All agency staff shall have a basic familiarity with LGBT issues as they pertain to services provided by the agency.
Standard 8:	All direct care staff shall routinely provide general care to LGBT clients. All direct care staff shall be competent to identify and address, within the scope of their field of expertise, specific health problems and treatment issues for LGBT clients and their families, to provide treatment accordingly, and to provide appropriate referrals when necessary.
Standard 9:	All case management and treatment plans shall include and address sexual orientation and gender identity where it is a necessary and appropriate issue in client care.
Standard 10:	The agency shall ensure the confidentiality of client data, including information about sexual orientation and gender identity issues. LGBT clients shall be informed about data collection that includes references to sexual orientation and/or gender identity, including in what circumstances such information may be disclosed, whether it may be disclosed as aggregate or individual information, whether personal identifiers may be disclosed, and how and by whom such information may be used.
Standard 11:	The agency shall provide appropriate, safe, and confidential treatment to LGBT minors unless the agency's services are inappropriate for all minors. All clients who are minors shall be informed of their legal rights and advised of the possibility and possible consequences of any statutory or otherwise mandated reporting.
Standard 12:	The agency shall include LGBT people and their families in outreach and health promotion efforts.
Standard 13:	The composition of the agency Board of Directors and other institutional bodies shall encourage representation from LGBT communities.
Standard 14:	Agency community benefits programs shall include LGBT people in the communities the agency serves.

in the GLMA report on LGBT health in the United States, which was made as a supplement to the national Healthy People 2010 policy initiative (GLMA, 2001). These Standards of Practice represent a comprehensive set of policies that health care organizations can implement to better serve LGBPs. They cover employment and staffing issues, confidentiality, intake and assessment procedures, and the rights of young LGBPs, among other topics pertinent of LGB health. Health care organizations that adopt the Community Standards of Practice are likely to have success in reaching and promoting health among all LGBPs, (member of an ethnic minority or otherwise). Currently, there are no estimates of the proportion of hospital, clinics, and/or physicians' offices that follow the Standards of Practice (J. Schneider, MD, GLMA, personal communication, January 21, 2005). However, the available data on experiences of antigay discrimination that LGBPs have in health care settings suggest that more work needs to be done to implement these standards in healthcare organizations.

4.1.3 Conducting Research in Healthcare Settings

To promote access to health care among ethnic minority LGBPs it is important for healthcare organizations to conduct in-house research, such as needs assessments and program evaluations. Hospitals, clinics, and other community-based health programs must make an effort to collaborate with researchers in designing research projects that aid in targeting ethnic minority LGBPs and developing effective and relevant health programs for men and women in the population. Likewise, it is imperative that researchers with expertise in working with ethnic minority LGB populations and conducting research in Community-based organizations (CBOs) and healthcare settings seek out healthcare organizations in an effort to create partnerships and foster collaborative relationships. Healthcare organizations should focus on not only treating health problems that may be unique to or most prevalent among ethnic minority LGBPs but also gaining broader knowledge of the health issues affecting African American, Latino, and API LGBPs. To provide a high level of care to LGBPs of color, healthcare professionals can review contemporary epidemiologic and other health research relevant to these populations and, through implementing needs assessments, collect data that can be used to describe the unique population of LGBPs in the communities in which they work. Similarly, periodic program evaluation ought to be an instrumental part of any health care program regardless of whether it takes the form of a freestanding intervention or is a component of a larger program in a hospital or clinic. It is important that when engaging in research work healthcare organizations are conscious of community attitudes toward health-based research work and employ sampling procedures that ensure all persons in the community have their voices heard, paying close attention to the representation of LGBPs of color. As has been suggested before, collaboration with community and social organizations when conducting needs assessments and program evaluations may be of particular importance. When conducting research, healthcare organizations must ensure that the assessment techniques and instruments employed do not disenfranchise ethnic minorities and/or immigrants, and they must put procedures in place that ensure the confidentiality of participants' personal information and data (Wheeler, 2003). Proper informed consent is of paramount importance for all research participants, but particularly ethnic minority LGBPs, who may be more distrustful of researchers than White LGBPs. Successful research projects implemented by health organizations are those that are conducted with LGBPs of color who feel comfortable participating in research studies, are completely clear about how their information will be used, and understand the purpose of the research project.

4.2 Community Responses

We suggest three actions that can be taken by community-level interventions to promote healthcare access among ethnic minority LGBPs: (1) increasing comfort and trust with the health care system; (2) taking into account folk models of "good health"; and (3) increasing the number of ethnic minority and LGB healthcare professionals.

4.2.1 Increasing Comfort and Trust in the Healthcare System

As indicated earlier, ethnic minority LGBPs are more likely to be distrustful with medical and mental health professionals and more apprehensive when receiving care from health care professionals they perceive to be racist and/or homophobic. Thus, it is important for interventions to address these concerns by working to increase comfort with and trust of the modern healthcare system and healthcare professionals. This can be achieved through promoting the disclosure of sexual behavior to health care providers and the utilization of available healthcare programs, as well as through increasing comfort in accessing services for LGB immigrants who are not citizens or are undocumented. It should be noted that these interventions cannot be effective if healthcare providers serving LGBPs of color are homophobic and/or racist. Encouraging the utilization of healthcare organizations that are insensitive to the needs of ethnic minorities and LGBP only exacerbates health disparities. Thus, institutional interventions that aim to train healthcare professionals to be culturally sensitive and competent in working with ethnic minorities and LGBPs must take place for community interventions to increase comfort and trust in the healthcare system successfully among ethnic minority LGBP.

For LGB ethnic minorities to receive high-quality health care, it is important for interventions to promote openness among ethnic minority LGBPs with regard to reporting their sexual behaviors and/or sexual orientation to their healthcare providers. Although it is a difficult task for interventions to change deep-rooted social norms and promote "coming out" in ethnic communities that may stigmatize homosexual behaviors, these interventions can encourage ethnic minority LGBPs to disclose their sexual behaviors in certain health contexts (e.g., to medical doctors and mental health professionals). When promoting openness about health-related behaviors (such as substance use and sex), it is important for LGB ethnic minorities to be aware of confidentiality policies regarding nondisclosure of information about their behavior to other people or institutions (Wheeler, 2003). Educational campaigns that work to help ethnic minority LGBPs understand the changes that have been made to the U.S. healthcare and research systems, such as laws surrounding the protection of human subjects and the promotion of ethical research, could be highly effective in reducing distrust of the system. Similarly, it is important for ethnic minority LGBPs to not feel like outsiders to the healthcare system. Interventions must aim to develop collaboration between health care organizations and community members and to foster relationships between healthcare organizations and ethnic minority LGBPs. This could be achieved by linking ethnic and/or LGB social groups to hospitals, clinics, and treatment centers, organizing community health fairs, and providing referrals for ethnic minority LGBPs to healthcare providers. By showing LGB ethnic minorities that there are contexts in which it is not only acceptable to discuss their sexual behavior openly but ultimately advantageous for their good or improved health, it is possible to address some of the discomfort those in this population may experience in being forthright with the healthcare professionals with whom they interact. Several mechanisms used in HIV/AIDS prevention interventions that have been shown to have community-level impacts may be useful to accomplish the goal of increasing ethnic minority LGBPs' comfort with the healthcare system and allow for greater openness among LGBPs of color and their health providers. These mechanisms include (1) enlisting community leaders to aid in bridging ethnic minority LGBPs and health organizations (e.g., the multisite AIDS Community Demonstration Projects) (Higgins et al., 1996); (2) employing media campaigns designed for ethnic minority LGBPs (Myrick, 1999); and (3) utilizing the "diffusion of innovations" theory (Rogers, 1995) in community settings by identifying opinion leaders and training them to deliver health- and prevention-related messages to members of their networks. Diffusion models have been effectively implemented in the form of popular opinion leader interventions taking place in gay bars (Kelly et al., 1997), low-income housing projects (Sikkema et al., 2000), and small communities of MSM in the United States (Kegeles et al., 1996) and Russia (Amirkhanian et al., 2003).

Many ethnic minority LGBPs are aware of health programs in which they may be able to participate, but they do not utilize these programs even when facing ailing health (Morales, 1990; Shedlin & Shulman, 2004). Therefore, community interventions must focus at least partially on promoting healthcare service utilization among ethnic minority LGBPs. Nonutilization of programs may stem from the expectation that the health care will be too costly, a lack of health insurance, or the perception of a minimal need for health-related advice from others, as well as a variety of other factors. Informational campaigns are needed that not only let ethnic minority LGBPs know about available health care programs and programs but make them aware of any costs or requirements associated with utilizing services. Furthermore, community-level interventions must help ethnic minority LGBPs engage in preventive care and facilitate relationship-building among healthcare professionals and patients, so ethnic minority LGBPs feel comfortable talking to healthcare professionals about their health and health-linked behaviors. Interventions must focus not only on the target population of LGBPs who are ethnic minorities but also their families, friends, and colleagues, who can help support their increased utilization of health care programs (Icard et al., 1992). Social marketing campaigns with health-based messages may prove themselves effective by building on existing networks of support. This is largely because ethnic minority LGBPs may be more likely to engage in health preventive behaviors and seek medical help before becoming very ill if they are told to seek care by respected others, not solely by the public health system. Interventions that aim to create awareness of available health care programs and encourage utilization of these programs could also be successful in promoting access to health care. The common saying "knowledge is power" applies here. By informing ethnic minority LGBPs about gay-friendly healthcare providers and programs that would be sensitive to their needs, interventions can enable ethnic minority LGBPs make good choices about their health care providers. The creation of regional guidebooks that list services targeted toward LGBPs and/or persons of color, and medical offices with staff who are ethnic minorities and/or LGBPs may be one good way to implement an effective information-based intervention at the community level.

When increasing the level of comfort of the ethnic minority LGBP experience when accessing health care, it is important to consider the needs of LGBPs of color who are immigrants. Immigrant LGBPs have unique needs with regard to the way they access and use health care. As noted in an earlier section, this group of LGBPs may experience major difficulties in accessing high-quality health care because of language difficulties and poor translation of health-focused prevention messages. Interventions are needed that can be effectively conducted in the languages of prominent immigrant groups in the United States, notably Spanish, Chinese dialects, Tagalog, Vietnamese, Korean, and other languages that are not as nationally prevalent but that are spoken by ethnic minority immigrants clustered in particular areas (e.g., Arabic, French, Portuguese, Japanese, Bengali, Hindi). To increase access to health care successfully, interventions targeted toward LGBPs who are immigrants may need to be carried out by similar others and must be modeled in such a way that they not only respect, but integrate, the culture and tradition of the immigrant group(s) targeted in their interventions. For example, because many APIs maintain a strict silence around sexuality (including topics related to sex, such as condom use and HIV/STIs), interventions aimed in reducing HIV-risk behaviors in this population have distributed condoms packaged in ways to make them resemble Chinese New Year gifts (i.e., wrapped in red packaging and with gold lettering), thereby making them more palatable to immigrant APIs (Chng et al., 2003; Yoshikawa et al., 2003). It is also important that interventions targeted toward immigrant LGBPs address the discomfort many may feel when accessing health-care programs based on their undocumented and/or illegal immigration status. For some immigrants, the history of discriminatory policies regarding immigration as well as the perception of negative national attitudes toward immigrants who come from countries that have been or are now considered political opponents of the United States (e.g., China, Vietnam, Cuba, Middle Eastern countries) may lead to distrust of the U.S. public health system (Chng et al., 2003). Immigrants who have not been granted citizenship may believe that accessing any government-sponsored program (such as low-cost health clinics, free HIV/STI screening) could make them a target for deportation (Yoshikawa & Lugo-Gil, 2004). Identification as gay, lesbian, or bisexual can cause further distress when accessing healthcare programs that may reveal one's undocumented immigration status. Many LGB immigrants seek asylum in the United States—they wish to live freely as GLB individuals, without the heightened stigma they may face by living in their home countries (Chng et al., 2003; Shedlin & Shulman, 2004). This may create heightened motivation to maintain anonymity and not access health care programs that they perceive could result in deportation. Thus, for interventions to be effective, they must promote comfort with the U.S. healthcare system for all persons.

4.2.2 *Taking into Account Folk Models of "Good Health"*

To promote access to health care among LGBPs who are ethnic minorities, it is important that community-level interventions acknowledge and account for the meaning of "good health" among ethnic minority populations. For some Americans, engaging in preventive health care is the norm. From vaccinations given to infants and children to cancer and high blood pressure screening for middle-aged adults, health care is as much about prevention as it is treatment. This may not be the case, however, for some ethnic minorities. Ethnic minority LGBPs are likely to have been raised in communities that apply alternative models of health promotion and disease treatment. For example, many Latinos believe in folk healing traditions. Notably, Parés-Avila & Montano-López (1994) highlight *Curanderism* as a common tradition among Latinos originally from countries with strong indigenous influences (e.g., Mexico). In *Curanderism*, prayers, massage, and herbs are used to treat physical and emotional ailments. Similarly, some API cultures employ non-Western medical techniques such as acupuncture and the use of natural medicines, herbs, and extracts to treat physical and mental ailments. Ethnic minorities are also more likely than Caucasians to utilize nontraditional forms of medical care and to access members of the community who may have not had medical training but are nonetheless considered erudite in their assessment and treatment of health problems. Based on the legacy of discrimination in the U.S. public health system, African Americans and other minorities may be more likely to trust nonmedically trained community members with their health care than medical professionals who are demographically different from them (Dowd, 1994). Community-level interventions would be ill-advised to disregard these traditions or attempt to remove or alter them, regardless of whether they can be empirically shown to be beneficial to the ethnic minorities employing them. Rather, interventions need to work with informal health providers within the target population community and integrate them into health-based interventions. Including respected community members who are understood to have expertise in health care (regardless of whether they were trained in Western-style educational settings) in health-based interventions not only acknowledges the importance of addressing the health of ethnic minority LGBPs from a cultural perspective but also gives the intervention a more trusted face, making ethnic minority LGBPs more likely to access the intervention and utilize the programs and services of the intervention (Brotman et al., 2002).

Many Latino and African American LGBPs place a strong focus on religion with regard to health and the treatment of illness. Based on their experience as stigmatized minority members, ethnic minority LGBPs may be more likely to rely on religious and spiritual beliefs during difficult times (Chatters et al., 1992). It is important that interventions encapsulate the spiritual and religious traditions of ethnic minority LGBPs into health-based interventions. For many people, prayer and spirituality represent much more powerful forms of treatment than visiting a doctor's office or taking medications. Many ethnic minorities speak with members of the clergy or other spiritual leaders before they talk to health care professionals when they are sick. Correspondingly, many LGBPs of color are likely to turn to religion upon receiving a poor health diagnosis, or they may choose to forego medical treatment as a matter of faith. By integrating a spiritual perspective into health-based interventions, ethnic minority LGBPs may be more likely to utilize services available to them. Health service organizations designed largely for White LGB populations may not be open to these spiritual and religious traditions because of how homophobic Christian religious institutions are perceived to be by their staff. Thus, it is important that community interventions targeted to ethnic minority LGBPs educate them about health risks and treatments in ways that respect religious beliefs. For these interventions to be effective, LGBPs of color cannot be made to feel that institutionalized health care and religion are mutually exclusive. Healthcare providers and religious officials need to endorse one another and work together in promoting health among ethnic minority LGBPs. Parish nursing programs, in which registered professional nurses are embedded in church congregations to provide health services and education to fellow parishioners (Anderson, 2004), represent prime examples of how religious and health organizations can collaborate to achieve the common goal of promoting health among ethnic minority LGBPs. Although churches with predominantly ethnic minority memberships have been shown to offer several social and health services, few have implemented programs that integrate formal healthcare services into the church setting (Blank et al., 2002) even though these programs are frequently perceived to be highly desirable among many minority parishioners (Madison & McGadney, 2000; Wallace et al., 2002). Thus, it would be wise for interventions to promoting parish nursing in congregations that may include ethnic minority LGBP members.

4.2.3 *Increasing the Number of Ethnic Minority and LGB Healthcare Professionals*

Community interventions aimed at increasing healthcare access among ethnic minority LGBPs could achieve this goal by aggressively recruiting ethnic minorities and/or LGBPs to work in the healthcare industry. Research has shown that ethnic minority patients are more likely to feel comfortable and report satisfaction with medical professionals who share their ethnic/racial background (Saha et al., 2003; Blanchard & Lurie, 2004). Ethnic minority healthcare providers allow many of their same-ethnicity patients to feel a sense of personal connection with their provider, which is important to the access to and utilization of health care. For example, a participant in Malebranche and colleagues' (2004) study of perceptions of healthcare organizations among African American MSM noted:

Black male doctors, because I am a Black male, have always been easier for me to relate to. My doctor now says, 'What have you been eatin'?' And I say, 'McDonalds.' He says, 'Brother, you need to cut that out.' You know, they get real with you. [p. 103]

Similarly, LGBPs report being more comfortable accessing healthcare programs when they are treated by other LGB medical professionals (Klitzman & Greenberg, 2002). Currently, there is a shortage of ethnic minority and LGBP health care professionals (Cooper & Powe, 2004), which affects ethnic minority LGBPs in two ways. First, the likelihood that LGBPs of color will access health care and/or build a relationship with a health care provider is diminished in the absence of a diverse group of medical professionals. Second, because minority healthcare providers are more likely than White physicians to serve minority patients and to work in underserved areas, ethnic minority LGBPs may have fewer opportunities to receive care (American Medical Association, 1999). Interventions are desperately needed to promote diversity among healthcare professionals. The American Association of Medical Colleges (2002) reported that the number of minority medical school graduates has steadily decreased over the past decade, most notably in states that have overturned affirmative action laws. Interventions to increase the number of minority healthcare professionals must take place at multiple levels—at the community, institutional, and policy levels. However, community interventions that mobilize ethnic minorities and LBGPs to enter medical professions, offer training to increase the probability of acceptance into educational programs, and provide access to scholarships or other forms of financial support for higher education may be most effective at helping to create a more diverse population of medical professionals in the United States.

4.3 Policy Responses

Major policy responses to racial or ethnic disparities in healthcare access among LGBPs, based on the evidence reviewed in this chapter, encompass health insurance and HIV/AIDS treatment policy. We discuss each of these in this section.

4.3.1 Reduce Disparities in Health Insurance Access

The federal welfare reform legislation of 1996 (the Personal Responsibility and Work Opportunity Reconciliation Act, or PRWORA) sharply restricted eligibility for federal means-tested programs for immigrants arriving in the United States after 1996. Guidelines differ by program (Capps et al., 2002; Singer, 2004). Postenactment immigrants are ineligible for Medicaid (except for Medicaid-funded emergency care and the State Children's Health Insurance Program, or SCHIP) for their first 5 years after coming to the United States. For SSI (Supplemental Security Income—cash assistance for low-income elderly and disabled persons), postenactment legal immigrants are simply ineligible, no matter how long they are in the United States. To receive Food Stamps, legal immigrants must prove that they have worked at least 10 years in the United States. A few select groups are not subject to these restrictions (refugees or asylees during the first 7 years after entry; children who arrived before 1996, and some elderly or disabled). States can provide their own funding to replace these programs for postenactment immigrants (Zimmerman & Tumlin, 1999).

To the extent that LGB communities of color have higher proportions of immigrants, as well as lower incomes, than White LGB communities, they have borne a greater share of the burden of government-directed exclusion from Medicaid and SSI. Although some states have been relatively generous in substituting their own programs, there is great variability among the 50 states (Zimmerman & Tumlin, 1999). This has created obvious inequities based solely on residence for LGB immigrants arriving after 1996. It is likely that PRWORA exacerbated racial/ethnic disparities among low-income citizens in health care access indicators, such as seeing a doctor in the last year. Ku and Waidmann (2003) found, for example, that 67% of low-income White U.S. citizens reported having seen a doctor during the last year compared to 49% for Latino noncitizens who spoke English as their primary language and an even lower 36% among Latino noncitizens who spoke Spanish. The 1996 law has had, according to some, a "chilling" effect on utilization of Medicaid and other means-tested benefits, even among those eligible (e.g., immigrants who arrived before 1996) (Capps et al., 2002). Recent studies of low-income immigrants have found that even those legal permanent residents who are eligible for benefits avoid using them for fear of future consequences for their applications for citizenship (Yoshikawa & Lugo-Gil, 2004). These fears are expressed despite current Immigration and Naturalization Service (INS) guidelines indicating that use of Medicaid and other government assistance programs cannot be a reason to deny a legal immigrant citizenship.

The picture of Medicaid eligibility for undocumented immigrants is, not surprisingly, more bleak than for legal immigrants. Undocumented persons are not eligible for any care under Medicaid except emergency care. LGB populations who are undocumented are thus likely to receive health care only when they are so sick they cannot work. Because LGB populations who are undocumented are more likely to be Latino or Asian than White, this federal policy almost certainly exacerbates racial/ethnic disparities in health outcomes among LGBPs.

As is the case with benefits for legal immigrants, states have to varying degrees stepped in with state-funded programs for which undocumented immigrants are eligible. For example, New York State allows them to receive prenatal and postnatal care in addition to emergency care. However, no state allows undocumented immigrants to receive the full range of Medicaid benefits, including HIV prophylaxis and treatment.

The simplest policy solution to state-level inequities in eligibility for Medicaid is to roll back exclusion of legal immigrants from federal means-tested benefits. This was accomplished for Food Stamps soon after passage of PRWORA owing to the outcry over the immigrant provisions of the law. However, the exclusion from Medicaid has not been addressed at the federal level. Rolling back exclusionary policies in the area of nutrition but not health does not make sense from a public health perspective. Disparities in healthcare utilization among low-income LGB communities of color would be most fundamentally addressed by extending Medicaid eligibility to all residents of the United States.

4.3.2 Address HIV/AIDS Prevention and Treatment Disparities
Disparities across racial/ethnic groups have been found in the use of federally funded HIV treatment programs. The disparities may be particularly strong among LGB populations owing to their higher incidence of HIV and AIDS. However, no studies have examined racial/ethnic differences in HIV treatment access among LGBPs. We therefore rely here on more general data across race/ethnicity, regardless of sexual orientation or identity.

The two major federally funded programs providing coverage of HIV treatments are the AIDS Drug Assistance Program (ADAP) and Medicaid. Both provide assistance in obtaining highly active antiretroviral treatment (HAART) and other advanced HIV/AIDS treatments, as well as prophylaxis. Medicaid coverage of HIV-related drugs is generally limited to low-income individuals relative to ADAP. National data from 1998 showed that HIV-positive African Americans are substantially less likely to make use of ADAP than HIV-positive members of other racial/ethnic groups (Morin et al., 2002). This may be because African Americans are more likely to have low income and therefore are more likely to receive HIV treatment through Medicaid. However, according to a review of studies dating back to 1985, non-White populations were less likely to use antiretroviral drugs than White populations in most of the studies (Palacio et al., 2002). These data suggest that disparities across racial/ethnic groups in treatment utilization are longstanding and occur regardless of the specific program being considered.

As we have seen, Medicaid eligibility for legal immigrants differs considerably across states. Medicaid coverage guidelines for HIV treatment also differ substantially. In an analysis performed in 2000 of policies regarding ADAP and Medicaid-funded AIDS treatment in the four largest states, Morin et al. (2002) found large differences in policy dimensions, such as the number of HIV treatment drugs covered for reimbursement. California and New York did not limit the number of drugs covered in any month for treatment. In contrast, Florida allowed only four HIV drugs per month and Texas three. As a result, in Florida and Texas, individuals with HIV and other co-occurring diseases reported finding it difficult to have their complete prescribed set of treatments covered by Medicaid. Eligibility guidelines also differed across these state policies. Florida, Texas, and California all required federal disability designation or welfare receipt as part of eligibility. New York did not have these requirements.

ADAP policies differed even more drastically among the four states. For example, ADAP drugs were available in 2000 at only 244 pharmacies in Texas, compared to more than 2000 in both California and New York (a huge disparity even taking into account differences in population among these states). California's ADAP program covered use of 110 HIV-related drugs and New York 395, but in Florida only 26 such drugs and in Texas only 19. Finally, income eligibility for ADAP in the four states ranged from 200% to 400% of the federal poverty threshold.

Thus, large inequities exist in state-level ADAP and Medicaid policies regarding HAART and other HIV treatments. These inequities may be implicated in state-level mortality disparities across racial/ethnic groups (in three of the four stated studied by Morin et al., declines in HIV/AIDS mortality across 1996 to 1998 were smaller among African Americans than in Whites). In addition, across the four states, the percentage of individuals with AIDS diagnoses covered by Medicaid or ADAP differed significantly, with New York covering more individuals through its two programs than the number of diagnosed (because of its coverage of prophylactic medications, for example), and Texas covering the smallest proportion (68%). As in the case of Medicaid eligibility for immigrants, the simplest policy solution is to make HIV treatment eligibility and drug coverage regulations equal across states through federal law. Such regulations should be created for each of the two major programs, ADAP and Medicaid.

In addition to policy regulation, federal support of community-based efforts to increase utilization of ADAP and Medicaid among individuals of color affected by HIV should be increased. For low-income individuals coping with HIV/AIDS, for example, a recent set of studies found that two policy steps are crucial for community-based outreach to communities of color affected by HIV/AIDS (Richards et al., 2002). The first is to ensure that the take-up of HIV-related services occurred at the critical juncture of the test result. Individuals who do not receive services at that point often do not reappear until they have symptoms of AIDS, at a point when prophylactic action is too late. The second is to acknowledge that for low-income people affected by HIV/AIDS problems with daily living and making ends meet often overwhelm health and health promotion. Embedding HIV/AIDS care in the context of other services that address the needs of the poor (e.g., income support, employment, education, child care, and other services) was critical in this study to the success of the HIV/AIDS care (Richards et al., 2002). Not surprisingly, states that were less generous in terms of eligibility and coverage of HIV/AIDS treatments were also less comprehensive in meeting the needs of low-income populations in general. Federal support of "one-stop" centers, such as those that have been implemented in the area of job training and work support, could be implemented to integrate health care coverage and services with other services for the populations most at risk for HIV infection, more frequent general poor health outcomes, and poverty. These persons are of course more likely to be populations of color, and such policies are likely to improve health outcomes among African American, Asian, and Latino LGB people.

5 Summary

We have examined access to health care among African American, API, and Latino lesbian, gay, and bisexual populations. Epidemiologic data show that ethnic minority LGBPs are more likely to experience physical and mental health problems than heterosexuals and Caucasian LGBPs. Indeed, ethnic LGBPs have higher rates of STIs, certain cancers, depression, and substance use than other populations. Although research explaining health disparities has been called for in U.S. government and community-based organizations, work specifically examining the needs of LGBPs of color has been scant. Nonetheless, the available relevant studies suggest three major factors involved in understanding ethnic minority LGBPs' heightened risk for poor health outcomes. They include the negative impact of discrimination on health and risk behavior, racism and homophobia in health care and research settings, and immigration experiences that may negatively affect health access and utilization. To be effective in reducing and eliminating health disparities between minority and nonminority populations in the United States it is of great importance that researchers, health organizations, minority and/or LGB community-based organizations, and policymakers make an effort to improve health care and healthcare accessibility among LGBPs of color.

There are several ways in which interventions can improve access to health care among LGBPs of color. These interventions may occur at various levels of the healthcare system: institutional, community, and policy levels. Institutional interventions are needed to reduce the isolation of healthcare programs from ethnic minority LGBPs, train healthcare professionals to be culturally sensitive to the needs of ethnic minority LGBPs, and promote research on LGB populations in healthcare settings. Community-level interventions that aim to increase ethnic minority LGBPs' comfort for accessing the healthcare system and trusting healthcare professionals, incorporate ethnic-centered models of the meaning of good health into their services and programs, and increase the number of ethnic minority and LGB healthcare professionals are likely to be successful in promoting improved health care for LGBPs of color. Finally, policy-level interventions are warranted that reduce disparities in health insurance access among ethnic minority LGBPs and improve access to HIV/AIDS prevention and treatment services among LGBPs of color.

Health care is commonly understood to be a human right in the United States; however, serious discrepancies in access to health care make the receipt of health-related services a luxury for many, notably those who belong to ethnic minorities. As research has shown, disparities in health care among LGBPs resemble those observed in the general U.S. population—they both fall along ethnic and racial lines. Thus, in our efforts to understand and promote health among all people who are lesbian, gay, and bisexual, our goal must be to improve access to high quality health care among African American, API, and Latino LGBPs. Achieving this goal not only will help eliminate health disparities in the United States, it will further the ultimate objective of making the receipt of high quality health care a right of all individuals.

References

American Association of Medical Colleges, Division of Community and Minority Programs. (2002) *Minority students in medical education: facts and figures XII.* American Association of Medical Colleges, Washington, DC.

American Medical Association (1999) *Board of Trustees report: diversity in medical education.* Report 15—A-99. American Medical Association, Chicago.

Amirkhanian, Y.A., Kelly, J.A., Kabakchieva, E., McAuliffe, T.L., Vassileva, S. (2003) Evaluation of a social network HIV prevention intervention program for young men who have sex with men in Russia and Bulgaria. *AIDS Education & Prevention* 15:205–220.

Anderson, C.M. (2004) The delivery of health care in faith-based organizations: parish nurses as promoters of health. *Heath Communications* 16:117–128.

Avery, A.M., Hellman, R.E., and Sudderth, L.K. (2001) Satisfaction with mental health services among sexual minorities with major mental illness. *American Journal of Public Health* 91:990–991.

Barbara, A.M., Quandt, S.A., and Anderson, R.T. (2001) Experiences of lesbians in the health care environment. *Women & Health* 34(1):45–62.

Blanchard, J., and Lurie, N. (2004) R-E-S-P-E-C-T: patient reports of disrespect in the health care setting and its impact on care. *Journal of Family Practice* 53:721.

Blank, M.B., Mahmood, M., Fox, J.C., and Guterbock, T. (2002) Alternative mental health services: the role of the Black church in the south. *American Journal of Public Heath* 92:1668–1672.

Broman, C.L. (1997) Race-related factors and life satisfaction among African-Americans. *Journal of Black Psychology* 23:36–49.

Brotman, S., Ryan, B., Jalbert, Y., and Rowe, B. (2002) Reclaiming space-regaining health: the health care experiences of two-spirited people in Canada. *Journal of Gay & Lesbian Social Services* 14(1):67–87.

Cabaj, R.P. (1992) Substance abuse in the gay and lesbian community. In: Lowinson, J.H., Ruiz, P., and Millman, R. (eds) *Substance abuse: a comprehensive textbook.* Williams & Wilkins, Baltimore, pp. 852–860.

Caldwell, S.A. (1994) Twice removed: the stigma suffered by gay men with AIDS. In: Caldwell, S.A., Burnham, R.A., and Forstein, M. (eds) *Therapists on the front line: psychotherapy with gay men in the age of AIDS.* American Psychiatric Press, Washington, DC. pp. 3–24.

Capps, R., Ku, L., and Fix, M. (2002) *How are immigrants faring after welfare reform? Preliminary evidence from Los Angeles and New York City.* The Urban Institute, Washington, DC.

Capps, R., Passel, J.S., Perez-Lopez, D., and Fix, M. (2003) *The new neighbors: a users' guide to data on immigrants in U.S. communities.* The Urban Institute, Washington, DC.

Centers for Disease Control (2002) *HIV/AIDS surveillance report 2002.* 14(7).

Centers for Disease Control (2003) HIV/STD risks in young men who have sex with me who do not disclose their sexual orientation—six U.S. cities, 1994–2000. *MMWR Morbidity and Mortality Weekly Report* 53:891–894.

Chatters, L.M., Levin, J.S., and Taylor, R.J. (1992) Antecedents and dimensions of religious involvement among older Black adults. *Journal of Gerontology* 47:269–278.

Chin, D., Takeuchi, D.T., and Suh, D. (2000) Access to health care among Chinese, Korean, and Vietnamese Americans. In: Houge, C., Hargraves, M.A., and Collins, K.S. (eds) *Minority health in America: findings and policy implications from the Commonwealth Fund minority health survey.* Johns Hopkins University Press, Baltimore, pp. 77–96.

Chng C.L., and Collins, J.R. (2000) Providing culturally competent HIV prevention programs. *American Journal of Health Studies* 16(1):24–33.

Chng, C.L., and Géliga-Vargas, J. (2000) Ethnic identity, gay identity, sexual sensation seeking and HIV risk taking among multiethnic men who have sex with men. *AIDS Education and Prevention* 12:326–339.

Chng, C.L., Wong, F.Y., Park, R.J., Edberg, M.C., and Lai, D.S. (2003) A model for understanding sexual health among Asian American/Pacific Islander men who have sex with men (MSM) in the United States. *AIDS Education and Prevention* 15(Suppl. 1):21–38.

Clark, R., Anderson, N.B., Clark, V.R., and Williams, D.R. (1999) Racism as a stressor for African Americans: a biopsychosocial model. *American Psychologist* 54:805–816.

Cochran, S.D., and Mays, V.M. (1994) Depressive distress among homosexually active African American men and women. *American Journal of Psychiatry* 151:524–529.

Cochran, S.D., Sullivan, J.G., and Mays, V.M. (2003) Prevalence of mental disorders, psychological distress, and mental health services use among lesbian, gay and bisexual adults in the United States. *Journal of Consulting and Clinical Psychology* 71:53–61.

Cooper, L.A., and Powe, N.R. (2004) *Disparities in patient experiences, health care processes, and outcomes: the role of patient-provider racial, ethnic, and language concordance.* Commonwealth Fund, New York.

Council of Scientific Affairs, American Medical Association. (1996) Health care needs of gay men and lesbians in the United States. *Journal of the American Medical Association* 275:1354–1359.

Dalton, H.L. (1989) AIDS in blackface. *Daedalus* 118:205–227.

Dean, L., Meyer, I.H., Robinson, K., Sell, R.L., Sember, R., Silenzio, V.M.B., Bowen, D.J., Bradford, J., Rothblum, E., White, J., Dunn, P., Lawrence, A., Wolfe, D., and Xavier, J. (2000) Lesbian, gay, bisexual, and transgender health: findings and concerns. *Journal of the Gay and Lesbian Medical Association* 4(3):102–151.

Díaz, R.M. (1998) *Latino gay men and HIV: culture, sexuality, & risk behavior.* Routledge, New York.

Díaz, R.M., and Ayala, G. (2001) *Social discrimination and health: the case of Latino gay men and HIV risk.* National Gay and Lesbian Task Force, New York.

Díaz, R.M., Ayala, G., and Bein, E. (2004) Sexual risk as an outcome of social oppression: data from a probability sample of Latino gay men in three U.S. cities. *Cultural Diversity & Ethnic Minority Psychology* 10:255–267.

Doutrich, D., and Storey, M. (2004) Education and practice: dynamic partners for improving cultural competence in public health. *Family and Community Health* 7:298–307.

Dowd, S.A. (1994) African-American gay men and HIV and AIDS: therapeutic challenges. In: Caldwell, S.A., Burnham, R.A., and Forstein, M. (eds) *Therapists on the front line: psychotherapy with gay men in the age of AIDS.* American Psychiatric Press, Washington, DC. pp. 319–338.

Eliason, M.J., and Schope, R. (2001) Does "don't ask, don't tell" apply to health care? Lesbian, gay, bisexual people's disclosure to health care providers. *Journal of Gay and Lesbian Medical Association* 5(4):125–134.

Gamble, V.N. (1993) A legacy of distrust: African-Americans and medical research. *American Journal of Preventive Medicine* 9:35–38.

Gay and Lesbian Medical Association. (2001) *Healthy People 2010 companion document for lesbian, gay, bisexual, and transgender (LGBT) health.* Gay and Lesbian Medical Association, San Francisco.

Gerbert, B., Maquire, B.T., Bleeker, T., Coates, T.J., and McPhee, S.J. (1991) Primary care physicians and AIDS: attitudinal and structural barriers to care. *Journal of the American Medical Association* 266:2387–2842.

Gilman, S.E., Cochran, S.D., Mays, V.M., Hughes, M., Ostrow, D., and Kessler, R.C. (2001) Prevalence of DSM-III-R disorders among individuals reporting same-gender sexual partners in the national co-morbidity survey. *American Journal of Public Health* 91:933–939.

Gomez, C.A., and Marin, B.V. (1996) Barriers to HIV prevention strategies for women. *The Journal of Sex Research* 33:355–362.

Greene, B. (1997) Ethnic minority lesbians and gay men: mental health and treatment issues. In: Greene, B. (ed) *Ethnic and cultural diversity among lesbians and gay men.* Sage, Thousand Oaks, CA, pp. 216–239.

Hawkeswood, W.G. (1996) *One of the children: gay black men in Harlem.* University of California Press, Berkeley.

Higgins, D.L., O'Reilly, K., Tashima, N., Crain, C., Beeker, C., Goldbaum, G., Elifson, C.S., Galavotti, C., and Guenther-Grey, C. (1996) Using formative research to lay the foundation for community-level HIV prevention efforts: the AIDS community demonstration projects. *Public Health Reports* 111 (Suppl.):28–35.

Holland, L., and Courtney, R. (1998) Increasing cultural competence with the Latino community. *Journal of Community Health Nursing* 15(1):45–53.

Icard, L., and Traunstein, D.M. (1987) Black, gay, alcoholic men: their character and treatment. *Social Casework: The Journal of Contemporary Social Work* May:267–272.

Icard, L.D., Schilling, R.F., El-Bassel, N., and Young, D. (1992) Preventing AIDS among Black gay men and Black gay and heterosexual male intravenous drug users. *Social Work* 37:440–445.

Jiang, W., Babyak, M., Krantz, D.S., Waugh, R.A., Coleman, R.E., Hanson, M.M., Frid, D.J., McNulty, S., Morris, J.J., O'Connor, C.M., and Blumenthal, J.A. (1996) Mental stress-induced myocardial ischemia and cardiac events. *Journal of the American Medical Association* 275:1651–1656.

Jones, J.H. (1993) *Bad blood: the Tuskegee syphilis experiment*, 2nd ed. Free Press, New York.

Kegeles, S.M., Hays, R.B., and Coates, T.J. (1996) The Mpowerment Project: a community-level HIV prevention intervention for young gay men. *American Journal of Public Health* 86:1129–1136.

Kelly, J.A., Murphy, D.A., Sikkema, K.J., McAuliffe, T.L., Roffman, R.A., Solomon, L.J., Winett, R.A., and Kalichman, S.C. (1997) Randomised, controlled, community-level HIV-prevention intervention for sexual-risk behavior among homosexual men in US cities. *The Lancet* 350:1500–1505.

Klitzman, R.L., and Greenberg, J.D. (2002) Patterns of communication between gay and lesbian patients and their health care providers. *Journal of Homosexuality* 42(2):65–75.

Klonoff, E., and Landrine, H. (1997) Distrust of Whites, acculturation, and AIDS knowledge among African Americans. *Journal of Black Psychology* 23(1):50–57.

Krieger, N. (1999) Embodying inequality: a review of concepts, measures, and methods for studying health consequences of discrimination. *International Journal of Health Services* 29:295–352.

Krieger, N., and Sidney, S. (1996) Racial discrimination and blood pressure: the CARDIA study of young Black and White adults. *American Journal of Public Health* 86:1370–1378.

Ku, L., and Waidmann, T. (2003) *How race/ethnicity, immigration status and language affect health insurance coverage, access to care and quality of care among the low-income population.* Kaiser Family Foundation, Washington, D.C.

Maccio, E.M., and Doueck, H.J. (2002) Meeting the needs of the gay and lesbian community: outcomes in the human services. *Journal of Gay & Lesbian Social Services* 14(4):55–73.

Madison, A., and McGadney, B. (2000) Collaboration of churches and service providers: meeting the needs of African-American elderly. *The Journal of Religious Gerontology* 11(1):23–38.

Malebranche, D.J., Peterson, J.L., Fullilove, R.E., and Stackhouse, R.W. (2004) Race and sexual identity: perceptions about medical culture and healthcare among Black men who have sex with men. *Journal of the National Medical Association* 96(1):97–107.

Mancoske, R.J. (1997) Rural HIV/AIDS social services for gays and lesbians. In: Smith, J.D., and Mancoske, R.J. (eds) *Rural gays and lesbians: building on the strengths of communities.* Haworth Press, Binghamton, NY. pp. 37–52.

Mays, V.M., Cochran, S.D., and Sullivan, J.G. (2000) Health care for African American and Hispanic women: report on perceived health status, access to care, and utilization patterns. In: Hogue, C., Hargraves, M.A., and Collins, K.S. (eds) *Minority health in America: findings and policy implications from the Commonwealth Fund minority health survey.* Johns Hopkins University Press, Baltimore, pp. 97–123.

Meyer, I.H. (1995) Minority stress and mental health in gay men. *Journal of Health and Social Behavior* 36:38–56.

Meyer, I.H., and Dean, L. (1995) Patterns of sexual behavior and risk taking among young New York City gay men. *AIDS Education and Prevention* 7(Suppl.):13–23.

Mills, T.C., Stall, R., Pollack, L., Paul, J.P., Binson, D., Canchola, J., and Catania, J.A. (2001) Health-related characteristics of men who have sex with men: a comparison of those living in "gay ghettos" with those living elsewhere. *American Journal of Public Health* 91:980–983.

Morales, E.S. (1990) HIV infection and Hispanic gay and bisexual men. *Hispanic Journal of Behavioral Sciences* 12:212–222.

Morin, S.F., Sengupta, S., Cozen, M., Richards, T.A., Shriver, M.D., Palacio, H., and Kahn, J.G. (2002) Responding to racial disparities in use of HIV drugs: analysis of state policies. *Public Health Reports* 117:263–272.

Myrick, R. (1999) In the life: culture-specific HIV communication programs designed for African American men who have sex with men. *The Journal of Sex Research* 36:159–170.

Neville, H.A., Heppner, M.J., Louie, C.E., Thompson, C.E., Brooks, L., and Baker, C.E. (1996) The impact of multicultural training on White racial identity attitudes and therapy competencies. *Professional Psychology: Research and Practice* 27:83–89.

Palacio, H., Kahn, J.G., Richards, T.A., and Morin, S.F. (2002) Effect of race and/or ethnicity in use of antiretrovirals or prophylaxis for opportunistic infection: a review of the literature. *Public Health Reports* 117:233–251.

Parés-Avila, J.A., and Montano-López, R. (1994) Issues in the psychosocial care of Latino gay men with HIV infection. In: Caldwell, S.A., Burnham, R.A., and Forstein, M. (eds) *Therapists on the front line: psychotherapy with gay men in the age of AIDS*. American Psychiatric Press, Washington, DC, pp. 339–362.

Peterson, J.L., and Carballo-Dieguez, A. (2000) HIV prevention among African-American and Latino men who have sex with men. In: Peterson, J.L., and DiClemente, R.J. (eds) *Handbook of HIV prevention*. Plenum, New York, pp. 217–224.

Phillip M. (1993) Gay issues: out of the closet, into the classroom, racism, fear of reprisals force black gays and lesbians to keep low profile on campus. *Black Issues In Higher Education* 9:20–25.

Richards, T.A., Vernon, K., Palacio, H., Kahn, J.G., and Morin, S.F. (2002) The HIV care continuum in publicly funded clinics. *Public Health Reports* 117:233–251.

Rogers, E.M. (1995) *Diffusion of innovations*, 4th ed. Free Press, New York.

Rumbaut, R.G. (1994) The crucible within: ethnic identity, self-esteem, and segmented assimilation among children of immigrants. *International Migration Review* 28:748–794.

Saha, S., Arbelaez, J.J., and Cooper, L.A. (2003) Patient-physician relationships and racial disparities in the quality of health care. *American Journal of Public Health* 93:1713–1719.

Semple, S.J., Patterson, T.L., and Grant, I. (2002) Motivation associated with methamphetamine use among HIV+ men who have sex with men. *Journal of Substance Abuse Treatment* 22:149–156.

Shatz, B., and O'Hanlon, K. (1994) *Anti-gay discrimination in medicine: results of a national survey of lesbian, gay, & bisexual physicians*. Gay & Lesbian Medical Association, San Francisco.

Shedlin, M.G., and Shulman, L. (2004) Qualitative needs assessment of HIV services among Dominican, Mexican and Central American immigrant populations living in the New York City area. *AIDS Care* 16:434–445.

Siegel, K., and Raveis, V. (1997) Perceptions of access to HIV-related information, care, and services among infected minority men. *Qualitative Health Research* 7(1):9–31.

Sikkema, K.J., Kelly, J.A., Winett, R.A., Solomon, L.J., Cargill, V.A., Roffman, R.A., McAuliffe, T.L., Heckman, T.G., Anderson, E.A., Wagstaff, D.A., Norman, A.D., Perry, M.J., Crumble, D.A., and Mercer, M.B. (2000) Outcomes of a randomized community-level HIV prevention intervention for women living in 18 low-income housing developments. *American Journal of Public Health* 90:57–63.

Singer, A. (2004) Welfare reform and immigrants: a policy review. In: Kretsedemans, P., and Aparicio, A. (eds) *Immigrants, welfare reform, and the poverty of policy*. Praeger, Westport, CT, pp. 21–34.

Stevens, P.E. (1998) The experiences of lesbians of color in health care encounters: narrative insights for improving access and quality. *Journal of Lesbian Studies* 2(1):77–94.

Thomas, S.B., and Quinn, S.C. (1991) The Tuskegee syphilis study, 1932 to 1972: implications for HIV education and AIDS risk education programs in the Black community. *American Journal of Public Health* 81:1948–1505.

Wallace, D.C., Tuck, I., Boland, C.S., and Witucki, J.M. (2002) Client perceptions of parish nursing. *Public Health Nursing* 19:128–135.

Wheeler, D.P. (2003) Methodological issues in conducting community-based health and social services research among urban Black and African American LGBT populations. *Journal of Gay & Lesbian Social Services* 15(1/2):65–78.

Williams, D.R. (2000) Race, stress, and mental health. In: Houge, C., Hargraves, M.A., and Collins, K.S. (eds) *Minority health in America: findings and policy implications from the Commonwealth Fund minority health survey.* Johns Hopkins University Press, Baltimore, pp. 209–243.

Williams, D.R., Spencer, M.S., and Jackson, J.S. (1999) Race, stress, and physical health: the role of group identity. In: Contrada, R.J., and Ashmore, R.D. (eds) *Self, social identity, and physical health: interdisciplinary exploration.* Oxford University Press, New York, pp. 71–100.

Wilson, P.A., and Yoshikawa, H. (2004) Experiences of and responses to social discrimination among Asian and Pacific Islander gay men: their relationship to HIV risk. *AIDS Education and Prevention* 16:68–83.

Wilson, P.A. (2005) The contexts of sexual risk-taking and drug use among Latino men who have sex with men (MSM). Oral presentation given at the American Psychological Association Convention, Washington, DC (April).

Woodyard, J., Peterson, J.L., and Stokes, J. (2000) Let us go into the house of the Lord: participation in African American churches by African American men who have sex with men (MSM). *Journal of Pastoral Care* 54:451–460.

Yoshikawa, H., and Lugo-Gil, J. (2004) How lower-income immigrant parents in New York City learn about and navigate programs and policies for families and children. Presented at the Radcliffe Institute for Advanced Study Conference "The Next Generation: Immigrant Children and Youth in Comparative Perspective." Harvard University, Radcliffe Institute for Advanced Study, Cambridge, MA.

Yoshikawa, H., Wilson, P.A., and Chae, D.H. (2002) Demographic, psychosocial and neighborhood predictors of HIV risk and testing among Asian/Pacific Islander men who have sex with men in the U.S. Poster presentation at the XIV International AIDS Conference, Barcelona.

Yoshikawa, H., Wilson, P.A., Chae, D.H., and Cheng, J. (2004) Do family and friendship networks protect against the influence of discrimination on mental health and HIV risk among Asian and Pacific Islander gay men? *AIDS Education and Prevention* 16:84–100.

Yoshikawa, H., Wilson, P.A., Hsueh, J., Rosman, E.A., Chin, J., and Kim, J.H. (2003) What frontline CBO staff can tell us about culturally anchored theories of behavior change in HIV prevention for Asian/Pacific Islanders. *American Journal of Community Psychology* 32:143–158.

Zimmerman, W., and Tumlin, K.C. (1999) *Patchwork policies: state assistance for immigrants under welfare reform.* The Urban Institute, Washington, DC.

26

Public Health and Trans-People: Barriers to Care and Strategies to Improve Treatment

Emilia Lombardi

1 Introduction

The first half of this chapter is intended to familiarize public health practitioners, researchers, and students with the central issues of concern for an often stigmatized and marginalized group of lesbian, gay, bisexual, and transgender (LGBT) individuals, that is, trans-people. The second half of the chapter suggests ways to improve their health and well-being. Note that use of the terms transgender and transsexual varies from person to person, regardless of a person's desires to use medical resources to transition from one social gender to another. Therefore, throughout this chapter *trans* is used as a shorthand term to refer to transgender and/or transsexual people. I also recognize that there is great diversity among trans-people. This chapter refers most specifically to those who have transitioned socially from one gender to another. When a trans-person does not identify as either a man or a woman, gender-neutral pronouns are used (e.g., sie and hir). I begin with a review of what is known about public health and trans-people from recent studies.

Results published in the peer-reviewed literature have consistently shown that most trans men and women have experienced some form of violence, prejudice, or discrimination. In a recent study, approximately 60% of a sample of trans-people in the United States had experienced some form of harassment and/or violence, and 37% had experienced some form of economic discrimination (Lombardi et al., 2001). In a study conducted in Los Angeles, 30% of a sample of trans-women reported being fired from their jobs, and 29% reported discrimination in housing (Reback et al., 2001a). A San Francisco study found that 83% of trans-women and 85% of trans-men had experienced some form of verbal harassment (Clements, 1999). Furthermore, trans-men experienced more job discrimination than trans-women (57% vs. 46%), whereas trans-women experienced more physical abuse than trans-men (37% vs. 30%) (Clements, 1999). These group-based experiences parallel individual trans-people's experiences in society, including within healthcare systems. Selected vignettes are provided below for further depth of understanding into the issues that trans-people encounter.

A revealing example of healthcare discrimination against a trans-person is the experience of Tyra Hunter (Fernandez, 1998). After being hit by a car, she was refused treatment by the paramedics who responded to the accident once they discovered that she had male genitals. She subsequently died from her injuries, and her mother was awarded $2.9 million in her wrongful death suit. Another trans-person, Leslie Feinberg, previously detailed the discrimination sie received when sie visited the emergency room (Feinberg, 2001). The physician examining hir ordered hir out of the emergency room even though sie had a temperature above 104 degrees, and told hir that hir fever was the result of hir being a very troubled person. Finally, the documentary film entitled *Southern Comfort* followed the last year in the life of Robert Eads. Eads was a trans-man who died of ovarian cancer when his attempts to find a medical provider failed as none of them wanted to treat a transgender patient (Davis, 2001).

Other trans-individuals face similar problems accessing health care. Although overt forms of discrimination such as those just described have been reported, other more insidious factors affect trans-people's access to heath care. Major issues for many trans-people involve having their identities validated and their lives seen as authentic by the people around them. Their appearances, legal identities, or even just the knowledge that a given person is trans may limit access to and the provision of quality care in health care facilities. The basis of discrimination against trans-people lies in social norms that identify individuals as either a man or a woman, as discussed below.

1.1 Genderism and Transphobia

In large part, societal beliefs concerning sex and gender underlie the problems experienced by trans-people. Certain definitions may help clarify the biases experienced by trans-people in society. *Heterosexism* is defined as "an ideological system that denies, denigrates, and stigmatizes any nonheterosexual form of behavior, identity, relationship, or community" (Herek, 1991 pp. 89). *Sexism* refers to the inequality that results when one gender (usually men) has privilege, power, or access to resources over another (usually women), combined with the rigid application of social norms to specific genders and the belief in the existence of two static genders. *Genderism* is defined as the ideology that people's physical sex and psychological, social, and legal genders are linked and binary, and that anything different from this condition is abnormal. Cope and Darke (1999) identified specific beliefs concerning trans-people based in genderism:

Biology is destiny. A person with a penis must be a man, and a person with a vagina must be a woman.
Trans-people are confused, if not mentally ill.
Trans-people are frauds.

Genderism is related to sexism and heterosexism but ought to be considered in addition to, and distinct from, these related forms of bias. All three forms of discrimination concern the changing societal norms with regard to sex, gender, and sexuality and the conflict that occurs between groups of people socially defined (Sakalli, 2002; Guindon et al., 2003). Politically, the groups organized around sexism and heterosexism tend to be allied with one another and against other groups (e.g., feminists and gay rights activists versus social and religious conservatives). Nonetheless, many of the same people who support the human rights of women and LGB individuals believe that physical sex (genitals) and gender are connected and immutable. Genderism lays the foundation for *transphobia*, which is defined as the hatred and unease people have toward those whose gender identity and/or presentation differs from the sex they were assigned at birth (Cope & Darke, 1999).

In sum, genderist rhetoric employs a belief in two distinct sexes and genders (usually ordained by some higher power) and a rigid coupling of biologic sex and social gender. Such rhetoric values a consistent, gendered life as well as a biologic deterministic viewpoint. Many people promote the idea that gender is based on one's physical sex at birth, whereas others focus on socialization. As Mantilla (2000) explains, "As a radical feminist, I believe that gender does not reside for the most part in our bodies—it resides in our heads, where gender socialization occurs." Nonetheless, Mantilla fails to recognize that to be socialized as a man or a woman in society, sie must first be identified via physical characteristics before undergoing distinct forms of socialization. Furthermore, these views fail to allow for individual agency or understanding. Such perspectives are genderist in that they allow for only two genders that are linked unequivocally with one's physical sex and can never be changed. Put another way, they do not allow for a trans-person's own sense of agency, how sie identifies, or how sie reacts to social experiences. Thus, trans-people live under the threat of having their lives devalued or outright negated by those who hold genderist beliefs, which results in transphobia and trans discrimination.

Individuals who voice problems with the appearance of trans-individuals often see them as disruptive and threatening. This is then used as justification to discriminate against trans-people. A legal example of transphobia is dissected below:

Ms. Cormier, in her notes, contemporaneous or otherwise, writes that she had determined that Ms. Nixon, based solely on her appearance, could not remain in the training group. [Reasons For Decision, Nixon v. Vancouver Rape Relief Society, Heather MacNaughton, Tribunal Chair Vancouver, British Columbia, January 17, 2002]

The Vancouver Rape Relief Society argued that because Ms. Nixon was not born female, she does not experience what it means to live as a woman in society, including encountering gender discrimination against women. Thus:

Rape Relief asserts that unless it can decide who is a woman for these purposes, its integrity as an organization devoted to promoting the interests and welfare of women will be so compromised that its right to be such an organization under s. 41 is rendered meaningless. [Vancouver Rape Relief Society v. Nixon et al. 2003 BCSC 1936 (2003)]

In Winchester City, California, a similar battle erupted over who gets to define people's gender but this time from a socially conservative point of view. The California state legislature and governor passed a law protecting trans-people from discrimination. Nonetheless, there were people who disagreed with this change and sought to limit its scope within their school districts.

Acting on a suggestion by Westminster City Councilman Kermit Marsh, he persuaded the board majority to rewrite the district policy in a way that satisfied O'Connell's office while still rejecting the idea that victims of discrimination may determine their own gender. Following Bucher's lead, the three trustees approved language that defines a person's gender as his or her biological sex or, in the case of discrimination, what it was perceived to be by an alleged discriminator. [Rubin, 2004]

The change was eventually allowed in the Winchester City school district. In both of the legal cases presented here, different groups argued that individuals cannot determine their own gender. Both deemed it important to protect certain groups of people from trans-people.

Note that the well-being and safety of trans-people were never considered in these decisions. The chair of the British Columbia Human Rights Tribunal wrote the following:

Following her expulsion from the Rape Relief training, Ms. Nixon said that the healing work that she had done with BWSS was undone and that she felt the same symptoms as she had following her abusive relationship. Her sense of herself and of her identity as a female was undermined. . . . I conclude that the impact of the actions of Rape Relief was exacerbated by the very difficult period of time that Ms. Nixon had experienced just prior to the incident. [MacNaughton, 2002]

Ms. Nixon's experience of transphobia resulted in her experiencing secondary victimization, that is, further victimization even as she was attempting to recover from her initial experience of violence. Ms. Nixon's own experiences of violence were not seen as legitimate by the members of Rape Relief. Similarly, the lives of trans-people were not seen as authentic by the Winchester City school board. The experiences of trans-people in these two legal cases are not uncommon. Many people in society—regardless of their social or political beliefs—do not understand or acknowledge the experiences or lives of trans-people. The idea that one's genital sex can be distinct from one's gender is very difficult for many people to accept, especially people whose beliefs are based on fixed ideas of male and female. It is these sorts of societal views that directly and indirectly affect the health and health care of trans-people.

1.2 Identification of Trans-People

Substantial variation exists in how trans-people choose to self-identify. For instance, Gutierrez (2004) interviewed trans-women of color and found that they resisted being labeled as transgender. While they viewed themselves as young women, they believed that placing themselves in a transgender category denied them authentic identities. As one young trans-woman stated, "We're women. We're not transgendered. We're who we are. That word transgender. It really does irk me" (Gutierrez, 2004, p. 72). The interviewee went on to say, "Transgender makes it sound like I'm a transformer or something, or a toy that could change into something to another. . . . I think if someone's gonna portray themselves as a woman they should be considered as a woman" (Gutierrez, 2004, p. 72). This same woman acknowledged that one reason some organizations seek to classify people like herself as transgender is to provide documentation for funding agencies or for other bureaucratic reasons.

Despite the variation in how trans-people choose to identify, the primary issue they face is that their identities and lives are not accepted in society or are accepted only under specific circumstances. This includes both trans-people who have more radical gendered lives as well as trans-people with more traditional gender identities. Ultimately, most trans-people have to deal with genderism and transphobia in virtually every aspect of their lives, including health care settings. Trans-people are subjected to both interpersonal and structural prejudice and discrimination, which in practice are very difficult to disentangle. In the absence of institutional guidelines, many health care professionals have only their personal beliefs to draw upon and are unprepared to treat trans men and women effectively, often to the detriment of the trans-people.

1.3 Treatment of Trans-People

Homeless and domestic violence shelters are contexts that are often gender-segregated and therefore likely to refuse services to trans-people. Instead of placement in facilities being based on social identities, placement of trans-people in facilities is often based on their genitals. In the case of domestic violence shelters, many trans-women are turned away because their presence is considered threatening to other women (Cope & Darke, 1999). This is done with little regard for the harm and threats that trans-women are experiencing.

A qualitative study conducted in Boston, Massachusetts exposed significant problems that trans-people encountered in accessing health care (GLBT Health Access, 2000). Findings from focus groups with trans-people revealed that health care providers blatantly refused to treat them or even to refer to them as the gender in which they lived their lives. Furthermore, providers were reported to lack the necessary information concerning routine health care of trans-people. From the participants' perspective, trans-people reported a reluctance to identify themselves as trans to their providers for fear of discrimination or over concern that their medical information might be disclosed to other sources (e.g., insurance companies), which might lead to them being denied benefits and entitlements, such as comprehensive health care coverage. In sum, fear of prejudice and discrimination from health care providers were behind many trans-people's reluctance to utilize many types of health care, including human immunodeficiency virus/acquired immunodeficiency syndrome (HIV/AIDS) education.

Focus groups conducted in San Francisco, California examined HIV/AIDS risks and health care issues for trans men and women (San Francisco Department of Public Health, 1997). Consistent with findings from Boston, participants in San Francisco reported problems accessing health care and discriminatory behavior on the part of providers. In particular, participants reported that HIV/AIDS prevention programs did not adequately represent their lives. Self-esteem issues were reported as having strong connections with unsafe sexual practices for trans-people. The need to have their lives and identities accepted was very important—so important that many trans-people placed themselves in risky situations to validate their identities. Some believed that insisting on condom use would lead to their rejection as sexual partners.

Trans-men felt especially invisible with regard to HIV/AIDS prevention programs, as many providers assume that they only have sex with nontrans-women. The reality is that many trans-men are at risk for HIV/AIDS because they identify as gay/bisexual and have sex with men, and/or because they are involved in intravenous drug use. Most HIV/AIDS programs are not explicitly designed for trans-people. Even those that include trans-women often neglect trans-men (Clements, 1999). As in health care settings, HIV/AIDS programs do not acknowledge the full lives of trans-people but focus exclusively on their genitals; for example, trans-women are categorized as men who have sex with men in HIV/AIDS surveillance programs. Again, prejudice and discrimination against trans-people can most often be traced to the notion that biologic sex and social gender are immutably linked.

The criminal justice system offers another setting where genderism and transphobia are institutionalized and result in harm to trans-people. Jails and prisons have policies similar to those of many domestic violence and homeless shelters: if someone has a penis, sie is housed with men, and if someone has a vagina, sie is housed with women, regardless of hir identity or other physical traits. For trans-women, such policies often lead to sexual assault and other forms of violence. When Kelly McAllister, a preoperative transsexual, was arrested for causing a public disturbance, she was placed in protective custody with a nontrans-man, who then sexually assaulted her (Libaw, 2003). If Ms. McAllister had been a postoperative trans-person, she would have been placed in a woman's facility. To be postoperative, however, requires resources (notably money and access to trans-specific services) that many trans-people lack, including those who are arrested for vagrancy if shelters refuse to admit them, prostitution if they cannot obtain other employment, or trespassing if people complain that they are using the wrong restroom.

A study of trans-women in prison found them to be more sexually active than other inmates (Stephens et al., 1999), in part because they trade sex for safety. Given that most prisons do not allow inmates access to condoms, trans-women who exchange sex for protection in prison are at risk for HIV/AIDS infection. With the imminent threat of violence, however, trans-women may not consider HIV/AIDS protection to be a priority.

Even among those who view themselves as accepting of trans-people, their acceptance can be problematic if it fails to encompass the actual lives of trans-people. Social scientists have been charged with using the information they gather about trans-people to support their theoretical viewpoints about gender while ignoring the specific lives of trans-people (Namaste, 2000). Namaste considers such work limited in scope, as it denies trans-people visibility and authenticity. As a case in point, Eyre et al. (2004) conducted a study on the lives of a community of African American male-to-female transgender adolescents and young adults. Although the authors stated that they deferred to their participants' meaning of transgender and used pronouns that their participants preferred in their article, they failed to present the lives of their participants in a manner that allowed them true authenticity. For instance, the authors mentioned that a specific style of dress used by young women in the community "had been *appropriated* (italics mine) as a popular look by transgenders at the time of the study" (Eyre et al., 2004, p. 151). Why *appropriated*? Why didn't the authors instead refer to a style of dress used by all feminine-identified individuals within a specific community? Eyre et al. (2004, p. 166) concluded by stating, "But hormones are not magic wands; both transgender and trade operate under a consensual illusion which may be less and less necessary to sustain as homophobia in the contextualizing culture diminishes." Their conclusion ignores the possibility—indeed likelihood—that their participants were expressing an identity that is as real to them as it is to other young women rather than a mechanism to protect themselves from homophobia.

1.4 Other Forms of Bias Against Trans-People

Knowledge about trans-people has greatly increased in recent years in the United States and other societies through books written by trans-people (see especially, *She's Not There: A Life in Two Genders*, by Jennifer Finney Boylan) and sympathetic representations of trans-people on television, radio, and other media. Such exposure can cause problems by creating a specific image of trans-people. Instead, trans-people have varied risks and experiences. Whereas the same social forces that affect nontrans-people also affect trans-people, such forces can both exacerbate and ameliorate the impact of transphobia on people's lives. Two primary stereotypes of trans-people exist: one of a white, middle-class, older trans-woman and the other of a young trans-woman of color involved in sex work. Trans-men are not usually thought about in discussions of transsexual or transgender issues. Even within trans-activism, much of the rhetoric comes explicitly from a U.S. perspective with its orientation toward a consumer health model (Namaste, 2000). Even studies that examine the health of trans-people (primarily trans-women) find that not all trans-people have the same risks, as discussed below.

Whereas trans-women have high reported prevalence rates of HIV/AIDS infection, trans-women of color, especially African American trans-women, have reported rates as high as 60% (Clements-Nolle et al., 2001; Reback, 2001b; Nemoto et al., 2004). An explanation for this finding is that, in addition to transphobia, many trans-people have to deal with racism, poverty, and other oppressions due to social structures and biases. Furthermore, access to both trans- and nontrans-related health care resources are curtailed for many trans-people because they cannot afford it or because facilities are biased against trans-people who do not fit a specific social image. Trans-women who are shunted to the margins of society may become involved in sex work as a way to earn their incomes, but this may hinder their access to even trans-related services because of biases against providing services to sex workers (Namaste, 2000).

A geographic bias also exists in that most services for trans-people exist in large cities. Those who live in rural areas are likely to face significant barriers to accessing any kind of health care, as per the experiences Robert Eads, which were thoughtfully documented in the film *Southern Comfort*. A political factor to consider at the national level is how a country's health care system is structured. Namaste (2000) analyzes how trans-activism mirrors the consumer-based health system in the United States. The U.S. focus on services on demand ignores those without the resources to purchase health care. Countries with nationalized health systems have other institutionalized forms of discrimination against trans-people. For instance, Namaste (2000) found that one type of gender clinic in Canada imposes a harsh system of rules and regulations on trans-people, with health care providers demonstrating exploitive behavior.

In sum, health care for most trans-people—especially those who are poor—is lacking for the reasons discussed above as well as others. The end result is that many trans-people either choose to go without health care or find alternatives to formal systems of care. An underground distribution of hormones and other services exist that trans-people use to shape their bodies to better resemble the gender in which they identify, but these alternatives may have other costs. In particular, sex hormones can be toxic at high levels; without medical supervision, their use can lead to serious health problems. Trans-people may also be at risk for HIV/AIDS infection through the sharing of needles and injecting equipment when administering hormones (Bockting et al., 1998; Nemoto et al., 1999; Sebastian, 1999; Wiessing et al., 1999). Trans-people have resorted to using back alley surgeons or cutting themselves out of desperation because they cannot access or afford health care (Murphy et al., 2001; Press, 1998). Trans-women have utilized liquid silicone to alter their bodies as a cheaper alternative to plastic surgery but often face serious health consequences as a result of this practice (Wiessing et al., 1999; Davis, 2004; Fox et al., 2004; Gaber, 2004; Rosioreanu et al.,

2004). Despite these risks, trans-people utilize alternative avenues rather than traditional health care services because they are less expensive, less discriminatory, and lack gate-keeping mechanisms.

I believe it is a mistake to base health and social policy on an image of a specific trans-person in the media or on a particular stereotype of a trans-person. For example, Jennifer Finney Boylan, the author of *She's Not There: A Life in Two Genders*, is in a privileged position both socially and economically, which no doubt abetted her transition from one gender to another. Few other trans-people have her resources. Health and social policy must be based instead on the range of resources available to most of the population. Requiring trans-people to have had expensive, difficult-to-attain medical procedures only adds to the problems experienced by those who are socially and economically disadvantaged. More supportive health and social policy will better enable trans-people to attain their goals of social integration without placing their lives at risk.

2 Summary and Solutions

As I have previously described, genderism is related to sexism and heterosexism. Together, these three forms of bias represent assumptions about gender, sex, and sexuality that are currently operating in the United States and other societies to oppress people, specifically trans-people. Genderism refers to how a person is ascribed a gender and to the response people have to any individual who fails to fit within their normative understanding of men and women. Genderism results in the policing of gender identities and expression. All members of society—not only trans-people—are constantly evaluated based on whether they look or act in a manner that is consistent with the gender they are identify as or present as. As entrenched as genderism might seem within the United States and other societies, the problems trans-people experience as a result of genderism are not insurmountable. What follows are some suggested solutions.

2.1 Identifying Trans-People

A first issue with which healthcare workers and organizations need to grapple when serving trans-people concerns labeling. In this chapter, I use trans as a short-hand notation for transgender and transsexual, even as this terminology may not be acceptable to everyone, especially when referring to a broad group of people (Valentine, 2002, 2003). Although the term transgender is generally accepted as a political label, is not widely accepted as an individual label. Gutierrez (2004) presented four young women who were transitioning from male to female and do not refer to themselves as transgender, but as women. Other recent studies have likewise found that many people who transition from male to female identify as women and not as transgender or even transsexual (Clements-Nolle et al., 2001; Reback, 2001b).

The connection with sexuality is equally problematic, as different groups identify in different ways. Valentine (2002) referred to one woman who identified as being gay (attracted to men), whereas Gutierrez (2004) referred to a young woman who identified as a lesbian (attracted to women). Both were identified as male at birth, both identified as women, both claimed to be homosexual, yet they were oriented toward different genders. Although this complexity does not mean that labels such as transgender, transsexual, or even trans cannot be used, it does mean that these labels are imprecise and should not be used to deny the identities and lives of anyone, including those seeking healthcare services.

Given a choice of male/man or female/woman, some people may make their decision based on how they identify (how they want staff to treat them), whereas others may base their decision on their current legal sex status. It is important for health care providers to decide what information is actually needed (e.g., identity, legal sex, genital status) and to be explicit and consistent in asking everyone for the required information, not only those they think might be trans-people. An explicit, open-ended option for any sex/gender information requested would be helpful, as it would allow people to be specific about their sex/gender status. Regardless, most people want to be referred to as the gender they are presenting as, and thus health care providers ought to use gendered pronouns based on the person's gender presentation. When in doubt, it is respectful to ask people politely which pronoun they prefer be used when referring to them.

2.2 Housing and Bathroom Facilities

Gender segregation creates problems for trans-people. In large part, the concern is whether trans-women can be housed with nontrans-women. As mentioned previously, conflict has resulted over the inclusion/exclusion of trans-women with other women in homeless, criminal justice, and bathroom facilities, even as the situation has also been described for substance-use treatment facilities and domestic violence shelters (Cope & Darke, 1999; Lombardi & vanServellen, 2000).

A spokesperson for a homeless shelter explained, "We can certainly handle inappropriate behaviour that might be aggression or alcoholism or anger management or those types of things. It's the other behaviour that relates to women feeling uncomfortable around pre-operative transgender clients, related to sexuality, that is the issue for us" (Benzie, 2004). Nonetheless, this same individual also stated, "Post-operative transgender women would continue to be welcomed at the centres" (Benzie, 2004). The main issue for most facilities is how to accommodate trans-women who have not had genital surgery, even as those in need of shelters seldom possess the resources for genital surgery.

While the previous discussion seems to imply that trans-women are somehow threatening to other women, the real issue may well be the shock that people experience when they discover that trans-people do not have the genitals they are expected to have. Two related issues that are all too often overlooked are the safety of trans-women in men's facilities and how best to accommodate trans-men in gender-segregated facilities (Libaw, 2003).

Solutions to accommodate trans-people may take many forms. An important principle underlying all of them is to acknowledge that trans-people are welcome and work with them to accommodate their needs rather than stigmatize them. There is no a priori reason to assume that trans-people behave any differently than nontrans-people. Thus, existing regulations concerning harassment and violence are adequate to deal with most situations involving trans-people as well as nontrans-people. Trans-people choose to use whatever facilities respect their gendered lives and are safe for them. In instances where assimilation is not possible or is unsafe for trans-people, alternatives include designating a private area for trans-people to sleep and creating gender-neutral bathrooms and shower areas. If bathroom and shower facilities are limited, staff might establish specific times to allow trans-people to use these facilities.

Trans-people ought to be expected to follow standard codes of appearance, but requiring them to wear any particular clothing or appear in any manner contrary to their gender identity is very distressing to them and may create or exacerbate existing problems. In other words, it is possible for trans-people to respect dress codes without the requirement that they appear as the gender associated with their biologic sex.

2.3 Education and Training of Staff

I believe it is critically important for all health personnel—administrative, research, and clinical staff alike—to be educated on trans issues, including transgenderism, transsexualism, and cross-dressing. Ambiguity causes problems for trans-people in health care settings. Thus, staff ought to be explicitly trained in how to deal with trans-people so they respect their identities and lives. In some geographic areas, there may be people available to conduct trans-issue education and training for staff at low or no cost. There may also be opportunities at professional meetings to provide trans-issue education and training to public health professionals and students. Furthermore, information is available on the Internet (Table 1) and published in peer-reviewed journals and books that can inform health care professionals about respectful strategies to ensure the safe inclusion of trans-people in health services.

Clients also need to respect the rights of trans-people. It is thus essential for health care providers to ensure that trans-people are treated fairly in their agencies and to make it known that discrimination against any client would not be tolerated. One strategy is to write and post nondiscrimination policies that refer to gender identity and expression and encompass a range of identities and behaviors among trans-people.

Table 1. Online Resource List for Trans Issues

Organization	Web site	Mission
The National Center for Transgender Equality (NCTE)	www.nctequality.org	A 501(c)3 social justice organization dedicated to advancing the equality of transgender people through advocacy, collaboration, and empowerment
Tom Waddell Health Center Transgender Team	www.dph.sf.ca.us/chn/HlthCtrs/ HlthCtrDocs/TransGendprotocols. pdf	To outline the clinic's protocol regarding the administration of hormones
Trans-Health	www.trans-health.com/	To provide an online magazine of health and fitness for transsexual and transgender people
Transgender Resource and Neighborhood Space (TRANS)	www.caps.ucsf.edu/TRANS/	To provide culturally and gender-appropriate substance abuse intervention, HIV prevention, and mental health services to transgender people in San Francisco
Gender Identity Project— New York LGBT Center	www.gaycenter.org/ program_folders/gip	To offer transgender-identified people an opportunity to discover who they are and to build communities in an atmosphere of self-acceptance
If You Are Concerned about Your Child's Gender Behaviors: A Parent Guide (educational booklet)	www.dcchildrens.com/dcchildrens/ about/subclinical/subneuroscience/ subgender/guide.aspx	To provide a resource for parents who want information and advice on a child with gender-variant behaviors
Transgender Law and Policy Institute	www.transgenderlaw.org/index.htm	A non-profit organization dedicated to engaging in effective advocacy for transgender people in our society
Trans Accessibility Project: Making Women's Shelters Accessible to Transgendered Women	http://www.queensu.ca/ humanrights/tap/	A manual to assist shelters for abused women make the changes required to provide transgender women with the respectful and supportive services (also useful for other settings involving housing and facilities usage)

In conclusion, it is important to communicate to trans-people that they are welcome within one's agency, as many have come to expect negative treatment from agency staff and clients. Having information available that states the agency's support for trans-people and gender variance helps convey to trans-people that they are in a safe space. Ensuring that health educational materials refer explicitly to trans-people helps overcome biases against them and ensures they are no longer invisible to staff, other clients, and society at large.

References

Benzie, T. (2004) *Charity bans trannies*. Retrieved August 15, 2004 from http://www.ssonet.com.au/display.asp?ArticleID=3406.

Bockting, W.O., Robinson, B.E., and Rosser, B.R. (1998) Transgender HIV prevention: a qualitative needs assessment. *AIDS Care* 10:505–525.

Clements, K. (1999) *The Transgender Community Health Project: descriptive results*. San Francisco Department of Public Health, San Francisco.

Clements-Nolle, K., Marx, R., Guzman, R., and Katz, M. (2001) HIV prevalence, risk behaviors, health care use, and mental health status of transgender persons: implications for public health intervention. *American Journal of Public Health* 91:915–921.

Cope, A., and Darke, J. (1999) *Trans accessibility project*. Violence Intervention and Education Workgroup, Ontario, Canada.

Davis, K. (2001) On *Southern Comfort*. HBO Theatrical Documentary.

Davis, K. (2004) Woman charged with injecting silicone into trans people. Retrieved August 6, 2004, from http://www.planetout.com/news/article.html?2004/08/06/2.

Eyre, S.L., Guzman, R.D., Donovan, A.A., and Boissiere, C. (2004) Hormones is not magic wands: ethnography of a transgender scene in Oakland, California. *Ethnography* 5:147–172.

Feinberg, L. (2001) Trans health crisis: for us it's life or death. *American Journal of Public Health* 91:897–900.

Fernandez, M.E. (1998) Death suit costs city $2.9 million; mother of transgendered man wins case. *Washington Post*, December 12, p. C1.

Fox, L.P., Geyer, A.S., Husain, S., Della-Latta, P., and Grossman, M.E. (2004) Mycobacterium abscessus cellulitis and multifocal abscesses of the breasts in a transsexual from illicit intramammary injections of silicone. *Journal of the American Academy of Dermatology* 50:450–454.

Gaber, Y. (2004) Secondary lymphoedema of the lower leg as an unusual side-effect of a liquid silicone injection in the hips and buttocks. *Dermatology* 208:342–344.

GLBT Health Access. (2000) *Access to health care for transgendered persons in greater Boston*. JSI Research and Training Institute, Boston.

Guindon, M.H., Green, A.G., and Hanna, F.J. (2003) Intolerance and psychopathology: toward a general diagnosis for racism, sexism, and homophobia. *American Journal of Orthopsychiatry* 73:167–176.

Gutierrez, N. (2004) Resisting fragmentation, living whole: four female transgender students of color speak about school. *Journal of Gay & Lesbian Social Services* 16:69–79.

Herek, G.M. (1991) The social context of hate crimes: notes on cultural heterosexism. In: Berrill, K.T. (ed) *Hate crimes: confronting violence against lesbians and gay men*. Sage, Newbury Park, CA, pp. 89–104.

Libaw, O. (2003) *Gender dilemma: inmates who look like women, housed with men.* Retrieved January 23, from http://www.abcnews.go.com/sections/us/ DailyNews/transgender030122.html.

Lombardi, E.L., and vanServellen, G. (2000) Building culturally sensitive substance use prevention and treatment programs for transgendered populations. *Journal of Substance Abuse Treatment* 19:291–296.

Lombardi, E.L., Wilchins, R.A., Priesing, D., and Malouf, D. (2001) Gender violence: transgender experiences with violence and discrimination. *Journal of Homosexuality* 42(1):89–101.

MacNaughton, H. (2002) *Nixon v. Vancouver Rape Relief Society, 2002 BCHRT 1,* retrieved from http://www.bchrt.gov.bc.ca/nixon_v__vancouver_rape__ relief_society_2002_bchrt_1.htm.

Mantilla, K. (2000) *Men in ewes' clothting: the stealth politics of the transgender movement.* Retrieved August 22, 2004 from http://www.rapereliefshelter. bc.ca/issues/menewes.html.

Murphy, D., Murphy, M., and Grainger, R. (2001) Self-castration. *Irish Journal of Medical Science* 170:195.

Namaste, V.K. (2000) *Invisible lives: the erasure of transsexual and transgendered people.* University of Chicago Press, Chicago.

Nemoto, T., Luke, D., Mamo, L., Ching, A., and Patria, J. (1999) HIV risk behaviours among male-to-female transgenders in comparison with homosexual or bisexual males and heterosexual females. *AIDS Care* 11:297–312.

Nemoto, T., Operario, D., Keatley, J., Han, L., and Soma, T. (2004) HIV risk behaviors among male-to-female transgender persons of color in San Francisco. *American Journal of Public Health* 94:1193–1199.

Press, T.A. (1998) *Former doctor charged with murder is accused of shoddy surgeries.* Retrieved October 15, 2004.

Reback, C.J., Simon, P.A., Bemis, C.C., and Gatson, B. (2001a) The Los Angeles transgender health study: community report. Unpublished manuscript, West Hollywood.

Reback, C.J., Simon, P.A., Bemis, C.C., and Gatson, B. (2001b) *The Los Angeles transgender health study: community report.* Van Ness Recovery House: Prevention Division, Los Angeles.

Rosioreanu, A., Brusca-Augello, G.T., Ahmed, Q.A., and Katz, D.S. (2004) CT visualization of silicone-related pneumonitis in a transsexual man. *AJR American Journal of Roentgenology* 183:248–249.

Rubin, J. (2004) New O.C. school lawyer's big win; Westminster trustees hired Mark Bucher to fight a rule offending their religious views. *Los Angeles Times,* April 21, p. 1.

Sakalli, N. (2002) The relationship between sexism and attitudes toward homosexuality in a sample of Turkish college students. *Journal of Homosexuality* 42(3):53–64.

San Francisco Department of Public Health. (1997) *HIV prevention and health service needs of the transgender community in San Francisco: results from eleven focus groups.* San Francisco Department of Public Health, AIDS Office, San Francisco.

Sebastian, C. (1999) Transgenderism and the AIDS epidemic. *Posit Aware* 10(3):57.

Stephens, T., Cozza, S., and Braithwaite, Rl. (1999) Transsexual orientation in HIV risk behaviours in an adult male prison. *International Journal of STD and AIDS* 10(1):28–31.

Valentine, D. (2002) We're "not about gender": the uses of "transgender." In: Lewin, E., and Leap, W.L. (eds) *Out in theory: the emergence of lesbian and gay anthropology.* University of Illinois Press, Chicago. pp. 222–245.

Valentine, D. (2003) The calculus of pain: violence, anthropological ethics, and the category transgender. *Ethnos* 68(1):27–48.

Vancouver Rape Relief Society v. Nixon et al. (2003) BCSC 1936, http://www.courts.gov.bc.ca/Jdb-txt/SC/03/19/2003BCSC1936.htm (Supreme Court of British Columbia 2003).

Wiessing, L.G., van Roosmalen, M.S., Koedijk, P., Bieleman, B., and Houweling, H. (1999) Silicones, hormones and HIV in transgender street prostitutes. *AIDS* 13:2315–2316.

HIV Prevention and Care for Gay, Lesbian, Bisexual, and Transgender Youths: "Best Practices" from Existing Programs and Policies

Joyce Hunter and Jan Baer

1 Introduction

A public health crisis in the United States is affecting youths, including gay, lesbian, bisexual, and transgender (GLBT) youths. At least half of the newly infected cases of human immunodeficiency virus (HIV) infection are under the age of 25. More than 126,000 young people have developed acquired immunodeficiency syndrome (AIDS) in their twenties (CDC, 2001a). The rate of HIV infection and high-risk behaviors among youth must be lowered. This can only be accomplished with a coordinated effort at community, state, and national levels to provide prevention and a continuum of care, from counseling, testing, and referral (CTRS) to therapeutic counseling and behavioral change prevention programs. The focus for public health has been keeping HIV-negative individuals negative. Now HIV-positive youth are also being targeted (Futterman et al., 2001).

1.1 Youth Vulnerability

The GLBT youths are among the most vulnerable. Sexual development in youths is integral to personal identity development (Udry, 1998), often proceeding more rapidly than cognition and the skills to handle sexual urges safely. Drug use, frequent in the teen years, can lead to lowered inhibitions and risky sexual behaviors (Hunter & Mallon, 1998). GLB youth are at risk for HIV infection, not only because of the high prevalence of HIV among potential sexual partners but also because of heterosexism and homophobia, causing them to hide their orientation and behavior, distorting the developmental processes, and creating isolation and related stresses and behaviors (Havens, 2002).

Young Black men who sleep with men (MSM) are now the population most highly affected (CDC, 2001b). In the Young Men's Survey, HIV infection was high among African Americans (6.3%), mixed or other (4.8%), and Latinos/as (2.3%). Unprotected sex during the prior

6 months was high (41%), and only 18% of the HIV-positive young men knew they were positive before participation in the study (Valleroy et al., 2000). One-fourth of this group reported having had unprotected sexual relations with both men and women, putting themselves and their partners at risk (CDC, 2000).

In a state-wide high school survey, 32% of sexually active GLBT youth reported they had been or had gotten someone pregnant compared with 12% of sexually active heterosexual youth (Massachusetts Department of Education, 1995). Many also report having sex with older partners (AIDS Action Council, 2001).

Youths of color who are LGB confront a tricultural experience: membership in their ethnic/racial community, the lesbian/gay community, and in the larger society (Hunter, 1995). To sustain themselves in three communities requires an enormous effort (Chau, 1989). Gender inequalities in society contribute to the risk for young women, including lack of access to information, decreased power to negotiate protection with partners, and unprotected sex without consent (Wingood & DiClemente, 2000).

Youths who identify as transgender have often been rejected by family, peers, and social institutions, including health care providers; as a result they have high levels of homelessness and denial of employment and education. Moreover, a largely hidden population, they often underutilize medical and social services (Israel & Tarver, 1997). Most HIV prevention messages do not reach, or are ignored by, transgender youth as not applicable to them (Dugan, 1998).

HIV-positive youth, including those who do not know their status, are at risk for secondary infection and for emotional and behavioral problems, including unsafe sexual and drug behaviors (Nicholas & Abrams, 2002). Youths who live in high-HIV incidence areas are also at risk, as are partners of HIV-positive youths (Hays et al., 1997).

1.2 Societal Influences on Sexual Health of Youths

Communities, parents, schools, religious institutions, and faith-based social services teach and influence youths. The law restricts or allows schools to teach sexual health, and funding influences what is taught (i.e., recent federal funding for abstinence-only-until-marriage curriculum). Health care professionals have opportunities, at regular checkups or times of health crisis, to address these issues with the youths (Hunter et al., 2005).

Peer influence among young people has been well documented, including pressure to engage in risk behaviors (Paikoff et al., 1997). Young people are also spending time on the Internet. Among young people ages 10 to 17, who use the Internet on a regular basis, one-fifth had been exposed to unwanted sexual solicitations or approaches through the Internet (Finkelhor et al., 2000).

1.3 Barriers to Successful HIV Prevention and Care Efforts

Major barriers to youths' access to care are lack of knowledge and discomfort among providers about the levels of risk behaviors in their clients and the need for raising issues, as well as social isolation in hard-to-reach youth populations (Surgeon General, 2001). No provision is made to take sexual and drug histories, inquire about level of risk, or suggest counseling and testing for HIV at many medical centers and clinics where youths go for regular or crisis care. For example, in a New York City study assessing health care of GLBT youths, only 17% were asked by a provider about their sexual identity, and 18% reported being afraid to tell a physician about their sexuality (Hunter et al., 2001).

It is difficult to link youths to CTRS and the follow-up services they need (Forum for Collaborative HIV Research, 2001). There is poor communication among providers, inability or lack of funding by agencies to provide the services needed, lack of vital drug treatment services, agency staff turnover, and a lack of trust by clients. Many at-risk youths are being overlooked.

Many who are diagnosed are not in care, and many are not diagnosed until AIDS symptoms appear (Forum for Collaborative HIV Research, 2001). The long incubation period of the virus adds to the general lack of awareness of HIV as a public health crisis among youth populations. At-risk youth may have survival stresses, or they may not know where to access youth-friendly testing and care (Kaiser Family Foundation, 2005). Lack of confidential testing, issues of partner notification, lack of health insurance, and mental health problems as a result of the virus, the diagnosis, and/or co-occurring factors (i.e., depression, substance abuse, sexual compulsivity, history of violence) are barriers to prevention and care (Havens et al., 2002).

Discrimination and stigmatization of HIV-positive individuals in rural areas is high. They often face poverty, isolation, lack of confidentiality, resources (i.e., transportation), and lack of accessible youth-friendly or GLBT-friendly health care services (National Association of Social Workers, or NASW, 2002). School sexuality education often begins too late, before initiation of sexual and drug-using behaviors that put them at risk for HIV (Bachanas et al., 2002). Most parents want comprehensive sex education (Sexuality Information and Education Council of the United States, or SIECUS, 2004).

School-based sex education and condom availability programs do not increase sexual activity among adolescents (Institute of Medicine, 2000). High numbers of youths begin sexual activity between 12 and 14 years of age (MARS Project, 2000), and many sexual health programs focus only on abstinence and delay of sexual activity. These programs are unrealistic and developmentally inappropriate (Hunter & Mallon, 1998). One study found that adolescent females who completed the abstinence-only program had more unsafe sexual behaviors than those who had completed an abstinence-plus program (Jemmott et al., 1998).

Effective outreach and care services for youths require extensive funding and programming to have an effect client behaviors. Government entities funding HIV prevention and care programs for youths now mandate or strongly recommend adoption of theory-based programs that have "demonstrated effectiveness" through randomized, controlled trials (RCTs). Several are included in the CDC's Compendium of Effective Interventions (CDC, 2001a), and a few, such as

Diffusion of Effective Behavioral Interventions (DEBI) (CDC, 2004), are being disseminated. Technical assistance is provided, but defined outcomes are expected, requiring capacity building in already underfunded agencies (Gilliam et al., 2003).

2 Best Program Principles: Intervention Theories

Intervention theories, based on beliefs, methods, and procedures that have been scientifically studied, help providers frame their programs and design evaluations. Although there are limitations to their proven effectiveness across settings, theories are an important beginning for developing programs to respond to community needs. Theories can apply to structural and policy levels, community-level collaboration, and program development processes, as well as to specific intervention programs for youths (i.e., individual counseling or group workshops). Several of the most widely accepted theories are described here (Gandelman & Freedman, 2002). No one theory or intervention is best for all young people or a specific population (Yoshikawa et al., 2003). Interventions often have many components, targeting by age, gender, sexual orientation, sexual experience, culture/ethnicity, behavioral risk, or even neighborhood (AIDS Action Council, 2001).

Adolescents need to personalize general knowledge into behavior change and develop skills to negotiate safer sex and change their risky sex or drug behaviors (Hunter & Schaecher, 1992). Behavioral change theories provide ideas on how and why young people can change their behavior (Herlocher et al., 1995). To be effective, individual or clinical approaches must take into account the contextual, relational, and interpersonal components that will make up the experience for its participants (Rapkin & Trickett, 2005). Following are several theories useful in various steps for providing effective programs for GLBT youths.

2.1 Social Support/Social Networks Theory

The social support/social networks theory refers to aid and assistance received from social relationships and support (Glanz et al., 1997). Lista Para Accion (Long Beach, CA), a skills-based program for Latino gay men, is based on social support and cognitive theories (Buitron et al., 1998).

2.2 Diffusion of Innovation Theory

The diffusion of innovations theory provides guidelines for the development and dissemination of programs into a community (Rogers, 1995). It has been found useful for developing, adopting, and disseminating intervention programs. Rogers' theory states that (1) peers who adopt an innovation can become social models whose behavior tends to be imitated by others; (2) adoptable prevention packages should meet successful diffusion standards: advantageous, compatible, simple, testable, and observable; (3) reinvention should be expected, encouraged, and assisted; and (4) change agents should have characteristics similar to those of individuals expected to adopt the innovation.

Popular opinion leaders serve as role models and can spread new ideas, a model developed by Kelly and colleagues at the Center for AIDS Intervention Research (CAIR), Medical College of Wisconsin, are a part of this theory (Rogers, 1995; Kelly, 2000).

2.3 Theory of Reasoned Action

The theory of reasoned action emphasizes intention as key to behavioral change. Developed by Ajzen and Fishbein, this theory assumes that people are rational and make systematic use of information available to them, considering their actions before they decide to or not to engage in certain behaviors. The theory of planned behavior was developed to account for behavior not fully within a person's control and includes the necessary component of belief in one's ability and opportunity to control the particular behavior (self-efficacy) (Fishbein & Middlestadt, 1989).

2.4 Theory of Gender and Power

The theory of gender and power views power dynamics, with gender roles as structures that produce inequalities and increase women's vulnerability to HIV. Developed by Connell, this social structure theory is based on sexual inequality and gender and power imbalances in divisions of labor and power, activities in which one is emotionally invested (cathexis) (Wingood & DiClemente, 2000).

2.5 Stages of Change

The transtheoretical model describes four transitions: precontemplation to contemplation, contemplation to preparation, preparation to action, and action to maintenance. This intervention combines individual (clinical) and population (public health) perspectives. Many interventions focus on the preparation–action transition, but some individuals are not be ready for that stage. This model has been used successfully for smoking cessation interventions and other health education activities, and it is being adapted for programs with youths in HIV prevention (Velicer et al., 1995).

2.6 Social Cognitive Theory/Cognitive Behavior Model

The social cognitive theory/cognitive behavior model includes both adopting behavior seen modeled (social learning theory) (Rogers, 1995) and self-efficacy—confidence that the person will be able to use that behavior in new settings (Bandura, 1994.) Skills-based training appears to be more effective than standard education (St. Lawrence et al., 1995). Components of this model are as follows: (1) information designed to increase awareness and knowledge of behavior consequences; (2) social and self-regulative skills development to act on that knowledge; (3) practice, with feedback, to build skills and self-efficacy; and (4) changes in social norms and social supports for behavior change

(Woods, 1998). The protection motivation theory (PMT), a social cognitive theory, uses cost-and-reward constructs to explain how intentions are formed to respond to threats in adaptive or maladaptive ways. Self-efficacy is balanced with barriers to form a response to a potential threat in an adaptive or a maladaptive manner (Stanton et al., 1996).

2.7 Health Belief Model

On the individual level, the health belief model includes the need for individuals to believe (1) they are at risk for a certain condition; (2) the condition is very serious; (3) there are benefits to changing behavior to avoid the condition; (4) The individual can understand and overcome barriers to change; (5) sufficient reason (i.e., symptoms of a close friend, intervention messages); and (6) self-confidence to make the changes necessary (Rosenstock et al., 1994).

2.8 Interpersonal Psychotherapy

Interpersonal psychotherapy (IPT), is a time-limited treatment for major depression. It has been tested and modified for various age groups, including youths, with various mental health issues internationally. As a promising treatment for depressed adolescents, it has been recommended for HIV-positive youths, most of whom have major mental health issues as a result of their diagnosis and co-occurring factors (Weissman, 1997).

2.9 Empowerment Education Theory

The empowerment education theory focus on the identification and discussion of problems for joint agreement and action (Wallerstein, 1992).

2.10 Harm Reduction Theory

The harm reduction theory is often used in drug treatment programs whose goal is to reduce negative effects of harmful behavior through a process of behavioral change (Brettle, 1991). Harm reduction can be utilized with users who do not seek traditional drug treatment options or in whom these treatments have been unsuccessful.

3 Best Processes in HIV Prevention and Care

"Both individual and community interventions are needed to defeat the epidemic in America's youth" (Kelly, 2000). Individual level interventions can change behavior but may not be sufficiently powerful for youth in populations with high prevalence of HIV infection, where there are complex needs and negative group norms (Green, 2001). Timing of interventions for youth readiness also matters. They are most effective when they reach the youths before they initiate sexual and drug-using behaviors that put them at risk for HIV (CDC, 1998). Also, HIV-positive youths need time to cope with their diagnosis. Counselors can assist them to determine readiness, the need for counseling, and referral to follow-up care (Crosby et al., 2000). Agencies serving GLBT youth typically offer multiple services to respond to complex client needs. Continuum of care for HIV-positive and at-risk youths cannot be done realistically by one program or one agency alone (Wandersman & Florin, 2003).

3.1 Focus on the Service Provider

Public health efforts must support the service provider in the local community. Often in collaboration with the local health department and other service providers, they are the first to see new populations, recognize new needs, and respond to the needs of their client populations.

3.1.1 Role of Agencies in the Community

Agencies must define their unique role in the community based on the needs of the community to build the groundwork for internal review and establishing relationships with other providers. Components of this planning process include needs assessment of the agency and client populations, defining program goals, planning for case management, program development and implementation, staff training and support, involvement of volunteers, and outreach activities.

3.1.2 Cultural Competence

Cultural competence is essential at both agency and community levels. Culturally appropriate refers to an unbiased attitude and an organizational policy that values cultural diversity in the population served. Cultural competence reflects an understanding of diverse attitudes, beliefs, behaviors, practices, and communication patterns that could be attributed to race, ethnicity, religion, socioeconomic status, historical and social context, physical or mental ability, age, gender, sexual orientation, or generational and acculturation status. It includes awareness that cultural differences may affect health and the effectiveness of health care delivery (Healthy People 2010, 1999; Multicultural Competency Self-Assessments, 2001a,b).

Cultural competence for staff in schools and community programs working with GLBT youths includes examining one's own values and biases, training on knowledge of the needs of GLBT youths, providing inclusive programs, comprehensive sexual health education, and community resources. Challenging homophobic remarks and advocating for GLBT youths are essential (Monahan, 1997).

3.1.3 Capacity

The local service provider must have resources to respond to this crisis. Within agencies, money, staff, time, and space are considered the main barriers to implementation of research-based risk-reduction interventions in agencies (DiFranceisco et al., 1999). Local communities can bring resources (i.e., information campaigns, funds, volunteers) to assist agencies. Local health departments, medical and social service provider collaborations, and state and federal agencies all play key roles in the fight against HIV by providing funding, training, and technical assistance to service providers. Whether initiated from local communities or from the "top down," these partnerships can assist in developing a successful continuum of care (Forum for Collaborative HIV Research, 2001). The CDC's intervention checklist is an example of a resource for local programs (CDC, 2001a).

Capacity building involves obtaining funding and services to strengthen the agency to achieve its mission. Many agencies serving LGBT youth have been created to address the issues of isolation and stigmatization that this population often experiences in the larger community. These community agencies vary in their capacity to respond to tight resources and changing requirements of funding agencies for accountability and outcomes. Capacity building includes both assistance from outside resources and developing capacity within and increasing agency staff skills in participation with other agencies, such as governmental and research institutions, in relation to programming and evaluation (Miller et al., 2003).

3.1.4 Needs Assessment Process

Decision making based on sound needs assessment is key to responding to client needs and developing, improving, or expanding the HIV/AIDS continuum of care. Results can be used by service providers/community-based organizations (CBOs), health departments, and advocates to improve programs and secure funding (Health Resources & Services Administration, or HRSA, 1998). Components of a needs assessment include gathering data from a variety of sources, both quantitative (i.e., epidemiologic data, questionnaires, agency databases) and qualitative (i.e., focus groups, key informants, community forums); analyzing the information to determine the current status and unmet needs of a defined population or geographic area and the resources available (HRSA, 1998); and active participation from the client populations, CBOs, and other community representatives. These components lay the groundwork for future planning and community acceptance.

When adopting an intervention program developed by others, areas of focus include identifying possible programs, examining characteristics of the current client population compared to populations of the original intervention (i.e., culture, risk behaviors), characteristics of the intervention (i.e., key components, appropriateness to population needs, feasibility), characteristics of the agency (i.e., mission, level of commitment, motivation for new program), implementation (i.e., balancing fidelity with tailoring to the current population) (Goldstein, 2001).

3.1.5 Program Development

Agencies wishing to adopt interventions need organizational support, appropriate staffing, and sufficient resources for adoption, adaptation and implementation, program support, and evaluation (CDC, 2001a). Implementation of individual and group interventions with youths involves collaboration with research for development, adoption, and adaptation of HIV intervention programs for specific populations (AIDS Action Council, 2001). Examples of model programs and their theory bases are discussed below.

3.1.6 Outreach

Innovative ways must be found to reach out successfully to at-risk or isolated youths residing in areas served by the agency. Outreach and youth involvement are vital to effective programs. GLBT peers can serve on the agency's Board and can act as advisors in program development and implementation and as outreach workers and peer educators, with incentives ranging from expenses paid to full time, paid positions. Including the youths' perspectives and ideas during program development and implementation increase the program's ability to reach these youths successfully (Rosenfeld et al., 2000). Empowerment, including peer-based programs, include shared leadership and collective decision-making, development of a group identity, skills development, and participation in important group tasks (Minkler, 1997). Adult mentoring is an additional way to empower GLBT youths.

3.1.7 Advocacy

Advocacy, a key to continuation and dissemination of programs for youths, is needed at both the agency and community levels. GLBT youths have few advocates. This is also true for HIV-positive youth (HRSA, 1997). The advocate role must be part of staff training. Local organizations can advocate for comprehensive sexuality and HIV prevention education in their local schools. If not successful, they can offer the programs themselves. They can outreach to out-of-school youths, who are at higher risk than in-school youths (Harper & DiCarlo, 1999). Communities can unite for a stronger advocacy voice. The scope of HIV intervention must be broadened to include the need for changing group norms and activities, including community mobilization in the effort to improve public health, and removing social barriers to risk reduction (Friedman et al., 1997).

3.1.8 Evaluation of Program Efficacy

"We are asking people to make lifelong changes," and we need to know what works (Forum for Collaborative HIV Research, 2001).

1. Evaluation is the systematic collection of information about activities, characteristics, and/or outcomes of programs to make judgments about and improve their effectiveness, and/or inform decisions about future programming/approaches (HRSA, 1998). Evaluation is an essential component of the design, implementation, and improvement of an intervention program.

2. The more the community, agency partners, and knowledgeable staff are involved from the beginning, the more useful the evaluation will be. Empowerment evaluation includes program participants and communities at all stages of the planning and carrying out of the evaluation process (Sullivan et al., 2005).

Adopting programs found effective in other settings brings about potential conflict between fidelity to the original program for purposes of comparison and the opportunity to adapt and increase effectiveness when implemented for currently targeted populations (Rapkin & Trickett, 2005). Although new approaches will have to be developed that allow evaluation of the dynamics of programs as they are adopted and adapted (Rapkin & Trickett, 2005), these approaches must occur at the policy and funding levels of government. "The road to greater success includes prevention science and newer community-centered models of accountability and technical assistance systems for prevention" (Wandersman & Florin, 2003).

Box 27.1. Alternatives to Randomized Controlled Trials

Designs must:

- Take into account the diversity inherent in the determinants of health and risk behavior.
- Recognize that different people can respond to the same intervention in different ways.
- Accommodate personal choice and preference.
- Anticipate nonindependence and significant potential benefits associated with contamination across arms (control vs. experimental groups).
- Avoid ethical dilemmas associated with substandard treatment of some participants.
- Be responsive to evolving understanding of this to best administer an intervention and to local innovations and ideas.
- Contribute to community capacity building and empowerment at every step of the research process.

(Rapkin & Trickett, 2005)

---

3. Evaluation is conducted at the program level to establish effectiveness of a program (Windsor et al., 1994).

- *Process evaluation (quality assurance review)* is used to assess activities during the process of program development and implementation. "What services are being delivered and to whom?" (National AIDS Fund, 1993). With staff input into objectives, process, and scope, this type of continuous feedback can provide valuable insights for ongoing program improvement (Rapkin & Trickett, 2005). Process evaluation is also an important tool for developing collaborative processes between agencies and in research–community collaborations.
- *Formative evaluation (assessing feasibility/efficacy)* can assist in reviewing the feasibility of program implementation (i.e., results of "field testing" of a health education program). Results can be used to choose one program over others and revise components of a program, from its duration or venue of intervention to the data-collection procedures.
- *Impact evaluation (effectiveness assessment)* is designed to evaluate the longer-term effectiveness of a particular program with a specific population. Frequently asked questions include the following: (1) Is

the intervention reaching the target population? (2) Is it being implemented in the ways specified? (3) Is it effective? (4) How much does it cost? (5) What are its costs relative to its effectiveness? Comparison with results from similar studies is a valuable aspect but may not be possible in all cases. Measuring the rate of change of HIV transmission in a particular population is a difficult challenge methodologically (National AIDS Fund, 1993).

• *Evaluation research (efficacy, long term)* seeks to document the potential impact of an intervention on a defined population at risk. This research seeks to measure behavioral impact and health outcomes under research conditions and can add to the knowledge base for dissemination. Owing to its complexity, evaluation research is usually done by specialized university-based research centers in collaboration with agencies and/or local collaborations (Hunter et al., 2001).

3.2 Research–Community Collaboration

Research–community collaboration provides resources to agencies and communities to measure the effectiveness of their interventions. Various collaborations are possible, from a CBO seeking consultation from a research institution about aspects of their program (i.e., needs assessment, evaluation design, procedures) to full partnership in a research study within the agency or community. In a collaborative partnership, shared decision-making and joint ownership can best begin with the joint development of study aims and proceed to collaborative design of research questions, development of outcome measures, research procedures (i.e., data collection, recruitment), implementation of the intervention, data analysis, and dissemination (Hunter & Lounsbury, 2005). Community-based participatory research (CBPR) is a method that seeks to articulate active community involvement in research and intervention, addressing social disparities in health (Northridge et al., 2000).

As most funding organizations now require demonstration of program efficacy, community participation can improve design and effectiveness and ultimately empower communities (Green, 2001). Active participation by community members in research activities can be structured in the research plan. Community members can serve on advisory or decision-making bodies, such as formal Community Advisory Boards (CABs). For community participation to be real, the research plan must include activities to facilitate participation, build skills and capacity, and train community members in their roles, responsibilities, and the research principles and implementation plans. Also, researchers need to learn about community expectations and perspectives (Cross-Network CAB Working Group Meeting, 2005).

3.2.1 *Waiver of Parental Permission/Consent/Confidentiality*
Issues of ethical and regulatory protections of minors in intervention research must be addressed by both research organizations and CBOs. Parental consent is required to ensure the protection of children as subjects. However, parental consent becomes a barrier for many youths

---

Box 27.2. Variations on "Best Practices"

- Consider "best practice" as a process rather than as packaged interventions.
- Emphasize control by practitioner, patient, client, community, or population.
- Emphasize local evaluation and self-monitoring.
- Conduct a more systematic study of the place, setting, and culture
- Research the tailoring process and new technologies.
- Consider the possibility of synthesizing research from sources other than randomized trials.

(Green, 2001)

(i.e., GLBT youths who would be "outed" and at risk of disclosure to their parent before they are ready to come out). Parental consent may be waived in cases where parental consent would not, in fact, protect the youth. The waiver must meet the following criteria: (1) The research involves only minimal risk; (2) the waiver would not adversely affect the welfare of the youth; (3) the research could not be carried out without a waiver; and (4) The youth is provided with additional pertinent information after participation. All youths who participate in research activity must give "informed consent," including information, comprehension, and free will, which must be formalized into a consent form. All states recognize the concept of emancipated minors not subject to parental consent laws (Santelli & Rogers, 2002).

Community partners can also participate in the dissemination process through participation in evaluation, conference presentations and training, newsletter articles, and writing of journal articles (Hunter et al., 2001). When dissemination of program efficacy is part of the research task (i.e., journal articles, conference presentations), communities can benefit from participation in the dissemination process. Program staff can present programs they represent for possible adoption by others, and they are able to use and develop their own skills in a broader venue and contribute to the dialogue (Hunter et al., 1999).

Confidentiality is absolutely necessary if youths are to access health care (White House, 2000). The debate over a client's right to privacy and health care versus a parent's or government's right to know continues at all levels, including in the courts. Federal law allows minors to make decisions about their health care. States vary in their laws and practices. Exceptions center around reproductive care services and mandatory reporting of HIV infection.

Confidentiality does give health care providers the responsibility to report behaviors usually defined as a genuine and immediate threat (e.g., when one is a danger to self or others, sexual abuse) and a "duty to warn," which dictates that providers must notify appropriate professionals when a client is at risk for harming themselves or others (Ryan & Futterman, 1997). Serious suicide ideation or attempts or homicidal threats must be examined and addressed. Less clearly a threat are risky sexual and drug behaviors of adolescents. Often the health care provider must make a judgment based on professional ethics and training and also on their own beliefs, value judgments, and experience with similar patients (Fisher, 2003). There is little agreement on what levels of intensity, frequency, and duration of sexual and drug behaviors constitute risk on the part of health care professionals. A major concern for the provider is losing the patient to care if confidentiality is broken.

Research–community collaborations involving programs for youth at CBOs must get permission from all institutions involved. Institutional Review Boards (IRBs) exist at universities with strict human subjects guidelines and requirements for the protection of anyone involved in a research study (Getz & Borfitz, 2002). Agencies have their own procedures as well. When the Working It Out Project applied for IRB approval at the New York State Psychiatric Institute to enter into a research project at nine CBOs, compliance with procedures to guarantee confidentiality of data and procedures for and content of consent forms to be reviewed with each interviewee and details of possible risks to the participants were all required (Hunter et al., 2001). In addition, as the participants were GLB youths, researchers and agencies all believed it could be hazardous to the youths' health for their parents to be informed of their participation in the study. A Confidentiality Certificate was granted from the National Institute of Mental Health allowing the adults to protect the confidentiality of the youth on the basis that "youth will be sharing information about their sexual lives . . . in a society that is hostile to homosexuality." Consent forms were reviewed with each participant at both before and after assessment interviews. Each agency designated a staff member to act "en loco parentis" for participants under age 18. The project had available a qualified crisis counselor in case any youth would become upset over questions asked regarding sexual and drug behaviors. Although this counselor was not needed, this service was important to have in place (www.hivcenternyc.org).

When planning HIV prevention and care, and best processes can be identified at agency and community levels and in school programs. Resources include state and national governmental agencies, universities, foundations, media health promotion campaigns, and the Internet.

3.3 Broader Community Collaboration

3.3.1 Forming Coalitions
Forming coalitions with other service agencies provides a continuum of care that could not be offered within any one agency. Resources (i.e., funds, staff) need to be devoted to the development of coalitions (Forum for Collaborative HIV Research, 2001). Establishing relationships and sharing information begin the process of formally linking strong community partnerships. These coalitions also make it possible for case managers to make appropriate referrals for competent, culturally sensitive care not offered internally. Also, formal linkages among medical and social services agencies for a continuum of care create

possibilities for effective program coordination and advocacy in a community. "Working at the level of community can sometimes lead to significant behavioral changes" (AIDS Action, 2001). Means to improve service integration need to focus on six areas: theory, infrastructure, support, training, indicators, and evaluation (Kolbe et al., 1999).

3.3.2 Community-Level Needs Assessment

The community-level needs assessment as a cooperative process is the necessary first step toward comprehensive program development to achieve the goal of a continuum of care. The process of assessing past planning activities and refining, improving, or expanding future planning is most effectively done at the local community level, where youths have access to care (HRSA, 1997). Service components of CTRS through follow-up can be reviewed and gaps in care identified (Healthy People 2010, 1999).

Comprehensive needs Assessment requires active participation of all involved and includes preplanning activities: timetable, budget, personnel, procedures, data needed, plan for analyzing data and writing reports, provision for confidentiality. The Needs Assessment includes gathering an epidemiologic profile of the epidemic in the local service area. Many at-risk youth populations are "hidden populations," and careful examination of these data is required. In addition, the long incubation period of the virus requires additional information about potential youths at risk. Clinicians and service providers can supply data from their experience with populations they serve, including (1) assessment of service needs, including barriers to care, from those in care and those not in care; (2) inventory of resources available; (3) review of the capacity of providers in the target area; and (4) assessment of gaps in service (HRSA, 1998).

3.3.3 Other Successful Joint Strategies

Other strategies include agencies jointly marketing services, cross-training of staff, co-locating services in a single site, and jointly securing funding for data analysis and evaluation activities (Forum for Collaborative HIV Research, 2001).

3.3.4 School-Based Education

Guidelines for comprehensive sexuality education curriculum developed by a broad-based task force of health and education professionals at the Sexuality Information and Education Council of the United States (SIECUS) includes information, attitudes/values/insights, relationship and interpersonal skills, and responsibility taught at appropriate developmental levels, kindergarten through grade 12. Sex education and HIV prevention education exist in most school programs, but many omit topics considered controversial, such as a balanced discussion of abstinence and safer sex (SIECUS, 2004). In 1997, the National Institutes of Health (NIH) announced that programs must include instruction in safer sex behavior, including condom use, a practice strongly supported by scientific evidence (National Institutes of Health, 1997).

Sexual health education needs to be taught earlier than high school for it to have a impact on youths' risk behaviors. Youths who participate in sex education programs before they become sexually active, stay abstinent longer and use protection when they do become sexually active (Kirby et al., 1991).

Knowledge alone is not enough to change behavior, and programs that give information and tell teens what they should and should not do have not worked (DiClemente, 1992). In a review of 23 studies of effective programs, social learning theories were chosen as a foundation for the programs, including recognizing social influences, changing values and group norms, and building social skills. These programs also focused on reducing sexual risk-taking behaviors, addressed social and media influences, and included experiential activities designed to personalize knowledge. Reinforcing clear values against unprotected sex and modeling and practice in communication, negotiation, and refusal skills were incorporated into the programs (Kirby et al., 1991).

Educators need to be both knowledgeable and comfortable with teaching sexuality education. The more knowledgeable they are, the more positive/supportive are the attitudes toward HIV/AIDS and persons with HIV/AIDS (Dawson et al., 2001). Programs that target behavioral change through role playing, games, and social skills exercises can work (Ubell, 1995). In addition, the use of HIV-positive speakers, when combined with multicomponent programs, have a positive impact on youths (Markham et al., 2000).

Most of the following programs can be characterized as comprehensive sexuality education, or "abstinence plus." Medical, social service, and school-based professionals largely endorse the policy of providing young people with accurate information and choices, as many are already sexually active. Effective programs include information about risks of unprotected sex, how to avoid those risks, and openness in discussing sexuality (UNAIDS, 1997). Skills for avoiding and resisting peer pressure to engage in risk-taking behaviors cannot be overlooked (Madison et al., 2000).

3.3.5 School-Based Clinics

School-based clinics comprise a model of care that, by offering confidential comprehensive services, provide a place where adolescents can go for their health needs. These clinics, usually serving a group of schools, have access to youths in school and contact with school staff, which facilitates referrals and consultations. The experience of many such clinics is that they also serve out-of-school youths and are able to provide confidential, age-appropriate services. Individual clinic visits with medical providers that focus on appropriate sexual and contraceptive behavior, including specific discussions about the client's behavior, can positively affect condom or contraceptive behavior (Kirby, 2002). Flexibility in hours, innovative billing systems, and offering services free of school control are all helpful to adolescents. Counseling and referral are important components of school-based clinics. As a number of sexually transmitted diseases (STDs) are asymptomatic,

STD/HIV screening at clinics can be an effective means of determining the infection status of at-risk youths and allowing them to obtain appropriate health care (Kirby, 2002). However, many clinics have had to limit the reproductive health services offered, including access to contraceptives. This model may be a promising way to provide care to traditionally difficult-to-reach populations. Additional research will yield more information on how effective school-based clinics are in meeting the needs of adolescents (Fothergill & Ballard, 1998).

3.3.6 Broad-Based HIV Prevention Health Media Campaigns Targeting Youth/Internet

HIV prevention health promotion media campaigns can be carried out in many ways, targeting specific geographic areas or nationally, to change social attitudes and inform people of risks, prevention, and resources. Safe–sex media campaigns have contributed to a reduction in teen-reported sexual activity and increased condom use (Alstead et al., 1999). Campaigns can be sustained over time or be conducted as one-time saturation. People living with HIV/AIDS, celebrities and others, sharing their life experiences through national and local media, can have a profound impact on both individuals and communities (AIDS Action Council, 2001). Youths reported that Magic Johnson's disclosure (the Magic Johnson effect) of his HIV status increased their awareness of AIDS (60%) and safer sexual practices (65.4%) and increased their resistance to peer pressure for having sexual intercourse (37.2%) (Brown et al., 1996).

Several strategies can be employed by health advocates using media to promote health, including mass media campaigns using social marketing and "edu-tainment," embedded messages, and "small media," (e.g., pamphlets, brochures, Internet) (Keller & Brown, 2002). The "HIV. Live With It. Get Tested!" campaign (discussed below) combined radio messages using hip hop language, an appealing design on palm cards, and a "Zine" to reach youths in several cities for HIV testing awareness.

Clear campaign goals, identified target audiences, media channels, and campaign strategy are important steps when planning a successful media campaign. Communities can design cost-effective approaches (e.g., transit cards, billboards, radio, pamphlets, the Internet) and can create news events, taking advantage of the mass media. Media organizations and experts can be called upon for assistance. Combining media and community strategies can be effective in bringing young people into programs, enlisting volunteers for local organizations, and reinforcing the instruction provided by schools and community agencies. Applying behavioral change models, increasing awareness, and then increasing knowledge and changing beliefs, teaching new skills, and reinforcing behavioral change is recommended. Evaluation, although complex, has been done on several media campaigns targeting youth (Bertrand & Kincaid, 1997; Alstead et al., 1999).

The Internet provides information on a need-to-know basis. This service is important for youths who are not connected to a health service or who lack transportation or access to health facilities.

Limitations include dissemination of inaccurate information, possible violations of privacy, and unwanted pornography; ironically, it is also limited by the increasing censorship of any sexually explicit information offered by libraries and school system software. Those most at risk may have access to the Internet (Keller & Brown, 2002). Internet chat rooms for youths, to be a positive influence, must be managed or supervised. Model programs, below, include community-level HIV prevention health campaigns.

3.4 Funding Resources

It is imperative that funding for at risk and HIV-positive youth continue.

3.4.1 State and Federal Agencies

State and federal agencies have been taking steps to integrate funding for HIV counseling and testing, care and treatment, and prevention. The Forum for Collaborative HIV Research, a coalition of representatives from five constituency groups, including government, industry, patient advocates, health care providers, and researchers, formed in 1997 and is jointly funded by the CDC, HRSA, and the Forum. A 2-day meeting held in October 2001 addressed linkage and integration of HIV testing, prevention, and care services (Forum for Collaborative HIV Research, 2001).

Simplification and coordination to support cross-agency linkages at the local and state levels have been recommended for use across services. Additional funding is needed for every aspect of outreach to difficult-to-reach youth. Recommendations have been made for federally funded programs to be funded for longer periods than the current practice of funding for 3-year periods, allowing for more successful outreach, delivery of prevention messages, and reinforcement of behavioral change on the part of clients. The need for additional funding for evaluation and program improvement has also been cited, as have joint evaluation guidelines by funding agencies for standard data and evaluation systems, coordinated technical assistance, and resources.

3.4.2 Foundations/Private Funders, National Organizations

Priorities include linking with foundations/private funders for funding needed programs and with national organizations for resources, technical support, and advocacy at the local, state, and national levels (i.e., Advocates for Youth, National Youth Advocacy Coalition, SIECUS, and other organizations listed in Online Resources, below).

4 Model Programs

Many programs offering medical and/or social services to youths are multidimensional. They are presented here in broad categories of school-based community-based (including continuum of care, outreach, and social service programs), and individual and group interventions, including model programs developed through research-community collaboration. The NIH, CDC, other federal agencies, and state and local health departments fund well designed evaluations of HIV prevention programs, and many of these programs are described in the scientific literature (White House, 2000).

Sustained interventions are more likely to lead to sustained behavioral change (risk reduction) (Collins, 1997; Kim et al., 1997), as are *more intense interventions* (Institute of Medicine, 2000). Information, skills building, and modification of social norms are more effective when presented together (St. Lawrence et al., 1995).

Some effective *tools* utilized by effective programs include youth-friendly environments, flexible hours of operation, utilization of popular opinion leaders and youth advisors/peer outreach and educators, and incentives (i.e., refreshments, bus tokens, T-shirts, money). Programs involving youths in community service are worthy of note, as there is evidence that sexual risk behaviors are reduced among youth who participate in them (Kirby, 2002). Components of establishing relationships with caring adults, fostering a sense of belonging, and activities that structure time and limit the amount of unsupervised time may contribute to lower sexual risk behaviors. These elements can be included in various ways in HIV prevention programs for youths (Kirby, 2002).

Peer education is found to be a highly effective strategy, "an approach, a communication channel, a methodology, and a philosophy" (UNAIDS, 1997). Peer support groups are a critical component of HIV prevention for youths across cultural and racial groupings and whether youth are GLBT or heterosexual. Being with their peers, youths can address common problems (i.e., school issues, relationship issues) and reduce their isolation, thereby building self-esteem and a support system.

Traditional programs may not be effective for some groups of youths. For example, a study soliciting recommendations from young MSM (YMSM) (age 12.2 years; range 10–16 years; 46% White, 32% African American, 10% Latino, 8% biracial, 4% Asian American/Middle Eastern) from a variety of social networks found that broad aspects of sexuality and emotionally intimate relationships in an environment accepting of all, regardless of sexual identity, need to be addressed to be effective. Suggestions for programming, particularly to hidden populations, include "rap sessions" at cafes, bars, and other venues where YMSMs congregate, in collaboration with HIV prevention providers. Topics could include "meeting partners," "maintaining relationships," and "making safer sex fun" (Seal et al., 2000). Here the venue becomes important in effective outreach to this population.

4.1 School-Based Models

In a review of sex education programs that work, Pamela DeCarlo (2002) cited examples of effective school-based programs. These programs either increased the numbers of youths who delayed sexual activity and/or reduced unprotected intercourse among students who became sexually active.

1. AIDS Prevention for Adolescents in School. This intervention for 9th and 11th graders in New York City schools, focused on teaching facts about AIDS, cognitive skills to appraise risk, correcting facts, increasing knowledge of resources, values clarification, understanding external influences, and skills development for delaying intercourse and/or consistently using condoms (Walter & Vaugh, 1993) (retrieved September 22, 2005 from www.advocatesforyouth/programs that work/).

2. Health Oakland Teens (HOT). In addition to units on basic sex and drug education, HOT utilized peer educators in interactive exercises on values, decision-making, communication, and condom-use skills (Ekstrand et al., 1996).

Additional school-based models are as follows:

3. BASE—Be Active in Self-Education. This program is in New York City sponsored by the HIV/AIDS Technical Assistance Project (TAP) and Atlanta, Kansas City, Los Angeles, Minneapolis, San Jose, Salt Lake City, and Albuquerque. A peer-education program, it helps high school students teach each other about HIV prevention through a student-designed and student-led grant-making program for the development of innovative prevention projects. Programs include a student advisory committee, consultation with foundation representatives and AIDS service providers, talk-show formats, interactive theater presentations, support groups, posters and murals, T-shirts and buttons, comic books, health fairs, conferences, mobile van displays, school assemblies, awards and scholarships, and community service projects. CBOs can partner with local schools to help them develop a BASE Program. Although funding is required, the program is also adaptable for use within CBOs (AIDS Action Council, 2001) (retrieved September 22, 2005 from www.youthbase.org).

4. Get Real About AIDS 1992. Based on the social cognitive theory and the theory of reasoned action, this intervention was carried out in 10 Colorado schools (average age of participants was 15). Teachers from health, science, physical education, and study skills fields attended a 5-day training program. The curriculum included HIV knowledge to reduce risk, teen vulnerability to HIV, risky behavior, condom use, and skills to help youth manage, avoid, or leave risky situations ($n = 2015$; males 51%, females, 49%; average age 15 years; 65% White, 21% Latino/a, 6% African Americans, 3% Asian; 44% were sexually active prior to the study). (Main et al., 1994) (retrieved September 22, 2005 from www.etr.org/recapp/programs.getreal.htm).

5. Harlem Health Promotion Center's School Health Promotion Initiative (SHPI). This initiative aims to connect youth with preventive care. The program is located at a Harlem high school. Youths, with parental permission, attend a series of three 2-hour weekly workshops led by trained facilitators, learning about the importance of getting a checkup, basic information about reproductive health, and how to talk to a health provider, as well as identification of youth-friendly health care resources in the community. Questions to expect from health care providers are discussed, and youths are encouraged to discuss any sensitive issues on their minds at their medical visits (i.e., substance use, smoking, sexual behaviors). Communication skills practice and role-playing with visiting health professionals help prepare the youths to take an active role in their health care. The program is being adapted for inclusion into the school's health curriculum and to be used as a potential model for other schools (Harlem Health Promotion Center Newsletter, 2001 (Fall)).

6. *Midwest AIDS Prevention Project (MAPP) Peer Education and Social Marketing Program.* This program was developed in conjunction with the Michigan Department of Community Health and targets students in middle and high school, including alternative schools and out-of-school youths. Using the Center for AIDS Intervention Research (CAIR) prevention science research on popular opinion leaders, teen educators are trained to provide HIV prevention information to their peers (MAPP's Teen Leadership Corp). MAPP counsels teachers and school counselors and advises CBOs on getting youth invested in HIV prevention. Included are workshops, outreach projects, theater programs presented at schools, and educational programs—all emphasizing self-esteem, self-reliance, communication skills, relationships to help young people make safe and healthy decisions, and a Teen ADAPT program for drug abuse prevention (AIDS Action Council, 2001).

7. *Reducing the Risk.* Based on social learning, social inoculation, and cognitive behavioral theories, 15 sessions were carried out as part of the 10th grade comprehensive health curriculum in 13 high schools in California. Volunteer teachers attended a 3-day training session. The curriculum included the development of strategies and skills, using role-playing and other practices, to resist social pressure and reduce sexual risk-taking. Decision making was emphasized, and students were encouraged to seek out health information at clinics and stores and were required to ask their parents their views on abstinence and birth control ($n = 758$; average age 15 years; males 47%, females 53%; 62% White, 20% Latino/a, 18% others; 37% were sexually experienced prior to the study) (DeCarlo, 2002) (retrieved September 22, 2005 from www2.edc.org/NTP/PTW/ptwrtrcurriculum.html).

8. *Safer Choices.* This is a multicomponent behavioral theory-based HIV, STD, and pregnancy prevention program instituted in 20 urban high schools. The program was evaluated 31 months after the intervention, with the results indicating fewer risky sexual behaviors and higher knowledge, attitudes, perceived norms, and self-efficacy (Basen-Engquist et al., 2001) (retrieved September 22, 2005 from www.etr.org/recapp/programs/saferchoices.htm).

9. *Gay-Straight Alliances.* These have served to de-isolate young people, provide safe spaces, and build awareness and support in the larger school community (Seal et al., 2000) (retrieved September 22, 2005 from www.centeryes.org).

4.2 Community-Based Models

The HRSA-funded Special Projects of National Significance (SPNS) Program funded 10 Adolescent Initiative projects for a 3-year period beginning in 1994 (HRSA, 1999). Lessons learned include the importance of collaboration among agencies, as one agency is rarely equipped to meet the diverse needs of HIV-positive and at-risk youth. Collaboration about referral and outreach programs was essential. The reality is that most CBOs serving this population are understaffed, making it difficult to maintain those linkages and provide the intensive case management needed when working with these populations.

Intervention/prevention programs may target by age, gender, sexual experience, ethnicity/cultural group, behavioral risk, or neighborhood. Programs must be culturally appropriate and provide confidentiality. Keeping youths in care requires establishment of trust. Peer-based outreach, counseling, and recreational and socialization activities are all essential. Youths were on staff at most of the 10 SPNS agencies, from peer outreach to program planning and management. Staff must provide added supervision and ongoing support for the youths on staff and allow opportunities for advancement to staff/management roles.

Challenges include addressing client needs (i.e., housing and food) so youths can focus on their care, reminders to clients of their appointments, possibly transportation, flexibility of evening and weekend hours at off-site locations, adapting programs to limitations of clients' ability to participate (i.e., self-contained sessions), and simplifying printed materials for some youths. Separate support groups for subpopulations of youths served may be needed (i.e., gay males, bisexual males). Psychological barriers to accepting care must be addressed (i.e., "HIV infection can't happen to me" or the opposite, hopelessness and fatalism, often accompanied by drug or alcohol abuse) (HRSA, 1999). Peer support groups, linking with substance abuse treatment programs for youths, and nonjudgmental support are also vital. Confidentiality and quality of care reflect respect for the client.

A continuum of care is essential for HIV-positive youths to help them deal with the complex issues of adherence to medication and interventions to address co-occurring grief and depression (Murphy et al., 2001). At-risk youth also need access to interdisciplinary care in primary care settings from late elementary school to middle school ages to encourage them to delay intercourse, practice safer sex, and avoid substance use (Bachanas et al., 2002).

1. Adolescent AIDS Program (AAP) at Montefiore Medical Center, Bronx, New York, is the country's first adolescent AIDS program and is a leader in the field of HIV prevention, care, and research. The program specializes in providing medical and counseling services to adolescents, including GLBT youth, who are infected with HIV or who are at risk for HIV infection. In addition to clinical services, the AAP provides specialized training to medical and mental health care professionals who treat adolescents, including GLBT youth. They design and implement innovative HIV prevention campaigns targeting at-risk youth, and they participate in groundbreaking HIV research on diverse adolescent patient populations (retrieved September 22, 2005, from www.adolescentaids.org).

2. Children's Hospital Los Angeles (CHLA), a comprehensive outreach and case management model for homeless and other high-risk youths, serves hidden youths, including GLBTs, gang-affiliated, intravenous drug users (IDUs) and their partners, and homeless or street youths, most of whom are Latino/a or African American. In addition to its extensive outreach, it has established a clinic at the Los Angeles Free Clinic that includes a case management system that links youths with primary care, substance abuse, and mental health services, including services for Spanish-speaking youths. Clients can access an automated referral service, the Computer Assisted Adolescent Referral System (CAARS). An SPNS Program of HRSA (Huba & Melchior, 1998) (contact: CHLA, 213-669-4604).

3. Huckleberry Youth Programs, Huckleberry House, and Cole Street Youth Clinic program addresses primary health care and psychosocial needs of homeless, runaway, and at-risk youth in San Francisco and Marin County, California. The program, which began as an emergency shelter 30 years ago, has expanded to include HIV prevention peer education initiatives, offering group sessions (one to six sessions) that address risk prevention, negotiating safer sex, and setting limits. Workshops are also offered in middle and high schools, through street outreach, and in community sites such as Planned Parenthood. Huckleberry also works with the Violence is Preventable (VIP) Girls Collaborative and the Highway 101 Program, serving youth in shelters. Extensive evaluation is being done to provide behavioral outcome measures and determine potential as a national model (AIDS Action Council, 2001) (retrieved September 22, 2005, from www.caps.ucsf.edu/capsweb/yabio.html).

4. Larkin Street Youth Center, in San Francisco, California, provides comprehensive care to address specific needs of homeless and runaway youths who are living with HIV. Outreach workers locate and assist youth on the streets, offer HIV prevention and education materials, invite the youths to the Center for services, where they would have access to food, showers, counseling, and case management services, as well as recreational and therapeutic activities in their Drop-In Center. In addition, Larkin Street runs a free confidential medical clinic in collaboration with the local health department. Mental health, substance abuse, a community art program, and housing assistance programs are also offered. The Diamond Youth Shelter provides emergency overnight shelter for young people ages 12 to 17. The Lark-inn for Youth provides emergency and interim housing for homeless and runaway youth ages 18–23. The Loft provides transitional housing for youth who cannot return home. The assisted residential care program for young people living with disabling HIV disease also provides medical and support services under one roof. Comprehensive Education and Employment Services The Institute for Hire Learn is a career-training program, part of HIRE UP (retrieved September 22, 2005, from www.larkinstreetyouth.org).

5. Project S.T.A.Y. (Services to Assist Youth) (Center for Community Health and Education, New York Presbyterian Hospital and Harlem Health Promotion Center, Mailman School of Public Health, Columbia University) is a client-centered model of integrated medical care that strives to identify assets and risk for the young person. The program weaves counseling, testing services (CTS) into an ambulatory care setting, providing thorough psychosocial assessment at intake and testing (when the youth is ready to do so), and referral within the linked coalitions, which include many youth-serving agencies. One such coalition is the Adolescent Initiative Project (AIP), a consortium of more than 60 agencies serving youths in northern Manhattan. Outreach is an important component of the program and the AIP, which sponsors community-wide events for at-risk youth. Other linkages are to the Gay Men of African Descent (GMAD); People of Color in Crisis (POCC); the Center Harlem and East Harlem HIV Care Networks; the Northern Manhattan Women and Children's HIV Project; Job Corp, The Door, a social service agency; and the Department of Health's STD clinics (Harlem Health Promotion Center Newsletter, Summer, 2002) (retrieved September 22, 2005, from www.checkoutthatbody.com and www.healthyharlem.org).

6. Streetwork, in New York City, is a comprehensive primary care program for street-based youths ages 24 and under. It is based partially on the harm reduction theory. The program provides daily living support (i.e., food, clothing, showers, advocacy for housing, counseling/educational/social groups, advocacy, referrals, legal services) as well as several health-related services, including HIV counseling and testing, primary care, acupuncture, wellness services, and confidential Syringe Exchange. Streetwork also operates two drop-in centers and two emergency housing programs, one on the lower East Side (LES), and one in Midtown Manhattan (retrieved September 22, 2005, from www.thebody.com/hud/streetwork.html).

7. YouthCare's Prevention, Intervention and Education Program, a model of care for HIV-positive, homeless, and at-risk youth in Seattle, Washington, maintains a youth shelter, a case management system for accessing youth to a continuum of care, including free confidential testing, risk-reduction counseling, and skills building programs. It has intensive outreach and linkages to social services and government agencies, including the juvenile justice system and the Housing Authority. Young people have been involved in developing an HIV testing protocol and participate as peer outreach workers and peer educators. It is an SPNS Program of HRSA (Huba & Melchior, 1998) (retrieved September 22, 2005, from www.youthcare.org)

4.3 Outreach and Social Service Programs

1. The Asian & Pacific Islander Coalition on HIV/AIDS (APICHA), a CBO, serves a rich diversity of Asian and Pacific Islanders in New York City. It offers bilingual programs through school-based workshops and one-to-one outreach at community centers, video arcades, pool halls, and other gathering places for young Asians (AIDS Action Council, 2001) (retrieved September 22, 2005, from www.apicha.org).

2. *Bay Area Young Positives* (*Bay Positives*). A peer-based program serving HIV-positive young people, both males and females, BAY Positives includes psychological support services, social and recreational services, advocacy training, and linkages to youth-sensitive providers. Two strong components include promoting youths into program positions of responsibility and providing support to staff and volunteers with the same quality as with clients. They have a monthly newsletter, *On The Plus Side*, and have begun an alumni program for those over age 25. They link with San Francisco General Hospital's adolescent clinic and several social services and drug treatment programs. It is an SPNS Program of HRSA (HRSA, 1997; Huba & Melchior, 1998) (retrieved September 22, 2005, from www.baypositives.org).

3. *Hetrick-Martin Institute* (*HMI*), New York City, has a wide range of programs to serve GLBT youths, including an extensive social services (i.e., individual, group, and family counseling) and after-school drop-in program, meals program, computer learning center, alternative high school program, the Harvey Milk High School, and GED program. Youth initiatives include the Peer Education Program and the Street Outreach Intern Program. HMI has adapted the Working It Out Project (WIO) for use in their Peer Education Program. Trained interns also serve in AIDS service organizations in the city through the Linking Lives Program. The HMI training institute provides training and technical assistance to parents groups, government agencies, businesses, schools, and youths in foster care. Project First Step is a comprehensive range of services to help all homeless and street-involved youths build a healthier life away from the streets, including its Project First Step's outreach distribution program of food, safer-sex kits, personal hygiene items, and referrals for housing and health care. Youth interns accompany staff for peer-to-peer outreach. Case managers act as primary resource people in linking youths to essential health care services, emergency housing, educational programs, and vocational training. A Youth Council and youth members of the Board of Directors also afford youth leadership experience (retrieved September 22, 2005, from www.hmi.org).

4. *Indiana Youth Access Program* (*IYAP*) links youths through the state-mandated reporting system. In partnership with the County Health Department and a hospital Adolescent Health Clinic, IYAP has developed a program for training social service providers to spur the development of a large, accessible network of providers knowledgeable about and available to GLB youth. A peer Youth Council and peer counselors and educators are integral to the program. It is an SPNS program of HRSA (1997) (retrieved September 22, 2005, from www.themeasurementgroup.com/documents/adolspns/resource/iyap.htm).

5. *La Raza's Latino Youth Peer-to-Peer HIV/STD Prevention Program* has developed presentations with male and female teens discussing the transmission of AIDS. The dialogue was developed by the teens and is available as a PowerPoint presentation for use by others in the field of

HIV prevention for youths (DHHS, 2001) (retrieved September 22, 2005, from www.omhrc.gov/OMH/aids/impact/spring2001.pdf).

6. *The Mpowerment Project.* Based on theories of peer influence and diffusion of innovations, this project's goal was to reach all young gay men in a Eugene, Oregon community to decrease unprotected sex among this population. The program, run by a "core group" of young gay men, consisted of formal and informal outreach in social settings and peer-initiated communications, peer-led small groups, and a publicity campaign through gay newspapers and outreach materials (*n* = 300; young gay men ages 18–29, average age 23 years; 81% White, 7% Asian or Pacific Islander, 6% Latino/a, 4% African American). This program is one of the CDC's Replicating Effective Programs (REP) Project, which identifies interventions with demonstrated effectiveness (Hays et al., 2003; CDC, 2005) (retrieved September 22, 2005, from http://hivinsite.ucsf.edu).

7. *Queercore Program, a project of Gay City*, Seattle, WA, is a community-based HIV prevention program for men under age 30. It blends grassroots organizing, marketing, and empowerment theories, social marketing, and diffusion of education to create programs (Kelly, 2000), including retreats, film nights, forums, a talk show held at the local community college, and theater pieces at local theaters. Evaluation is part of the ongoing program, from postevent questionnaires to follow-up telephone surveys (AIDS Action Council, 2001) (retrieved September 22, 2005, from www.gaycity.org).

8. *University of Minnesota Youth and AIDS Project (YAP)* reaches out to HIV-positive youths, ages 13 to 21 identified through the state-mandated HIV reporting system. Through the program, youth receive early intervention and case management services, including a health care assessment, referrals, help with scheduling and transportation, risk-reduction counseling, and partner notification. YAP sponsored a Community AIDS Network, a coalition of 116 youth-serving organizations, collaborating with local and state agencies, including the state Department of Health, to serve this population. It is an SPNS Program of HRSA (1997) (Remafedi, 2001) (retrieved September 22, 2005, from www.peds.umn.edu/peds/gpah/programs/youthaids/home.html).

9. *Walden House Young Adult HIV Program*, serving multidiagnosed youths, provides risk assessment, pretest and posttest counseling, and HIV test access to all young adults, including GLBTs, at the Walden House residential substance abuse treatment program in San Francisco. Case management, peer counseling, and support programs have been developed for all youths. Some program staff members are graduates of the Walden House program. Medical and other services for a continuum of care are arranged for, and transportation is provided to, services outside the agency. It is an SPNS Program of HRSA (Huba & Melchior, 1998) (retrieved from www.waldenhouse.org).

10. *The WEHO Lounge*, Los Angeles, California, a coffee house and HIV testing and information center, offers free confidential oral HIV testing, community forums, peer counseling, drug adherence support groups, condom distribution, and a youth and HIV resource library, as

well as coffee drinks. It is located near two popular gay discos and has been highly successful with clients (Weinstein et al., 1998) (retrieved September 22, 2005, from www.wcities.com/en/record/71,35570/44/record.html).

11. *Youth Enrichment Services (YES Program)*, LGBT Community Center, New York City, is a multifaceted program offering support groups and socials, computer laboratory work, youth-centered leadership, school advocacy programs, and art and performance art programs for GLBT and questioning youths. The Working It Out Project (WIO) for GLB youth (discussed below) and an adapted WIO curriculum for transgender youths are part of the ongoing program. Self-expression through the arts is a program that reaches out to schools and other organizations regarding performance. The YES Program's website includes the SIGNS Project, working to help youth organize gay–straight alliances in schools, and it addresses homophobia and harassment youths face in schools (retrieved September 22, 2005, from www.centeryes.org).

4.4 Individual and Group Interventions

1. *Act Safe* was a program for HIV-positive youth ages 13 to 24, in Los Angeles, Miami, New York City, and San Francisco. It consisted of 11 small-group counseling sessions conducted over 3 months with the goal of reducing the minter of additional infections and the transmission of HIV to others. Sessions addressed ways to identify and change substance abuse and sexual risk behaviors. Although many youths found it difficult to attend consistently, the intervention was effective. Alternative ways to deliver messages (i.e., individual sessions, phone sessions) are being developed as a result of the experience (National Institute on Drug Abuse, 2002).

2. *Be Proud! Be Responsible!* is a program whose goal is reduction in HIV risk-associated sexual behaviors among African American male adolescents, was offered to 157 youths at one-time 5-hour Saturday morning sessions led by African American men and women with backgrounds in sexuality education, nursing, social work, and group facilitation. Leaders received 6 hours of training. Videos, games, role plays, exercises, Uncle Bill's Advice Column, and other activities focused on information about risks (i.e., IDU and specific sexual activities) and how to implement safer-sex practices including abstinence and correct use of condoms: A Discovery Approach to Science Enhancement (DASH) Program (Jemmott et al., 1992) (retrieved September 22, 2005, from www.cdc.gov/healthyyouth).

3. *Street Smart.* The social learning theory was the basis for this series of group sessions (10 group sessions, 3 times per week, repeated every 4 to 6 weeks; and one individual counseling session), for runaway and homeless youths ages 11 to 18. The primary components was (1) HIV-related knowledge; (2) social skills; (3) access to resources; and (4) personalized beliefs, attitudes, and norms. Group activities included video and art workshops where youths developed soap opera dramatizations, public service announcements, and commercials.

Assertiveness and coping skills, using the "feeling thermometer," were employed. Participants visited a comprehensive health and mental health center. Incentives were food and $1 for carrying condoms and arriving at the program on time ($n = 312$; male 51%, female 49%; runaway and homeless youths; average age 16 years; 57% African American, 22% Latino/a, 21% white/other) (Rotheram-Borus et al., 1991) (retrieved September 22, 2005, from www.cdc.gov/hiv/projects/rep/runaway.html).

4. *Working It Out* (WIO), a video-based manualized intervention program for lesbian, gay, and bisexual (LGB) adolescents, was developed jointly by researchers, representatives from CBOs, and youths. It is based on cognitive behavior and social learning theories. WIO, a 14-session group intervention curriculum with GLB youth, was designed to help youths develop skills to address stressful life events encountered during the coming-out process, deal with stigma, and manage developing social and sexual roles in a healthy way (Miller et al., 1996). Group facilitators participate in a 3-day training program, gaining skills to lead intervention groups at their agencies.

Each session focuses on a video vignette depicting real-life issues that youths must confront (i.e., suicide ideation, getting thrown out of the house, peer pressure to use drugs/alcohol, negotiating safer sex). Tools used include role-playing, the feeling thermometer, thanks, journals, Dear Abby letters, and other skills-building activities. Dissemination and adaptation activities are discussed below (see section 4.6) (Lesbian, Gay, Bisexual & Transgender Community Services Center Newsletter, 1997/1998, www.gaycenter.com; Hunter et al., 1998; Pratt, 2002) (retrieved September 22, 2005, from www.hivcenternyc.org).

4.5 Social Health Promotion/Social Marketing Media Campaigns

National, regional, and one-time saturation campaigns can all influence communities and individuals, combat stigma, and disseminate important health information (Futterman et al., 2001). Communities can utilize small media in many ways to disseminate sexual health messages. Model programs (below) have used such diverse campaigns as volunteers handing out condoms and bleach kits at strategic locations, putting signs on bus stops, chatting in chat rooms on the Internet to influence peers' norms regarding risky behaviors and HIV prevention, and using targeted websites with information and resources.

Two model Internet sites for youth include that of the American Social Health Association (www.iwannaknow.org) and Rutgers University of New Jersey's Network for Family Life Education's website (www.sxetc.org). Community-based organizations can also provide information on their programs as well as general health information and important Internet links, on their own websites. An example, above, is the LGBT Community Center of New York's Youth Enrichment Program's (YES Program) (retrieved September 22, 2005, from www.centeryes.org).

1. AIDS Community Demonstration Project. This intervention is based on the transtheoretical model of behavior change, a stage-based theory. The intervention was carried out in Dallas, Denver, Long Beach, New York City, and Seattle in street, public sex, and other community venues over a 3-year period. Using peer outreach workers from each community, model stories were developed from real-life experiences of target populations and were then distributed with condoms and bleach kits by peer volunteers. Interviews were conducted with 15,205 IDUs or their female partners, sex workers, MSMs, high-risk youth, and residents of high-STD neighborhoods (CDC, 1999) (retrieved September 22, 2005, from www.cdc.gov/hiv/projects/acdp/acdp.htm).

2. Community Awareness Network (C.A.N), NO/AIDS C.A.N. Project, outreaches to MSMs through the Internet, targeting community norms. Several staff and volunteers log on to MSM chat rooms, providing information and giving others the chance to think and talk about the choices they make. Working with the Office of Minority Health, USDHHS, a draft of best processes and procedures was prepared as guidelines for staff and volunteers who "chat" online. Some evaluation strategies have also been developed (DHHS, 2001) (retrieved September 22, 2005, from www.omhrc.gov/omh/sidebar/archivedhiv.htm#2).

3. HIV. Live with it. Get Tested! is a social marketing project to promote HIV testing to adolescents, speaks to youth in their language, asking through print and broadcast media if they're "Doin' it?" or "Gettin' Busy?" and then replies that if they are they should "Do it Safe. Get Tested"—familiar language that provokes their attention, invoking: "If you're sexually active, you should 'get tested!' to know your HIV status and make responsible choices regarding your health and sexual behaviors." The campaign's marketing materials have been researched and crafted with language and visual images that attract the attention of urban youths. The campaign further utilizes community mobilization and coalition building with other adolescent health programs, youth organizations, schools, and faith organizations to enhance outreach. The participation of young people is central to the program's success. Community visibility is created using paid advertising, public service announcements, street marketing, and public relations as components of an integrated communications program to get messages onto the streets and the airwaves that drive youths to get tested (Futterman et al., 2001) (retrieved September 22, 2005, from www.adolescentaids.org/healthcare/outreach.htm).

4. Youth Guardian Services, Manassas, Virginia, is a youth-run non-profit organization that provides support services through Internet-based projects, targeting GLBTQ youths and HIV-positive youths, as well as providing Internet services to other nonprofit agencies. (www.youth-guard.org) (DHHS, 2001). (retrieved September 22, 2005, from www.whatkidscando.org)

4.6 Research–Community Collaboration

It is often difficult to get agencies to adopt new and innovative programs (Rogers, 1995). Research–community collaboration is an important tool for the development, adoption, evaluation, and dissemination of effective intervention programs for youths. CBOs' service needs must be the focus for entering into collaboration with the researchers' plans (Rapkin & Trickett, 2005). CBOs and researchers can collaborate on the development of a program based on sound theory and the appropriateness for the populations to be served. One model draws on the work of Thompson, who suggested that researchers and CBOs analyze the domains, power, interdependencies, and legitimacy and, then, based on that framework, develop a cooperative partnership strategy, engaging the popular opinion leaders within the agency (Kelly, 2000).

Best processes for researcher–community collaboration include choosing partners carefully, verifying the support and capacity of agency/agency staff and directors, defining the roles in and responsibilities of goal setting, design, methods, evaluation of the process, planning adequate time for collaboration and meetings, addressing conflict, and allowing flexibility in the scope of research (Community-Campus Partnerships for Health, 1998; Israel et al., 1998). Flexibility is needed at each step (i.e., expect staff turnover and a need for retraining, provide alternative research questions for new interventions). Planning the dissemination activities, jointly monitoring research, and securing adequate resources and support for intervention and evaluation are also essential (Allman et al., 1997; Goldstein et al., 2000).

Barriers to overcome in research–community collaboration range from institutional and financial constraints to partners' lack of trust or understanding of each other's roles and priorities. The importance of both entities having ownership of the project in the increased credibility and dissemination of the project (Lewando-Hundt & Zaroo, 2000).

1. *Center for AIDS Prevention Studies (CAPS)*, a University of California, San Francisco (UCSF) and San Francisco AIDS Foundation collaboration, examined why gay and bisexual men were continuing to become HIV-infected. It resulted in two ongoing programs, Gay Life and Black Brothers Esteem (Goldstein et al., 2001). In this collaboration, CAPS provided funding, training, supervision, technical assistance, and researcher–CBO pairing for program evaluation (Bey et al., 2000) (retrieved September 22, 2005, from www.caps.ucsf.edu).

2. *Working It Out Project (WIO)*, described above, was developed by a close collaboration of HIV Center for Clinical and Behavioral Studies/NYSPI researchers and representatives from New York metropolitan area agencies serving this population. A video of 14 vignettes depicting scenes from the lives of LBG youths was originally developed with agency staff and youth feedback through focus groups. Then, with additional funding, six agency representatives and researchers worked together over a 15-week period to develop a manual, identified themes from the video vignettes, and developed skills-building activities to increase coping skills and reduce high risk behaviors. Based on diffusion of innovation and popular opinion leaders theories, the process of collaboration began as a joint research–community joint venture, with the program-

ming, evaluation, and dissemination planned together from the beginning.

Nine community agencies serving this population participated in implementing the program, each agency offering 14 weekly 2-hour WIO intervention group sessions with youths. WIO was adopted into the agencies' ongoing program in the original seven social service agencies and has been disseminated and adopted by additional agencies in New York, Massachusetts, Washington, DC, and Utah through community centers, health departments, and schools. WIO has been adapted for various client populations, including a peer training program for young adult MSMs of color in a New York inner-city community health center, as curriculum for peer training and train the trainer programs, WIO alumni groups, and transgender youths at a community center in New York City. WIO has also been presented in schools and on local cable TV; and it was a featured program in a CDC satellite broadcast to health departments in 2001. Training new staff and original agencies, staff at new agencies, and conference presentations co-presented by the principal investigator and the community partners have taken place. Community partners also participate in its dissemination through agency newsletters, networking activities, and interviews (Hunter et al., 1999) (retrieved September 22, 2005, from www.hivcenternyc.org).

5 Future Directions: Effective HIV Prevention and Care Programs

Agencies serving GLBT youth offer a rich array of programs to respond to their clients' needs, most often delivered by dedicated professionals and volunteers in small CBOs, some with links to clinics in cities across the country. During an era of shrinking resources, we must be able to identify those programs or components of programs that work. How do we do that?

- Response to the complex issues facing this population must combine individual- and community-level interventions that have built-in mechanisms for continuous program improvement to promote more responsive, sustainable approaches to HIV prevention (Rapkin & Trickett, 2005).
- Communities, including LGBT youths, must be partners in programs serving them.
- Community-initiated programs may not be able to demonstrate proven effectiveness; agencies need assistance to be able to evaluate their programs to ascertain their effectiveness by scientific standards. They must find ways to build their capacities in relation to program evaluation and accountability.
- Community-based organizations, research/academic institutions, and government and other funders must partner to bring all their diverse resources to this task.

- We must find/develop scientific measures that are capable of measuring beyond arbitrary outcome measures against which the entire population is measured—both grassroots and "top down" interventions. "The current reliance on randomized controlled trials ... to measure program effectiveness is not adequate to the task of evaluating program effectiveness" (Rapkin & Trickett, 2005).

References

AIDS Action Council (2001) What works in prevention for youth. Website: The body: an AIDS and HIV information resource. Retrieved September 22, 2005 from www.thebody.com; www.thebody.com/aac/sitemap.htm.

Allman, D., Myers, T., and Cockerill, R. (1997) *Concepts, definitions and models for community-based HIV prevention research in Canada*. HIV Social, Behavioral and Epidemiological Studies Unit, Faculty of Medicine, University of Toronto, Toronto.

Alstead, M., Campsmith, M., Halley, C.S., Hartfield, K., Goldbaum, G., and Wood, R.W. (1999) Developing, implementing, and evaluating a condom promotion program targeting sexually active adolescents. *AIDS Education and Prevention* 11:497–512.

Bachanas, P.J., Morris, M.K., Lewis-Gess, J.K., Sarett-Cuasay, E.J., Flores, A.L., Sirl, K.S., and Sawyer, M.K. (2002) Psychological adjustment, substance use, HIV knowledge, and risky sexual behavior in at-risk minority females: development differences during adolescence. *Journal of Pediatric Psychology* 27:373–384.

Bandura, A. (1993) Perceived self-efficacy in cognitive development and functioning. *Educational Psychologist*, 28(2):177–148.

Bandura, A. (1994) Social cognitive theory and exercise of control over HIV infection. In: DiClemente, R.J. (ed) *Preventing AIDS: theories and methods of behavioral interventions*. Plenum, New York.

Basen-Engquist, K., Coyle, K.K., Paracel, G.S., Kirby, D., Banspach, S.W., Carvajal, S.C., and Baumler, E. (2001) Schoolwide effects of a multicomponent HIV, STD, and pregnancy prevention program for high school students. *Health Education and Behavior* 28:166–185.

Bertrand, J., and Kincaid, D.L. (1997) *Evaluating information, education, and communication in family planning*. The Evaluation Project, Chapel Hill, NC. Cited in Keller and Brown (2002).

Bey, J., Durazzo, R., Headlee, J., Howard, G., Crosby, M., and Williams, A.W. (2000) *Prevention among African American gay and bisexual men*. Presented at the 8th International AIDS Conference, Durban, South Africa. Abstract WePeD4523. Cited in Goldstein et al. (2001).

Brettle, R.P. (1991) HIV and harm reduction for injection drug users. *AIDS* 5:125–136.

Brown, B.R., Jr, Baranowski, M.D., Kulig, J.W., Stephenson, J.N., and Perry, B. (1996) Searching for the Magic Johnson effect: AIDS, adolescents, and celebrity disclosure. *Adolescence* 31:253–264.

Buitron, M., Corby, N., and Rhodes, F. (1998) Creating a culturally appropriate behavioral prevention intervention for Spanish speaking gay men from an existing risk-reduction program. Presented at the International Conference on AIDS, Geneva, Abstract 335553. Cited in Gandelman and Freedman (2002).

CDC (1998) Patterns of condom use among adolescents? The impact of mother–adolescent communication. Centers for Disease Control and Prevention, Atlanta, GA.

CDC (2000) Prevention press briefing, HIV trends in U.S. highlight need for expanded prevention. Presented at the XIII International AIDS Conference, Durban, South Africa.

CDC (2001a) Compendium of HIV prevention interventions with evidence of effectiveness (including intervention checklist: elements of successful programs, a tool for assessment of local HIV/AIDS interventions). Retrieved September 22, 2005 from www.cdc.gov/hiv/projects/rep/compend.htm.

CDC (2001b) *HIV/AIDS—United States, 1981–2000.* MMRW Morbidity and Mortality Weekly Reports 50(No. RR-9). Retrieved September 5, 2005 from www.cdc.gov/YRBSS/.

CDC (2004) Diffusion of effective behavioral interventions project. Retrieved September 22, 2005 from www.effectiveinterventions.org/documents/DEBI-Overview.pdf.

CDC (2005) Replicating effective programs plus. Retrieved September 22, 2005 from www.cdc.gov/hiv/projects/rep/default.htm.

Centers for Disease Control and Prevention (CDC) (1999) AIDS community demonstration projects research group: community-level HIV intervention in five cities: final outcome data from the CDC AIDS community demonstration projects. *American Journal of Public Health* 89:336–345.

Chan, C.S. (1989) Issues of identity development among Asian-American lesbians and gay men. *Journal of Counseling and Development* 68:16–20.

Chau, K.L. (1989) Sociocultural dissonance among ethnic minority populations. *Social Casework* 70:224–230.

Collins, C. (1997) *Dangerous inhibitions: how America is letting AIDS become an epidemic of the young.* Monograph series occasional paper no. 3. Center for AIDS Prevention Studies (CAPS), University of San Francisco. Retrieved September 22, 2005 from www.caps.ucsf.edu.

Community-Campus Partnerships for Health. (1998) Principles of good community–campus partnerships, 1998 Conference. Retrieved September 22, 2005 from http://depts.washington.edu/ccph/principles:html#principles.

Crosby, R.A., DiClemente, R.J., Wingood, G.M., Sionean, C., Cobb, B., and Harrington, K. (2000) Correlates of unprotected vaginal sex among African American female adolescents: importance of relationship dynamics. *Archives of Pediatric and Adolescent Medicine* 154:893–899.

Cross-Network CAB Working Group (2005) *Defining best practices for community representative involvement in HIV clinical research networks.* National Institute of Allergy and Infectious Diseases (NIAID), Division of AIDS (DAID), Washington, DC.

Dawson, L.J., Chunis, M.L., Smith, D.M., and Carboni, A.A. (2001) The role of academic discipline and gender in high school teachers: AIDS-related knowledge and attitudes. *Journal of School Health* 71(1):3–8.

DeCarlo, P. (2002) Does sex education work? Center for AIDS Prevention (CAPS), University of California at San Francisco. Retrieved September 22, 2005 from www.caps.ucsf.edu/sexedtext.html.

DHHS (2001) Newsletter of the Office of Minority Health. Retrieved September 22, 2005 from www.omhrc.gov/OMH/sidebar/archivedhiv.htm#2.

DiClemente, R.J. (1992) Psychosocial determinants of condom use among adolescents. In DiClemente, R.J. (ed) *Adolescents and AIDS: A generation in jeopardy.* Sage Publications, Thousand Oaks, CA, 34–51.

DiClemente, R.J., and Peterson, J.L. (1994) Changing HIV/AIDS risk behaviors: the role of behavioral interventions. In: DiClemente, R.J., and Peterson, J.L. (eds) *Preventing AIDS: theories and methods of behavioral interventions.* Plenum, New York.

DiFranceisco, W., Kelly, J.A., Otto-Salaj, L., McAuliffe, T.L., Somlai, A.M., Hackl, K., Heckman, T.G., Holtgrave, D.R., and Rompa, D.J. (1999) Factors influencing attitudes within AIDS service organizations toward the use of research-based HIV prevention interventions. *AIDS Education and Prevention* 11:72–86.

Dugan, T. (1998) Transgendered people. In: Smith, R.A. (ed) *Encyclopedia of AIDS: a social, political, and scientific record of the HIV epidemic.* Fitzroy Dearborn, Chicago.

Ekstrand, M.L., Siegel, D., Nido, V., Faigeles, B., Krasnovsky, F., Battle, R., Cummings, G., Chiment, E., and Coates, T.J. (1996) Peer-led AIDS prevention delays sexual debut among U.S. junior high school students. Presented at the XI International Conference on AIDS, Vancouver, Canada.

Finkelhor, D., Mitchell, K.J., and Wolak, J. (2000) *Online victimization: a report on the nation's youth.* National Center for Missing and Exploited Children, Washington, DC. Retrieved September 22, 2005 from www.UNH.edu/ccrc/projects/internet_survey.html.

Fishbein, M., and Middlestadt, S.E. (1989) Using the theory of reasoned action as a framework for understanding and changing AIDS-related behaviors. In: Wasserheit, J.N. (ed) *Primary prevention of AIDS: psychological approaches.* Cited in Gandelman & Freedman (2002).

Fisher, C.B. (2003) Adolescent and parent perspectives on ethical issues in youth drug use and suicide survey research. *Ethics & Behavior* 13(4):303–332.

Forum for Collaborative HIV Research. (2001) Linkage and integration of HIV testing, prevention, and care services. Project of CDC, HRSA, and the Forum for Collaborative Research. Retrieved September 22, 2005, from www.hivforum.org/publications/SummaryLinkRprt.pdf.

Fothergill, K., and Ballard, E. (1998) The school-based health center: a promising model of community-based care for adolescents. *Journal of Adolescent Health* 23:29–38.

Friedman, S.R., Curtis, R., Jose, B., Neaigus, A., Zenilman, J., Culpepper-Morgan, J., Borg, L., Kreek, J., Paone, D., and DesJarlais, D.C. (1997) Sex, drugs, and infections among youth: parentally and sexually transmitted diseases in a high-risk neighborhood. *Sexually Transmitted Diseases* 24:322–326.

Futterman, D.C., Peralta, L., Rudy, B.J., Wolfson, S., Guttmacher, S., Rogers, A.S., and Project Access Team of the Adolescent Medicine HIV/AIDS Research Network. (2001) The ACCESS (Adolescents Connected to Care, Evaluation, and Special Services) project: social marketing to promote HIV testing to adolescents, methods and first year results from a six city campaign. *Journal of Adolescent Health* 29S:19–29.

Gandelman, A., and Freedman, B. (2002) What is the role of theory in HIV prevention? Center for AIDS Prevention (CAPS), University of California at San Francisco. Retrieved September 22, 2005 from www.caps.ucsf.edu.

Getz, K., and Borfitz, D. (2002) *Informed consent: a guide to the risks and benefits of volunteering for clinical trials.* CenterWatch, Boston. Retrieved September 22, 2005 from www.centerwatch.com.

Gilliam, A., Barrington, T., Davis, D., Lacson, R., Uhl, G., and Phoenix, U. (2003) Building evaluation capacity for HIV prevention programs. *Evaluation and Program Planning* 26:133–142.

Glanz, K., Marcus Lewis, F., and Rimer, B.K. (eds). (1997) Theory at a glace: a guide for health promotion practice, In: *Health behavior and health education: theory, research and practice*, 2nd ed. Jossey-Bass, San Francisco.

Goldstein, E. (2001) Finding, selecting, implementing HIV/AIDS prevention programs. Retrieved September 22, 2005 from www.caps.ucsf.edu/collaboration.html.

Goldstein, E., Freedman, B., Richards, A., and Grinstead, O. (2000) *The Legacy Project: lessons learned about conducting community-based research*. Science to Community Series. AIDS Research Institute, University of California, San Francisco. Cited in Goldstein et al. (2001).

Goldstein, E., Freedman, B., and Wohlfeiler, D. (2001) *How can service providers and researchers collaborate in HIV prevention?* Center for AIDS Prevention (CAPS), University of California, San Francisco. Retrieved September 22, 2005 from www.caps.ucsf.edu.

Green, L.W. (2001) From research to "best practices" in other settings and populations. *American Journal of Health Behavior* 25:165–178.

Harlem Health Promotion Newsletter. (2001, Fall) Retrieved September 22, 2005 from www.healthyharlem.org.

Harlem Health Promotion Newsletter. (2002, Summer).

Harper, G.W., and DeCarlo, P. (1999) *What are adolescents' HIV prevention needs?* Center for AIDS Prevention (CAPS), University of California, San Francisco. Retrieved September 22, 2005 from www.caps.ucsf.edu/adolrev.html.

Havens, J., Mellins, C.A., and Hunter, J. (2002) Psychiatric aspects of HIV/AIDS in childhood and adolescence. In: Rutter, M., and Taylor, E. (eds) *Child and adolescent psychiatry*, 4th ed. Blackwell Science, London.

Hays, R.B., Kegeles, S.M., and Coates, T.J. (1997) Unprotected sex and HIV risk-taking among young gay men within boyfriend relationships. *AIDS Education and Prevention* 9:314–329.

Hays, R.B., Rebchook, G., and Kegeles, S.M. (2003) The Mpowerment Project: community-building with young gay and bisexual men to prevent HIV. *American Journal of Community Psychology* 31:301–312.

Healthy People 2010. (1999) *Educational and community-based programs*, conference edition, No. 7. Centers for Disease Control and Prevention (CDC), Atlanta; Health Resources and Services Administration (HRSA), Bethesda.

Henshaw, S.K. (1999) *Teenage pregnancy statistics with comparative statistics for women aged 20–24*. Alan Guttmacher Institute, New York. Retrieved September 22, 2005 from www.guttmacher.org/pubs/fb_teen_sex.html.

Herlocker, T., Hoff, C., and DeCarlo, P. (1995) *Can theory help in HIV prevention?* Center for AIDS Prevention (CAPS), University of California, San Francisco. Retrieved September 22, 2005 from www.caps.ucsf.edu.

Howard, M., and McCabe, J. (1990) Helping teenagers postpone sexual involvement. *Family Planning Perspectives* 22:21–26.

HRSA, U.S. Department of Health and Human Services. (1997) Self Assessment Modules: *Comprehensive HIV Services Planning, 1997; Developing and Pursuing the Mission; and Continuum of Care*, Bethesda, MD.

HRSA, U.S. Department of Health and Human Services. (1998) *Using data to assess HIV/AIDS service needs*. HIV/AIDS Evaluation Monograph, Report No. 2. HRSA, Bethesda.

HRSA, U.S. Department of Health and Human Services. (1999) *HRSA Care-ACTION: providing HIV/AIDS care in a changing environment*. HRSA, Bethesda.

Huba, G.J., and Melchior, L.A. (1998) A model for adolescent-targeted HIV/AIDS services: conclusions from 10 adolescent-targeted projects funded by the Special Projects of National Significance Program of the Health Resources and Services Administration. *Journal of Adolescent Health* 23S:11–27.

Hunter, J. (1995) At the crossroads: lesbian youth. In: Jay, K. (ed) *Dyke life*. Basic, Books, New York, pp. 50–60.

Hunter J., and Lounsbury, D. (2005) So you want to work with researchers? Negotiating effective community–research partnership. Skills Building Workshop presented at the Conference on Biopsychosocial Aspects of HIV Infection, Capetown, South Africa.

Hunter, J., and Mallon, G.P. (1998) Adolescents. In: Smith, R.A. (ed) *Encyclopedia of AIDS: a social, political, and scientific record of the HIV epidemic*. Fitzroy Dearborn, Chicago, pp. 41–43.

Hunter, J., and Schaecher, R. (1992) Adolescents and AIDS: coping issues. In: Ahmed, P.I. (ed) *Living and dying with AIDS*. Plenum, New York, pp. 35–45.

Hunter, J., Baer, J., and Williams, S. (2001) Adoption and dissemination of an HIV risk reduction program for lesbian, gay, and bisexual adolescents: a joint researcher-community program. Presented at the AIDS Impact Biopsychosocial Conference, Brighton, UK.

Hunter, J., Cohall, R., Castrucci, B., and Ellis, J. (2001) Lesbian, gay, bisexual, transgender, and questioning adolescent perceptions of medical providers. Presented at the Annual Meeting of the American Public Health Association, Atlanta, GA.

Hunter, J., Cohall, A., Mallon, G., Moyer, M.B., and Riddel, J. (2005) Health care delivery and public health related to LGBT youth and young adults. In: Shankle, M.D. (ed) *Handbook of lesbian, gay, bisexual, and transgender public health: a practitioner's Guide to Service*. Haworth Press, Binghamton, NY.

Hunter, J., Miller, S., Hughes, B., and Brown, C. (1999) Coping with stress in the lives of lesbian, gay and bisexual youth. Skills building workshops I and II at the 4th International Conference on the Biopsychosocial Aspects of HIV Infection, Ottawa, Canada.

Institute of Medicine. (2000) No time to lose: getting more from HIV prevention. Report to Congress. National Academy Press, Washington, DC.

Israel, B.A., Schulz, A.J., Parker, E.A., and Becker, A.B. (1998) Review of community-based research: assessing partnership approaches to improve public health. *Annual Review of Public Health* 19:173–202.

Israel, G.E., and Tarver, D.E. (1997) *Transgender care: recommended guidelines, practical information, and personal accounts*. Temple University Press, Philadelphia.

Jemmott, J.B., Jemmott, L.S., and Fong, G.T. (1992) Reductions in HIV risk-associated sexual behaviors among Black male adolescents: effects of an AIDS prevention intervention. *American Journal of Public Health* 82:372–377.

Jemmott, J.B., Jemmott, L.S., and Fong, G.T. (1998) Abstinence and safer sex HIV risk-reduction interventions for African-American adolescents: a randomized controlled trial. *Journal of the American Medical Association* 279:1529–1536.

Kaiser Family Foundation (2005) Teen sexual activity. Kaiser, Menlo Park, CA. Retrieved September 22, 2005 from www.kff.org.

Keatley, J., and Clements-Nolle, K. (2001) What are the HIV prevention needs of male-to-female transgender persons (MTFs)? Centers for AIDS Prevention (CAPS), University of California, San Francisco. Retrieved September 22, 2005 from www.caps.ucsf.edu.

Keller, S.N., and Brown, J.D. (2002) Media interventions to promote responsible sexual behavior. *Journal of Sex Research* 39:67–72.

Kelly, J.A. (2000) *Mobilizing community strengths to prevent AIDS*. Center for AIDS Intervention Research, Milwaukee.

Kim, N., Stanton, B., Li, X., Dickersin, K., and Galbraith, J. (1997) Effectiveness of the 40 adolescent AIDS risk reduction interventions: a quantitative review. *Journal of Adolescent Health* 20:204–215.

Kirby, D.J. (2002) The impact of schools and school programs upon adolescent sexual behavior. *Journal of Sex Research* 39:27–33.

Kirby, D.J., Barth, R., Leland, N., and Fetro, J.V. (1991) Reducing the risk: a new curriculum to prevent sexual risk-taking. *Family Planning Perspectives* 23:253–263.

Kolbe, L.J., Talley, R.C., and Short, R. (1999) Integrating education, health and social services for young people: current status and future directions. *Journal of Educational & Psychological Consultation* 10:297–313.

Lesbian and Gay Community Services Center (1997, December/1998 January) *HIV prevention for youth*. LGCSC, New York.

Lewando-Hundt, G., and Zaroo, S.A. (2000) Evaluating the dissemination of health promotion research. In: Thorogood, M., and Coombes, Y. (eds) *Evaluating health promotion: practice and methods*. Oxford University Press, London, pp. 151–162.

Lin, Y.G., Melchiono, M.W., Huba, G.J., and Woods, E.R. (1998) Evaluation of a linked service model of care for HIV-positive, homeless, and at-risk youths. *AIDS Patient Care and STDs* 12:787–796.

Lyon, M.E., and Richmond, D. (1995) Is sexual abuse in childhood or adolescence a predisposing factor for HIV infection during adolescence? *Pediatric AIDS HIV Infection* 6:271–275.

MacKellar, D.A., Valleroy, L.A., Secura, M.G., Bartholow, B.N., McFarland, W., Shehan, D., Ford, W., LaLota, M., Celetano, D.D., Koblin, B.A., Torian, L.V., Perdue, T.E., and Janssen, R.S. (2002) Repeat HIV testing, risk behaviors, and HIV seroconversion among young men who have sex with men: a call to monitor and improve practice of prevention. *Journal of Acquired Immune Deficiency Syndromes* 29:76–85.

Madison, S.M., McKay, M.M., Paikoff, R., and Bell, C.C. (2000) Basic research and community collaboration: necessary ingredients for the development of a family-based HIV prevention program. *AIDS Education and Prevention* 12:281–298.

Main, D.S., Iverson, D.C., McGloin, J., Banspach, S.W., Collins, J.L., Rugg, D.L., and Kolbe, L.J. (1994) Preventing HIV infection among adolescents: evaluation of a school-based education program. *Preventive Medicine* 23:409–417.

Markham, C., Baumler, E., Richesson, R., Parcel, G., Basen-Engquist, K., Kok, G., and Wilkerson, D. (2000) Impact of HIV-positive speakers in a multicomponent, school-based HIV/STD prevention program for inner-city adolescents. *AIDS Education and Prevention* 12:442–454.

MARS Project (Strack, R.W., Alexander, C., Weston, C., Tomoyasu, N., and Solomon, L.). (2000) *Report of the Monitoring Adolescents in Risky Situations (MARS) project: findings from the 1999 out-of-home youth survey*. CDC, Atlanta.

Massachusetts Department of Education. (1995) *Massachusetts youth risk behavior survey*.

Miller, R.L., Bedney, B.J., Guenther-Grey, C., and the CITY Project Study Team. (2003) Assessing organizational capacity to deliver HIV prevention services collaboratively: tales from the field. *Health Education and Behavior* 30:582–600.

Miller, S., Hunter, J., Haymes, R., Kilmnick, D., Hughes, B., Schneider, B., Scarella, J., and Schreibman, J. (1996) *Working it out, an intervention manual for lesbian, gay, and bisexual youth*. HIV Center for Clinical & Behavioral Studies/NYSPI, New York (www.hivcenternyc.org).

Minkler, M. (ed). (1997) *Community organizing and community building for health*. Rutgers University Press, Piscataway, NJ.

Monahan, N. (1997) Making the grade: responding to lesbian, gay and bisexual youth in schools. In: Schneider, M.S. (ed) *Pride & prejudice: working with lesbian, gay and bisexual youth*. Central Toronto Youth Services, Toronto.

Multicultural Competency Assessment for Organizations. (2001a, Spring) Wisconsin HIV Prevention Community Planning Council, Nara Smith Cox, PhD,

Consultant. In: *HIV Impact*, Newsletter of the Office of Minority Health (USDHHS).

Multicultural Competency Self-Assessment for Prevention Service Providers. (2001b, Winter) Wisconsin HIV Prevention Community Planning Council, Nara Smith Cox, PhD, Consultant. In: *HIV Impact*, Newsletter of the Office of Minority Health (USDHHS).

Murphy, D.A., Wilson, C.M., Durako, S.J., Muenz, L.R., and Belzer, M. (2001) Antiretroviral medication adherence among the REACH HIV-infected adolescent cohort in the USA. *AIDS Care* 13(1):27–40.

National AIDS Fund. (1993) *Evaluating HIV/AIDS Prevention Programs in Community-Based Organizations*. Communications Sciences Group, National AIDS Fund, Washington, DC.

National Association of Social Workers. (2002, October) Rural social workers embrace challenge. *NASW Newsletter*. NASW, Washington, DC.

National Institute on Drug Abuse. (2002) Prevention programs for HIV-positive youths reduces risks of further HIV transmission. In: *NIDA Notes*. Newsletter, NIH, USDHHS. Retrieved September 22, 2005 from www.drugabuse.gov.

National Institutes of Health. (1997) *Consensus development conference statement*. NIH, Rockville, MD. Retrieved September 22, 2005 from www.advocatesforyouth.org.

Nicholas, S.W., and Abrams, E.J. (2002) Boarder babies with AIDS in Harlem: lessons in applied public health [editorial]. *American Journal of Public Health* 92:163–165.

Northridge, M.E., Vallone, D., Merzel, C., Greene, D., Shepard, S., Cohall, A.T., and Healton, C.G. (2000) The adolescent years: an academic-community partnership in Harlem comes of age. *Journal of Public Health Management and Practice* 6:53–60.

Paikoff, R.L., Holmbeck, G.N., Parfenoff, S.H., Bhorade, A., and Gillming, G. (1997) *Family, peer, and social problem solving factors and risk for HIV exposure among urban African American adolescents*. Cited in Madison et al. (2000).

Pratt, D. (2002) Working it out: scenes from the lives of gay and lesbian youth. In *Body Positive Magazine* 15(6):7–12. Retrieved September 22, 2005 from www.thebody.com/bp/nov02/working_it_out.html.

Rapkin, B., and Trickett, E.J. (2005) Comprehensive dynamic trial designs for behavioral prevention research with communities: overcoming inadequacies of the randomized controlled trial paradigm. In: Trickett, E.J., and Pequenaut, W. (eds) *Community interventions and AIDS*. Oxford University Press, New York.

Reback, K., and Lombardi, E.L. (1999) HIV risk behaviors of male-to-female transgenders in a community-based harm reduction program. *International Journal of Transgenderism* 3:1–2.

Remafedi, G. (2001) Linking HIV-seropositive youth with health care: evaluation of an intervention. *AIDS Patient Care STDs* 15:147–151.

Rogers, A.S., Miller, S., Murphy, D.A., Tanney, M., and Fortune, T. (2001) The TREAT (Therapeutic Regimens Enhancing Adherence in Teens) program: theory and preliminary results. *Journal of Adolescent Health* September:30–38.

Rogers, E.M. (1995) *Diffusion of innovations*, 4th ed. Free Press, New York.

Rosenfeld, S.L., Keenan, P.M., Fox, D.J., Chase, L.H., Melchiono, M.W., and Woods, E.R. (2000) Youth perceptions of comprehensive adolescent health services through the Boston HAPPENS program. *Journal of Pediatric Health Care* 14:60–67.

Rosenstock, I.M., Strecher, V.J., and Becker, M.H. (1994) The health belief model and HIV risk behavior change. In: DiClemente, R.J. (ed) *Preventing AIDS: theories and methods of behavioral interventions*. Plenum, New York.

Rotheram-Borus, M.J., Koopman, C., Haignere, C., and Davies, M. (1991) Reducing HIV sexual risk behaviors among runaway adolescents. *Journal of the American Med Association* 266:1237–1241.

Ryan, C., and Futterman, D. (1997) Lesbian and gay youth: care and counseling. *Adolescent Medicine: State of the Art Reviews* 8:207–374.

Santelli, J., and Rogers, A.S. (2002) Parental permission, passive consent, and "children" in research [letter]. *Journal of Adolescent Health* 31:303–304.

Schmitt, S. (2001) *Five steps to effective AIDS advocacy, test positive aware network*. Retrieved September 22, 2005 from www.thebody.com.

Seal, D.W., Kelly, J.A., Bloom, F.R., Stevenson, L.Y., Coley, B.I., Broyles, L.A., and the Medical College of Wisconsin CITY Project Research Team. (2000) *HIV prevention with young men who have sex with men: what young men themselves say is needed*. AIDS Care 12(1):5–26.

Sexuality Information and Education Council of the United States (SIECUS). (2004) *Guidelines for comprehensive sexuality education, K-12*. 3rd ed. Retrieved September 22, 2005 from www.siecus.org/pubs/guidelines/guidelines.pdf.

Stanton, B.S., Li, X., Ricardo, I., Galbraith, J., Feigelman, S., and Kaljee, L. (1996) A randomized, controlled effectiveness trial of an AIDS prevention program for low-income African-American youths. *Archives of Pediatric and Adolescent Medicine* 150:363–372.

St. Lawrence, J.S., Brasfield, T.L., Jefferson, K.W., Alleyne, E., O'Bannon, R.E., and Shirley, A. (1995) Reducing the risk: cognitive-behavioral interventions to reduce African-American adolescents' risk for HIV infection. *Journal of Consulting and Clinical Psychology* 63:221–237.

Sullivan, M., Bhuyan, R., Senturia, K., Shiu-Thornton, S., and Ciske, S. (2005) Participatory action research in practice: a case study in addressing domestic violence in nine cultural communities. *Journal of Interpersonal Violence* 20:977–995.

Surgeon General. (2001) The Surgeon General's call to action to promote sexual health and responsible sexual behavior (www.surgeongeneral.gov/library/sexualheath). Retrieved December 30, 2004.

Ubell, E. (1995) Sex education programs that work—and some that don't. *Parade Magazine*, February 12, pp. 18–20.

Udry, J.R. (1998) Biological predispositions and social control in adolescent sexual behavior. *American Sociological Review* 53:709–722. Also in: Hyde, J.S., and DeLamater, J.D. (eds) *Understanding human sexuality*, 7th ed. McGraw-Hill, Boston 2000.

UNAIDS. (1997) *Impact of HIV and sexual health education on the sexual behavior of young people: a review update*. In: *CAPS: Fact sheet: what are adolescents' prevention Needs?* 1999. Retrieved September 22, 2005 from www.caps.ucsf.edu.

Valleroy, L.A., MacKellar, D.A., Karon, J.M., Rosen, D.H., McFarland, W., Shehan, D.A., Stoyanoff, S.R., LaLota, M., Celentano, D.D., Koblin, B.A., Theide, H., Katz, M.H., Torian, L.V., and Janssen, R.S., for the Young Men's Survey Study Group. (2000) HIV prevalence and associated risks in young men who have sex with men. *Journal the American Medical Association* 284:198–204.

Velicer, W.F., Fava, J.L., Prochaska, J.O., Abrams, D.B., Emmons, K.M., and Pierce, J. (1995) Distribution of smokers by stage in three representative samples. *Preventive Medicine* 24:401–411.

Wallerstein, N. (1992) Powerlessness, empowerment and health: implications for health promotion programs. *American Journal of Health Promotion* 6:197–205.

Walter, H.J., and Vaugh, R.D. (1993) AIDS risk reduction among a multi-ethnic sample of urban high school students. *Journal of the American Medical Association* 270:725–730.

Wandersman, A., and Florin, P. (2003) Community interventions and effective prevention. *American Psychologist* 58:441–448.

Weinstein, M., Farthing, C., Portillo, T., et al. (1998) Taking it to the streets: HIV testing, treatment information and outreach in a Los Angeles neighborhood coffee house. Abstract 43125. Presented at the XII World AIDS Conference, Geneva. In: CAPS: fact sheet: what are adolescents' prevention needs? 1999. Retrieved September 22, 2005 from www.caps.ucsf.edu.

Weissman, M.M. (1997) Interpersonal psychotherapy: current status. *Keio Journal of Medicine* 46(3)105–110.

White House (2000) White House Report, 2000. Office of National AIDS Policy, Washington, DC.

Wilitsky, R., for the Seropositive Urban Men's Study Group. (1999) Rethinking primary prevention to meet the needs of gay and bisexual men living with HIV (no. 184). Presented at the National HIV Prevention Conference, Atlanta. Cited in Remien, R., Senterfitt, W., and DeCarlo, P. (2002) *What are HIV+ persons HIV prevention needs?* Center for AIDS Prevention (CAPS), University of California, San Francisco. Retrieved September 22, 2005, from www.caps.ucsf.edu.

Wilson, C.M., Houser, J., Partlow, C., Rudy, B.J., Futterman, D.C., Friedman, L.B., and the Adolescent Medicine HIV Research Network. (2001) *Journal of Adolescent Health* 29S:8–18.

Windsor, R., Baranowski, T., Clark, N., and Cutter, G. (1994) *Evaluation of health promotion, health education, and disease prevention programs*, 2nd ed. Mayfield Publishing, Mountain View, CA, pp. 15–23.

Wingood, G.M., and DiClemente, R.J. (2000) Application of the theory of gender and power to examine HIV-related exposures, risk factors and effective interventions for women. *Health Education and Behavior* 27:539–565.

Woods, E.R. (1998) Overview of the special projects of national significance program's 10 models of adolescent HIV care. *Journal of Adolescent Health* 23(Supplement):5–10.

Yoshikawa, H., Wilson, P., Hsueh, J., Rosman, E., Chin, J., and Kim, J. (2003) What front-line CBO staff can tell us about culturally anchored theories of behavior change in HIV prevention for Asian/Pacific Islanders. *American Journal of Community Psychology* 32:143–158.

Online Resources

Adolescent Trials Network for HIV/AIDS Interventions: prevention and care for today's youth (www.atnonline.org). Retrieved September 22, 2005.

Advocates for Youth: www.advocatesforyouth.org. Additional sponsored Web sites: www.ambientejoven.org (for Latino GLBTQ youth); www.themediaproject.com (for the entertainment industry; www.mysistahs.org (for young women of color); and www.youthresource.com (for gay, lesbian, bisexual, transgender, and questioning (GLBTQ) youth).

AIDS Alliance for Children, Youth, Families. Retrieved September 22, 2005, from www.aids-alliance.org.

American Psychological Association's Healthy LGBT Students Project (www.apa.org/ed/hlgb.html). Retrieved September 22, 2005.

American Social Health Association's website for teens (www.ashastd.org). Retrieved September 22, 2005.

Gay/Lesbian/Straight Education Network (GLSEN): Safe schools action network; resources; directory of local chapters (www.glsen.org). Retrieved September 22, 2005.

Health Resources Administration (HRSA), AIDS Education Training Centers (AETCs): For clinicians on care and treatment (www.hab.hrsa.gov). Retrieved September 22, 2005.

Minnesota Department of Health: A professional's guide to GLBT youth health, Minnesota adolescent health action plan, 2002 (www.mnschoolhealth.com). Retrieved September 22, 2005.

National Minority AIDS Council (www.nmac.org). Retrieved September 22, 2005.

National Native American AIDS Prevention Center (NNAAPC): prevention programs, national case management network, technical assistance (www.nnaapc.org). Retrieved September 22, 2005.

National Youth Advocacy Coalition (NYAC): Improving the lives of lesbian, gay, bisexual, and transgender youth (www.nyac@nyacyouth.org). Retrieved September 22, 2005.

Parents, Families and Friends of Lesbians and Gays (P-FLAG): English/Spanish website (www.pflag.org). Retrieved September 22, 2005.

Planned Parenthood (www.plannedparenthood.org). Retrieved September 22, 2005.

28

Fenway Community Health's Model of Integrated, Community-Based LGBT Care, Education, and Research

Kenneth H. Mayer, Matthew J. Mimiaga, Rodney VanDerwarker,
Hilary Goldhammer, and Judith B. Bradford

1 Overview and History of Fenway Community Health

Fenway Community Health (FCH) was founded by local activists in 1971 in the Fenway area of downtown Boston, Massachusetts, as a primary care neighborhood health center serving diverse local populations. FCH quickly developed expertise in caring for lesbian, gay, bisexual, and transgender (LGBT) populations, reflecting the demographics of the staff and clients; and within a decade FCH rapidly expanded its medical and mental health services for gay men in response to the acquired immunodeficiency syndrome (AIDS) epidemic. As part of a growing recognition of the need to develop expertise and cultural competence in lesbian, bisexual, and transgender health concerns to better serve the full spectrum of the LGBT community, clinical services were expanded to include culturally sensitive programs to address substance use, parenting issues, and domestic and homophobic violence as well as specialized medical care programs for lesbians, bisexuals, and transgendered individuals.

FCH began as a grassroots neighborhood clinic. In 1975, the center recorded about 5000 patient care visits. In 2003, FCH's clinical departments recorded 61,983 visits by 11,154 individuals, including more than 1000 individuals receiving medical care for human immunodeficiency virus (HIV) infection. In 2004, a total of 11,799 individuals received services at FCH (Table 1, Fig. 28.1). The Center now has more than 170 staff responsible for clinical programs, community education, research, administration, planning, and development. Over the past few years, FCH's annual budget has exceeded $12 million.

The specific mission of FCH has been to enhance the physical and mental health of the local general community, with an emphasis on the

Table 1. Fenway Community Health Patient Demographics, 2004

Parameter	Female	Male	Total
Race/ethnicity			
Black/African American	239	359	598
Hispanic/Latino	136	364	500
Asian	315	299	614
White/Caucasian	2,615	5,813	8,428
Other/unknown	620	1,039	1,659
Total	3,925	7,874	11,799
Age (years)			
<18	3	4	7
18–19	72	52	124
20–29	1,891	1,957	3,848
30–39	965	2,270	3,235
40–49	573	2,268	2,841
50–59	313	999	1,312
60–69	71	262	333
>70	35	62	97
Unknown	2	0	2
Total	3,925	7,874	11,799

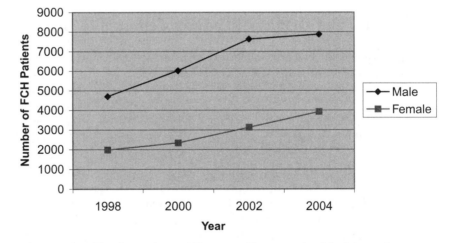

Figure 28.1 Total number of Fenway Community Health patients per year by gender.

provision of services for LGBT individuals. The Health Center also seeks to improve the overall health of the larger community—locally, nationally, internationally—through education and training, policy and advocacy, and research and evaluation. FCH is one of only seven LGBT-specific community health centers in the United States. FCH's services include primary medical care and specialty HIV/AIDS, gynecology, gerontology, podiatry, and nutritional counseling; mental health and addiction services; complementary therapies including chiropractic, massage, and acupuncture; health promotion programs, community education programs, programs for the prevention of domestic and homophobic violence, and parenting programs; and family planning services that include alternative insemination and same-sex marriage clinics. FCH received accreditation from the Joint Commission on Accreditation of Healthcare Organizations (JCAHO) in the spring of 2000 and was reaccredited in 2003.

FCH has established standards for improved cultural competence about LGBT health issues for other health providers and has developed programs to educate health professionals, as well as the general community, about specific LGBT health concerns. This Health Center may provide a model of comprehensive LGBT health services that have a local, as well as a broader, public health impact. FCH has developed unique programs for community health education and promotion, community-based research, health policy advocacy, and leadership in ongoing and emerging LGBT health care coalitions. These programs have been evaluated by external monitors, including federal agencies, and have been replicated elsewhere in the United States. FCH has also developed an active professional educational program, participating in the training of medical students, residents, social workers and other mental health interns, nurses, and allied health professionals; and many staff have appointments at local professional schools.

FCH developed one of the nation's first community-based research programs. The program has been conducting prospective epidemiologic studies to delineate factors associated with HIV transmission and prevention, as well as the natural history and treatment of HIV infection since 1985. Research is both informed by, and informs, clinical services at FCH to provide high-quality LGBT health care.

2 Medical Care

Although FCH offers a diverse array of clinical services, and defines health care broadly, incorporating preventive services and complementary therapy, the provision of comprehensive primary, and relevant subspecialty, care is at the core of its mission. As of 2004, the Medical Department employed 12 primary care staff physicians who are boarded in Internal or Family Medicine; many are also certified in a subspecialty. The Medical Department also has a gynecologist and a family practitioner trained in pediatrics. Medical staff physicians have admitting privileges at Beth Israel Deaconess Medical Center, a Harvard-affiliated hospital; and FCH physicians hold faculty appointments at Harvard Medical School.

To augment health center-wide communications and further improve quality of care in its clinical departments, FCH began using Logician (now known as Centricity EMR), an electronic medical record system, in 1997. The electronic record system enhances the comprehensiveness and integration of care by allowing providers who share patients to easily access reports, medication lists, and diagnoses scripted by other providers (including medical, mental health, and complementary therapy providers) and to notify relevant staff of critical chart notes immediately.

2.1 Primary Care

The Medical Department is the largest FCH clinical department. Physicians are teamed with other primary care providers (nurse practitioners, physician's assistants, registered nurses, licensed practical nurses) and medical social workers, who deal with issues ranging from health insurance access to housing and provide triage for mental health services. Primary care providers can readily refer clients to on-site mental health and other prevention services, including stress reduction programs, nutritional counseling, and substance abuse treatment.

Every medical patient at FCH works with a primary care team. Patients may select a primary care provider at the Health Center or at a freestanding, affiliated satellite practice. Depending on the patients' preferences, their primary care provider may be a physician, physician's assistant, or nurse practitioner. Patients may also request a female provider or a Spanish-speaking provider. The medical provider serves as a team leader and coordinates all routine medical care: examinations, laboratory tests, medical imaging, diagnosis, and treatment. In addition, providers can make referrals to other professionals within FCH who can promote wellness measures, such as stress reduction, nutritional education, and substance abuse counseling or to programs to help decrease sexual risk-taking behavior. FCH has also developed specialty clinics to address unique community needs, ranging from an anal dysplasia clinic, which provides high-resolution anoscopy and specially trained staff to manage complex lesions, to premarital screening clinics for same-sex couples.

2.2 Urgent Care/Hospitalization

For patients who are facing a medical or mental health crisis, FCH offers 24-hour emergency coverage 7 days a week. During office hours, patients may contact a member of their physician's team directly, who then directs them to the right resources. Depending on the situation, FCH staff arranges for them to be seen at the Health Center or the Beth Israel Deaconess Medical Center emergency room.

2.3 Case Management

For patients with complex health problems—such as HIV infection and other chronic illnesses—FCH offers comprehensive case management services. Registered nurses and medical social workers help clients understand and access the many resources available to them. For chronically ill patients, the primary care nurse assumes the additional role of case manager, assisting and supporting patients throughout the course of their illness. The primary care nurse helps patients understand the disease process and the impact it is likely to have on their health.

In addition, medical social workers are available to help patients cope with the practical and emotional aspects of their care and help them access mental health services. A medical social worker can help patients apply for Medicare or Medicaid and access community-based services such as financial, housing, and legal assistance programs and pastoral counseling; coordinate and facilitate communication among multiple service providers; and make referrals to various other services. To help patients deal with the profound disruptions—physical, emotional, financial—that serious illness or injury can bring, medical social workers also provide short-term, focused counseling and education to patients and their families.

2.4 Pharmacy

In 2003, FCH established its own freestanding pharmacy, and after 1 year of opening it dispenses more than 2700 prescriptions per month. The pharmacy is staffed by two pharmacists, who provide culturally sensitive patient education in addition to enhancing the "one-stop shopping" goal of FCH for facilitating comprehensive health care while minimizing barriers to care.

2.5 Senior Services

FCH has a long-standing relationship with the many seniors who live in the Fenway neighborhood. Senior patients make extensive use of the Center's board-certified geriatricians, a staff nutritionist, a podiatrist, and medical social workers. In addition, providers may make "house calls" for homebound patients, provide blood pressure screening, flu shot clinics, and educational information.

2.6 Specialty Care

FCH has a broad spectrum of on-site specialists, including clinicians trained in infectious diseases, gynecology, psychiatry, gerontology, nutrition, and podiatry. If a required specialty is not available at FCH, medical providers refer their patients to a specialist at Beth Israel Deaconess Medical Center or through its affiliated CareGroup network.

2.7 Women's Health

FCH offers medical and mental health care that is sensitive to the needs of women, particularly lesbians. Women's health at Fenway addresses the whole woman—from primary care, gynecology, and mental health to complementary therapies and substance abuse treatment (Carroll et al., 1999). The Health Center provides services that include a wide range of women-specific medical issues, including breast cancer, menopause, and osteoporosis. FCH also has providers on staff who specialize in helping women who are lesbian or bisexual address mental health issues. A comprehensive chart review of mental health services to sexual minority women resulted in changes to diagnostic procedures and greater standardization for assessment and referral (Rogers et al., 2003).

FCH also holds women-only and lesbian-only workshops and support groups that encompass a range of health concerns. Knowledgeable, skilled, and compassionate, FCH's staff has created a climate where all women can feel comfortable seeking care regardless of sexual orientation, race, or economic status.

2.8 Family and Parenting Services

In addition to having developed one of the nation's largest alternative insemination (AI) programs for nontraditional families, FCH provides support, information, and educational services to LGBT families, including educational presentations where parents can network. Support and counseling groups for lesbians and gay men considering parenting, childbirth classes for lesbians, and resources for prospective LGBT parents are also offered. Since 1983, FCH has been an international pioneer in helping lesbians and gay men claim their rights to parenthood. FCH was one of the first in the nation to offer AI services to lesbians and has assisted in more than 300 live conceptions. When the Massachusetts Supreme Judicial Court declared in May 2004 that same-sex couples had an equal right to marry, FCH responded quickly. The Health Center provided same-sex premarital screening appointments for more than 1000 patients from April 2004 to December 2004. FCH staff co-sponsored community forums to educate community members about the implications of this historic decision, and testimony was provided at statewide and national meetings about the impact of marital rights on personal and family health.

2.9 Transgender Health Program

In 1998, FCH served about 50 transgender patients. By 2004, the number of transgender patients had grown to almost 200. As a result of this growth, FCH formed the Transgender Health Program (THP), whose mission is to provide excellent comprehensive care in a comfortable, safe, respectful environment. A clinical committee that is co-led by medical and mental health providers who have significant experience working with transgender patients oversees the THP. The THP developed an extensive protocol for the prescription of hormone therapy, including guidelines for mental health and medical providers, visit timelines, medication recommendations, and consent forms. Additionally, the co-chairs of the committee oversee training within various departments at FCH to foster a welcoming environment for transgender patients.

2.10 Complementary Therapies

Complementary therapies (also known as holistic or alternative medicine) play an integral role in patient care at FCH. The complementary therapies program at FCH was founded in 1989 in direct response to community needs, particularly those of HIV-infected patients. Currently, FCH offers massage therapy, chiropractic medicine, and acupuncture treatment to both its HIV-infected and uninfected patients seeking acute and preventive care. During 2004, there were 318 massage therapy visits, 380 chiropractic therapy visits, and 197 acupuncture therapy visits at FCH. Most of the complementary therapy clients seek assistance with managing chronic and acute musculoskeletal issues. Some of these clients are music, dance, and voice students from the nearby performing arts colleges who use FCH as their primary health care facility. Other reasons for complementary therapy visits include acupuncture for irritable bowel syndrome, anxiety, fertility treatment, and nausea related to chemotherapy after breast cancer treatment. FCH also operates a free Acupuncture Detoxification daily walk-in clinic (see Section 3.1).

Both massage and acupuncture have also been used to help HIV-infected patients with medication and disease-related symptoms, such as nausea, digestion, and neuropathy. Massage also helps promote emotional well-being in HIV patients who may lack the benefit of physical touch and validation in their everyday lives.

Complementary therapy practitioners work in conjunction with medical and mental health providers to determine how chiropractic, acupuncture, and massage can benefit patients. All providers share the same facilities, including access to electronic patient medical records, allowing ease of communication and continuity of care across disciplines.

2.11 HIV Testing Services Program

One of the largest confidential test sites in Massachusetts, FCH provides HIV antibody testing, as well as pretest and posttest counseling to help patients deal with the issues that surround one's decision to test and the impact of knowing one's HIV status. Confidential testing is available for clients who want documentation of their HIV antibody test results. The HIV Testing Services Program (HTSP) was initiated in 1985 and is presently funded by the Massachusetts Department of Public Health AIDS Bureau. The HTSP has three full-time and two half-time staff and offers testing by both scheduled appointments and drop-in hours. From July 2003 to June 2004, the HTSP at FCH tested 1600 clients for HIV antibodies. Of these patients, 1200 identified as male, of which 1000 were men who have sex with other men (MSM). The remaining 600 patients described their HIV risks as heterosexual sex, injection drug use, and occupational exposure. Thirty individuals were confirmed to be HIV-infected, and more than 90% were triaged into other services at FCH.

The HTSP also offers a variety of short-term intervention groups for people newly found to be HIV-infected, those with an HIV-infected partner, and HIV-negative individuals who are at risk of infection. During 2004, approximately 200 individuals accessed these groups.

FCH was one of the first testing sites in Massachusetts to provide rapid HIV testing services to the community; this test enables us to produce results for the patient in about 20 minutes. Rapid testing began in December 2003; and since its inception the HTSP has performed more than 1000 tests. In addition, the HTSP offers hepatitis B and C testing as well as hepatitis A and B vaccinations.

3 Mental Health and Addiction Services

Staff psychiatrists, psychologists, and social workers offer a wide range of mental health services, including individual, group, couples, and family therapy as well as psychiatric medication evaluation and management; they also offer 24-hour beeper coverage to handle emergencies. At FCH, mental health intakes consist of a 1- to 3-hour clinical intake interview conducted by a psychologist or clinical social worker to determine the client's therapeutic program. Also, as part of HIV primary care at FCH, patients usually meet with a medical case manager. This case manager assesses mental health needs and makes referrals for mental health treatment when deemed necessary or when requested by the patient. Additionally, some individuals present for mental health treatment at FCH who receive their primary care elsewhere. Between July 2004 and December 2004, on average, the Mental Health Department had the following number of visits: 1494 for individual therapy per month, 163 for group therapy per month, and 196 for psychopharmacology per month. For a complete list of support/therapy groups offered by the Mental Health Department, see Table 2.

3.1 Addiction Services

Outpatient substance abuse treatment and acupuncture detoxification are an integral component of FCH's primary health services. Clients have access to recovery groups, including an onsite 12-step Alcoholics Anonymous (AA) program, HIV risk reduction education, primary care and referral services, and a variety of community support networks. The acupuncture detoxification and relapse prevention program offers daily walk-in clinic treatment 6 days per week. Counseling is offered on-site as part of the treatment model. Clients are required to participate in a series of HIV psychoeducational groups and often receive referrals to the HIV counseling and testing program. The outpatient-counseling program is available for those in various stages of recovery as well as their families and partners. In 2003, a total of 383 individuals received services in the acupuncture detoxification program and about 20% of them were from communities of color. Crystal methamphetamine addiction currently accounts for about 25% of the detoxification clients.

3.2 Crystal Methamphetamine Use Among MSM

The number of people seeking treatment for crystal methamphetamine addiction at FCH has increased over a 2-year period. From February 2003 through January 2004, FCH had 361 new patients in its substance abuse treatment program, 45 (12%) of whom reported crystal methamphetamine as their primary drug of concern. From February 2004 to December 2004, of 266 new patients 52 (20%) reported crystal methamphetamine as their primary drug of concern.

Table 2. Current Ongoing Support/Therapy Groups Available at
Fenway Community Health

Group	Description
Mental health	
Coming Out/ questioning	Short-term group (10 weeks) for men and women who are in the process of coming out or questioning their sexuality.
Compulsive sexual behavior therapy	Ongoing group for gay and bisexual men to develop skills to address their out-of-control sexual behavior.
Gender identity— biologic male	Ongoing group for people who have grown up being viewed as biologically male. Issues around gender, gender expression, and sexuality are discussed. Group members may identify, dress, and express their gender in any way they wish, including changing their expression, without any expectations that members identify or dress in any particular way.
FTX—biologic female	A gender queer/gender questioning group for people born into female bodies who are looking for a place to explore a broad range of gender journeys.
Gay men's mood disorder	Ongoing group for gay men who struggle with mood disorders such as major depression, anxiety, and bipolar illness. This group offers a supportive environment for members to share and cope with life issues that are affected by living with a chronic mood disorder.
Gay men's intimacy	Ongoing group focusing on helping members develop deeper and more intimate relationships.
Gay men's general issues	Ongoing group for gay men who want to explore relationship issues, which may include intimacy, trust, and self-esteem. Men have the opportunity, through the group process, to gain insight into how to have healthier, more meaningful relationships.
60+ Support	Ongoing group to discuss the challenges and rewards associated with LGBT aging, including relationships, social isolation, sexuality, health and illness, loss of friends and family, and reduced income.
Transgender partner	10-Week group for people who are partnered with someone who is exploring or has changed in some aspect of gender identity.
Navigating trauma	12-Week group designed to explore the impact that physical and sexual abuse, neglect, and other forms of trauma have on current lives, sense of self, and relationships with other people. The group focuses on making connections and developing strengths.
LGBT considering parenting	8-Week support group for LGBT people both single and in a couple, to discuss issues and concerns about parenting.
Partners of lesbians with cancer	Ongoing free support group that offers a space for self-care for those who are dealing with the impact of their partner's illness.
Lesbians with cancer	Ongoing free support group for those who want to discuss the impact of this disease and its treatments on their lives.
HIV	
3 Weeks HIV–	Reactions to testing negative, maintaining one's health and staying negative, safer sex in the real world, relationships with HIV-positive friends and partners, and handling the stresses of living in an epidemic.
3 Weeks HIV+	A place to talk about the first steps. A chance to talk about whom to tell, medical information, safer sex information, and community resources.
Long-term survivors with HIV	Ongoing to provide people living with HIV support around issues such as family, relationships, work, and health.
Partners of people with HIV	Ongoing support group that allows individuals with HIV-positive partners to discuss issues surrounding the virus in every aspect of their lives.

Table 2. *Continued*

Group	Description
Addiction services	
Orientation	Drop-in discussion and education group focusing on differentiating between substance abuse and addiction. Explores the place that alcohol and/or other drugs occupy in one's life and supports members in setting individual goals for reduced use, moderation, or abstinence from any substance the individual determines to be problematic.
Contract	Ongoing group for people committed to abstinence from all mood-altering substances except prescribed psychotropic medications, which are being taken as prescribed.
Recovery	Ongoing group for LGBT men and women in recovery from substance dependence. Focus is on maintaining recovery, dealing with past trauma, childhood and family-of-origin issues, self-esteem, intimacy, and establishing social support. Participants must have at least 3 months of clean and sober time.
Women's group	Ongoing group for women that focuses on reducing behaviors that are self-destructive and looks at current or past substance use.
Crystal meth	Ongoing group designed for gay/bisexual men who have goals of abstinence from crystal meth. The group is process-oriented that utilizes relationships, experiences, and support from group members to address issues related to their crystal meth addiction.
Violence Recovery Program	
Survivors of domestic violence	Free 12-week group for LGBT survivors of domestic violence. Provides an opportunity for participants to come together to learn about the dynamics of abuse and gain support from each other. Members may still be in an abusive relationship, trying to leave the relationship, or simply want to talk about a past relationship. Location is confidential.
Male survivors of adult sexual assault	Free 10-week group for adult men of all sexual orientations who have experienced a rape or sexual assault as an adult or as a child. The group provides male survivors an opportunity to discuss the impact of the sexual assault/rape on their lives and relationships. Special emphasis is placed on effective coping strategies. The group is run in collaboration with the Boston Area Rape Crisis Center.
Trauma education	Free 12-week group for LGBT people who have experienced abuse, violence, or other trauma. Discussions focus on the effects and symptoms of trauma in general, rather than each individual's traumatic story or memories. Group members learn how trauma affects one physically and emotionally; ways to cope with symptoms related to trauma; how to find support and heal from traumatic experiences; and ways to increase personal safety and improve self-care.

All of the new patients were MSM who frequented nightclubs and used Internet sites for soliciting sex. The rise in crystal methamphetamine use and its detrimental effects on the health of MSM prompted FCH to organize a public forum, held on March 17, 2003. As a result, a local chapter of Crystal Methamphetamine Anonymous was initiated. Initially, the group started with weekly meetings but soon increased its meetings to twice per week. FCH offers space free of charge for the group to meet.

In July 2004, FCH began a public awareness campaign regarding its services related to crystal methamphetamine. Palm cards and posters were printed and placed in community venues. Advertisements were placed in public transportation stations near places where high concentrations of MSM live. Additionally, advertisements were placed on www.manhunt.net (Manhunt), one of the most popular Internet sex sites used by local MSM, and web pages were developed and hyperlinked to the FCH website (www.fenwayhealth.org). The web page includes information about crystal methamphetamine, the connection between crystal methamphetamine and risky sexual behavior, personal stories of former users, and staff who oversee FCH services and area resources.

FCH currently offers two ongoing groups for people whose primary drug use problem is crystal methamphetamine. For those who have questions or concerns about their use, FCH offers a free of charge, weekly drop-in group that provides risk reduction information, referrals, short-term counseling, and support.

3.3 Violence Recovery Program

The Violence Recovery Program (VRP) at FCH was founded in 1986 and provides counseling, support groups, advocacy, and referral services to LGBT victims of bias crimes, domestic violence, sexual assault, and police misconduct. In 2003 and 2004, the VRP saw 158 and 151 clients, respectively. The program also compiles statewide statistics on antigay hate crime and same-sex domestic violence; and in collaboration with the National Coalition of Anti-Violence Programs, it releases annual reports based on these statistics. In 2003, the VRP documented 81 hate crime incidents and saw 75 victims of domestic violence at FCH. VRP staff members frequently give presentations at training sessions for police, court personnel, and human service providers regarding LGBT crime survivor issues. Other services include a support group for LGBT domestic violence survivors, the region's only support group for male survivors of rape and sexual assault, advocacy with the courts and police, and assistance with victim compensation. Via its toll-free number (800-834-3242), the VRP provides assistance to crime survivors statewide and provides short-term counseling to survivors and their families and referrals to longer-term counseling through FCH's Mental Health Department.

3.4 Peer Listening Line/Gay, Lesbian, Bisexual, and Transgender Helpline

FCH maintains the largest LGBT help and crisis intervention telephone hotlines in New England. The Peer Listening Line (toll-free: 800-399-PEER) is staffed by volunteers age 25 and under who provide anonymous psychosocial, health, and informational support to LGBT youths aged 13 to 25. The Gay, Lesbian, Bisexual, Transgender Helpline (toll-free: 888-340-4528) volunteers provide these services to all callers, regardless of age. Both lines are operated seven nights per week by a staff of about 90 volunteers. In 2004, the Helpline received almost 4000 calls, 40% of which were for general support; more than 22% were regarding coming-out issues. Altogether, 65% of Helpline calls came from outside Massachusetts. The Peer Listening Line received more than 1000 calls, 45% of which were for general support, and more than 31% were regarding coming-out issues. Almost 80% of these calls came from outside Massachusetts.

4 Wellness Programs and Community Education

Over the years, FCH has developed a program of community education and health promotion. A variety of programs and services are in place to provide accurate, up-to-date information on health and wellness topics important to the LGBT community and to build skills needed to maintain and/or improve one's health. These programs and services were developed to complement the clinical care of current patients and to assist with connecting more difficult to reach populations (e.g., communities of color and non-gay-identified MSM) in need of the clinical services to FCH.

Today, as the largest provider of HIV and AIDS care in New England, FCH prevention programs focus on both helping HIV-negative individuals stay healthy and dealing with the emotional impact that HIV has on self, family, friends, and community. Other programs assist HIV-positive clients, their loved ones, and caregivers to deal with the medical, emotional, social, financial, and legal aspects of HIV and AIDS.

4.1 Living Well

Living Well is a series of seven health education programs held throughout the year that seek to create a stronger gay and bisexual male community by providing men with a comfortable, friendly, supportive space to discuss and explore some of the most challenging personal and social issues in the age of HIV/AIDS. Living Well sponsors workshops, forums, and lectures on topics such as sexually transmitted diseases, substance abuse, stress management, and body image. Most programs are directed toward men regardless of their HIV status, but some are directed specifically toward HIV-infected or uninfected men. Attendance ranges from 10 to 100 people per session depending on the format and topic.

4.2 Boundless

Boundless is a series of four health education events held throughout the year promoting holistically healthy lesbian, bisexual women, and transgender communities. Boundless sponsors workshops, forums, and lectures on topics such as adjustments to midlife, bisexuality, alternative insemination, and sexual communication. Attendance ranges from 10 to 50 people per session depending on the format and topic.

4.3 HotMale

HotMale is an Internet-based outreach program that provides information, referrals, and psychosocial support to men through chat sites where men seek other men for sex or dating. HotMale allows FCH staff to reach isolated men who may not frequent other outreach venues such as nightclubs and bars. In 2003, HotMale staff contributed 587 hours conducting online outreach and served 635 individuals.

4.4 Color Me Healthy

Color Me Healthy is a prevention and education program for Latino and African American gay, bisexual, and transgender people. Brothaz Orchestrating Safer Sex (BOSS), part of the Color Me Healthy program, offers 4-week and 6-week groups geared toward promoting healthier life-styles within this community. In collaboration with the HotMale program, FCH held several "Safety Net" parties at BOSS group member's homes. "Safety Net" party hosts volunteer to invite friends to participate in a conversation about safer sex over a meal that the BOSS staff provide. Another program of Color Me Healthy is called the "Down Low." This program holds a series of group meetings for HIV-positive men of color, designed to help keep this community healthy and strong.

4.5 Safer Sex Education Team

The Safer Sex Education Team (SSET) consists of a variety of health promotion programs. The largest program, the Virus and Infection Protection (VIP) Crew consists of a volunteer team of men, women, and transgender people of diverse sexual, racial, and ethnic backgrounds. The VIP Crew conducts outreach about safer sex in Boston area bars, nightclubs, and local hangouts primarily serving the LGBT community. The volunteer team reaches more than 4000 people at risk for HIV per year, and they distribute more than 10,000 condom packets annually to those at risk for HIV and other sexually transmitted infections. The SSET's trained staff members also offer individual risk reduction sessions for those most at risk. Additionally, a group tailored to bisexual and bi-curious men is held monthly at Fenway, serving about 30 men per quarter year.

5 Research and Evaluation Programs

FCH initiated one of the nation's first community-based AIDS research programs in 1983 and received its first state and federal funding in 1984. The first AIDS diagnosis among Fenway patients was made in 1981, and prospective epidemiologic studies soon followed (Groopman et al., 1985). The first estimates of HIV prevalence and incidence in New England were derived from Fenway studies (Mayer et al., 1986). For a complete list of FCH research studies, study sponsors, and collaborators, see Table 3.

FCH has been a site for more than 200 research studies since 1984, when the initial longitudinal cohorts of HIV-infected MSM were enrolled (Groopman et al., 1985; Mayer et al., 1986). Since then, FCH has successfully participated in more than 40 clinical trials of anti-HIV therapeutics (Ruff, 1991), enrolling several hundred participants from the medical clinic. FCH has also been a leader in testing biologic

Table 3. Contracts in Fenway Community Health's Research and Evaluation Department and The Fenway Institute, 2004–2005

Contract	Sponsors	Collaborators
Research and Evaluation Department		
HIV Prevention Trials Network	NIAID	The Miriam Hospital (Providence, RI); YRG CARE (Chennai, India)
HIV Vaccine Trial Network	NIAID	Harvard Medical School and Brigham and Women's Hospital (Boston, MA); The Miriam Hospital (Providence, RI)
Center for AIDS Research (CFAR)	NIAID	Harvard Medical School Division of AIDS (Boston, MA)
CFAR Network of Integrated Clinical Systems	NIAID	University of California—San Francisco (San Francisco, CA)
Acute HIV Infection and Early Disease Research Program	NIAID	Massachusetts General Hospital (Boston, MA)
Understanding and Improving Adherence in HIV Disease	NIMH	New England Medical Center (Boston, MA)
Cognitive Behavioral Therapy for Depression and HIV Medication Adherence	NIAID	
HIV Primary Prevention for Persons with HIV	NIAID	University of Minnesota (Minneapolis, MN)
Enhancing HIV Prevention Among High-Risk HIV Infected Men in Primary Care	NIMH	
Client-Level Data Project	HRSA	
The Phoenix Project: A Contextual Model of Microbicide Acceptability	NIMH	Centers for Behavioral and Preventative Medicine/The Miriam Hospital (Providence, RI); Sociomedical Research Associates (Westport, CT, New York, NY)
STD surveillance projects	Massachusetts Department of Public Health and CDC	
Topical Microbicide Acceptability Study	NICHD	Columbia University (New York, NY)
Safer Sex Education Team	Massachusetts Department of Public Health	
Peer-to-Peer Project	HRSA	
Nonoccupational post-exposure prophylaxis studies	Gilead Sciences	
Clinical trials	Examples: Merck, GlaxoSmithKline, Boehringer Ingelheim, Saliva Diagnostic Systems	

Table 3. *Continued*

Contract	Sponsors	Collaborators
The Fenway Institute		
LGBT Smoking Cessation Project	American Legacy Foundation	The LGBT Center (Los Angeles, CA); Howard Brown Health Center (Chicago, IL)
Patient Retention Project	HRSA	
Positive Connections: Health System Navigation Project	HRSA	Multicultural AIDS Coalition, Living and Recovery Community at Victory Programs, and SPAN, Inc (Boston, MA)
Social Networks Demonstration Project	CDC	Multicultural AIDS Coalition (Boston, MA)
Ecstasy and Other Club Drug Prevention	SAMHSA	Bureau of Substance Abuse Services, Massachusetts Department of Public Health, Boston Public Health Commission, and AIDS Action Committee (Boston, MA)
Community Promise Plus	CDC	AIDS Action Committee

NIAID, National Institute of Allergies and Infectious Diseases, National Institutes of Health; NIMH, National Institute of Mental Health, National Institutes of Health; HRSA, Health Resources and Services Administration; CDC, Centers for Disease Control and Prevention; NICHD, National Institute of Child Health and Human Development, National Institutes of Health; SAMHSA, Substance Abuse and Mental Health Services Administration.

interventions to prevent HIV transmission, having been the first site in New England to test therapeutic and preventive HIV vaccines (DeMaria et al., 2000; Belshe et al., 2001). FCH studies were among the first to determine the relative efficiency of HIV transmission between MSM (DeGruttola et al., 1989) and to describe the effects of HIV disease progression and antiretroviral therapy on HIV in genital secretions (Anderson et al., 1992; Mayer et al., 1999). FCH behavioral research studies have focused on the interactions of substance use and risk taking (Seage, 1992, 1998) and sexual risk among younger MSM (Seage, 1997) and bisexual men (Wold, 1998). FCH collaborations have assessed community interest in HIV vaccines and risk factors for HIV serocon-version among MSM (Gross, 1996; Seage, 2001) as well as attitudes about other modes of HIV prevention (e.g., oral chemoprophylaxis) (Gross, 2000).

Recent FCH studies of sexually transmitted disease (STD) incidence, risk-taking behavior among Massachusetts MSM, and utilization of nonoccupational postexposure prophylaxis for HIV have been supported by the Centers for Disease Control and Prevention (CDC) (Mayer, 2002). FCH is the first National Institutes of Health (NIH)-funded site to look at the acceptability of rectal microbicides among high-risk men and women, in collaboration with researchers from Columbia University. FCH is a lead site for the National Institute of Allergies and Infectious Diseases (NIAID)-funded HIV Prevention Trials Network (HPTN), coordinating multiple HIV prevention studies at sites in Boston, Providence, and Chennai, India (Mayer et al., 2001, 2003; Chesney et al., 2003; Koblin et al., 2003; Chin-Hong et al., 2004; EXPLORE Study Team, 2004; Mimiaga et al., 2004b). Qualitative and quantitative studies of MSM are in development and in progress with collaborators in Chennai, India (Safren et al., 2004a,b,c, 2005; Kumarasamy et al., 2005).

FCH researchers have analyzed medical record information to examine the mental health concerns of lesbian and bisexual women (Rogers et al., 2003), gay and bisexual men (Mimiaga et al., 2002; Berg et al., in press), and HIV-infected gay and bisexual men (Berg et al., 2004; Mimiaga et al., 2004a) as well as to examine nonadherence to medical appointments in relation to increased plasma HIV RNA and decreased CD4 cell counts (Berg et al., 2005; Safren et al., 2005).

Along with its increased expertise in studying the health care concerns of MSM, FCH has increased the range of lesbian research studies and developed a formalized structure and agenda for lesbian health research that is commensurate with the expansion of clinical programs for women and reflecting the community's interest and support. Studies have ranged from the assessment of lesbians' access to care (Bradford and Norman, 2003) to a study of STDs among lesbians to the evaluation of techniques for alternative insemination (Carroll et al., 1997; Carroll & Palmer, 2001).

The Research and Evaluation Department employs more than 40 staff, including research physicians, nurses, psychologists, epidemiologists, data analysts, survey methodologists, and clinical research associates.

FCH has a freestanding institutional review board as well as a community advisory board that help the research staff evaluate the responsiveness of the current research agenda to community needs and expectations.

6 The Fenway Institute

As Healthy People 2010 documents were prepared at the end of the 1990s, community advocates and prominent national advocacy organizations argued successfully for inclusion of "persons defined by sexual orientation" as a population experiencing health disparities (Dean et al., 2000; Gay and Lesbian Medical Association, 2001). Additionally, various limitations of the current knowledge about LGBT populations has raised serious concerns. Among them are that data on LGBT persons of different race and ethnicity are insufficient, that few studies focus on transgender individuals, and that research studies are inconsistent in their definition and measures of sexual orientation and gender identity (Sell, 1997; Boehmer, 2002). Based on these concerns, The Fenway Institute (TFI) was established in 2000 to build on FCH's 30 years of innovative LGBT clinical initiatives and its research, education, and advocacy activities to (1) disseminate culturally sensitive best practices; (2) educate the LGBT community, healthcare providers, and public health officials; and (3) create a "think tank" to incubate new ideas to promote LGBT health. TFI has been dedicated to creating a national, interdisciplinary center of excellence to ensure the best healthcare standards for the diverse LGBT community. This is achieved through the development of research to understand better the health needs of the community, with the creation of programs and policies based on this knowledge. TFI formulates sociologic and epidemiologic questions and collaborates with expert researchers to uncover the answers; it uses the information gathered to develop policies and advocates for their adoption at the local, state, and national levels; it shares the information with others such as medical and mental health providers, government agencies, and community-based leaders (Bradford and Mayer, 2003); and it creates programming models to put the information into practice—and then assists in replicating it through other community-based organizations.

Development of TFI has provided a foundation from which to expand the scope and diversity of FCH research and evaluation studies and to translate results into education and practice. A core strength of TFI is the focus on development of a population research program using the most rigorous methods available to develop generalizable data about LGBT health and to evaluate the effectiveness of interventions. Since the initiation of TFI in 2000, we have been able to attract new researchers to work with us, further broadening our expertise in population-based research.

7 Program Support and Sustainability

FCH started as a free clinic, supported partially through donations by clients and partially through subsidies from the city of Boston. Over the past three decades FCH has become a sophisticated multidisciplinary center that is supported through a variety of sources, including patients' private insurance as well as Medicare and Medicaid for the payment of medical and mental health services (see Figures 28.2 and 28.3 for FCH's revenue and expenses for fiscal year 2004). In 2002, FCH was designated a part of the Community Health Center Program, a

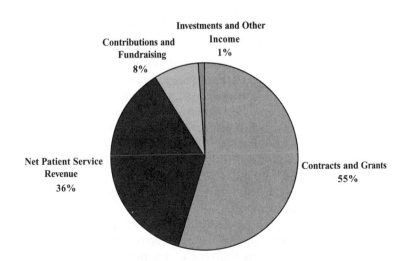

Figure 28.2 Fenway Community Health FY04 revenue.

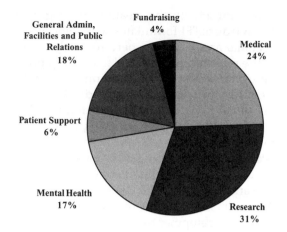

Figure 28.3 Fenway Community Health FY04 expenses.

program funded under Section 330 of the Public Health Service Act to provide for primary and preventive health care services in medically underserved areas. Other government-sponsored programs are available for individuals who qualify for specific programs so no individual is turned away because of the inability to pay.

The health education, service evaluation, and research components of the Health Center are usually funded by federal grants, including grants from the CDC, the Health Resources and Services Administration, the NIH, and the Substance Abuse and Mental Health Services Administration, and by the Massachusetts Department of Public Health. However, there is a substantial shortfall in funding for FCH's wide array of programs, and the Health Center continues to solicit independent donors, corporations, and foundations and to conduct fund-raising activities. Presently FCH benefits from three annual community fundraising events—the Men's Event, the Women's Dinner Party, and the Harbor to the Bay Ride, which had about 1400, 1200, and 100 attendees in 2004, respectively. In addition, FCH has close to 2000 individual donors per year.

8 Next Steps

FCH has evolved over the past three decades from a community health center to a model demonstrating how community-based LGBT services can be integrated with other innovative and culturally specific programs. The infrastructure that evolved to respond to the complex biopsychosocial challenges of AIDS helped to jump-start the development of a large number of activities that addressed the other health concerns of the LGBT community. Although other communities may not choose to replicate or be able to provide all of the programs that are available at FCH, we hope this chapter encourages local discussions that facilitate the development of comparable programs in other settings. The premise of FCH is not that LGBT individuals cannot receive competent care from heterosexual health care providers or in settings where LGBT patients are not a primary focus. Rather, FCH's unique, culturally specific programs can serve as models of care for LGBT individuals in other settings throughout the country. The goal is for LGBT individuals, wherever they are, to receive the most culturally competent and clinically proficient services possible.

In the future, FCH will continue to disseminate information learned during the establishment of its unique programs and to train health care providers and administrators in other settings to establish programs similar to those that FCH has proven successful in addressing the specific health care needs of LGBT individuals.

Acknowledgments: We acknowledge the hard work of dedicated staff, board members, and volunteers of Fenway Community Health, particularly those who gave their talents, time, and energy during the early years. We also acknowledge and thank all of the following FCH staff who have contributed and shared their expertise to help develop this chapter: Jon Appelbaum, Beth Belinky-Cohen, Gail Beverley, Steve Boswell, Frank Busconi, Phyllis Dixon, Nan Dumas, Eleni Eliades, Jerry Fensterman, Phillip Finch, Niamh Foley, Chris Grasso, Will Halpin, Henia Handler, Susan Johnson, Randi Kaufman, Hugo Lopez, Aaron Miller, Emily Pitt, Steven Safren, Peter Stein, Chris Viveiros, Lisa Whittemore, and Ian Wilson.

References

Anderson, D.J., O'Brien, T.R., Politch, J.A., Martinez, A., Seage, G.R., Padian, N., Horsburgh, R., and Mayer, K.H. (1992) Effects of disease stage and zidovudine therapy on the detection of human immunodeficiency virus type 1 in semen. *Journal of the American Medical Association* 267:2769–2774.

Belshe, R.B., Stevens, C., Gorse, G.J., Buchbinder, S., Weinhold, K., Sheppard, H., Stablein, D., Self, S., McNamara, J., Frey, S., Flores, J., Excler, J.L., Klein, M., El Habib, R., Duliege, A., Harro, C., Corey, L., Keefer, M., Mulligan, M., Wright, P., Celum, C., Judson, F., Mayer, K., McKirnan, D., Marmor, M., and Woody, G. (2001) Safety and immunogenicity of a canarypox-vectored human immunodeficiency virus type 1 vaccine with or without gp120: a phase 2 study in higher- and lower-risk volunteers. *Journal of Infectious Diseases* 183:1343–1352.

Berg, M.B., Mimiaga, M.J., and Safren, S.A. (2004) Mental health concerns of HIV infected gay and bisexual men seeking mental health services: an observational study. *AIDS Patient Care and STDs* 18:635–643.

Berg, M.B., Mimiaga, M.J., and Safren, S.A. (in press) Mental health concerns of gay and bisexual men seeking mental health services: a retrospective chart review. *Journal of Homosexuality.*

Berg, M.B., Safren, S.A., Mimiaga, M.J., Grasso, C., Boswell, S., and Mayer, K.H. (2005) Nonadherence to medical appointments is associated with increased plasma HIV RNA and decreased CD4 cell counts in a community-based HIV primary care clinic. *AIDS Care* 17:902–907.

Boehmer, U. (2002) Twenty years of public health research: inclusion of lesbian, gay, bisexual and transgender populations. *American Journal of Public Health* 92:1125–1130.

Bradford, J., and Mayer, K. (2003) Fenway Community Health's core data project: building a foundation for health services research. Presented at the Annual Conference of the Gay and Lesbian Medical Association, Miami.

Bradford, J., and Norman, N. (2003) Barriers faced by pregnant and parenting African American lesbians. Presented at the Annual Conference of Women in Medicine, Monterrey, CA.

Carroll, N., and Palmer, J.R. (2001) A comparison of intrauterine versus intracervical insemination in fertile single women. *Fertility and Sterility* 75:656–660.

Carroll, N., Goldstein, R.S., Lo, W., and Mayer, K. (1997) Gynecological infections and sexual practices of Massachusetts lesbian and bisexual women. *Journal of Gay and Lesbian Medical Association* 1:15–23.

Carroll, N., Linde, R., Mayer, K., Lara, A.M., and Bradford, J. (1999) Developing a lesbian health research program: Fenway Community Health Center's experience and evolution. *Journal of the Gay and Lesbian Medical Association* 3:145–152.

Chesney, M.A., Koblin, B.A., Barresi, P.J., Husnik, M.J., Celum, C.L., Colfax, G., Mayer, K.H., McKirnan, D., Judson, F.N., Huang, Y., Coates, T.J., and the EXPLORE Study Team (2003) An individually tailored intervention for HIV prevention: baseline data from the EXPLORE study. *American Journal of Public Health* 93:933–938.

Chin-Hong, P.V., Vittinghoff, E., Cranston, R.D., Buchbinder, S., Cohen, D., Colfax, G., Da Costa, M., Darragh, T., Hess, E., Judson, F., Koblin, B., Madison, M., and Palefsky, J.M. (2004) Age-specific prevalence of anal human papillomavirus infection in HIV-negative sexually active men who have sex with men: the EXPLORE study. *Journal of Infectious Diseases* 190:2070–2076.

Dean, L., Meyer, I.H., Robinson, K., Sell, R.L., Sember, R., Silenzio, V.M.B., Bowen, D.J., Bradford, J., Rothblum, E., Scout, White, J., Dunn, P., Lawrence, A., Wolfe, D., and Xavier, J. (2000) Lesbian, gay, bisexual and transgender health: findings and concerns. *Journal of the Gay and Lesbian Medical Association* 4:101–151.

DeGruttola, V., Seage, G.R., Mayer, K.H., and Horsburgh, C.R. (1989) Infectiousness of HIV between male homosexual partners. *Journal Clinical Epidemiology* 42:849–856.

DeMaria, A., Jr., Kunches, L., Mayer, K., Cohen, C., Epstein, P., Werner, B., Day, J., DeCristofaro, J., Landers, S., Tang, Y., Coady, W., and the Massachusetts gp160 Working Group. (2000) Immune responses to a recombinant human immunodeficiency virus type 1 (HIV-1) gp160 vaccine among adults with advanced HIV infection. *Journal of Human Virology* 3:182–192.

EXPLORE Study Team. (2004) Effects of a behavioural intervention to reduce acquisition of HIV infection among men who have sex with men: the EXPLORE randomised controlled study. *The Lancet* 364:41–50.

Gay and Lesbian Medical Association, LGBT health experts. (2001) Healthy People 2010 companion document for lesbian, gay, bisexual and transgender (LGBT) health. http://wwwglmaorg/policy/hp2010/. Retrieved April 12, 2001.

Groopman, J.E., Mayer, K.H., Sarngadharan, M.G., Ayotte, D., DeVico, A.L., Finberg, R., Sliski, A.H., Allan, J.D. and Gallo, R.C. (1985) Seroepidemiology of HTLV-III among homosexual men with acquired immunodeficiency syndrome or generalized lymphadenopathy and among asymptomatic controls in Boston. *Annals of Internal Medicine* 102:334–337.

Gross, M., Holte, S., Marmor, M., Mwatha, A., Koblin, B., and Mayer, K.H., for the HIVNET Vaccine Preparedness Study 2 Protocol Team. (2000) Anal sex among HIV-seronegative women at high risk of HIV exposure. *Journal of Acquired Immune Deficiency Syndromes* 24:393–398.

Gross, M., Seage, G.R., Mayer, K.H., Goldstein, R.S., Losina, E., and Wold, C. (1996) Interest among gay/bisexual men in greater Boston in participating in clinical trials of preventive HIV vaccines. *Journal of Acquired Immune Deficiency Syndromes and Human Retrovirology* 12:406–412.

Koblin, B.A., Chesney, M.A., Husnik, M.J., Bozeman, S., Celum, C.L., Buchbinder, S., Mayer, K.H., McKirnan, D., Judson, F.N., Huang, Y., Coates, T.J., and the EXPLORE Study Team. (2003) High-risk behaviors among men who have sex with men in 6 US cities: baseline data from the EXPLORE study. *American Journal of Public Health* 93:926–932.

Kumarasamy, N., Safren, S., Krishnan, A.K.S., Raminani, S., Pickard, R., James, R., Solomon, S., and Mayer, K.H. (2004) A qualitative study of cultural dimensions regarding adherence to antiretroviral therapy among patients with HIV in Chennai, India. Poster presented at the XV International AIDS Conference, Bangkok.

Kumarasamy, N., Safren, S., Raminani, S.R., Pickard, R., James, R., Krishnan, A.K., Solomon, S., and Mayer, K.H. (2005) A qualitative study of cultural dimensions regarding adherence to antiretroviral therapy among patients with HIV in Chennai, India. *AIDS Patient Care and STDs* 19:526–537.

Mayer, K.H., Ayotte, D., Groopman, J., Stoddard, A., Sarngadharan, M., and Gallo, R. (1986) Association of HTLV-III antibodies with sexual and other behaviors in a cohort of homosexual men from Boston with and without generalized lymphadenopathy. *American Journal of Medicine* 80:357–363.

Mayer, K.H., Boswell, S., Goldstein, R., Lo, W., Xu, C., Tucker, L., DePasquale, M.P., D'Aquila, R., and Anderson, D.J. (1999) Persistence of human immunodeficiency virus in semen after adding Indinavir to combination antiretroviral therapy. *Clinical Infectious Diseases* 28:1252–1259.

Mayer, K.H., Karim, S.A., Kelly, C., Maslankowski, L., Rees, H., Profy, A.T., Day, J., Welch, J., and Rosenberg, Z., for the HIV Prevention Trials Network (HPTN) 020 Protocol Team. (2003) Safety and tolerability of vaginal PRO 2000 gel in sexually active HIV-uninfected and abstinent HIV-infected women. *AIDS* 17:321–329.

Mayer, K., MacGovern, T., Golub, S., Lo, W., Singal, R., Kwong, J., Cohen, D., and Smith, D. (2002) Trends in the use of non-occupational post-exposure prophylaxis (NPEP) in Massachusetts (MA). Presented at the XIV AIDS Conference, Barcelona.

Mayer, K.H., Peipert, J., Fleming, T., Fullem, A., Moench, T., Cu-Uvin, S., Bentley, M., Chesney, M., and Rosenberg, Z. (2001) Safety and tolerability of BufferGel, a novel vaginal microbicide, in women in the United States. *Clinical Infectious Diseases* 32:476–482.

Mimiaga, M.J., Berg, M., and Safren, S.A. (2002) Sexual minority men seeking services: a retrospective study of the mental health concerns of men who have sex with men (MSM) in an urban LGBT community health clinic. Poster presented at the 36th annual convention for the Association for Advancement of Behavioral Therapy (AABT), Reno, NV.

Mimiaga, M.J., Berg, M., and Safren, S.A. (2004a) Mental health concerns of HIV-positive gay and bisexual men seeking mental health services. Poster presented at the 2004 Society of Behavioral Medicine Annual Meeting & Scientific Sessions (SBM), Baltimore.

Mimiaga, M.J., Safren, S.A, Benet, D.J., Manseau, M., DeSousa, N., and Mayer, K.H. (2004b) MSM in HIV prevention trials are sexual partners with each other: an ancillary study to the EXPLORE intervention. *AIDS and Behavior* 10:27–34.

National Forum for Centers of Excellence in Women's Health. (2003) Sexual minority women of color: a summit to develop health priorities. Vienna, VA.

Rogers, T.L., Emanuel, K., and Bradford, J. (2003) Sexual minorities seeking services: a retrospective study of the mental health concerns of lesbian and bisexual women. *Journal of Lesbian Studies* 7:127–146.

Ruff, M.R., Smith, C., Kingan, T., Jaffe, H., Heseltine, P., Gill, M.A., Mayer, K.H., Pert, C.B., and Bridge, T.P. (1991) Pharmacokinetics of peptide T in patients with AIDS. *Progress in Neuro-Psychopharmacology and Biological Psychiatry* 15:791–801.

Safren, S.A., Berg, M., Mimiaga, M.J., Grasso, C., Boswell, S., and Mayer, K.H. (2005) Adherence to medical appointments and medical outcome in a community based HIV primary care clinic. Poster presented at the 2005 Society of Behavioral Medicine Annual Meeting & Scientific Sessions (SBM), Boston.

Safren, S.A., Hendriksen, E.S., Mayer, K., Mimiaga, M.J., Pickard, R., and Otto, M.W. (2004a) Cognitive-behavioral therapy for HIV medication adherence and depression. *Cognitive and Behavioral Practice* 11:415–423.

Safren, S., Kumarasamy, N., James, R., Raminani, S., and Mayer, K.H. (2004b) ART adherence, demographic variables, and CD4 outcome among HIV-positive patients on antiretroviral therapy in Chennai, India. Poster presented at the XV International AIDS Conference, Bangkok.

Safren, S., Kumaraswamy, N., James, R., Raminani, S., Solomon, S., and Mayer, K.H. (2005) ART adherence, demographic variables, and CD4 outcome among HIV-positive patients on antiretroviral therapy in Chennai, India. *AIDS Care* 17:853–862.

Safren, S.A., Martin, C., Menon, S., Mimiaga, M.J., Solomon, S., and Mayer, K. H. (2004c) A survey of MSM outreach workers in Chennai, India. Poster presented at the XV International AIDS Conference, Bangkok.

Seage, G.R., III, Holte, S.E., Metzger, D., Koblin, B.A., Gross, M., Celum, C., Marmor, M., Woody, G., Mayer, K.H., Stevens, C., Judson, F.N., McKirnan, D., Sheon, A., Self, S., and Buchbinder, S.P. (2001) Are US populations appropriate for trials of human immunodeficiency virus vaccine? The HIVNET Vaccine Preparedness Study. *American Journal of Epidemiology* 153:619–627.

Seage, G.R., III, Mayer, K.H., Horsburgh, C.R., Holmberg, S.D., Moon, M.W., and Lamb, G.A. (1992) The relationship between nitrite inhalants, unprotected receptive anal intercourse, and the risk of HIV infection. *American Journal of Epidemiology* 135:1–11.

Seage, G.R., III, Mayer, K.H., Lenderking, W.R., Wold, C., Gross, M., Goldstein, R., Cai, B., Heeren, T., Hingson, R., and Holmberg, S. (1997) HIV and hepatitis B infection and risk behavior in young gay and bisexual men. *Public Health Reports* 112:158–167.

Seage, G.R., III, Mayer, K.H., Wold, C., Lenderking, W.R., Goldstein, R., Cai, B., Gross, M., Heeren, T., and Hingson, R. (1998) The social context of drinking, drug use, and unsafe sex in the Boston Young Men Study. *Journal of Acquired Immune Deficiency Syndromes and Human Retrovirology* 17:368–375.

Sell, R.L. (1997) Defining and measuring sexual orientation: a review. *Archives of Sexual Behavior* 26:643–658.

Wold, C., Seage, G.R., III, Lenderking, W.R., Mayer, K.H., Cai, B., Heeren, T., and Goldstein, R. (1998) Unsafe sex in men who have sex with both men and women. *Journal of Acquired Immune Deficiency Syndromes and Human Retrovirology* 17:361–367.

Index

Printed in the United States of America.